Clinical Laboratory Pearls

Upon your graduation.
Congratulations. May this book
serve you well. Go forth, and do
great things.COL Eric Berg,
MDMedical DirectorPA student phase
II Ft Campbell, Kentucy

MAY 1 9 2006

Clinical Laboratory Pearls

Editor

Steven L. Jones, M.D.
Department of Pathology
Dukes Memorial Hospital
Peru, Indiana

LIPPINCOTT WILLIAMS & WILKINS
A **Wolters Kluwer** Company
Philadelphia · Baltimore · New York · London
Buenos Aires · Hong Kong · Sydney · Tokyo

Acquisitions Editor: *Ruth W. Weinberg*
Developmental Editor: *Sara H. Fitz-Hugh*
Production Editor: *Emily Lerman*
Manufacturing Manager: *Colin J. Warnock*
Cover Designer: *Mark Lerner*
Compositor: *Circle Graphics*
Printer: *R.R. Donnelley, Crawfordsville*

© **2001 by LIPPINCOTT WILLIAMS & WILKINS**
530 Walnut Street
Philadelphia, PA 19106 USA
LWW.com

Library of Congress Cataloging-in-Publication Data

Clinical laboratory pearls / editor, Steven L. Jones.
    p.cm.
  Includes bibliographical references and index.
  ISBN 0-7817-2579-8 (alk. paper)
    1. Diagnosis, Laboratory—Handbooks, manuals, etc. I. Jones, Steven L., M.D.
RB38.2 .C558 2000
616.07′56—dc21   00-061818

10 9 8 7 6 5 4 3 2

For Jill

Contents

4. Chemistry

5. Immunology

6. Special Topics

Contributing Authors

Patricia I. Bader, M.D., *Associate Professor, Department of Medical and Molecular Genetics, Indiana University School of Medicine, 2101 Coliseum Boulevard East; Medical Director, Cytogenetics Laboratory, Parkview Hospital, 2200 Randallia Drive, Fort Wayne, Indiana 46805*

Barbara J. Bain, F.R.C.Path, F.R.A.C.P., *Reader in Haematology, Division of Investigative Sciences, Imperial College of Science, Technology and Medicine; Consultant, Department of Hematology, St. Mary Hospital, Praed Street, London W21NY, England*

Thomas D. Batiuk, M.D., Ph.D., *Assistant Professor, Department of Medicine, Indiana University School of Medicine, 1120 South Drive, Indianapolis, Indiana 46260*

John F. Bohnsack, M.D., *Professor and Associate Chair for Clinical Affairs, Department of Pediatrics, University of Utah Health Sciences Center, 50 North Medical Drive, Salt Lake City, Utah 84132*

Michael S. Brown, M.D., *Pathology Consultants, P.C., Yellowstone Pathology Institute, Inc., 2900 12th Avenue North, Billings, Montana 59101*

Paul I. Brown, B.S., M.T. (A.S.C.P.), *Technical Supervisor, Department of Clinical Toxicology, ARUP Laboratories, 500 Chipeta Way, Salt Lake City, Utah 84108*

D. Joe Chaffin, M.D., *4616 West 23rd Street, Greeley, Colorado 80634*

Constance F. M. Danielson, M.D., Ph.D., *Clinical Associate Professor, Department of Pathology and Laboratory Medicine, Indiana University School of Medicine, 635 North Barnhill Drive; Director, Department of Transfusion Medicine, Wishard Health Services, 1001 West 10th Street; Director, Blood Bank and Coagulation Laboratories, R.L. Roudebush VAMC, 1481 West 10th Street, Indianapolis, Indiana 46202*

Darrell D. Davidson, M.D., Ph.D., *Clinical Assistant Professor, Department of Pathology and Laboratory Medicine, Indiana University School of Medicine, 550 North University Boulevard; Cytopathologist, Department of Pathology and Laboratory Medicine, Clarion Health Partners, Methodist Hospital, 1701 North Senate Boulevard, Indianapolis, Indiana 46202*

Elizabeth L. Frank, Ph.D., *Clinical Chemistry Fellow, Department of Pathology, University of Utah School of Medicine, 50 North Medical Drive; Assistant Medical Director of Toxicology, ARUP Laboratories, 500 Chipeta Way, Salt Lake City, Utah 84108*

John Freedman, M.D., F.R.C.P.C., *Professor, Department of Laboratory Medicine and Pathobiology, University of Toronto, Banting Institute, 100 College Street; Director, Department of Transfusion Medicine, St. Michael's Hospital, 30 Bond Street, Toronto, Ontario M5B 1W8, Canada*

Jerome Goddard, Ph.D., *Clinical Assistant Professor, Department of Preventive Medicine, University of Mississippi Medical Center, 2500 North State Street, Jackson, Mississippi 39216*

Martin C. Gregory, B.M., B.Ch., D.Phil., *Professor, Department of Medicine, University of Utah School of Medicine, 50 North Medical Drive, Salt Lake City, Utah 84132*

Nancy Higgins, M.T., *Methodist Hospital, Wile Hall, 1701 North Senate Boulevard, Indianapolis, Indiana 46202*

Harry R. Hill, M.D., *Professor, Department of Clinical Immunology, University of Utah School of Medicine, 50 North Medical Drive, Salt Lake City, Utah 84132*

Jerry W. Hussong, D.D.S., M.D., *Director of Hematology Laboratory and Flow Cytometry, Department of Pathology, Laboratory Medicine Consultants, Ltd., Sunrise Hospital and Medical Center, 3186 South Maryland Parkway, Las Vegas, Nevada 89109*

Steven L. Jones, M.D., *Department of Pathology, Dukes Memorial Hospital, 275 West 12th Street, Peru, Indiana 46970*

Joseph A. Knight, M.D., *Professor, Department of Pathology, University of Utah, School of Medicine, 50 North Medical Drive, Salt Lake City, Utah 84132*

Gabor Komaromy-Hiller, Ph.D., *Technical Director, Automated Chemistry, RIA, Special Chemistry, and Trace Elements, Specialty Laboratories, Inc., 2211 Michigan Avenue, Santa Monica, California 90404*

Elmer W. Koneman, M.D., *Professor Emeritus, Department of Pathology, University of Colorado Health Science Center, 4200 East 9th Avenue, Consultant, Department of Pathology, Centura St. Anthony Hospital Central, 4231 West 16th Avenue, Denver, Colorado 80204*

Timothy R. La Pine, M.D., *Department of Clinical Immunology, University Hospital, 50 North Medical Drive, Salt Lake City, Utah 84132*

Alan H. Lazarus, M.D., *Department of Transfusion Medicine, St. Michael's Hospital, 30 Bond Street, Toronto, Ontario M5B 1W8, Canada*

Diane S. Leland, Ph.D., *Professor, Department of Pathology and Laboratory Medicine, Indiana University School of Medicine; Unit Director, Serology / Virology Laboratories, Indiana University Medical Center, 702 Barnhill Drive, Indianapolis, Indiana 46202*

Christine M. Litwin, M.D., *Associate Professor, Department of Pathology, University of Utah School of Medicine, 50 North Medical Drive, Salt Lake City, Utah 84132*

Leo J. McCarthy, M.D., F.R.C.P. Edin.Ire., *Professor, Department of Pathology and Laboratory Medicine, Indiana University School of Medicine, 635 North Barnhill Drive; Director, Transfusion Medicine, Department of Pathology and Laboratory Medicine, Indiana University Hospital, 550 North University Boulevard, Indianapolis, Indiana 46202*

Ann T. Moriarty, M.D., *3643 Delaware Common South Drive, Indianapolis, Indiana 46220*

Brent A. Neuschwander-Tetri, M.D., *Associate Professor, Department of Internal Medicine, St. Louis University, 3635 Vista Avenue, St. Louis, Missouri 63110*

William D. Odell, M.D., *Formerly Division of Endocrinology, University Hospital, 50 North Medical Drive, Salt Lake City, Utah 84132*

James C. Overall, Jr., M.D., *Professor Emeritus, Department of Pediatrics, University of Utah School of Medicine, 50 North Medical Drive, Salt Lake City, Utah 84132*

Sherrie L. Perkins, M.D., Ph.D., *Medical Director, Hematopathology Section and Associate Professor, Department of Pathology, University of Utah Health Science Center, 50 North Medical Drive, Salt Lake City, Utah 84132*

Elizabeth M. Petty, M.D., *Associate Professor, Department of Internal Medicine and Department of Human Genetics, University of Michigan 4301 MSRB III, 0638, Ann Arbor, Michigan 48109*

Bruce S. Rabin, M.D., Ph.D., *Professor, Department of Pathology, University of Pittsburgh; Director, Division of Clinical Immunopathology, Department of Laboratory Medicine, University of Pittsburgh Medical Center, 200 Lothrop Street, Pittsburgh, Pennsylvania 15213*

Neilsen J. Schulz, M.A., R.C.P., R.R.T., R.P.F.T., *MEA Program Chair, Health and Human Services, Ivy Tech State College, 104 West 53rd Street, Anderson, Indiana 46013; Pulmonary Function Lab Coordinator, Department of Respiratory Care, Wabash County Hospital, 710 North East Street, Wabash, Indiana 46992*

Richard B. Thompson, Jr., Ph.D., *Department of Pathology and Lab Medicine, Evanston Northwestern Healthcare, 2650 Ridge Avenue, Evanston, Illinois 60201*

Francis M. Urry, Ph.D., *Associate Professor, Department of Pathology, University of Utah School of Medicine, 50 North Medical Drive; Medical Director of Toxicology, ARUP Laboratories, 500 Chipeta Way, Salt Lake City, Utah 84108*

Ronald L. Weiss, M.D., M.B.A., *Professor, Department of Pathology, University of Utah School of Medicine, 50 North Medical Drive; Director of Laboratories, ARUP Laboratories, 500 Chipeta Way, Salt Lake City, Utah 84108*

James T. Wu, Ph.D., *Professor, Department of Pathology, University of Utah School of Medicine, 50 North Medical Drive; Director, Special Chemistry, ARUP Laboratories, 500 Chipeta Way, Salt Lake City, Utah 84108*

Lily L. Wu, Ph.D., *Research Associate Professor, Department of Pathology Internal Medicine, University of Utah School of Medicine, 50 North Medical Drive; Lab Director, Cardiovascular Genetic Clinics, University of Utah and ARUP Reagent Lab, 500 Chipeta Way, Salt Lake City, Utah 84108*

Preface

The purpose of *Clinical Laboratory Pearls* is to help medical students and house staff solve the most common laboratory-related diagnostic problems, and to help them use laboratory tests in the most effective way possible. Each topic in this text has already been covered in great detail by a number of excellent reference works. However, due to the exponential increase in the amount of information related to each topic, it is sometimes hard to "see the forest for the trees." This book was conceived as a pocket-sized guide to emphasize the most important concepts in laboratory medicine in the spirit of the famed architect Mies van der Rohe, who once said that "less is more."

Acknowledgments

I am deeply grateful for the mentors, colleagues, and friends whose influences have led to the creation of this text. First and foremost, I am grateful for the invaluable assistance of Jill Pulsipher Jones in the preparation of the manuscript and in a variety of administrative tasks, and without whose help the book would never have been completed. I am appreciative of the help that Betty A. Jones gave in the preparation of the manuscript, as well as support from my sister Patricia Essary and my brother Craig A. Jones.

I thank the following pathologists, who were or currently are associated with Ball Memorial Hospital (Muncie, Indiana): Dr. James Baldwin, Dr. George Branam, Dr. Tarik Elsheikh, Dr. Dan House, Dr. Victor Jolgren, Dr. Thomas Kocoshis, Dr. Richard Pearson, Dr. Ronald Schuen, Dr. David Soper, Dr. Joseph Tisone, Dr. Douglas Triplett, Dr. Joe Willman, and Dr. Howard Wu, for their encouragement and commitment to the quality education of residents. Dr. Greg Cameron, also at Ball Memorial Hospital, provided many practical insights regarding general approaches to writing. I am also indebted to the following pathologists at Indiana University Medical Center: Dr. O. "Bill" Cummings, Dr. Mary Davis, Dr. Philip Faught, Dr. John Henley, Dr. Meredith Hull, Dr. Helen Michael, Dr. Laurence Roth, Dr. Thomas Ulbright, and Dr. Moo-Nahm Yum, for their support and for the love of medicine that they inspire in others.

My partners, Dr. James Duncan, Dr. J. Dean Gifford, and Dr. Marvin Dziabis, deserve special thanks for their patience and their graciousness in arranging our schedules so that I could have the necessary time to complete this project. I am also appreciative of the invaluable interactions I have had with the laboratory personnel at Ball Memorial Hospital, Wabash County Hospital, and Dukes Memorial Hospital.

I express my appreciation for the following people at Lippincott Williams & Wilkins: Mary Beth Murphy, Senior Development Editor, for her consistent encouragement; Ruth Weinberg, Senior Editor, whose practical advice was always welcome; and Anne Patterson, Vice-President and Publisher, whose belief and confidence in the book's concept gave me the desire to persevere.

Most of all, I thank my wife Jill Pulsipher Jones, and our sons and daughters, Lori A. Hedquist, Ryan D. Jones, Jeff M. Jones, Megan Jones, Scott F. Jones, Erin E. Jones, and Kevin M. Jones, for all of the sacrifices they have made while I worked on "the book," and for their long-suffering, good humor, and love.

Steven L. Jones, M.D.

Introduction to Laboratory Testing

Steven L. Jones and Barbara J. Bain

I. Introduction

Laboratory tests are some of the most important tools available to clinicians. As with all tools, these tests have strengths and limitations, and are best used by one who understands both their strengths and their limitations. Before discussing the major fields of laboratory medical testing in the remainder of this book, it is important to review a few key principles.

A. Always interpret a laboratory result in the context of the patient's clinical condition, and try to anticipate what the appropriate physiologic response should be to that condition. For example, a "normal" reticulocyte count would be distinctly abnormal in the setting of severe anemia, because it would indicate an inadequate bone marrow response.

B. Always relate a test result to the appropriate normal range given by the specific laboratory that is doing the testing. Some tests, such as the white blood cell count (WBC), should give the same results in every laboratory. Other tests, such as the serum lactate dehydrogenase level (LDH), give results that vary depending on the instrument and the methods used (e.g., based on whether lactic acid or pyruvic acid is measured, at what temperature the reaction occurs).

C. Remember that laboratory test results are static representations of dynamic processes. For example, a "normal" test value, such as a normal haptoglobin level, could represent a stable, healthy condition. On the other hand, the test value could be part of an increasing trend (which could occur in inflammatory states, as haptoglobin is an acute phase reactant) or could be part of a decreasing trend as would occur in intravascular hemolysis. **Serial testing often provides more information about dynamic processes than does a single test result.**

A "normal" test value could also be the result of two **processes that are influencing the test value in different directions**. For example, iron deficiency in a menstruating patient would lead to microcytic red blood cells. However, if the female patient were also taking antiseizure medications, which tend to cause macrocytosis, the resulting *average* mean cell volume (MCV) could be normal.

D. Any process that involves human or machine occasionally involves errors. In cases of a glaring inconsistency between the patient's clinical situation and the laboratory test results, consider retesting the patient before making any serious clinical treatment decisions.

E. The following questions and principles are quite useful when assessing laboratory test results.

1

1. Does the result fall outside the laboratory's normal range?
2. If the result is outside the normal range, is it nevertheless likely to be normal for that particular individual?
3. If the result is within the normal range, is any reason seen to suspect that it is nevertheless abnormal for that individual? Are there records of previous results that would indicate that a significant change has occurred?
4. Is the detected abnormality likely to be clinically significant?
5. Is the detected abnormality expected and easily explicable? Are the known clinical circumstances consistent with the results? If so, no further investigation is usually warranted. For example, neutrophil counts rise and lymphocyte counts fall after major surgery. However, if the abnormal test result is unexplained, further investigation is warranted.

F.   When several laboratory values are abnormal, first consider the most common single cause that could explain all of the findings ("when you hear hoofbeats, think of a single horse"). If a single cause does not explain the findings, consider the possible presence of two or more common disorders, particularly if the patient is elderly. Finally, consider uncommon causes ("zebras also have hooves").

G.   Avoid the Ulysses syndrome. Ulysses was the main character in Homer's epic poem the *Odyssey*. His extensive wanderings were costly in many ways, and caused great suffering to the men for whom he was responsible. The Ulysses syndrome refers to the extensive investigations that can be triggered by an abnormal laboratory test value. The workups can be very costly and even entail some risk to the patient, but the cause is either insignificant or the "abnormal" laboratory value is actually normal for that patient.

To illustrate the probability of obtaining isolated "abnormal" test values, consider laboratory tests that are performed on a healthy person. If a 95% normal reference range is given for a particular test, then 5% of the normal population will by definition have a value that is outside of the reference range. If 20 tests are performed on a healthy person, the probability of at least one "abnormal" value is $1-(0.95)^{20}$ or 64%. Thus, 64% of healthy individuals who undergo 20 tests will have at least one "abnormal" test result, which in fact is a normal value for that person.

H.   Explain why tests are being done, and obtain the patient's implied or written informed consent.

I.   Tests should not be ordered unless the clinician has considered what the test results will signify, and how the results will be used.

II.   Normal reference ranges

A.   The best "normal" reference range in most situations is the patient's own baseline study. It is important, therefore, to obtain baseline laboratory values as soon as possible when an illness is suspected, and to correlate current test results with previous test results in the patient's medical record.

B.   A specific patient's test result may fall within the normal reference range, and yet nevertheless still be quite abnormal compared to that patient's baseline val-

ues. For example, a frail elderly patient may have a baseline serum creatine kinase (CK) value of 20 U/L, which could increase eightfold to a value of 160 U/L during an acute myocardial infarction, and yet still be within the "normal" reference range.

C.   Most laboratories list normal reference ranges that represent the range of values seen in 95% of a healthy population. Therefore, by definition, 2.5% of healthy subjects will have test results above the normal range and another 2.5% will have test results below the normal range. Ideally, each laboratory should create normal reference ranges for its own population, and should stratify those ranges based on gender, age, and time of day (when appropriate). For example, the average male hemoglobin level is higher than that of the average premenopausal woman. Likewise, a red blood cell MCV of 72 fL is normal for a 1-year-old child, but would be distinctly abnormal for an adult. In a healthy individual, serum cortisol is significantly higher at 8 AM than at 8 PM. Race should also be kept in mind when interpreting some laboratory tests. For instance, healthy blacks can have a lower neutrophil count than healthy whites.

D.   Pediatric populations. Many laboratory tests have reference ranges that are quite different for pediatric populations and for newborns, in particular. Please see the Appendix for representative pediatric reference ranges in selected chemistry and hematology tests.

E.   "Normal" reference ranges may not be helpful in situations where a high percentage of the population has values that are associated with disease. For example, a "normal" or "average" reference range for serum cholesterol is not as useful as a cholesterol reference range that is associated with good health.

F.   Some tests (e.g., blood alcohol, poisons, number of blasts in the peripheral blood) **have no normal reference range because the presence of the item in question is abnormal in any amount**.

III.   Key test characteristics

A.   Sensitivity refers to the test positivity when disease is present ("how many people who have the disease will the test identify?").

B.   Specificity refers to the test negativity when disease is absent ("how many people who do not have the disease will the test exclude?").

C.   Predictive values refer to the value of the test in assessing disease presence.

   1.   Positive predictive value. "If the test result is positive, what is the probability that the patient actually has the disease?"

   2.   Negative predictive value. "If the test result is negative, what is the probability that the patient does not have the disease?"

Unlike sensitivity and specificity, which are innate characteristics of each test, predictive values are markedly affected by disease prevalence in the population being tested. If a high percentage of the individuals tested has the disease in question, a positive test result has more meaning than if the disease is very rare in the population tested (consider the hypothetical situations where 100% of the population have the disease, or where 0% of the population have the disease). For example, a positive human immunodeficiency virus (HIV) test result has more meaning if the individuals being tested are adults with high-risk lifestyles than if the individuals being tested are children with no risk factors. Although this concept may seem obvious, its logical extension is that **clinicians can influence the predictive values of the tests they order**. In other words, if clinicians exercise sound medical judgment in analyzing the data before them (e.g., history and physical examination), develop a short differential diagnosis, and order tests for the most probable diseases, a resultant positive test result is likely to represent true disease. This is in contrast to a clinician who orders panels of ETKTM ("every test known to mankind") to "see if anything turns up positive." In the latter case, a positive test result is much less likely to represent true disease, and is more likely to represent a false-positive result related to inherent errors in testing methods and statistical interpretation.

D.   Units. Ideally, test results should be expressed in SI units [e.g., WBC count: $10 \times 10^9/L$ (SI) rather than 10,000/μL (conventional)].

IV.   Situations and substances that alter test values

A.   Inflammation. Several laboratory test values, such as acute phase reactants, are increased in inflammatory states (e.g., infection, inflammatory disorders, inflammation associated with carcinoma). These tests include α_1-antitrypsin, α_1-antichymotrypsin, amyloid-A-precursor protein, complement factor C3, C-reactive protein, ceruloplasmin, coagulation factor VIII, ferritin, fibrinogen, haptoglobin, plasminogen, and platelet counts.

B.   Pregnancy. Changes in laboratory test values associated with pregnancy include increases in serum alkaline phosphatase, glomerular filtration rate, leukocyte counts, and serum levels of several proteins produced by the liver; decreases often occur in blood urea nitrogen (BUN), serum albumin, sodium, hemoglobin, and osmolality.

C.   Vigorous exercise. Strenuous exercise can cause elevations in total creatine kinase, lactate dehydrogenase, potassium, BUN, uric acid, and leukocyte counts.

D.   Meals. Several tests may be elevated after a large meal, including potassium, serum lipids (i.e., triglycerides), and alkaline phosphatase. Diets that are high in protein can cause elevations in BUN, ammonia, and uric acid. Diets that include large quantities of tomatoes, bananas, and pineapple can cause elevations in 5-hydroxyindoleacetic acid (5-HIAA). Caffeine and theophylline can increase catecholamine levels.

E.   Time of day. The normal physiologic levels of several substances are affected by the time of day. Several tests peak in the morning hours (e.g., 8 AM), such as corticotropin, cortisol, lymphocyte count, and total WBC count. Several tests peak in the late afternoon hours, such as serum creatinine, triglycerides, BUN, and transferrin. Growth hormone levels peak 1–2 hours after the onset of sleep. Test results should always be interpreted relative to appropriate normal reference ranges. For example, a serum cortisol level drawn at 8 AM will appear to be inappropriately high if compared with reference ranges for 6 PM.

F. Drugs. A wide variety of drugs can influence laboratory tests, and the extent of their influence is well beyond the scope of this text. Laboratory personnel have access to test method descriptions that include potential drug interferences. Two of the most common drug influences are **alcohol** and **oral contraceptives**. Alcohol can elevate γ-glutamyl transferase (GGT), uric acid, lactic acid, and triglycerides, and with chronic use can elevate alanine aminotransferase (ALT), aspartate aminotransferase (AST), alkaline phosphatase, bilirubin, and the MCV of red blood cells. Folate is often decreased by alcohol. Oral contraceptives can elevate levels of thyroxine-binding globulin, total T4, α_1-antitrypsin, triglycerides, iron, ALT, and GGT. Oral contraceptives may cause albumin levels to decrease.

G. Venipuncture technique. Hemolysis from traumatic venipuncture can cause elevations in lactate dehydrogenase, AST, potassium, total creatine kinase, bilirubin, and magnesium. Antibody screens performed for blood transfusion testing can also be affected by hemolysis (causing false-negative results). Prolonged tourniquet application and hand clenching can cause elevations in potassium and lactic acid, and can decrease pH.

H. Fibrin clots in the collection tube, hyperbilirubinemia, and hyperlipidemia all can have various significant effects on a wide variety of tests.

I. Drawing blood. Blood drawn from an indwelling catheter or from an extremity with an intravenous infusion site can cause various errors because of dilutional effects, caused by the composition of the intravenous solution or the presence of an anticoagulant within the catheter.

J. Transfusions. Clinicians should exercise common sense in requesting laboratory tests for a patient who has recently been transfused. For example, hemoglobin electrophoresis, assay of red cell folate, and tests for glucose-6-phosphate dehydrogenase deficiency will be invalidated by a recent transfusion.

BIBLIOGRAPHY

Henry JB. *Clinical diagnosis and management by laboratory methods*, 19th ed. Philadelphia: WB Saunders, 1996.

Jacobs DS, Editor-in-Chief. DeMott WR, Grady HJ, Horvat RT, Huestis DW, Kasten BL Jr. *Laboratory test handbook*, 4th ed. Hudson (Cleveland), OH: Lexi-Comp, Inc., 1996.

Rang M. The Ulysses syndrome. *Can Med Assoc J* 1972;106:122–123.

Blood Bank

Blood Collection

D. Joe Chaffin

I. **Types of blood collection**
A. **Simple phlebotomy is the nonspecific removal of whole blood via a single venipuncture. The product can then be saved for future transfusion, or can be discarded as a therapeutic measure.**
    1. **Donations for future transfusion.** Whole blood can be transfused or centrifuged and separated into different components (e.g., red blood cells, platelets, plasma). Donors can donate for themselves ("**autologous**") or for someone else ("**allogeneic**").
    2. **Therapeutic collections**
       a. Done for various diseases in which removal of blood is beneficial for the patient (e.g., **hemochromatosis** and **polycythemia vera**).
       b. Requires a request by the patient's primary physician and approval by Blood Bank physician.
       c. By current standards, this blood is not to be used for transfusion.
B. **Apheresis (hemapheresis) is the specific removal of only a portion of the blood, using an apheresis machine** (see chapter 1.6, *Hemapheresis*, for more details). Apheresis is an automated process that can be done with a single venipuncture (using current technology). Whole blood is withdrawn and enters the apheresis machine. The whole blood is then separated into components, usually by centrifugation. Finally, the desired component is harvested and the remainder is returned to the patient. Platelets, plasma, white cells, or red cells can be targeted for removal.
II. **Whole blood collection**
A. **Primary anticoagulant and preservative solutions (AP solutions)**
    1. **Citrate phosphate dextrose (CPD)**
       a. Very commonly used, but not usually by itself (see "additive solutions" below).
       b. Red blood cells (RBCs) stored in CPD alone have a 21-day shelf life.
       c. A variant of CPD (CP2D) is identical in composition, but has twice as much dextrose; however, RBCs still have a 21-day shelf life).
    2. **Citrate phosphate dextrose adenine-1 (CPDA-1)**
       a. Until the mid 1990s, CPDA-1 was the most commonly used AP solution.
       b. CPDA-1 has a little more dextrose than CPD, but most importantly, also contains adenine. Adenine is a building block for adenosine triphosphate (ATP) generation in red cells. The ATP level in stored red cells is the best predictor of post-transfusion survival.

    c.   **Red cells in CPDA-1 have a 35-day shelf life.**

    3.   **Older solutions that are no longer used** include "anticoagulant citrate dextrose" (ACD, a.k.a. acid citrate dextrose), and heparin.

B.   Additive solutions

    1.   **General principle.** Blood is collected into a primary anticoagulant solution (see section II.A above). Red cells are separated via centrifugation, and an additive solution (100 mL) is then added. All of the additive solutions described below **extend the shelf life of red cells to 42 days**.

        a.   The shelf life is extended because of the additional adenine and dextrose, as well as mannitol (in AS-1 and AS-5; see below).

        b.   In neonatal transfusions, some concern has been raised that the extra adenine and mannitol in additive solutions may cause renal toxicity. However, most studies support the use of additive solutions in neonates unless a massive or exchange transfusion is performed.

    2.   **AS-1 (Adsol) and AS-5 (Optisol).** The primary anticoagulant is CPD. AS-1 and AS-5 contain mannitol, which enhances red cell viability (the purpose of the mannitol is not for diuresis).

    3.   **AS-3 (Nutricell).** The primary anticoagulant is CP2D. AS-3 does not contain mannitol.

C.   Amount of blood drawn during a donation. The current standard is to draw up to **10.5 mL/kg body weight of blood**, including testing samples (a 70-kg donor could theoretically donate >700 mL of blood!). The most common donation amount is approximately **450 mL** ± 10%.

III.   Donor screening. The collection facility physician is the person who is primarily responsible for protecting donors and recipients, not the ordering physician. The collection facility physician must ensure that the procedure will not unduly endanger the donor, and that donor factors will not unduly endanger the recipient. If this standard is not met, the donor must be deferred.

A.   Deferrals to protect the donor

    1.   **Deferrals based on donor's history**

        a.   **Less than 8 weeks since last whole blood donation, or less than 48 hours since last apheresis procedure** (platelet or plasma donation). When blood is needed for a particular patient, exceptions to this rule can be made with physician approval and informed consent.

        b.   **Poor health**, including significant cardiopulmonary disease, bleeding disorders, cancer, and so on. Exceptions require approval by the donor center physician.

        c.   **Pregnancy** (during and up to 6 weeks after). An exception can be made when donating for the donor's own fetus or neonate.

        d.   **Previous significant complications of donation**

    2.   **Deferrals based on donor's physical examination**

        a.   **Pulse < 50 or > 100 beats/minute.** Pulse rates > 100 can be permitted with physician approval. Pulse rates < 50 are permitted if the donor is a well-trained athlete.

   b. Blood pressure > 180/100
   c. Note: current standards do not establish a minimal body weight for donation (a change from past standards)
   3. Defer donation if donor's hemoglobin < 12.5 g/dL (or hematocrit < 38%).
B. Deferrals to protect the recipient
   1. Deferrals based on donor's history
      a. Permanent or indefinite deferrals
         (1) Clinical or laboratory evidence of viral diseases
            (a) Viral hepatitis (any form) after 11th birthday
            (b) Positive hepatitis B surface antigen (HBsAg), anti-human immunodeficiency virus (HIV), anti-human T-cell lymphotrophic virus (HTLV), or anti-hepatitis C virus (HCV) testing any time in the past (including childhood, or with current donation)
            (c) Positive anti-hepatitis B core antigen (HBc) on more than one occasion
         (2) Risk of Creutzfeldt–Jakob disease (CJD): family history of CJD; corneal or dura mater transplant recipient; human pituitary growth hormone injection recipient
         (3) Receiving money or drugs for sex
         (4) High-risk behavior for HIV: intravenous (IV) drug use; male homosexual intercourse
         (5) Babesiosis or Chagas' disease
         (6) Leukemia or lymphoma
      b. Three-year deferrals
         (1) Malaria survivors or patients who have lived in a malaria-endemic area
      c. One-year deferrals
         (1) Blood (or intimate) contact (or potential contact) with another individual in the following settings: blood transfusion; needle sticks/scalpel injuries; mucus membrane exposure to foreign blood; intimate contact with a person with known HIV, hepatitis, or high-risk behavior; rape victims; incarceration for >72 hours; tattoo placement
         (2) Paying for sex, or having venereal disease
         (3) Syphilis, gonorrhea, or both
         (4) Travel to a malaria-endemic area
         (5) Intranasal cocaine use
      d. Deferrals because of donor medications. Most drug deferrals are for the protection of the donor (clinical judgment is required; the medication is usually a clue to the donor's state of health), except for the following medications which are potential teratogens:
         (1) Etretinate (Tegison): permanent deferral
         (2) Acitretin (Soriatane): 3-year deferral
         (3) Isotretinoin (Accutane) and Finasteride (Propecia, Proscar): 30-day deferral
         Note: If the donor will be the sole source of platelets for a recipient and has taken **aspirin**, the blood donation should be **deferred for 36 hours** (this is a change from previous standards).

    e.   Deferrals because of donor immunizations
      (1)   Killed, toxoid, or recombinant vaccines require no deferral if the donor is asymptomatic.
Examples include hepatitis A and B (Heptavax); polio (Salk); influenza; diphtheria, pertussis, and typhoid (DPT); anthrax; and cholera vaccines.
      (2)   Four-week deferrals: rubella or varicella vaccinations
      (3)   Two-week deferrals: measles (rubeola), mumps, oral polio, typhoid, yellow fever
    f.   Miscellaneous: donors must be deferred for 72 hours after nonroutine dental work.
  2.   Deferrals based on donor's physical examination
    a.   Donor temperature >**99.5°F (37.5°C)**
    b.   Defer in cases of suspicious lesions on either arm or any other evidence of IV drug use

IV.   Complications of blood donation
A.   Vasovagal reactions are, overall, the most common donor reaction (occurs in <5% of transfusions). Signs and symptoms include **bradycardia, hypotension**, syncope (not always), incontinence (not always), and nausea and vomiting (not always). Treatment for vasovagal reactions is supportive.
B.   Hypotensive reactions are much less common than vasovagal reactions. Signs and symptoms include **tachycardia** (helps distinguish this reaction from vasovagal reactions), **hypotension,** and **loss of consciousness**. The treatment is immediate IV fluid resuscitation.
C.   Hyperventilation is the most common reaction in first-time donors and in children. Signs and symptoms include **shortness of breath and facial twitching**. Treatment is reassurance and rebreathing (into a paper bag).
D.   Severe reactions are reactions that require hospitalization (approximately 1/200,000 blood donations). The causes vary, and include cardiac, hypovolemic, severe vasovagal, and so forth.
E.   Apheresis-related reactions
  1.   "Citrate effect" from the citrate used as an anticoagulant; it binds calcium and causes perioral tingling and rarely tetany. Treat with oral calcium and slow the infusion rate.
  2.   Hypotension can occur when >15% of the patient's blood volume is extracorporeal.

V.   Testing of donated blood
A.   Infectious disease testing (as of Spring, 2000)
  1.   Seven tests are required
    a.   HIV: HIV-1 antigen (p24 antigen) and anti-HIV 1/2
    b.   Hepatitis viruses: HBsAg, anti-HBc, anti-HCV
    c.   HTLV: anti-HTLV I/II
    d.   Serologic test for syphilis
  2.   Approved for research protocols: nucleic acid testing (NAT) for HIV and HCV. Polymerase chain reaction (PCR) testing can reduce the "window period" between

actual infection and laboratory detection by current screening methods.

B. Blood typing and screening

   1. ABO grouping

   2. Rh typing (including "weak D" testing if D-negative; see below)

   3. Screening for significant non-ABO donor antibodies

VI. Autologous blood collection and transfusion: collection of donor blood for future transfusion to the same donor

A. General criteria. Autologous donations must be ordered by the donor's physician, approved by the collection facility physician, and preceded by informed consent by the donor. They are most commonly done before elective surgery or other procedure. The criteria that the donor must meet are more lenient than the criteria for allogeneic blood donors (blood donations to be used by someone other than the donor; see Table 1-1)

B. Infectious disease issues. Donors with a history of hepatitis or HIV may be acceptable as autologous donors. The issue is controversial because of the potential exposure to collection center workers and the possibility of transfusion errors (giving an autologous unit to the wrong patient); however, a recent US Supreme Court ruling will likely force more acceptance of HIV-positive autologous blood donors.

C. Other forms of autologous blood collection

   1. Isovolemic hemodilution. Blood is collected intraoperatively into blood collection bags, and replaced by saline. This means that the patient will bleed more dilute blood if further bleeding occurs during the procedure. Collected blood is returned at or near the end of the procedure (≤8 hours after collection).

   2. Intraoperative blood salvage. Blood is collected intraoperatively and washed ("cell saver"). The blood is returned to the patient within 6 hours. Do not use this procedure if the operating field is contaminated with bacteria or malignant cells.

   3. Postoperative blood salvage. Blood is collected from postoperative drains, and has a 6-hour shelf life.

Table 1-1. Comparison of criteria for autologous vs. allogeneic donors

Parameter	Allogeneic (Volunteer)	Autologous
Minimum interval between donations	8 wk	72 h
Hemoglobin or hematocrit	>12.5 g/dL or 38%	>11 g/dL or 33%
Infectious disease screening	Required	Not required (unless shipped)

VII.   Criteria for apheresis donation of platelets
   A.   Donors must meet the same history and physical requirements as whole blood donors. Donors **should not have had aspirin within 36 hours** of the donation.
   B.   Interval between donations may be as short as 48 hours; however, the procedure must not be performed more than twice a week or 24 times a year, unless approved by the collection center physician in unusual circumstances.
   C.   Preprocedure platelet count must be >150,000/μL; however, this criteria does not apply for the donor's first donation, or if >4 weeks have passed since a previous donation.

1.2

Blood Component Therapy

D. Joe Chaffin

I. Introduction

Most patients needing transfusion do not require whole blood to improve their clinical situation. **"Component therapy" is the concept of using only specific portions of the blood** to meet the patient's particular needs. For example, an anemic patient needs only red cells, a thrombocytopenic patient needs only platelets, and so on. This chapter focuses on each of the blood components and their respective uses.

II. Whole blood

A. Definition. Unmodified blood (~ 450 mL) is suspended in anticoagulant or preservative (AP) solution. Its use is rarely indicated, but the frequency of its use has been slightly increasing. Its shelf life is **35 days at 1°C to 6°C**.

B. Potential uses (none are particularly common today)

    1. Massive blood loss (e.g., trauma)

        a. Advantage: reduces the exposure to multiple donors. (Patients with massive blood loss who receive individual blood components are receiving large amounts of red cells and plasma from different donors.)

        b. Disadvantages

            (1) ABO considerations because of the large amount of plasma. Antibodies in group-O donor whole blood may hemolyze the red cells in non–group-O recipients because of **incompatible plasma** (not a great concern with group-O packed red cells).

            (2) Limited availability in most blood banks

    2. Exchange transfusions in neonates (combinations of red cells and plasma are more commonly used).

    3. Autologous transfusions (at physician's request). Some physicians prefer whole blood.

III. Red blood cells ("packed" RBCs and additive solution red blood cells): the most commonly used blood component

A. Manufacture. Freshly collected whole blood is centrifuged ("hard spin" = $5,000g \times 5$ minutes), which separates red cells from plasma. Approximately 225–250 mL of plasma is then removed to make "packed RBCs" (PRBCs) with a hematocrit between 70% and 80%. Then, 100 mL of additive solution (AS-1, AS-3, or AS-5) can be added to make a product with a hematocrit between 50% and 60% (AS-RBCs). PRBCs have a shelf life of 35 days (in CPDA-1) or **42 days (e.g., in AS-1, -3, -5) at 1°C to 6°C**. If frozen, they have a shelf life of **10 years at – 65°C, and 24 hours at 1°C to 6°C after thawing**.

B. Contents

    1. PRBCs (total volume = 250 mL): **red cells (200 mL)**, plasma (50 mL), white blood cells (~10^8) and platelets. **Note that 1 mg of iron is also present in each milliliter of RBCs.**

2.   **Additive solution RBCs** (total volume = 350 mL). Are the same as PRBCs, with an additional 100 mL of additive solution.

C.   **Indication for use. The need for increased oxygen-carrying capacity**. All reasons for transfusion of RBCs should be based on this rationale, and include, for example, acute hemorrhage >20% of a patient's blood volume, lack of production of red cells, destruction of red cells (hemolysis), symptomatic chronic anemias, and cardiopulmonary disorders in association with any of the above. The need for RBCs can be assessed by invasive techniques (e.g., mixed venous O_2 saturation, cardiac index), or by evaluation of clinical and laboratory data (more common). The **expected effect of transfusing one unit of PRBCs is to raise the hemoglobin by 1 g/dL and the hematocrit by 3%** (may take 24 hours to be evident). **Compatible fluids for the transfusion include normal saline, ABO-compatible plasma, and 5% albumin (not lactated Ringer's, 0.45% normal saline, antibiotics, total parenteral nutrition, for example.).**

D.   **Contraindications for use**
1.   **Hemoglobin and hematocrit thresholds for transfusion**. The traditional "automatic" threshold of 10 g/dL hemoglobin (30% hematocrit) for red cell transfusion has been discredited in the literature from the areas of surgery, anesthesiology, and transfusion medicine. **Decisions for transfusion should be based on an individual patient's need**, not on a physician's "level of comfort cutoff." General guidelines from the literature state that patients with **hemoglobin levels >10 g/dL rarely need transfusion, whereas those with levels <6 g/dL almost always need transfusion**.
2.   **Nutritional anemias**. Patients who can tolerate correction via iron, folate, or B_{12} replacement should be managed in that manner.
3.   **In general, hemorrhage of <20% of a patient's blood volume** (crystalloids are a better choice)

IV.   **Platelet concentrate and apheresis platelets**
A.   **Platelet concentrate (a.k.a., "Whole Blood-Platelet Concentrate" or WB-PC)**
1.   **Manufacture**. In the United States, whole blood is centrifuged ("soft spin") to separate **"platelet-rich plasma" (PRP)** from red cells. The PRP is then centrifuged at a higher speed ("hard spin") to separate platelets from plasma by creating a platelet button, which is then resuspended in ~50 mL of donor plasma. In Europe, platelets are harvested from buffy coat layers. The shelf life is **5 days at 20°C to 24°C with gentle agitation**.
2.   **Contents**. Current American Association of Blood Bank (AABB) standards (19th edition) require at least **5.5 × 10^{10} platelets** in 75% of PC units tested. The product also contains 50 mL of donor plasma and 10^7 white blood cells.
3.   **"Standard" dosage**. Most clinicians use **between 6 and 10 bags of** PC as a "dose" of platelets. A general guideline is to use **one bag per 10 kg body weight** (for neonates, use 10–15 mL/kg body weight). Multiple bags are usually "pooled" together for ease of transfusion.

4. Indications for use
   a. Thrombocytopenia (decreased platelet count). "Absolute thresholds" are controversial and are often institution-specific. **Thresholds should be as individualized as possible**, taking into account the clinical situation. Given thrombocytopenia, additional risk factors that can increase the likelihood of bleeding include fever, sepsis, major surgical procedures, a patient who is **already** bleeding, and thrombocytopathy. General guidelines for when to give platelets include:

- **No risk factors (listed above): give platelets if <10,000– 15,000 platelets/μL**
- **With other risk factors: give platelets if <20,000 platelets/μL**
- **With surgery or ongoing bleeding: give platelets if <50,000 platelets/μL**

   The expected effect (in reality, this is usually not achieved) of transfusing platelets is to **increase the platelet count 5,000–10,000 per bag of platelets in a 70-kg adult**.
   b. Thrombocytopathy (platelets that function abnormally). The key to deciding whether to transfuse is to recognize that **the clinical situation is the most important factor**, and that **the actual platelet count has little bearing on the decision**. Several types of thrombocytopathies exist:
     (1) Acquired thrombocytopathies (more common and transient), including, for example, aspirin or other drug ingestion, cardiopulmonary bypass procedures.
     (2) Primary (inherited) thrombocytopathies, including Glanzmann's thrombasthenia, Bernard–Soulier disease, and von Willebrand's disease.
5. Contraindications for use
   a. Thrombotic thrombocytopenic purpura (TTP). A platelet-consumptive disorder caused by abnormal von Willebrand's factor, leading to platelet thrombi and microangiopathic hemolytic anemia. Transfused additional platelets contribute to the formation of platelet-fibrin thrombi, which is thought to worsen the clinical situation.
   b. Heparin-induced thrombocytopenia (HIT). The pathophysiology is different than that of TTP, but the rationale for not transfusing platelets is the same.
   c. Immune (idiopathic) thrombocytopenic purpura (ITP). A relative contraindication, as platelets will not actually harm the patient, but will not be of much benefit either. Platelets can be transfused in situations of life-threatening bleeding.
B. Apheresis platelets: prepared from one donor. In many centers, apheresis platelets are used preferentially over platelet concentrates.
   1. Contents. AABB standards (19th edition) require at least 3.0×10^{11} **platelets** in 75% of apheresis units tested. The plasma volume is usually 100–200 mL.
   2. Indications for use. Normal indications for platelets detailed above for PC. In addition, apheresis platelets reduce

donor exposures (1 donor exposure with apheresis vs. 6 to 10 with PC). **HLA antigen-matched or cross-matched apheresis platelets may also be useful in patients who are "refractory" to platelet transfusion** (i.e., post-transfusion counts do not increase adequately). Refractoriness to platelets may be caused by nonimmune [e.g., disseminated intravascular coagulation (DIC), fever, splenomegaly, drug reactions] or immune factors such as anti-HLA or anti-platelet antibodies. A platelet antibody screen using chloroquine may be useful in differentiating the anti-HLA from the anti-platelet antibodies (think "HLA goes away"). HLA-matched apheresis platelets are most useful in patients with anti-HLA antibodies; however, 25% to 40% of HLA-matched platelets will also fail to raise the platelet count. **Cross-matched apheresis platelets are usually more successful than HLA-matched platelets.**

   3.   **Myths about apheresis platelets**
      a.   "They work better than platelets in platelet concentrates." **In truth, platelet function is not significantly different between the two.**
      b.   "They prevent HLA antigen alloimmunization." This commonly held misbelief is based on a theoretic decrease in the risk of immunization if fewer foreign donor exposures occur. The TRAP study clearly refutes this myth ("Trial to Reduced Alloimmunization to Platelets," published in *The New England Journal of Medicine*, 1997). Increased risk of **immunization is associated with exposure to foreign white blood cells** (regardless of the number of donors), so **leukoreduction is better** than using apheresis platelets to prevent immunization (see below).

V.   Modifications to red cells and platelets
   A.   Leukocyte reduction. Reduces the risk of HLA antigen alloimmunization and the risk of cytomegalovirus (CMV) transmission, and decreases the risk of febrile, nonhemolytic transfusion reactions (especially for RBCs). Important things to remember:
      1.   Red cells and platelets may both be leukoreduced, but not by the same filter (the filters are not interchangeable between products).
      2.   CMV-seronegative products and leukocyte-reduced products have been shown to have about the same risk.
      3.   Leukoreduction can limit the immunosuppressive effects of transfusion, but the practice is not universally accepted.
      4.   Leukoreduction has not been proved to reduce the risk of Creutzfeldt–Jakob disease from transfusion.
      5.   Current **fourth generation filters are the method of choice** to reduce leukocytes, and remove 99.99% of the white cells. Other less efficacious methods include microaggregate filters and washing, freezing red cells, or both.
   B.   Irradiation prevents transfusion-associated graft-versus-host disease (TA-GVHD). Important things to remember:
      1.   Transfused lymphocytes react against host tissues that are not HLA identical; in susceptible patients, this can lead to a catastrophic, nearly always fatal TA-GVHD.

2. Patients potentially at risk for TA-GVHD:

a. Patients with primary T-cell immunodeficiencies (e.g., DiGeorge's syndrome, severe combined immunodeficiency)

b. Bone marrow or stem cell transplant recipients (before and after)

c. Markedly lymphopenic patients (the absolute threshold is unclear, but probably is ~500/μL)

d. Fetuses and premature newborn babies

e. Patients receiving blood from a first-degree relative or HLA-matched transfusion (recipients that share many, but not all, HLA antigens with the donor are at increased risk).

3. Gamma irradiation at 25 Gy makes transfused lymphocytes incapable of dividing or attacking host tissues.

C. Freezing (primarily for red cells) allows the storage of red cell units of special value, and is also useful for patients with hypersensitivity to plasma proteins (e.g., antibodies to IgA) or who have repeated febrile nonhemolytic transfusion reactions. Important things to remember:

1. Glycerol is used as the cryopreservative.

2. The shelf life is at least **10 years at – 65°C** (with 40% glycerol concentration)

3. Thawing and deglycerolizing is not an instantaneous process; it requires coordination between the transfusionist and the blood bank.

4. Once deglycerolized, the product has a shelf life of **24 hours at 1°C to 6°C**.

5. Platelets can also be frozen, but the technology and effective platelet recovery is poor.

D. Washing allows the removal of plasma from red cells, which is useful for patients with hypersensitivity to plasma proteins (e.g., antibodies to IgA) or who have repeated febrile, nonhemolytic transfusion reactions. Washed maternal platelets may also be useful in neonates who have neonatal alloimmune thrombocytopenic purpura (caused by maternal *anti-PL*[A1]). Important things to remember:

1. Washed red cells have a shelf life of 24 hours at 1°C to 6°C; washed platelets have a shelf life of 4 hours at 20°C to 24°C

2. The classic cause of plasma hypersensitivity in a recipient is a nearly complete IgA deficiency. These recipients typically have antibodies against IgA, and when exposed to IgA in a donor's plasma, can develop cataclysmic anaphylactic reactions. Washed RBCs are useful for these patients. Deglycerolized red cells (frozen red cells that have been thawed) are an equally effective option. Still another option is to use blood from an IgA-deficient donor.

3. Washing does not prevent GVHD.

E. Rejuvenation takes an expired unit of red cells and makes it available for immediate transfusion or preservation (freezing). Important things to remember:

1. Red cells can be rejuvenated up to **3 days** after expiration (platelets cannot be rejuvenated).

2. Rejuvenating solution replenishes 2,3-diphosphoglycerate (2,3-DPG) and adenosine triphosphate (ATP) to near initial levels.

3. Rejuvenated units require washing before transfusion because of inosine in the solution, which may be toxic.

VI.   **Fresh frozen plasma (FFP)**

A.   **Manufacture**. Two common methods of preparation:

1.   **Method 1**. Whole blood undergoes "hard spin" centrifugation, after which the plasma is expressed off of the red cells and frozen at −18°C within 8 hours of collection. This yields PRBCs and FFP.

2.   **Method 2**. Whole blood undergoes "soft spin" centrifugation, after which the PRP is expressed off the red cells; PRP then undergoes "hard spin" and the plasma is expressed off of platelets and frozen as above. This yields PRBCs, platelet concentrate, and FFP (less than in method 1)

3.   **Preparation for transfusion**. FFP is thawed at 30°C to 37°C (usually in a water bath) and can be stored at **20°C to 24°C for up to 24 hours**.

B.   **Contents** (200 mL plasma). All coagulation factors [1U/mL International Unit (IU) of plasma; therefore, **200 IU of each coagulation factor** per bag], and approximately **400 mg of fibrinogen** per bag.

C.   **Indications for use**

1.   **Deficiencies of multiple coagulation factors**, such as in hepatic failure or dilutional coagulopathy from massive transfusions (when the patient receives >10 units of red cells within 24 hours). Providing 15% to 20% of most coagulation factors is often sufficient to treat the coagulopathy.

2.   Deficiencies of a single coagulation factor (e.g., antithrombin) when no factor-specific concentrate is available.

3.   **Emergency reversal of the effects of warfarin (Coumadin); vitamin K takes hours** to fully reverse warfarin, even when given intravenously (IV).

4.   Plasma replacement for **exchange transfusions** in certain diseases (e.g., **TTP**; see chapter 1.6, *Hemapheresis*, for more details).

D.   **Contraindications**

1.   Prophylactic replacement in mild prothrombin time (PT) or partial thromboplastin time (PTT) elevations

2.   **Reversal of heparin effect** (the antithrombin in FFP prevents it from neutralizing heparin, and **protamine should be used** instead).

3.   Wound healing, general well-being, or other unproved philosophies

E.   **Other options**

1.   **Solvent detergent-treated plasma (SDP)**: approved in 1998 for use in the United States.

a.   **Manufacture**. FFP from up to 2,500 donors of a single ABO type is pooled, then treated to eliminate enveloped viruses, and finally packaged in 200-mL bags.

b.   **Benefits**

(1)   The process removes enveloped viruses such as human immunodeficiency virus (HIV), human T-cell lymphotrophic virus (HTLV), hepatitis B virus, and hepatitis C virus.

(2)   Uniform volume and factor concentration

(3) May be useful in TTP exchange transfusions (the processing of SDP removes the large von Willebrand factor (vWF) multimers that cause TTP).

c. **Concerns**

(1) Some blood-borne viruses (that are nonenveloped) remain in the product (e.g., hepatitis A virus and parvovirus B19); however, "neutralizing antibodies" from previously exposed donors in the pool may limit the danger.

(2) Cost is nearly **double** that of regular FFP.

2. Donor-retested plasma (DRP) serves as an alternative to SDP.

a. **Concept and manufacture**. Most transfusion-transmitted infections result from "window-period" infections, wherein the donor actually has the disease but is not yet testing positive for it. DRP is manufactured by collecting donor plasma, performing infectious disease testing, making FFP, and then storing the plasma (the unit is not immediately available for transfusion). The donor returns at least 16 weeks later, donates again, and gets tested again for infectious diseases. If infectious disease testing is still negative, plasma from the first donation is released, whereas plasma from the second donation is held as above.

b. **Concerns:** decreased availability of product because of the waiting time, logistical difficulties in mobile donor pools (especially military), and more potential for error because of increased clerical tasks.

VII. Cryoprecipitate (CRYO). CRYO is an infrequently used and commonly misunderstood product.

A. Manufacture. CRYO is made from FFP. **FFP is thawed slowly** at 1°C to 6°C (NOT at 30°C to 37°C as when preparing it for transfusion). Cryoprecipitate adheres to the sides of the bag. Most of the liquid plasma is then removed, and the remaining product (CRYO) is refrozen and stored at −18°C or below.

B. Contents. Fibrinogen, factor VIII, vWF, factor XIII, and fibronectin. AABB standards (19th edition) require at least **150 mg fibrinogen** per bag tested, and at least **80 IU of factor VIII** per bag tested. The total volume is 15 to 20 mL.

C. Pretransfusion preparation. As with FFP, CRYO is thawed at 30°C to 37°C. Unlike FFP, CRYO is stored at room temperature. Most CRYO is "pooled" (multiple units combined into a single bag) for transfusion efficiency. If pooled, the shelf life of CRYO is **4 hours**; if not pooled, the shelf life is 6 hours. The normal adult dose is 10 bags. See section VIII below for more details.

D. Indications for use

1. Fibrinogen deficiency. CRYO is very efficient because of the high fibrinogen content in a small volume.

2. Uremic thrombocytopathy. Renal failure leads to a mysterious platelet defect that increases the risk of bleeding. Adding vWF (e.g., CRYO) seems to transiently correct the deficit. Other options include the use of desmopressin analogues (e.g., DDAVP), which also increases vWF levels, and the use of conjugated estrogen therapy, which works through a mechanism other than vWF and for 2 weeks after a 5-day course of therapy.

3.   Component of "fibrin glue" for local bleeding control. CRYO is mixed with bovine thrombin and "painted" onto raw surgical surfaces for bleeding control. This technique will probably be replaced by new "fibrin sealants," which are treated to remove viruses and use human rather than bovine thrombin.

E.   **Myths and misconceptions about CRYO**

1.   "Cryoprecipitate and FFP are interchangeable." In truth, **CRYO is a mere shadow of FFP** (it contains only a few of the coagulation factors found in FFP). In treating a patient with multiple coagulation deficiencies, it is wrong to use CRYO in place of FFP just because the patient is volume sensitive, unless specifically treating fibrinogen deficiency.

2.   "There is more fibrinogen in CRYO than in FFP." In truth, this is impossible because CRYO is made from FFP and has less total fibrinogen (some is lost in the processing). However, it is true that fibrinogen is **more concentrated in CRYO** (150 mg in 15 mL) than in FFP (400 mg in 200 mL).

VIII.   **Calculating coagulation factor replacement**

A.   **General information**. The Blood Bank, which is often the site of coagulation factor replacement storage, is frequently requested to calculated proper dosages. The same basic principle of calculation can be used for specific coagulation factors, vWF, CRYO, and Rh immune globulin dosages (Table 1-2).

Table 1-2.   Calculating factor replacement and Rh immune globulin dosages

For coagulation factors (e.g., factor VIII, factor IX, von Willebrand factor)

A. Calculation Steps:

1. **Calculate the blood volume:** Multiply the patient's weight in kilograms by 70 mL/kg
2. **Calculate the plasma volume:** Multiply the blood volume by (1-hematocrit [as a decimal])
3. **Calculate the total factor units needed:** Start with the present factor activity level, and subtract it from the desired factor activity level (in general, 100% for surgery and 50% for hemophiliac–related bleeding). Multiply the result times the plasma volume, yielding the total factor units needed.
4. **Calculate the number of replacement factor vials needed:** Divide the total factor units needed by the number of units in one vial, and round up. The number of units per vial varies from product to product (and even from each lot to lot), and is listed on each vial.

B. Example: 80 kg hemophiliac patient has factor VIII activity of 5%. The desired activity level is 50%. The patient's hematocrit is 40%. The factor VIII product has 500 IU per vial.

1. **Calculate the blood volume:**
     $(80 \text{ kg}) \times (70 \text{ mL/kg}) = 5600 \text{ mL}$
2. **Calculate the plasma volume:**
     $(5600 \text{ mL}) \times (1 - 0.4) = 3360 \text{ mL}$

Table 1-2. *Continued*

3. **Calculate the total factor units needed** (note that the activity levels are in decimal form):
   $0.50 - 0.05 = 0.45$
   $0.45 \times (3360 \text{ mL}) = 1512$ units needed[a]
4. **Calculate the number of replacement factor vials needed:**
   1512 / 500 units factor VIII per vial = 3.02 vials needed, rounded up to 4 vials

For RH immune globulin (RhIG) dosages

A. **Calculation steps:** First perform the Kleihauer–Betke test (acid elution test), which yields the percentage of red cells in the mother that are from the fetus; flow cytometry is an alternative method. Next perform one of the following two calculations:

   Method 1: Calculate the maternal blood volume (see step 1 under coagulation factors). Multiply the maternal blood volume by the percentage of fetal red cells (in decimal form), yielding the amount of the fetal bleed. Then divide the amount of the fetal bleed by 30 to obtain the number of RhIG vials to give (if the result is a decimal <0.5, round *up*; if the decimal is >0.5, round up and then *round up again*)

   Method 2 (Original Kleihauer formula): Multiply the percentage of fetal red cells by 50, then divide by 30 to obtain the number of RhIG vials to give (round up as described in Method 1).

B. **Example (Method 2):** 70 kg woman with 3% fetal red cells in her blood.
   Step 1: $3 \times 50 = 150$
   Step 2: $150 \div 30 = 5.0$, rounded up to 6 vials of RhIG.

---

[a] **For factor IX only: double this amount** (for several reasons, including a redistribution phenomenon, only 50% of factor IX replacement doses actually end up in the circulation)

Blood Groups

D. Joe Chaffin

I. Introduction. Blood group antigens exist on the cytoplasmic membrane of red cells. Many of the antigens have a similar core structure, with the only difference in some cases being a single sugar molecule. In the Blood Bank, antigens are generally viewed in terms of their significance. **Antigens are considered significant if antibodies to the antigen are capable of causing either hemolytic transfusion reactions (HTR) or hemolytic disease of the newborn (HDN).** Antibodies are often described in terms of their behavior at different temperatures, because this is a major determinant of their significance:

- **"Warm" antibodies react best at body temperature (37°C) and are usually IgG.** IgG antibodies usually require exposure to foreign antigens before they are produced and, therefore, are also called **"acquired" antibodies.** This exposure usually occurs through either pregnancy or previous transfusions. **Most clinically significant blood group antibodies are IgG** (except the ABO IgM antibodies described below). IgG antibodies can coat red cells at body temperature and lead to removal by macrophages (**extravascular hemolysis**). **Some IgG subclasses (IgG$_1$ and IgG$_3$) are capable of fixing complement and causing intravascular hemolysis,** although this does not occur nearly as frequently as with IgM antibodies. Maternal **IgG antibodies can also cross the placenta and attack fetal red cells.**
- **"Cold" antibodies react best at temperatures below body temperature (e.g., 25°C or colder) and are usually IgM.** IgM antibodies usually exist in humans regardless of whether they have been pregnant or transfused and, therefore, are also called **"naturally occurring" antibodies.** This occurs because some foodstuffs and bacteria have antigens that are very similar to blood group antigens, and people are exposed to these antigens very early in life. **Most IgM antibodies are not clinically significant, with the major exception being the ABO IgM antibodies.** When significant (i.e., when IgM antibodies are able to coat red cells at body temperature), IgM antibodies are very efficient at fixing complement, and cause **intravascular hemolysis.** Maternal IgM antibodies, because they are pentamers (and five times larger than IgG), are **not able to cross the placenta.** The most common cold antibodies are against the ABO, P, I/i, Lewis, and some Lutheran antigens [think "for a **m**assive (Ig**M**) **cold**, take **A PILL**"].

Blood group antigens can also be classified based on how they react with antibodies after incubation with enzymes (e.g., papain, pepsin). **Blood group antigens are enhanced, weakened, or unchanged by enzymes** (Table 1-3).

Table 1-3. The relationship
of blood group antigens to enzymes

Enhanced by Enzymes	Decreased by Enzymes	Unchanged by Enzymes
ABO family (ABO,Lewis, I/i, P) Rh Kidd	MNSs Duffy	Kell

II. ABO family of antigens. Includes ABO, Lewis, I/i, and P.

A. ABO blood group

1. Biochemistry

a. Basic backbone chain. All of the antigens in the ABO family (including ABO, Lewis, I/i, and P) have the same core backbone, a carbohydrate called a "paragloboside." The final antigens differ by the addition of one or more sugar molecules. Two types of backbone chains exist—called type 1 and type 2—that differ in their bonds. The chains also differ in that **type 1 chains are found primarily in secretions, whereas type 2 chains are found primarily on red cells.** Both type 1 and type 2 chains can host an H antigen, which is the precursor to the A and B antigens.

b. H antigen. The H antigen is made by adding a fucose (a five-carbon sugar) to either the type 1 or 2 backbone chains (Fig. 1-1). The fucose is added by enzymes that both the *Se* and the *H* genes can create. The *Se* gene (for "secretor"; **80% of the population have this gene and they are called "secretors") creates the H antigen in secretions by the addition of fucose to type 1 chains. The H gene creates the H antigen on red cells by the addition of fucose to type 2 chains. After (and only after) the H antigen is made, A or B antigens can be added.** The A and B antigens functionally mask the H antigen, so that the more A or B that is made, the less H is present. Type O cells have no A or B and so express the most H antigen. The lectin *Ulex europaeus* agglutinates (and hence can identify) cells carrying the H antigen.

- Relative amount of H in major blood types: $O > A_2 > B > A_2B > A_1 > A_1B$

c. A and B antigens. A and B antigens are created by adding a sugar onto the H antigen. If no sugar is added to the H antigen, the red cells are called type O.

(1) Group A. Formed by the addition of *N*-acetyl-galactosamine (GalNAc) to the H antigen. Of the US population, **40% are group A** (varies with race).

(a) Genotypes *AA* or *AO*

(b) Patients who are type A have **naturally occurring, clinically significant, predominantly IgM antibodies (with a small amount of IgG) against type B.** Reminder: ABO antibodies are the exception

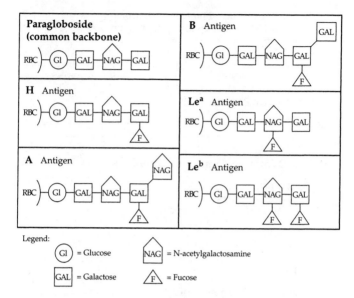

Legend:

- (Gl) = Glucose
- (NAG) = N-acetylgalactosamine
- (GAL) = Galactose
- (F) = Fucose

Fig. 1-1.   Relationship of the common backbone chain to the H, A, B, and Lewis antigens. RBC, red blood cell; Le^a, Lewis a antigen; Le^b, Lewis b antigen.

to the general rule that IgM antibodies are clinically insignificant. **ABO-incompatible transfusions are the main cause of Blood Bank fatalities, and clerical errors are the main cause of ABO-incompatible transfusions**.

(c)   The A antigen has subgroups, called A$_1$ and A$_2$. A$_1$ has more of the A antigen than has the A$_2$ subgroup. Of group A individuals, 80% are classed as A$_1$, whereas almost all of the remaining 20% are A$_2$. Occasionally, **people with A$_2$ may make antibodies against the A$_1$ subgroup**. Rarer additional subgroups of A exist, which are beyond the scope of this book.

(d)   A$_1$ and A$_2$ can be distinguished by using a lectin called **Dolichos biflorus**, which agglutinates A$_1$ and not A$_2$.

(2)   Group B. Formed by the addition of galactose (Gal) to the H antigen. Of the US population, **10%** are type B (varies with race).

(a)   Genotypes *BB* or *BO*

(b)   Patients who are type B have **naturally occurring, clinically significant, predominantly IgM antibodies (with a small amount of IgG) against type A** cells.

(3)   Group O. Of the US population, **45%** are type O (varies with race).

(a)   Genotype *OO* (**"universal donors"**)

(b)   Patients who are type O have **naturally occurring, clinically significant, very high titer, anti-**

A, anti-B, and anti-A,B antibodies. Anti-A,B is a strong antibody that reacts with the A antigen, the B antigen, and a separate and distinct antigen that occurs when A and B are both present. **Maternal anti-A,B is an IgG antibody, and can cross the placenta to cause hemolytic disease of the newborn.**

(c)   Group O cells have the most H antigen (see above). The lectin of *Ulex europaeus* agglutinates cells with abundant H antigen, including group O cells.

(4)   **Group AB.** Fewer than 5% of the US population are type AB.

(a)   Genotype *AB*

(b)   Patients who are type AB **have no ABO antibodies ("universal recipients").**

(c)   Very little H antigen is expressed (see above), depending on the subtype of A.

2.   **Testing**

a.   **"Forward" grouping** (also called "cell" typing). Uses commercial anti-A and anti-B versus patient red cells.

b.   **"Reverse" grouping** (also called "serum" or "back" typing). Uses patient serum versus commercial A_1 and B red cells, and is based on the principle that a person who is type A will have antibodies against the type B antigen, and so on.

c.   Interpretation (Table 1-4)

(1)   Note that forward reactions are the opposite of reverse reactions; if not, then an "ABO discrepancy" has occurred, and must be resolved. **Common causes of ABO discrepancies:**

(a)   **Abnormal antigens**

(i)   Person has an A_2 **blood group** with anti-A_1 formation.

(ii)   **"Acquired B" phenotype.** Seen in group A patients with exposure to gram-negative bacteria by way of intestinal obstruction or perforation, colon cancer, or gram-negative sepsis. Some bacteria have enzymes that can remove the *N*-acetyl group from the group A terminal *N*-acetylgalactosamine. The resulting galactosamine is similar to the group B terminal galactose and will react with reagent anti-B. This ABO discrepancy usually presents as a weak B antigen on forward grouping, along with a strong anti-B

Table 1-4.   ABO Typing

Forward Typing		Reverse Typing		
Anti-A	Anti-B	A_1 Cells	B Cells	**ABO Group**
4+	0	0	4+	**A**
0	4+	4+	0	**B**
4+	4+	0	0	**AB**
0	0	4+	4+	**O**

The numbers refer to the reaction (agglutination) between the serum antibodies and the red cells.
0, no reaction; 4+, the strongest reaction.

in the person's serum on reverse grouping. It can be resolved by the fact that acidified serum with anti-B does not recognize this "acquired B" antigen.

(iii) Polyagglutination (unusual antigens that cause agglutination with most sera)

(b) Abnormal antibodies or a lack of appropriate antibodies

(i) Non-ABO antibodies (e.g., polyagglutinins, multiple myeloma, monoclonal antibodies) are present that cause agglutination of test red cells.

(ii) Severe immunodeficiency or other low antibody states (AIDS, newborns, elderly)

3. Bombay (O_h) phenotype. A very rare condition wherein patients lack the H gene and, therefore, cannot make H, A, or B antigens on their red cells. These patients type as an "O" with strong reactions against all of the cells in antibody screens (the red cells in antibody screens are type O (with lots of H). These patients have very strong anti-H, anti-A, and anti-B antibodies, and can only receive red cells from a Bombay donor.

B. Lewis blood system

1. Biochemistry

a. The most common Lewis antigens, called Le^a and Le^b, are built on type 1 backbone chains (found primarily in secretions; see section II.A.1.a above). Unlike the terminology of many other blood groups, Le^a and Le^b do not reflect two different alleles, but are the product of a single Lewis gene and gene product (an enzyme that adds fucose to the *sub*terminal sugar of the type 1 chain). **Le^a antigen is the product of the Lewis gene. Le^b antigen refers to the combination of the Le^a antigen and the H antigen on the same type 1 chain** (the H antigen in secretions is controlled by the *Se* gene product, which adds a fucose to the terminal sugar of the type 1 chain). If the patient has the Lewis gene and is a secretor (in other words, has the *Se* gene which 80% of us have), the addition of another fucose by the *Se* gene product to the terminal sugar of the backbone chain creates the Le^b antigen *at the expense of the Le^a antigen* (think "Le^a for **a** fucose, and Le^b for **b**oth fucoses"). The Le^b antigen outcompetes with the Le^a antigen for binding sites on red cells, and so individuals with both Le^a and Le^b in their secretions will have Le^b only on their red cells (Table 1-5). **Most adults have both *Le* and *Se* genes and, thus, have both Le^a and Le^b [Le (a+b+)] in their secretions, and red cells with only Le^b [Le(a−b+)].**

b. Antigens and antibodies

(1) Lewis antigens are called a "system" (rather than a "group") because, unlike the other blood groups, the Lewis antigens are made by tissues other than red cells, and are found on type 1 chains found in secretions. The **Lewis antigens are then *adsorbed* onto the surface of red cells**.

(2) Lewis antibodies are **naturally occurring, cold-reactive, IgM antibodies** (like ABO), and are gener-

**Table 1-5. Lewis and secretor genes,
with their relationship to secretions and red cells**

Genes (Lewis and Secretor)	Secretions	Red Cells
le se	*Le* (a– b–); no H, A, or B antigens (controlled by *Se* gene)	*Le* (a– b–); H,A, and B antigens can be present (controlled by H gene, not the Se gene)
le Se	*Le* (a– b–); H,A, and B antigens can be present	*Le* (a– b–); H, A, and B antigens can be present
Le se	*Le* (a+ b–); no H, A, or B antigens	*Le* (a+ b–); H, A, and B antigens can be present
Le Se	*Le* (a+ b+); H,A, and B antigens can be present	*Le* (a– b+); H, A, and B antigens can be present

Capital letter in gene represents dominant gene.

ally *clinically insignificant* (unlike ABO), and cannot cross the placenta to cause hemolytic disease of the newborn (think "**L**ewis **l**ives and **K**ell **k**ills").

(3)   Lewis antibody activity is *neutralized* by **mixing serum with saliva from a secretor** (contains Le^a and Le^b antigens)

(4)   Lewis (a–b+) persons do not make anti-Le^a, because these persons have Le^a in their own secretions (but not on their red cells).

(5)   Many more blacks than whites lack Lewis antigens completely [22% of blacks are Le(a–b–), versus only 6% of whites].

C.   **I/i blood group**

1.   **Biochemistry**. The I/i antigens are created by adding sugars to the same backbone chains on red cells used to make ABO antigens. The final chains are very simple and unbranched in infancy—called the "i" antigen. They become more complex as the person ages and are then called the "I" antigen. These antigens are first seen after age 18 months and persist through adulthood. Remember: **"Big 'I' in big people, little 'i' in little people"**).

2.   **Antibodies. These are cold-reacting, naturally occurring IgM antibodies that are usually insignificant. The auto-anti-I is associated with cold agglutinin disease and *Mycoplasma pneumoniae* infections. The auto-anti-i is associated with infectious mononucleosis**.

D.   **P blood group**

1.   **Biochemistry**. Antigens are created from the same basic backbone chains on red cells that are used to create the ABO antigens.

2.   **Antigens and antibodies**

a.   The most common antigens are P_1 **(most frequent)**, **P, and** P^k.

b.   **Anti-P_1 is usually a cold-reacting, naturally occurring IgM that is clinically insignificant**. Mixing the patient's serum with **hydatid cyst fluid** or **pigeon egg fluid** neutralizes anti-P_1, which may be useful in its identification.

c.   **Anti-PP_1Pk is rare but significant**. It is rare because very few people lack all three antigens. It is significant because it causes **spontaneous abortions** and **acute hemolytic transfusion reactions**.

d.   Antibodies against P antigens are associated with **paroxysmal cold hemoglobinuria** (PCH), an acute hemolytic anemia caused by **auto-anti-P**. PCH is usually associated with a preceding viral illness. The antibody is an **IgG** (unlike most P antibodies) called a **"Donath-Landsteiner biphasic hemolysin."** These antibodies bind well to red cells at cold temperatures, and then hemolyze them *after* they are warmed up.

e.   **Parvovirus B19** gains entry into red cells via the P antigen.

III.   **Rh blood group system**

A.   **Biochemistry and terminology**. The Rh group of antigens is a complex blood group with >50 described antigens. The antigens are lipoproteins that form an integral part of the red cell membrane. **Five *major* antigens and genes exist: D, C, c, E, and e**. The phrase **"Rh positive" really means "D positive,"** and the phrase "Rh negative" means "D negative" (D negative is designated in genotypes by the letter "d," although no such antigen exists). These five genes can combine in eight different configurations (four being D-positive and four being D-negative), with a shorthand method used to describe each configuration (Table 1-6).

B.   **Antigens and antibodies**

1.   "The **Big Four**" antigens. Of the configurations listed in Table 1-6, four have by far the highest frequency: R^1, R^2, R^0, and **r** (>97% combined frequency).

2.   Relative frequencies of the Rh antigens for blacks and whites are important to remember:

- **White:** $R^1 > r > R^2 > R^0$
- **Black:** $R^0 > r > R^1 > R^2$

Table 1-6.   Shorthand notations for Rh antigens

R^1 = Dce	r′ = dCe
R^2 = DcE	r″ = dcE
R^0 = Dce	r = dce
R^z = DCE	r^y = dCE

The left column is all D–positive, whereas the right column is all D–negative. R = D; r = d; 1 or prime (′) = C; 2 or double prime (″) = E; 0 or blank, = ce; z or y = CE.

Clues: R^0 is most common in blacks and least common in whites, r is always the second most common, and R^1 always comes before R^2.

3. Rh antibodies are **warm-reacting, exposure-requiring IgG antibodies that are clinically significant**. Rh antigens (especially D) are potent immunogens. Of D-negative patients, 80% will develop an anti-D when transfused with a single unit of D-positive blood.

4. Rh antibodies can cause **significant acute and delayed hemolytic transfusion reactions, as well as classic, severe hemolytic disease of the newborn**.

5. Weak D phenotype. Most D-positive patients have easily detectable D antigens, whereas others have weakly expressed D antigens that require more sensitive testing to detect (e.g., an indirect antiglobulin test—IAT). Because of this, **all apparently D-negative blood donors must have a weak-D** test to avoid false classification. D-negative **recipients do not** automatically get a weak D test (although D-negative pregnant women should get one), and are just given D-negative blood.

6. Rh-$_{null}$ phenotype. These patients have a **total lack of all Rh antigens**, which can be associated with a **hemolytic anemia with stomatocytes** on the peripheral smear.

7. Unusual and compound Rh antigens

    a. G antigen. This is a specific antigen that may be present when either C or D antigen is present.

    b. f antigen. The f antigen is a compound antigen that represents the c and e genes when they are next to each on the same chromosome (i.e., with R^0 or r haplotypes).

IV. Kidd blood group

A. Biochemistry. The Kidd antigens are membrane proteins.

B. Antigens and antibodies. Jk^a and Jk^b are the two major antigens.

1. Anti-Jk^a and anti-Jk^b are **warm-reacting, exposure-requiring, and clinically significant IgG antibodies**.

2. Antibodies show marked **"dosage"**: for example, anti-Jk^a reacts much stronger against the Jk^a antigen in someone whose genotype is Jk^a/Jk^a ("homozygous" for Jk^a) than in someone who carries Jk^a/Jk^b ("heterozygous"). **Dosage is also prominent in the Duffy and MNSs systems, as well as in non-D Rh groups**.

3. Antibodies show variable titers over time, and may even completely disappear ("kids like to hide"). This emphasizes the importance of **prior record checks**, as well as asking the patient about a history of antibodies or previous transfusion reactions.

4. Kidd antibodies can cause delayed hemolytic transfusion reactions. This occurs when the antibodies "disappear" over time (as described above), making them undetectable in pretransfusion screening tests, and the patient is then re-exposed to the Kidd antigens through another transfusion. The anamnestic response leads to a surging tide of antibody that hemolyzes circulating cells in the weeks following transfusion. Although the Kidd antibodies are **IgG**, these antibodies are very capable of fixing complement and can cause **severe intravascular hemolysis**, which is unusual for IgG.

V. MNSs blood group system

A. Biochemistry. MNSs antigens are found on long glycoprotein chains called "glycophorins," the most common of which are called glycophorin A and glycophorin B.

1. Glycophorin A forms the foundation of the **M** and **N** antigens, which are found near the end of the glycophorin chain. The lectin **vicea graminea** agglutinates red cells with the N antigen.

2. Glycophorin B forms the foundation of the **S, s,** and **U** antigens. The U antigen is a common core that is shared by the Ss antigens (think of it as "Universal"). In addition, all glycophorin B chains carry a segment at the end of the chain that is identical to the N antigen ("N-like antigen"). This makes everyone who has glycophorin B (the vast majority of people), appear to have small amounts of the actual N antigen.

B. Antigens and antibodies

1. Antibodies to M, N, S, s, and U antigens fall into two polar, opposite groups:

- **Anti-M and anti-N: cold-reacting, naturally occurring, and usually clinically insignificant IgM**, although IgG examples are seen.
- **Anti-S, -s, and -U: warm-reacting, exposure-requiring, and clinically significant IgG**. These IgG antibodies show a strong **dosage effect** (see IV.B.2 above).

2. Antibodies to N are associated with hemodialysis. Formaldehyde sterilization of dialysis equipment can lead to a modification of the N antigen, with subsequent formation of anti-N.

3. Racial differences. Glycophorin B is absent in < 1% of blacks but never absent in whites. A lack of glycophorin B means that the S, s, and U antigens cannot form (see above). When these patients are exposed to red cells with glycophorin B (and S, s, and U antigens), they will make antibodies against U, and from that time forward, it becomes very difficult to find compatible donors (who also are lacking glycophorin B).

4. Glycophorin A (with the M antigen) may be the receptor that allows some virulent *Escherichia coli* strains to invade the urinary bladder. **Glycophorins A** and **B** (with antigens M, N, S, or s) may be the receptors that allow *Plasmodium falciparum* (malaria) to invade red cells.

VI. Duffy blood group

A. Biochemistry. The Duffy antigens are glycoproteins.

B. Antigens and antibodies. Fy^a and Fy^b are the main antigens.

1. Fy(a–b–) phenotype (lack of both main antigens) is very common in blacks (68%), but very rare in whites.

2. Anti-Fy^a and -Fy^b are **warm-reacting, exposure-requiring, clinically significant IgG** antibodies (can cause hemolytic transfusion reactions and HDN).

3. Anti-Fy^a and -Fy^b have a strong **dosage effect** (see IV.B.2 above).

4. Anti-Fy^a and -Fy^b can cause **severe acute and delayed hemolytic transfusion reactions.**

5. Anti-Fy^a and -Fy^b, as with Kidd antibodies, **can fade over time** and become undetectable until the patient is re-exposed to the antigens.

6. The lack of Duffy antigens conveys **resistance to infection by *Plasmodium vivax*** (malaria). *Plasmodium vivax* enters red cells via Fy^6, a Duffy antigen that is present when either Fy^a or Fy^b are present. Of black patients, 68% lack Fy^a and Fy^b and, therefore, Fy^6. Other common malarial parasites are unaffected by Duffy antigen absence.

VII. Kell blood group system

A. Biochemistry. Kell antigens are glycoproteins that can interact with structural proteins in red cell membranes.

B. Antigens and antibodies. The common Blood Bank issues involve the K, k, Kx, Kp^a/Kp^b, and Js^a/Js^b antigens.

1. **The K antigen**
   a. K is a relatively **low-frequency antigen** (9% in whites, 2% in blacks).
   b. The K antigen is **unaffected by proteolytic enzymes alone**, but is destroyed by thiol reagents such as dithiothreitol and ZZAP.
   c. Anti-K is a **very common, warm-reacting, exposure-requiring, clinically significant IgG**.
   d. Anti-K causes **significant acute and delayed hemolytic transfusion reactions, and HDN.**

2. **The k antigen (also known as "cellano" antigen)**
   a. The k antigen is a **high-frequency antigen** (99.8% of the population has it).
   b. Anti-k, although very uncommon because of the high antigen frequency, is similar in most other aspects to anti-K.

3. **The K$_x$ antigen** was formerly thought to be a precursor antigen, but is now known to be a separate antigen. It is probably a structural component of Kell antigens and red cell walls.

4. **McLeod phenotype**
   a. Defined as the **absence of the K$_x$ antigen**
   b. Patients may develop **hemolytic anemia with acanthocytes** on the peripheral smear.
   c. The most famous association is with **x-linked chronic granulomatous disease (CGD)**. CGD is characterized by a lack of nicotinamide adenine dinucleotide phosphate (NADPH) oxidase, which normally helps granulocytes kill ingested organisms. Patients with CGD are susceptible to repeated infections by catalase-positive organisms (especially *Staphylococcus aureus*).

5. **Other Kell system antigen pairs**
   a. Kp^a (low frequency) and Kp^b (high frequency)
   b. Js^a (low frequency) and Js^b (high frequency)

6. **Kell null phenotype**
   a. **Total lack of all Kell system antigens, except K$_x$ (which is increased)**

b.   Patients develop anti-Ku ("Kell universal") with exposure to red cells with K antigens. Anti-Ku reacts against all Kell system antigens, and finding compatible blood donors is a very difficult.

VIII.   High-titer, low-avidity antibodies (HTLA). The HTLA antibodies are composed of a group of antibodies that weakly react with high frequency antigens. These weak reactions typically occur with a broad spectrum of reagent cells in the antibody screens (the entire panel shows 1+ reactions). The most common are **Chido** and **Rodgers** types, which are clinically insignificant.)

Transfusion-Related Testing

Constance F. M. Danielson and Leo J. McCarthy

I. Introduction

A. Goals. The goals of transfusion-related testing are to **identify clinically significant antigens** (Ags) **on red blood cells** (RBCs), **identify plasma antibodies** (Abs) to RBC antigens, and to detect antibodies and complement bound to RBCs.

B. Antibodies of the immunoglobulin M (**IgM**) and **IgG** classes comprise 80% of the circulating Abs and are the **most significant** Abs for transfusion-related testing.

C. IgM is large and has 10 potential antigen-binding sites. IgM molecules can bind to Ags on adjacent RBCs ("bridging"), forming a lattice or clump (**agglutination**).

D. IgG is much smaller and has only two antigen-binding sites. Therefore, IgG usually binds to antigens on a single RBC, and is unable to bridge RBCs and cause agglutination.

E. RBCs that have Ab, complement, or both bound to their surfaces are referred to as **"sensitized."**

F. To detect Ab (particularly IgG) or complement bound to RBC, **anti-human globulin reagent** (AHG—Abs that bind to human IgG or complement) also referred to as **"Coombs reagent"** can be added. This causes bridging of adjacent sensitized RBCs and results in agglutination.

G. Agglutination (clumping) of RBCs is the end result of testing, which indicates a positive reaction.

II. The antiglobulin test (Coombs' test)

A. History. The antiglobulin test (AT) described by Coombs, Mourant, and Race in 1945, remains the most important single test in Ab detection. It is often referred to as the "Coombs' test" or "Coombs' phase" of the cross match.

B. Principle. Red blood cells sensitized by IgG or complement can be made to agglutinate by adding anti-human globulin. The **direct antiglobulin test (DAT)** detects RBCs that have already been sensitized with IgG or complement *in vivo* (Fig. 1-2). The **indirect antiglobulin test (IAT)** detects Abs (to RBC antigens) in the patient's serum.

C. Major uses of the antiglobulin test. To detect hemolytic disease of the newborn (HDN), hemolytic transfusion reactions, autoimmune hemolytic anemia (AIHA), drug-induced hemolytic anemias, and in the final Coombs' phase of typing, screening, and cross-matching blood.

III. Red blood cell (RBC) typing

A. Introduction. The **ABO blood group antigens** were discovered by Karl Landsteiner in 1900 and remain the most significant. **The second most important group of RBC antigens is the Rhesus (Rh)** blood group system. Although it is made up of more than 40 antigens, the **D antigen is the most clinically significant**. Approximately **85%** of the general population are Rh (D antigen) positive. The remaining **15% are Rh**

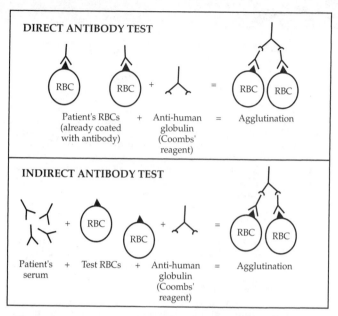

Fig. 1-2. Direct and indirect antiglobulin testing (Coombs' tests).

negative—capable of forming anti-D if exposed to the D antigen by transfusion or pregnancy. Approximately 70% to 80% of Rh-negative individuals who are transfused with Rh-positive blood will form anti-D. Therefore, it is important that **Rh-negative women capable of childbearing are transfused with only Rh-negative RBCs.**

Many bacteria, yeast, and foodstuffs possess structures similar to the A and B antigens. Consequently, **people are exposed early in life to A- and B-like antigens, and develop "naturally occurring" ABO Abs (isoagglutinins)** to the antigens which their own red cells do not express. Therefore, a group A person will form anti-B, a group B person will form anti-A, a group AB person will not form Abs to either A or B, and so forth. **Acquired RBC Abs are Abs that people develop after being exposed to foreign antigens by blood transfusions, tissue transplants, or pregnancy (e.g., anti-D).**

B. Procedure for RBC Typing

1. Forward typing. **Typing the red cells** is often referred to as "forward typing" or "front typing." A commercially obtained **monoclonal antibody reagent** (anti-A, anti-B, anti-A,B, or anti-D) is mixed separately with one drop of suspension containing the **red cells to be tested**, centrifuged, and then observed for agglutination. The **presence of agglutination is a positive test** (the red cells possess the antigen or are of the type for which the monoclonal Abs

Table 1-7. Forward typing (patient red cells and commercial antisera)

Patient's Blood Type	Commercial Antisera		
	Anti-A	Anti-B	Anti-A,B
A	+	0	+
B	0	+	+
O	0	0	0
AB	+	+	+

+, the commercial antisera agglutinates the patient's red cells; 0, the commercial antisera does not agglutinate the patient's red cells.

are specific), whereas the absence of agglutination is a negative test (Table 1-7).

　　2.   Back typing is testing a **person's serum with commercial red cells of known types** (Table 1-8).

　　3.   Forward typing can be used to detect other antigens present on the patient's RBCs (**RBC phenotype**), by using antisera with known specificity. Nearly 400 RBC antigens have been discovered, which vary greatly in clinical significance. Commercial human antisera are available to identify the more common ones, such as antigens of the **Kell, Duffy, Kidd, MNSs,** and **Lewis blood group systems**. For typing less common blood group antigens, sera must be obtained from individuals who have formed the corresponding Abs, and may or may not be available.

IV.   Detection of antibodies to RBC antigens ("screening" for antibodies)

　　A.   Tube testing—the most commonly used method

　　　　1.   The patient's serum is mixed with a suspension of commercial reagent RBCs (cells with known antigens). After mixing and centrifugation at **room temperature**, the RBC button is gently resuspended and examined for agglutination (agglutination indicates that the patient's serum

Table 1-8. Back typing (patient serum reactions with various types of commercial red cells)

Patient's Serum Blood Type	Commercial red cells of known types		
	A Cells	B Cells	AB Cells
A	0	+	+
B	+	0	+
O	+	+	+
AB	0	0	0

+, the patient's serum agglutinates the commercial red cells; 0, the patient's serum does not agglutinate the commercial red cells.

contains Ab attached to the RBCs). **Agglutination at this point indicates a positive test in the immediate spin phase of testing**.

   2. In addition to the patient's serum and the reagent RBCs, **an enhancing substance can be added** [e.g., albumin, low-ionic strength solution (LISS), polyethylene glycol (PEG)]. The patient's serum, reagent RBCs, and enhancing substance are then mixed, incubated at **37°C**, and centrifuged. The RBC button is gently resuspended and examined for agglutination (referred to as the "37°C reading").

   3. After the 37°C reading, the RBCs are washed with saline, and **anti-human globulin reagent (Coombs' reagent) is then added**. After mixing and centrifugation, the RBC button is again gently resuspended and examined for agglutination. **Agglutination indicates a positive test in the anti-globulin phase**. Agglutination in any phase of testing indicates that the patient's serum contains Abs to the RBCs.

   B.   Effects of temperature on antibodies. Different types of Abs display optimal reactivity at different temperatures. **IgM Abs usually react best at $\leq 22°C$**; they are referred to as **"cold antibodies"** and are often **detected in the immediate spin phase of testing** (performed at room temperature). **IgG Abs usually react optimally at 37°C**; they are referred to as **"warm antibodies"** and are often **detected in the anti-human globulin phase of testing**. Antibodies that do not react at body temperature are usually not clinically significant (Fig. 1-3).

V	Rh Antigens					Lewis		Kell		Duffy		Kidd		V	Results			
	D	C	c	E	e	Le^a	Le^b	K	k	Fy^a	Fy^b	Jk^a	Jk^b		IS	37°	AHG	FIC
1	o	+	o	+	o	o	+	+	+	+	o	+	+	1	O	4+	4+	1+
2	+	+	o	+	o	o	+	+	o	o	+	o	+	2	O	O	O	O
3	o	o	+	o	+	+	o	o	o	+	+	+	o	3	O	3+	3+	O
4	o	+	+	o	+	o	o	o	+	o	o	+	o	4	O	O	O	O
Patient autocontrol															O	O	O	O

STEP #1: check autocontrol: results are negative; therefore, there is no autoantibody. Procede to Step #2.

STEP #2: look at the vials with no agglutination ("O" under the "Results" column: Vials #2 and #4—the shaded rows), and cross out the antigens that are present in each of the vials (there is no agglutination, so the antibodies must not be against the antigens in these two vials).

STEP #3: Look at the antigens that are not yet crossed off (Lewis^a [Le^a] and Duffy^a [Fy^a]), and note that Fy^a best fits the agglutination pattern (each vial with Fy^a shows agglutination; compare to Le^a which is absent in vial #1 and yet there is agglutination).

STEP #4: The finding of an antibody against Fy^a is consistent with the fact that the agglutination occurs only at 37°C and is decreased by the enzyme ficin, both of which should occur with warm antibodies against Duffy (vs. anti-Lewis antibodies which are cold antibodies that show increased agglutination after enzyme treatment).

Fig. 1-3. **Example of how to identify an unknown antibody.** AHG, anti-human globulin; FIC, ficin (an enzyme from the fig tree); IS, immediate spin; V, vial; +, antigen is present in the vial mixture; o, antigen is absent in the vial mixture; (in the "Results" column), no agglutination; numbers with plus signs, agglutination occurred.

Table 1-9.   Recipient red cell types (Ag) with normally expected recipient serum Antibodies (Ab)

Recipient Red Cell Type	Expected Recipient Serum Antibodies
A	Anti-B
B	Anti-A
AB	None
O	Anti-A, Anti-B, Anti-A,B

C.   Nontraditional testing methods

1.   Flow cytometry. These techniques are useful to identify two populations of RBCs (e.g., transfused RBCs, fetal-maternal hemorrhage) or extremely low levels of IgG bound to RBCs.

2.   Solid-phase adherence can identify antigens or antibodies.

3.   Gel-test is useful for antigen or antibody identification and cross matching.

V.   Pretransfusion testing

A.   Type and screen. A blood specimen from the intended recipient (a single specimen can be used for up to 3 days) is tested in the following manner.

1.   Type. Determine patient's ABO and Rh type; both forward and back ABO typing are required. Expected results of ABO typing are listed in Table 1-9. **Any discrepancies must be resolved**. Most discrepancies result from **clerical** or **technical mistakes**. Some causes of true discrepancies are listed in Table 1-10.

Table 1-10.   Potential causes and methods of handling ABO typing discrepancies

Potential causes of ABO discrepancies:
1. **An expected back type (antibody) reaction is missing**, caused by immunodeficiencies (newborns, elderly, leukemias, AIDS, immunosuppression drugs.)
2. **An expected forward type (antigen) reaction is missing**, because of the presence of **A or B subgroups, leukemias** (may cause altered antigens), **blood–group–specific–soluble substances** (BGSS; found in some cancers; they bind and neutralize the reagent antibodies), and "acquired B" phenomenon. The **acquired B phenomenon** occurs when a patient with type A cells appears to have B antigens in the forward typing test; this is usually due to **gram–negative sepsis** by organisms (e.g., *Escherichia coli, Klebsiella sp.*) that have enzymes capable of cleaving the A antigen, leaving a residue that mimics the B antigen.
3. **Plasma proteins** (e.g., monoclonal immunoglobulins in multiple myeloma) may interfere with the tests.
4. **Autoantibodies** may interfere with the tests.

AIDS, acquired immunodeficiency syndrome.

2.   Antibody screen. Test serum or plasma to detect antibodies to RBC antigens. This is preformed by **adding the patient's serum to two or three different types of RBCs (with known antigenic phenotypes),** followed by the addition of anti-human globulin reagent.

3.   If unexpected RBC antibodies are detected, their specificity should be determined.

B.   **Type and cross match. Includes the testing for a type and screen as well as the following tests.**

1.   Donor RBC typing. RBCs from the unit to be transfused (donor RBCs) should be typed for **ABO, Rh,** and **any additional significant antigens for which the recipient has Ab** (if unexpected Abs are indeed discovered in the recipient).

2.   Major cross match. The recipients serum should be mixed directly with donor RBCs to ensure compatibility. For recipients with no current or past history of unexpected RBC antibodies, an "immediate spin cross match" may be performed (the antiglobulin phase of the cross match is omitted). This reduces the time it takes to do the cross match from approximately 40 minutes to 10 minutes, allowing blood or blood products to be released more quickly.

1.5

Transfusion Reactions

Constance F.M. Danielson and Leo J. McCarthy

I.   Introduction. A transfusion reaction, as defined here, refers to any adverse event that occurs as a result of infusing blood or blood components. Acute reactions occur within minutes to 24 hours of the transfusion. **Delayed reactions** develop days to months to even years after the transfusion. Fig. 1-4 is a simplified algorithm that may assist in the differentiation of acute transfusion reactions. For example, during transfusion of RBCs, a patient's temperature increases 1°C with only minor changes in other vital signs. A post-transfusion blood and urine specimen is collected from the recipient with the remainder of the transfused unit sent to the Blood Bank. A clerical check is repeated and the blood and urine checked for hemolysis. The patient's physician meanwhile has been evaluating the patient for evidence of respiratory distress and hypotension. If neither is present, blood for culture and Gram's stain should still be obtained and the Blood Bank should culture and perform the Gram's stain on the returned unit. All testing may be negative. In this case, symptoms and findings are most suggestive of a nonhemolytic febrile transfusion reaction (NHFTR).

II.   Acute transfusion reactions

A.   Clinical presentation. Several types of acute transfusion reactions occur. They vary in severity, but **may share some similar signs and symptoms** (Table 1-11). **Fever** (defined as a ≥1°C increase in temperature) is present in several of the reactions; however, patients taking antipyretics (e.g., acetaminophen, aspirin) may have a blunted or absent febrile response. **Chills, nausea, flank pain, hypotension,** and **shortness of breath** can also occur in some acute reactions.

B.   Responses to suspected transfusion reactions

1.   The initial response, regardless of the cause of the reaction, should be to:

a.   Stop the transfusion

b.   Keep the intravenous (IV) line open with 0.9% saline

c.   Notify the patient's physician and the Blood Bank

2.   Secondary responses should include obtaining **vital signs,** performing a **brief physical examination,** beginning O_2 and obtaining a chest x-ray study if pulmonary symptoms are present, and obtaining **post-transfusion blood and urine specimens.** Laboratory analyses that may be needed include tests for hemoglobinemia (free plasma hemoglobin), hemoglobinuria, direct antiglobulin test (DAT), and confirmatory ABO groupings. (Note: the partially transfused unit must be returned to the blood bank.) The hemoglobin and hematocrit should also be checked, along with serum haptoglobin, lactate dehydrogenase (LDH), and indirect (unconjugated) bilirubin if hemolysis is still suspected but unproved.

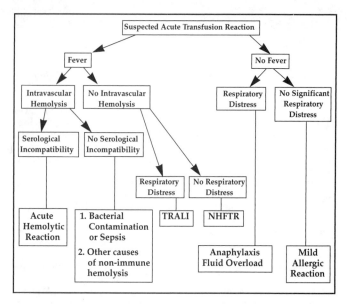

Fig. 1-4. Algorithm for suspected acute transfusion reactions. NHFTR, nonhemolytic febrile transfusion reaction; TRALI, transfusion-related acute lung injury.

Coagulation tests and platelet counts should be ordered if disseminated intravascular coagulation (DIC) is suspected. Electrolytes, especially potassium, should be monitored. If the differential diagnosis includes bacteremia or sepsis, specimens from the patient and from the partially transfused unit should be Gram stained and cultured.

C. Acute hemolytic transfusion reactions (AHTR)

1. **Hemolysis is defined as the lysis or accelerated removal of red blood cells (RBCs). AHTR has an incidence of 1 case per 25,000 units transfused.**

    a. **Intravascular hemolysis**, when immune mediated, is caused by rapid **complement activation by IgM** antibodies (less commonly, by IgG_1 or IgG_3). Nonimmune mechanisms include bacterial contamination, incompatible fluids (e.g., hypotonic, calcium-containing), temperature extremes during storage or administration, mechanical trauma (e.g., small needles or high pressures), intrinsic RBC or Hgb abnormalities in either blood product or recipient (e.g., glucose-6-phosphate dehydrogenase [G6PD] deficiency, Hgb SS)

    (1) **Laboratory findings include hemoglobinemia and hemoglobinuria** (the free hemoglobin causes both plasma and urine to appear red), **decreased serum haptoglobin,** and **increased lactate dehydrogenase.**

    (2) **Transfusion of ABO-incompatible blood is the most common cause of AHTR and is usually the result of clerical error!**

Table 1-11. Common signs and symptoms of acute transfusion reactions

Signs and Symptoms	Types of Acute Transfusion Reactions					
	Circulatory Overload	AHTR	FNHTR	Allergic Mild/Severe	TRALI	Bacterial Contamination
Fever	–	+	+	–/–	+	+
Chills	–	+	+	–/–	+	+
SOB	+	+	+	–/+	+	–
Hypotension and shock	–[a]	+	–[b]	–/+	+	+
DIC	–	+	–	–/–	–	+
N & V	–	+	+	–/+	–	+
Hgb–emia	–	+	–	–/–	–	+
Hgb–uria	–	+	–	–/–	–	+
DAT	–	+	–	–/–	–	–

AHTR, acute hemolytic transfusion reaction; DAT, direct antiglobulin test; DIC, disseminated intravascular coagulation; FNHTR, febrile non-hemolytic transfusion reaction; Hgb–emia, hemoglobinemia; Hgb–uria, hemoglobinuria; N/V, nausea and vomiting; SOB, shortness of breath; TRALI, transfusion related acute lung injury.

[a] Circulatory overload is associated with *hyper*tension and signs of congestive heart failure.

[b] Hypotension is unusual in FNHTR.

   b.   Extravascular hemolysis is usually caused by **IgG antibodies that coat the RBCs** and lead to their increased removal by macrophages of the reticuloendothelial system. Laboratory findings can include **spherocytes** on blood peripheral smears, **increased lactate dehydrogenase,** and **increased unconjugated (indirect) bilirubin**.

   c.   Symptoms associated with intravascular hemolysis tend to be severe and can even be life-threatening; however, both intravascular and extravascular hemolysis occur in most AHTR.

   2.   Clinical presentation. Signs and symptoms develop during or shortly after transfusion. They include **fever, chills, pain, nausea, hypotension, tachycardia**, and less frequently shortness of breath. DIC can develop and cause excessive bleeding in surgical patients. Renal failure is a serious complication.

   3.   Evaluation and initial response. Follow the steps listed in section II.B.

   4.   Treatment and prevention

   a.   To maintain intravascular volume, give IV fluids (0.9% saline) and, if necessary, dopamine 1–5 µg/kg/min.

   b.   Monitor and maintain urine output at ≥100 mL/h using diuretics (furosemide or mannitol) in addition to fluids.

   c.   Treat hyperkalemia and, if present, increased bleeding caused by DIC.

   d.   Prevention relies on error elimination, and requires **accurate identification of specimens, transfusion products,** and **intended recipients**.

D.   Bacterial contamination. Reactions caused by bacterial contamination are most commonly associated with transfusions of **platelets** (because they are stored at 20°C to 24°C for up to 5 days) or **RBCs** (stored at 1°C to 6°C for up to 42 days).

   1.   Clinical presentation. Signs and symptoms typically develop during, or within 3 hours of, the transfusion. They include **fever, chills, hypotension, nausea and vomiting, shortness of breath,** and **diarrhea**. Associated complications include DIC, renal failure, shock, and death.

   2.   Evaluation and initial response. Perform the three standard initial steps (see section II.B). Then perform **Gram's stain, and culture** the partially transfused unit and a blood specimen from the recipient. Organisms that have been implicated include *Yersinia enterocolitica, Salmonella, Bacillus, Campylobacter, Staphylococcus, Streptococcus, Serratia, Treponema pallidum* (syphilis), and diphtheroids.

   3.   Treatment and prevention

   a.   Broad spectrum antibiotic therapy should be quickly initiated on an empiric basis (Gram's stain results may be helpful but are negative in one third of cases). Provide supportive care as needed, including fluids, oxygen, and vasopressors.

   b.   To minimize risk, adhere to proper procedures for collecting, storing, and handling blood components. Inspect all components before transfusing. If appearance is abnormal (e.g., clots present, hemolyzed, darker, or discolored) do not transfuse. Unfortunately, not all contaminated components appear abnormal.

E. Allergic reactions can be caused by **recipient antibodies against donor plasma antigens** (e.g., an IgA-deficient recipient who has antibodies against **donor IgA**), **anaphylatoxins** (e.g., C3a and C5a) in the blood product, or **IgE antibodies in the blood product** that react with recipient antigens. The end result of all the above mechanisms is the activation of recipient mast cells or basophils.

 1. **Clinical presentation**

 a. **Mild allergic reactions. Pruritus and localized urticaria (hives)** during, or shortly after, the transfusion complicates approximately 1% of transfusions.

 b. **Severe allergic or anaphylactic reactions**. Symptoms can include generalized **urticaria, angioedema, respiratory distress** from bronchospasm or laryngeal edema, **gastrointestinal symptoms** (e.g., nausea and vomiting, cramps, diarrhea), **profound hypotension**, and possible loss of consciousness. These reactions, which are rare, tend to develop quickly, usually occurring **within 1 hour** of starting the transfusion.

 2. **Evaluation and initial response. Perform the three standard initial steps (see section II.B)**. Additional evaluation will depend on the severity of the reaction.

 a. **Mild reactions**. No additional investigation is necessary.

 b. **Severe or anaphylactic reactions**. Use history, including known food and drug allergies, to identify allergens if possible. If appropriate, test recipient for presence of IgA and anti-IgA antibodies.

 3. **Treatment and prevention**

 a. **Mild allergic reaction** (pruritus and localized urticaria only). Administer an antihistamine (e.g., diphenhydramine 25–50 mg IV or orally). If symptoms resolve, transfusion may be cautiously continued. Before future transfusions, diphenhydramine 25–50 mg PO or IV may be helpful.

 b. **Anaphylactic reaction**

 (1) Administer epinephrine subcutaneously (0.3–0.5 mL of a 1:1000 solution), which can be repeated in 20–30 minutes × 2.

 (2) Give O_2.

 (3) Diphenhydramine [50 mg intramuscularly (IM) or IV]; can be repeated × 1.

 (4) Crystalloids (either normal saline or Ringer's lactate solution) to maintain blood volume and blood pressure. If hypotension persists, give epinephrine IV (5–10 mL of a 1:10,000 solution), which can be repeated; continue crystalloid infusion; begin dopamine infusion (1–5 µg/kg/min).

 (5) Aminophylline—loading dose (6 mg/kg IV) then 0.5–1 mg/kg/h to reduce bronchospasm. If severe respiratory distress occurs, intubate and begin mechanical ventilation or perform tracheostomy in cases of severe laryngeal edema.

      c. **Prolonged reactions**. Consider hydrocortisone (up to 500 mg IV every 6 h) and monitor patients closely (at least 6 h) for recurrent symptoms.

      d. **Prevention of severe allergic reactions**

        (1) If possible, determine the allergen (e.g., does the patient have anti-IgA) and use blood products lacking the antigens.

        (2) Premedicate before transfusion if allogeneic plasma must be transfused which is not allergen free. One possible premedication regimen: 13, 7, and 1 hours pretransfusion, give prednisone (50 mg); in addition, 1 hour before transfusion give diphenhydramine (50 mg) and ephedrine (25 mg)[1].

        (3) Predeposit autologous blood or components before elective surgeries.

        (4) Provide washed allogeneic cellular components.

F. **Transfusion-related acute lung injury (TRALI)**. Caused by **donor antibodies to recipient leukocyte antigens** that results in complement activation and clustering of granulocytes in the recipient's pulmonary microvasculature. This is followed by endothelial damage and capillary leakage. **TRALI is similar to adult respiratory distress syndrome** except that the pulmonary lesion in TRALI appears more reversible.

    1. **Clinical presentation**. Signs and symptoms include **acute respiratory distress** resulting from severe bilateral pulmonary edema, hypoxemia, fever, tachycardia, hypotension, and cyanosis. These symptoms typically develop **1–6 hours after transfusion of plasma-containing blood components**. Chest x-ray study reveals patchy infiltrates or the classic **"white-out" of both lungs**. The central venous and pulmonary **wedge pressures remain normal**, ruling out circulatory overload.

    2. **Evaluation and initial response. Perform the three standard initial steps (see section II.B)**. Then obtain a chest x-ray study to confirm pulmonary edema. Rule out other causes of respiratory distress and pulmonary edema, including circulatory overload (invasive hemodynamic monitoring may be helpful), sepsis, and myocardial infarction. The donor plasma can be tested for HLA, granulocyte-specific antibodies, or both, but this is seldom indicated.

    3. **Treatment and prevention**. Oxygen should be provided, and mechanical ventilation is frequently required. Maintain adequate levels of hemoglobin to increase oxygen delivery. Specific mechanisms for prevention of TRALI are not available; however, use of solvent/detergent treated plasma (plasma-S/D) as an alternative to fresh frozen plasma (FFP) may be beneficial. Close monitoring of the transfused patient is always needed.

G. **Febrile nonhemolytic transfusion reactions (FNHTR)**. These reactions are most commonly associated with platelet transfusions, but can also occur with RBC transfusions. They complicate 0.5% to 1.5% of transfusions. Causes of FNHTR include **antibodies in the recipient that react with donor leukocytes** (causing subsequent cytokine release), and the accumulation during storage of pyogenic soluble factors (e.g., IL-1, IL-6, IL-8, tumor necrosis factor, complement fragments).

1. **Clinical presentation**. Signs and symptoms include **fever, chills (rigors), nausea and vomiting**, and uneasiness or discomfort, which typically develop **during or within 1–2 hours** of the transfusion.

2. **Evaluation and initial response. Perform the three standard initial steps (see section II.B)**. Rule out other potentially more serious transfusion reactions (e.g., bacterial contamination, immune hemolysis) and underlying clinical conditions.

3. **Treatment and prevention**. The following medications may be helpful in treating current symptoms or in preventing recurrent reactions: acetaminophen 650 mg PO (for fever); meperidine IV 50–75 mg (for chills); IV diphenhydramine 25–50 mg IV or PO (for allergic symptoms). For recurring FNHTR (~15% of FNHTR will recur), prestorage leukocyte-reduced RBCs and platelets should be provided.

H. **Other acute transfusion-related complications**

1. **Circulatory overload. Infants, the elderly, and severely anemic patients are at increased risk**. Signs and symptoms include **shortness of breath, tachycardia, increased blood pressure, headache, and edema**. Evaluation includes the standard three initial steps (see section II.B), followed by excluding other causes of respiratory distress. Treatment includes oxygen and diuretics. Administer future transfusions very slowly. Half-units or aliquots from the Blood Bank may need to be requested so that the entire amount can be infused within the maximal allowed time of 4 hours.

2. **Electrolyte abnormalities, and others**. Transfusions, especially when massive, can be associated with **hypocalcemia, hypomagnesemia, hyper- or hypokalemia, metabolic alkalosis, hypothermia**, and **dilutional coagulopathy** (with transfusion of RBCs equal to more than one or two blood volumes). Patients receiving massive transfusions must be closely monitored, and any abnormalities that develop should be corrected as quickly as possible.

III. **Delayed transfusion reactions**

A. **Delayed hemolytic transfusion reactions (DHTR)**. These reactions are typically caused by **IgG antibodies against RBC antigens** that developed in response to a previous transfusion or pregnancy, but which are no longer detectable because of very low titers. Following a repeat RBC transfusion, the anamnestic response causes the antibodies to quickly increase in titer and then coat the RBCs, and then the RBCs are removed by macrophages (**extravascular hemolysis**).

1. **Clinical presentation**. Signs and symptoms are **often mild, but can include fever, chills, pain, hyperbilirubinemia, anemia (with spherocytes in the peripheral smear)**, and **renal failure**.

2. **Evaluation**. Perform direct and indirect antiglobulin tests. Hemoglobin, hematocrit, indirect bilirubin, blood urea nitrogen (BUN), and creatinine may also be checked.

3. **Treatment and prevention**. Usually, no treatment is needed other than the possible transfusion of antigen-negative, compatible RBCs. If symptoms are severe, follow the guidelines for treatment of AHTR (see section II.B–C). Document the

unexpected RBC antibody in the patient's medical record. Communicate this information to the patient or guardian verbally and in writing, if possible.

B. Infectious disease transmission. Several infections are transmissible by transfusion, including **hepatitis B** (HBV) and **hepatitis C** (HCV) viruses, **human immunodeficiency virus** (HIV), **human T-cell lymphotrophic virus** (HTLV), **cytomegalovirus** (CMV), **Epstein-Barr virus** (EBV), **malaria, babesiosis, Chagas' disease, syphilis,** and **toxoplasmosis**. Although unproved, concern also exists over the possibility of transmitting Creutzfeldt–Jakob disease (CJD). All blood donors are currently tested for the viruses listed in Table 1-12. However, for a short period after becoming infectious, a donor's serologic tests may be nonreactive (the "window" period), resulting in a small risk for transfusion-transmitted disease. CMV and HTLV persist in leukocytes; transmission of these two agents can be prevented by providing leukocyte-reduced RBCs and platelets (WBC $<5 \times 10^6$). The evaluation of any patient with a potential transfusion-transmitted disease should include a transfusion history if no other likely source of the infection (i.e., IV drug use, sexual transmission) is found. If a transfusion-transmitted disease is probable, the Blood Bank should be notified and steps taken to notify and retest the potential donors.

C. Transfusion-associated graft-versus-host disease (TA-GVHD). This disease is caused by **T lymphocytes in donor blood products** that engraft in immunocompromised recipients and **mount an immune response against the recipient**.

  1. Clinical presentation. Signs and symptoms, which typically develop **1–2 weeks after transfusion**, include a macular or papular **rash** that progresses from the trunk to the extremities, watery **diarrhea, nausea and vomiting, fever, elevated liver function tests,** and **pancytopenia** of the bone marrow.

  2. Evaluation. Diagnosis requires a high index of suspicion as symptoms can mimic a viral infection or drug reaction. For definitive diagnosis, **donor-derived lymphocytes must be demonstrated in the recipient's tissues**. Biopsy of skin, liver, or bone marrow may be helpful. Flow cytome-

Table 1-12. Estimated risks of viral transmission in blood products

Virus	Estimated Risk from Blood Components
HBV	1 : 63,000
HCV	1 : 103,000
HIV	1 : 493,000
HTLV	1 : 641,000

HBV, hepatitis B virus; HCV, hepatitis C virus; HIV, human immunodeficiency virus; HTLV, human T-cell lymphotrophic virus.
(From Schreiber et al. *N Eng J Med* 1996; 334:1685–1690.)

try with HLA typing may also help to identify donor lymphocytes in the patient's blood.

 3.   Treatment and prevention. No effective treatment is available, although various agents have been tried, including glucocorticoids, cyclophosphamide, cyclosporine, and anti–T-cell antibodies. Recipients at risk for TA-GVHD (e.g., immunocompromised recipients, recipients receiving RBCs/platelets from a blood relative or HLA-compatible donor, newborns) should receive gamma-irradiated cellular blood components (2,500 cGy).

 D.   Other delayed transfusion reactions. Other reactions that may develop include **alloimmunization** to RBC, platelet, and HLA antigens, and **iron overload** (one unit of packed RBCs has more iron than a person would normally absorb in 6 months).

BIBLIOGRAPHY

Greenberger DA. Plasma anaphylaxis and immediate type reactions. In: Rossi EC, Simon TL, Moss GS, Gould SA, eds. *Principles of transfusion medicine*, 2nd ed. Baltimore: Williams & Wilkins, 1996: 765–771.

Schreiber GB, Busch MP, Kleinman SH, Korelitz JJ. The risk of transfusion-transmitted viral infections. *N Engl J Med* 1996;334: 1685–1690.

Hemapheresis

Constance F. M. Danielson

I. **Introduction**
A. **"Hemapheresis" or "apheresis."** These terms usually refer to automated procedures that **remove whole blood** from a patient, anticoagulate the blood with citrate, **separate out one or more components** by filtration or centrifugation, and **return the remainder** to the patient. Apheresis procedures can separate out plasma (plasmapheresis), platelets (platelet-pheresis), leukocytes (leukapheresis), or red blood cells (RBC apheresis).
B. **"Exchange procedures."** These are hemapheresis procedures that not only separate out blood components, but **replace the retained component with a similar substance** (e.g., plasma exchange).
II. **Use of apheresis for blood component collection.** Apheresis allows the specific collection of a desired component. A maximum of 10.5 mL of blood (or components) per kilogram of donor weight may be collected.
A. **Plasma**. For fresh frozen plasma (FFP), the quantity = approximately **500 mL**.
B. **Platelets**
1. **Quantity $\geq 3 \times 10^{11}$ platelets** per procedure (5–10 times the amount obtained from one unit of whole blood)
2. **Uses**
a. **HLA-matched platelets** for patients with anti-HLA antibodies (who are refractory to random donor platelets).
b. **Maternal platelets for newborns with neonatal alloimmune thrombocytopenia**, where maternal anti-platelet IgG antibodies (most commonly **anti-PL^{A1}**) cross the placenta and cause neonatal thrombocytopenia. Maternal platelets (lacking the causative antigen) are collected, washed, irradiated [to prevent graft-versus-host disease (GVHD)], and given to the baby until the titer of passively acquired maternal antibodies decreases.
C. **Leukocytes**
1. **Granulocytes**
a. Quantity $\geq 1 \times 10^{10}$ granulocytes per procedure.
b. Use. Rarely needed, but may be beneficial in patients with infections unresponsive to antibiotics, **and** who have <500 polymorphonuclear leukocytes/mm^3 **and** reversible marrow hypoplasia. The donor receives corticosteroids and/or granulocyte colony-stimulating factor (G-CSF) before apheresis and heta or penta hydroxyethyl starch is added during the procedure, all to increase the yield.
2. **Peripheral blood progenitor cells (PBPC or hematopoietic stem cells). PBPCs are an alternative to bone marrow transplants** for patients with marrow failure or suppression. PBPCs are highly enriched in the mononuclear

cell population that express the **CD 34** antigen. PBPCs can be collected from patients of all sizes and ages. In adults, one to three collections are usually performed, each of which involves three to six blood volumes (15–30 L) and takes 3 to 5 hours. Donors may receive chemotherapy or growth factors [G-CSF or granulocyte-macrophage colony-stimulating factor (GM-CSF)] to increase the yield of PBPCs. The minimal dose of PBPCs is $2-5 \times 10^6$ CD 34+ cells per kilogram of recipient body weight to obtain rapid hematopoietic reconstitution.

D. Red cells. Quantity = approximately 400 mL.

III. Therapeutic apheresis procedures. Therapeutic apheresis procedures are used to reduce the concentration of a pathologic substance in the blood or to replenish (through an exchange procedure) a substance that is lacking in the blood (Table 1-13).

A. Therapeutic cytapheresis. Cytapheresis is a term that encompasses plateletpheresis, leukapheresis, and erythrocytapheresis.

1. Plateletpheresis. Platelet counts >10^6/mm³ can paradoxically cause bleeding (because of platelet dysfunction) or thromboses (e.g., cerebrovascular insufficiency). Plateletpheresis can temporarily reduce the platelet count until cytotoxic or other therapies begin working.

2. Leukapheresis. Leukostasis may occur when white cell blast count is >100,000/mm³. Leukostasis is most common in acute nonlymphocytic leukemia, and leads to hypoxia and organ dysfunction (particularly in the lungs and the brain). Leukapheresis can temporarily reduce the blast count until chemotherapy starts, as well as reduce the risk of tumor lysis syndrome.

3. Erythrocytapheresis can be used to treat polycythemia rubra vera, hemochromatosis, and porphyria. However, it is expensive, and most patients choose simple phlebotomy as an alternative therapy.

B. Red blood cell exchange. This exchange is most commonly used to treat complications of **sickle cell disease**. The sickled cells can reduce blood flow and oxygen perfusion, leading to **acute chest syndrome, stroke, acute multiorgan failure syndrome, priapism,** and **hepatic crises.** RBCs lacking Hgb S are used for replacement, the usual goal being reduction of HbS to <30%. Some patients with sickle cell disease receive chronic transfusions to keep Hgb S levels low, but RBC exchange allows greater control of blood volume and viscosity, and has less risk of iron overload.

C. Plasma exchange

1. General information. Plasma exchange has been used, often as adjunctive therapy, to successfully treat a variety of neurologic, metabolic, autoimmune, and renal disorders. In most of these situations, the goal is to remove an offending antibody. Plasma exchange usually is performed with replacement with an equivalent amount of 5% human serum albumin (HSA) or a combination of 0.9% normal saline and HSA.

2. Common disorders treated

a. Thrombotic thrombocytopenic purpura (TTP). TTP is a systemic disorder classically characterized by thrombocytopenia, microangiopathic hemolytic anemia,

Table 1-13.   Disorders for which therapeutic apheresis is considered generally accepted or standard therapy

Disease	Procedure
Renal and metabolic diseases	
Anti–glomerular basement membrane antibody diseases	Plasma exchange
Rapid progressive glomerulonephritis	Plasma exchange
Familial hypercholesterolemia	Selective adsorption, plasma exchange
Phytanic acid storage disease	Plasma exchange
Autoimmune and rheumatic diseases	
Cryoglobulinemia	Plasma exchange
Idiopathic thrombocytopenic purpura	Immunoadsorption
Rheumatoid arthritis	Immunoadsorption, lymphoplasma-pheresis
Hematologic diseases	
ABO incompatible marrow transplant	Red cell removal (marrow), plasma exchange (recipient)
Erythrocytosis/polycythemia vera	Phlebotomy/erythrocytapheresis
Leukocytosis and thrombocytosis	Cytapheresis
Thrombotic thrombocytopenic purpura	Plasma exchange
Post-transfusion purpura	Plasma exchange
Sickle cell diseases	Red cell exchange
Myeloma/paraproteins/hyperviscosity	Plasma exchange
Myeloma/acute renal failure	Plasma exchange
Coagulation factor inhibitors	Plasma exchange
Aplastic anemia/pure red cell aplasia	Plasma exchange
Cutaneous T–cell lymphoma	Photopheresis
Neurologic disorders	
Chronic inflammatory demyelinating polyradiculoneuropathy	Plasma exchange
Acute inflammatory demyelinating polyradiculoneuropathy	Plasma exchange
Lambert–Eaton myasthenia syndrome	Plasma exchange
Myasthenia gravis	Plasma exchange
Acute central nervous system inflammatory demyelinating disease	Plasma exchange
Demyelinating polyneuropathy with IgG/IgA	Plasma exchange
Sydenham's chorea	Plasma exchange
Polyneuropathy with IgM (± Waldenström's)	Plasma exchange
Cryoglobulinemia with polyneuropathy	Plasma exchange
PANDAS	Plasma exchange

(Modified from a chart in McLeod BC, ed. *Introduction to the third special issue. Clinical applications of therapeutic apheresis. J Clin Apher* 2000;15:1–5, with permission.)

fever, neurologic abnormalities, and renal dysfunction. In some cases, an **IgG autoantibody is directed against metalloprotease** (which normally degrades large von Willebrand factor multimers), causing **large von Willebrand factor multimers to accumulate** at sites of vascular damage. This leads to platelet and fibrin **thrombi deposition** that causes multiorgan ischemia. **The treatment of choice for TTP is immediate plasma exchange, using FFP, solvent/detergent treated plasma (plasma-S/D)**, or cryoprecipitate-depleted plasma for the replacement fluid. The exchange not only removes the antibody inhibitor but also replaces the metalloprotease. Plasma exchanges **continue daily** (often along with corticosteroids and aspirin therapy) until platelet counts have normalized. **Note: do not give platelet transfusions!** (they can cause increased thrombi formation).

    b. **Goodpasture's syndrome** is associated with **antibodies directed against renal glomerular and pulmonary alveolar basement membranes**, and can lead to acute renal failure and pulmonary hemorrhage. **A short series of plasma exchanges** (along with immunosuppressive therapy) can be helpful, especially in limiting pulmonary hemorrhage.

    c. **Myasthenia gravis, Guillain–Barré syndrome, and Eaton–Lambert syndrome** are usually treated with a **short course of daily or alternate day procedures, exchanging** 1–1½ plasma volumes. Patients with chronic inflammatory demyelinating polyneuropathy usually receive a longer series of exchanges.

    3. **Important points to remember about plasma exchange**

    a. Plasma exchange is much **more effective in removing IgM than IgG**, because IgM is large and primarily confined to the intravascular space, whereas most of IgG is in the interstitial spaces.

    b. Ideally, **one volume exchange should remove about 60%** of a pathologic substance, whereas **two exchanges remove 85% to 90%, and three exchanges remove 95%**. In reality, multiple factors lead to **variable results**.

    c. **The production of an offending antibody is likely to continue unless the antigenic stimulus is removed** or immunosuppressive or cytotoxic therapy initiated.

    d. Calculating the patient's whole blood, RBC, and plasma volumes is necessary in planning several of the apheresis techniques (Table 1-14).

D. **Apheresis-related procedures**. The cells or plasma collected by apheresis are sometimes **treated** and **then returned to the patient**, such as in the following two examples.

    1. **Immunoadsorption of plasma** uses **staphylococcus protein-A filled columns, which bind the Fc portion of IgG** (except IgG_3), removing IgG as well as soluble Ag-IgG complexes. Through uncertain mechanisms, this can cause immunomodulation or suppression, and has been used to treat immune thrombocytopenic purpura (ITP) and rheumatoid arthritis.

Table 1-14.   Calculating patient blood volumes

1. **Multiply the adult patient's weight (in kg) by 70 mL/kg to yield the whole blood volume.**
   Example: 70 kg patient × 70 mL/kg = 4,900 mL of whole blood
2. **Multiply the whole blood volume by the patient's hematocrit to estimate the RBC volume, or by (1-Hct) to estimate the plasma volume.**
   Examples (in a patient with hematocrit of 40%)
   −4,900 mL of whole blood × 0.40 = 1,960 mL RBC in the patient
   −4,900 mL of whole blood × (0.60) = 2,940 mL plasma in the patient.

RBC, red blood cell.

    2.   **Photopheresis**. Leukocytes are collected, treated with **8-methoxypsoralen** (which binds to DNA), exposed *in vitro* to **ultraviolet-A irradiation**, and reinfused into the patient. Irradiation activates the drug, causing covalent pyrimidine **cross-linking in the DNA**, and the altered leukocytes cause **immunomodulation** or **suppression**. This has been successfully used to treat **cutaneous T-cell lymphoma and Sézary syndrome**, and may have possible benefit in treating patients with GVHD and transplant rejection.
IV. **Complications of hemapheresis**
  A.   **Citrate toxicity**. This is the **most frequent** complication of hemapheresis.
    1.   **Cause**. Citrate is used as an anticoagulant, and causes **hypocalcemia**.
    2.   **Symptoms**
      a.   **Mild**: numbness or tingling around the mouth and face (**circumoral paresthesia**), sneezing
      b.   **Moderate**: **paresthesia** progressing to hands, feet, or chest; **chills; nausea and vomiting**; mild hypotension; restlessness
      c.   **Severe**: **muscle cramps**, severe abdominal cramping, neuromuscular irritability, blurred vision, **confusion** or loss of consciousness, **seizures, hypotension, cardiac arrhythmias**
    3.   **Treatment**
      a.   **Slow down** the infusion rate of anticoagulant, or temporarily stop the procedure.
      b.   If symptoms persist, give calcium carbonate PO (e.g., **Tums**).
      c.   If symptoms still persist, give 10% solution of **calcium gluconate IV** (usually one ampule—90 mg/10 mL ampule of elemental calcium).
  B.   **Allergic reactions**
    1.   Not infrequent, especially in patients receiving **plasma replacement fluid**.
    2.   Treat with **diphenhydramine (Benadryl)** (25–50 mg IV in adults) and premedicate if patient has had previous reactions.

C. Volume alterations

1. **Cause**. Different procedures or machines can cause **hypo- or hypervolemia**. Hypovolemia can occur because of the amount of patient's blood that is extracorporeal (in the machine) at any given time.

2. **Prevention**

a. In general, closely monitor the patient's **"Ins and Outs"** and adjust fluids.

b. **Avoid apheresis in patients taking angiotensin-converting enzyme (ACE) inhibitors** because severe volume alterations have been reported.

c. In anemic or small pediatric patients, it may be necessary to **prime the tubing set** with compatible RBCs rather than the usual saline. This allows RBCs to be immediately infused as the patient's blood is being removed.

D. Therapeutic drug alterations. Plasma exchange can lower the blood concentration of many drugs, including antibiotics and anticonvulsants. **Adjust dosing schedules so that the drug is administered after completion** of the apheresis.

E. Hemolysis

1. Caused by malfunctioning equipment, administration of hypotonic fluids, and infusion of incompatible blood products.

2. Discontinue the procedure until the cause is corrected.

BIBLIOGRAPHY

McLeod BC. Introduction to the third special issue. Clinical applications of therapeutic apheresis. *J Clin Apher* 2000;15:1–5.

Blood Bank Inspections

Constance F. M. Danielson and Leo J. McCarthy

I. Introduction. The collection, processing (manufacturing), and transfusion of blood is assessed both by regulatory agencies (legally required) and by accrediting organizations (for voluntary certification). The most important organizations and the activities on which they focus are discussed below.

II. Food and Drug Administration (FDA). The FDA is responsible for ensuring the safety and adequacy of the nation's blood supply. Satisfactory completion of inspection by any of the following organizations, except the Food and Drug Administration, can enable blood banks and transfusion services to be certified to perform testing on human specimens under the Clinical Laboratory Improvement Amendment of 1988 (CLIA '88).

A. FDA registration is required for all manufacturers of drugs (including blood components).

B. FDA licensure is required for all manufacturers shipping blood products across state lines.

C. Transfusion services do not manufacture blood products and do not need to be FDA registered or licensed.

D. All blood facilities (A–C above) are required to follow the applicable statutes in part 200 (drugs) and part 600 (biologics) of title 21, Code of Federal Regulations (CFR), including adherence to Current Good Manufacturing Practices (CGMP).

E. Inspections of FDA registered or licensed facilities are performed by the FDA. The Health Care Financing Administration (HCFA) inspects transfusion services.

F. Fatal complications. All blood facilities must report any fatal complication of blood collection or transfusion to the Center for Biologics Evaluation and Research (CBER) **within 1 business day**: phone: (301) 827-6220, fax: (301) 443-3874, e-mail: fatality@cber.fda.gov. A written report must follow within 7 days.

III. American Association of Blood Banks (AABB)

A. Mission. The mission of the AABB is to promote the highest standard of care for blood banking and transfusion medicine.

B. Accreditation. Facilities who meet the current "AABB Standards for Blood Banks and Transfusion Services" can be accredited. The accreditation is based on an assessment of the facility's Quality and Operational Programs by specially trained peers on a biennial basis (once every 2 years).

C. AABB membership. Membership is voluntary; however, all institutional members must participate in AABB's Accreditation Program.

IV. College of American Pathologists (CAP)

A. Goal. The goal of the CAP Laboratory Accreditation Program is voluntary continual laboratory improvement (includes blood bank and transfusion service).

B.   Assessment. On-site assessment by peers using checklist questions is performed biennially. Most checklist questions applicable to the Blood Bank are based on "AABB's Standards for Blood Banks and Transfusion Services."

C.   Testing. A Proficiency Testing (PT) Program is maintained by CAP. Successful PT performance is required under the Clinical Laboratories Improvement Act (CLIA) '88 Regulations for Accreditation.

V.   Joint Commission on Accreditation of Healthcare Organizations (JCAHO)

A.   Standards. The JCAHO hospital standards stress evaluation of the entire transfusion process.

B.   Assessment. On-site assessment occurs once every 3 years.

C.   "Sentinel" events. All "sentinel" events, including acute hemolytic transfusion reactions, must be reported to the JCAHO **within 5 business days**. A root-cause analysis must be performed and reported within 30 days.

2

Hematology

Red Blood Cells

Sherrie L. Perkins and Jerry W. Hussong

I. Red cell kinetics and basic biology

A. Red cell kinetics

1. Bone marrow. Red blood cell (RBC) precursors proliferate and differentiate for approximately 5–7 days, concluding with extrusion of the nucleus. **Erythropoietin** regulates red cell development.

2. Peripheral blood. Red cells circulate for an average of **120 days**.

3. Cell destruction. Red cells are most commonly removed by extravascular lysis, as macrophages in the spleen or reticuloendothelial system recognize signs of cell senescense (decreased deformability and altered surface proteins).

B. Red cell structure

1. Red cell membranes are permeable to water and anions but impermeable to cations. Cell volume is controlled by an adenosine triphosphate (ATP)-dependent Na+/K+ pump. Membranes are composed of lipid, protein, and carbohydrate.

  a. Lipid bilayer (40%): composed of equal amounts of **phospholipids** and **cholesterol**.

  b. Proteins (50%).

   (1) Integral proteins span the membrane; they include **glycophorins**, ion and water transporters, glucose transporters, and antigenic determinants (e.g., Rh complex).

   (2) Cellular cytoskeleton forms a latticelike pattern on the inner membrane, and includes **spectrin, actin**, ankyrin, and protein band 4.1. These proteins allow cellular deformability, which permits the red cells to pass through capillaries and the spleen.

  c. Carbohydrates (10%) are linked to proteins to form sialoglycoproteins, and so on.

2. Red cell cytoplasmic enzymes control cellular metabolic functions.

  a. Glycolytic pathway converts glucose to lactate to produce **ATP**, which maintains intercellular volume and general cellular function. Also forms 2,3 diphosphoglycerate (**2,3 DPG**), which enhances the unloading of oxygen from hemoglobin.

  b. Hexose monophosphate shunt generates nicotinamide adenine dicluceotide phosphate (**NADPH**) and **glutathione**, which detoxify oxidants.

3. Hemoglobin (Hgb or Hb) makes up 90% of the red cell's dry weight, and functions to transport oxygen (O_2) to tissues and to remove carbon dioxide (CO_2). **Each hemoglobin molecule is composed of four globin (protein) chains and four heme molecules.**

  a. Globins. Each **chromosome 16** has one zeta gene (an embryonic globin) and two α-genes (which produce globins during fetal and adult life). Therefore, **four α-alleles are found in each cell**. Each **chromosome 11** has one ε-gene (another embryonic globin), one γ-gene (fetal globin), one δ-gene (adult globin), and one β-gene (adult globin) (Fig. 2-1). Therefore, **two β-alleles** are found in each cell. Each molecule of hemoglobin has four globin chains, consisting of two α-chains and two non-α—chains. In newborns, the non-α—chains are primarily γ-chains, and form fetal hemoglobin (**Hb F**). In adults, the non-α—chains are primarily β-chains (forming **Hb A**) and a small percentage of δ-chains (forming **Hb A$_2$**). The amino acid sequence of the globin chains, which is essential for stability and function of the hemoglobin molecule, provides sites of interaction with 2,3 DPG and heme.

    b. **Heme**. Each molecule of heme is composed of a **protoporphyrin IX** protein and iron (**Fe^{2+}**).

II. **Red cell analysis in the complete blood count (CBC)**

A. **Complete blood count: red cell indices**. Measurement of specific red cell parameters by automated hematology analyzers provides essential data for classifying red cell disorders, and should be correlated with blood smear morphology.

    1. **Red blood cell (RBC) counts** (normal reference range: male $4.6–6.0 \times 10^6/\mu L$; female $4.1–5.4 \times 10^6/\mu L$). Erythrocytes and white blood cells are enumerated together, but the 500 times excess of RBCs makes the error caused by the inclusion of white cells insignificant. White blood cell counts (WBC) >50,000/μL, or large platelets can introduce significant errors. Very small RBCs (that are below exclusion levels) and agglutination (caused by autoantibodies) can lead to spuriously decreased RBC counts.

    2. **Hemoglobin concentration** (**Hb**; normal reference range: male 14–18 g/dL; female 12–16 g/dL) is measured spectrophotometrically; therefore, increased sample turbidity from

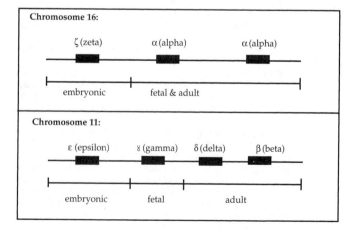

Fig. 2-1. **Globin gene locations.**

paraproteins, lipids, abnormal hemoglobins, or nucleated cells can lead to erroneously high results.

3. **Mean corpuscular volume** (**MCV**; normal reference range: 80–100 fL): **average measurement of red cell volume** or size. Warm or cold agglutinins causing red cell clumping and osmotic abnormalities (e.g., patient hyperglycemia or hypernatremia) can spuriously elevate the MCV. The MCV represents an average value and may not identify mixed cell populations (which are best shown in histograms).

4. **Hematocrit** (**Hct**; normal reference range: male 40%– 50%; female 37%–47%): **percentage of blood volume occupied by RBCs**. Calculated by multiplying RBC number by MCV; an alternative centrifugation method may show errors because of plasma trapping. Overdilution of the sample by anticoagulant or hemoconcentration caused by prolonged tourniquet application can also cause errors.

5. **Mean corpuscular hemoglobin** (**MCH**; normal reference range: 27–31 pg). Average amount of hemoglobin per cell. Calculated by dividing Hb (g/L) by RBC count (/L).

6. **Mean corpuscular hemoglobin concentration** (**MCHC**; normal reference range: 32–36 g/dL): **hemoglobin concentration in the cells**. Calculated by dividing Hb concentration (g/dL) by Hct and multiplying by 100. Represents an average value and may not identify mixed cell populations. Usually better than the MCH for identifying hypochromasia. MCHC is increased in spherocytosis and decreased in microcytic or hypochromic anemias. Can be affected by conditions that spuriously affect Hb measurements, such as hyperlipidemia or increased white cell counts.

7. **Red cell distribution width** (**RDW**; normal reference range: 11.5%–14.5%): measurement of **anisocytosis (differences in cell size)**; RDW reflects a coefficient of variation of red cell volumes divided by MCV. Elevated RDW may indicate mixed cell populations, and is helpful in characterizing anemias.

B. **Peripheral blood smear morphology** (Fig. 2-2).

III. **Anemia**

A. **Definition. Too few RBCs, or decreased Hgb** in the complete blood count (CBC) indicate anemia. Patients with significant anemia will have evidence of tissue hypoxia.

B. **Classification**. Anemia can be characterized by either morphologic or pathophysiologic criteria. Many classifying schemes combine both approaches (Fig. 2-3).

1. **Morphologic criteria is the use of CBC data, particularly MCV (cell size) to classify anemias as microcytic, normocytic, or macrocytic**. Microcytic anemias typically have a MCV <80 fL; normocytic 80–100 fL; macrocytic >100 fL. Mixed cell populations (microcytic and macrocytic) can result in a normal average MCV value, but are indicated by an increased RDW.

2. **Pathophysiologic criteria**. Classifies anemia **based on the underlying mechanisms (e.g., hypoproliferation vs. increased destruction). The reticulocyte count is a useful initial mechanistic indicator**: reticulocytes are increased when red cells are lost or destroyed (i.e., hemorrhage

(*text continues on page 66*)

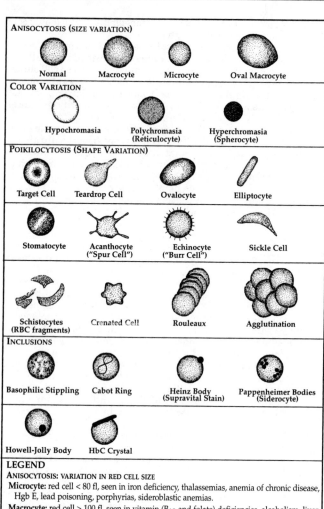

ANISOCYTOSIS (SIZE VARIATION)

Normal   Macrocyte   Microcyte   Oval Macrocyte

COLOR VARIATION

Hypochromasia   Polychromasia (Reticulocyte)   Hyperchromasia (Spherocyte)

POIKILOCYTOSIS (SHAPE VARIATION)

Target Cell   Teardrop Cell   Ovalocyte   Elliptocyte

Stomatocyte   Acanthocyte ("Spur Cell")   Echinocyte ("Burr Cell")   Sickle Cell

Schistocytes (RBC fragments)   Crenated Cell   Rouleaux   Agglutination

INCLUSIONS

Basophilic Stippling   Cabot Ring   Heinz Body (Supravital Stain)   Pappenheimer Bodies (Siderocyte)

Howell-Jolly Body   HbC Crystal

LEGEND

ANISOCYTOSIS: VARIATION IN RED CELL SIZE

Microcyte: red cell < 80 fl, seen in iron deficiency, thalassemias, anemia of chronic disease, Hgb E, lead poisoning, porphyrias, sideroblastic anemias.

Macrocyte: red cell > 100 fl, seen in vitamin (B_{12} and folate) deficiencies, alcoholism, liver disease, myelodysplastic syndromes, hemolytic anemia (reticulocytes) various drugs (e.g., anti-convulsants).

Fig. 2-2. Red cell morphology.

FIGURE 2. LEGEND continued

VARIATION IN COLOR:

Normochromic: normal red cell color (MCHC is normal), with 3µm area of gradual central pallor (sharply defined areas of central pallor are drying artifacts from humidity).

Hypochromic: pale red cells (MCHC is decreased), with > 4µm area of central pallor, seen in iron deficiency, thalassemias, anemia of chronic disease.

Hyperchromic: dark red cells (MCHC is increased), with <2µm area of central pallor, seen in spherocytes of hemolytic anemias, hereditary spherocytosis.

POIKILOCYTOSIS: variation in red cell shape

Acanthocyte: asymmetric, unequal long projections from the red cell surface, often with small bulbous ends; seen in liver disease, abetalipoproteinemia, lipid abnormalities, McLeod blood group.

Crenated cell: "scalloped" cell; seen as an EDTA artifact; also in hyperosmolality.

Echinocyte ("burr cell"): symmetric, short, sharp projections from the red cell; seen in iron deficiency, uremia.

Elliptocyte: "pencil cells", seen in iron deficiency, hereditary elliptocytosis, thalassemias.

Ovalocyte: oval red cell; enlarged cells (oval macrocytes) are seen in B_{12} and folate deficiencies, myelodysplasia.

Polychromatic: large, pale-blue cells, due to increased cytoplasmic RNA; represent reticulocytes.

Schistocytes: red cell fragments (helmet cells, triangle cells, bizarre shapes, etc.); seen in microangiopathic hemolytic anemias (e.g., disseminated intravascular coagulation, hemolytic uremic syndrome, thrombotic thrombocytopenic purpura, HELLP syndrome, etc.), and in hereditary pyropoikilocytosis (HPP).

Sickle cell: curved cell with sharp ends; seen in hemoglobinopathies (Hb S, Hb I, Hb C, Hb O^{Arab}).

Spherocyte: dark red cells with no areas of central pallor. Microspherocytes (MCV<70 fl) are seen in hemolytic anemias, burns, hypophosphatemia, drug (oxidant) injuries, etc.; near-normal sized spherocytes are seen in hereditary spherocytosis.

Stomatocyte: elongated area of central pallor ("stoma" = mouth); seen in EDTA artifacts, Rh null cells, alcoholism, hereditary stomatocytic elliptocytosis.

Target cell: red cell with central dark area ("bull's eye"); seen in lipid disorders, liver disease, hemoglobinopathies (e.g., thalassemias, Hb S, D, E, and particularly C), hyposplenism.

Teardrop cell: rounded cytoplasmic projection (vs. sharp projection in the axis of the smear that represents smear artifact); seen in iron deficiency, myelofibrosis.

INCLUSIONS*:

Basophilic stippling: composed of RNA; fine stippling seen with increased red cell production; coarse stippling seen in lead poisoning, thalassemias, unstable hemoglobins, myelodysplasia.

Cabot ring: figure-8 cytoplasmic structure that is a remnant of microtubules; non-specific.

Crystals: rod-shaped ("Washington Monument-like") cytoplasmic crystals in cells with Hb C.

Heinz body: peripheral, pale inclusions that push out the cell membrane, composed of hemoglobin; requires supravital stain (e.g., new methylene blue, brilliant cresyl blue, etc.).

Howell-Jolly body: single, large, round, dark purple remnant of nucleus: seen in splenectomy, myelodysplasia, megaloblastic anemia.

Pappenheimer body: multiple, small, peripheral, grape-like purple clusters of iron; Prussian blue stain confirms them (when confirmed as iron, they are called siderotic granules; red cells are siderocytes; red cell precursors with nuclei are sideroblasts; if granules extend > 3/4 around the circumference of the nucleus = ringed sideroblasts); seen in splenectomy, iron overload, sideroblastic anemia.

Reticulocyte: young red cell with cytoplasmic RNA (requires supravital stain [e.g., new methylene blue] to see; on regular Wright Giemsa smears, the cells appear diffusely pale blue [polychromatic]).

*Note that a wide variety of the shape variations and cell inclusions described above may be seen in myelodysplastic syndromes, and a variety of inclusions may be seen in patients who are hyposplenic or asplenic.

Fig. 2-2. Continued.

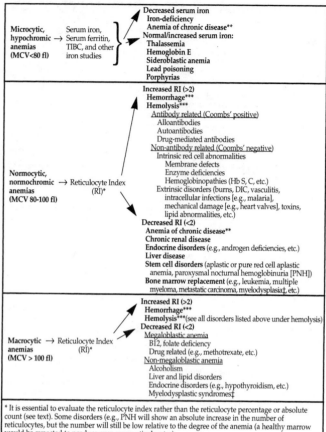

Fig. 2-3. Overview of anemias.

and hemolysis), and are insufficiently increased (or decreased) in anemias because of marrow hypoproliferative disorders (e.g., vitamin deficiencies, myelodysplasia).

IV.   Microcytic hypochromic anemias. Microcytic anemias are characterized by a **MCV of <80 fL**, and are often hypochromic. The microcytic hypochromic anemias **represent quantitative defects in hemoglobin synthesis,** with normal DNA synthesis. These anemias can be divided into **three groups: disorders of iron metabolism** (e.g., iron deficiency); **disorders of heme synthesis** (e.g., sideroblastic anemias), and **disorders of globin protein synthesis** (e.g., thalassemias).

A. Iron-deficiency anemia. Iron-deficiency anemia is the **most common disorder of iron utilization**, and is the **most common dietary deficiency** in the world.

    1. Causes

      a. Increased blood loss (by far, the most common cause of iron deficiency in adults). Usually results from menstruation, and gastrointestinal or urinary tract bleeding in men and postmenopausal women.

      b. Insufficient dietary intake. Infants maintained on mother's milk are at increased risk, as are children and adolescents during growth spurt periods, and women who are menstruating.

      c. Pregnancy and lactation. Iron requirements are markedly increased during pregnancy ($\cong$1,000 mg) because of expansion of the mother's blood volume as well as diversion of iron to the fetus; lactation also expends significant amounts of iron.

      d. Malabsorption of iron is a rare cause of iron deficiency. Gastric, duodenal, or jejunal resections lead to malabsorption.

    2. Iron absorption and stages of iron-deficiency anemia

      a. Iron absorption and utilization. Of the iron ingested in the diet, 5% to 10% is absorbed. Dietary iron is in the ferric state (Fe^{3+}) and must be converted to ferrous iron (Fe^{2+}) by stomach acid to allow absorption by the duodenum and jejunum. The body normally uses **1 mg/d of iron, and has approximately 1,000 mg of storage iron**.

      b. Stages of iron-deficiency anemia. Iron deficiency and the development of anemia occur in stages:

         (1) Iron depletion. Iron stores are depleted, represented by a decrease in serum ferritin.

         (2) Iron-deficient erythropoiesis. Inadequate iron for hemoglobin synthesis results in hypochromia. This is accompanied by decreased serum iron, decreased percent of transferrin saturation, increased free erythrocyte protoporphorin (FEP), and increased total iron-binding capacity (TIBC). Frank anemia is not present.

         (3) Iron-deficiency anemia. Development of hypochromic and microcytic anemia. Hgb, Hct, RBC count, and MCV are all decreased. Serum-soluble transferrin receptor levels are increased.

    3. Laboratory testing for iron status. In addition to the CBC, a number of serum tests are readily available to evaluate iron status.

      a. Serum iron (normal reference range: 50–150 µg/dL). **Iron circulates bound to transferrin**. It has a diurnal variation and is typically measured in a morning blood draw.

      b. Total iron-binding capacity (normal reference range: 250–450 µg/dL): **indirect measure of transferrin**; TIBC equals the sum of serum iron plus empty (unbound) transferrin sites.

      c. Percent transferrin saturation (normal reference range: 20%–50%): calculated by dividing serum Fe by the TIBC $\times$ 100; transferrin is normally 33% saturated.

Increases are seen in sideroblastic anemias, and decreases are seen in iron deficiency and anemia of chronic disease.

d.   Serum ferritin (normal reference range: male 20–250 ng/mL; reproductive-aged female 10–120 ng/mL; females >40 years of age: 10–260 ng/mL): **correlates with iron stores**; however, it is also an **acute phase reactant** that is elevated in infection, inflammation, neoplasia, etc.

e.   Free erythrocytic protoporphyrin (normal range varies with patient age and method). Free protoporphyrin normally combines with iron to form heme. FEP is increased with iron deficiency, anemia of chronic disease, some sideroblastic anemias, lead poisoning, and porphyrias.

f.   Serum-soluble transferrin receptor. The serum-soluble transferrin level is **increased with iron deficiency. Levels are not affected by inflammatory states**, and testing is particularly useful in cases of borderline iron deficiency.

4.   Clinical findings. Fatigue, irritability, headache, and dyspnea are commonly seen when the anemia is severe. Pallor, **glossitis**, stomatitis, pica (cravings for inorganic matter), and **koilonychia** (spooning of nails) may also be present. Iron deficiency is associated with **Plummer–Vinson syndrome** (esophageal webs). Patients with slowly developing anemia may have few symptoms because of compensatory mechanisms.

5.   Laboratory findings. RBC count, Hgb, Hct, MCV, MCH, **serum iron, serum ferritin** and percent transferrin saturation **are decreased** with iron deficiency; **RDW, TIBC**, FEP, and soluble-serum transferrin receptor levels are **increased** (Table 2-1 and Fig. 2-4).

6.   Morphologic findings. Anisocytosis is followed by microcytosis and hypochromasia. Hypochromic **elliptocytes** ("pencil cells"), burr cells, and tear-drop cells may also be seen. Bone marrow specimens stained with Prussian blue reveal decreased reticuloendothelial and sideroblastic iron.

B.   Anemia of chronic disease (ACD). Anemia of chronic disease is also a disorder of iron utilization. ACD can be microcytic and hypochromic, but is usually normocytic and normochromic (see section V.B.1, Table 2-1, and Fig. 2-4).

C.   Sideroblastic anemia. The sideroblastic anemias are a group of disorders characterized by ineffective erythropoiesis, **increased levels of serum and tissue iron, and increased numbers of marrow-ringed sideroblasts**. The MCV varies, and may be low, normal, or increased. The key finding is a dual **(dimorphic) population** of red cells (microcytic, hypochromic cells, and normocytic to macrocytic cells), with a high RDW. Sideroblastic anemias can be inherited or acquired, but all result in **abnormal deposition of iron within the mitochondria** of erythroid precursors. In some cases, this is caused by enzyme deficiencies (or toxins that affect such enzymes) related to protoporphyrin synthesis.

1.   Etiology

a.   Inherited. The **x-linked** variant is most common; autosomal recessive forms also exist.

Table 2-1.   Comparison of indices and features in anemia of chronic disease, iron deficiency anemia, sideroblastic anemia, and thalassemia

Findings	Anemia of Chronic Disease	Iron Deficiency Anemia	Sideroblastic Anemia	Thalassemia
COMPLETE BLOOD COUNT (CBC)				
Red blood cell count[a]	Decreased	Decreased	Decreased	Normal/increased
Hemoglobin concentration	Decreased	Decreased	Decreased	Decreased
Hematocrit	Normal/decreased	Decreased	Variable	Normal/decreased
Mean corpuscular volume	Normal/decreased	Decreased	Variable	Decreased[b]
Red cell distribution width[a]	Usually normal	Increased	Normal/increased	Normal[c]
Mean corpuscular hemoglobin	Normal/decreased	Decreased	Variable	Variable
Mean corpuscular hemoglobin concentration	Normal/decreased	Decreased	Variable	Variable
Reticulocyte count	Decreased	Decreased	Decreased	Decreased
OTHER SERUM STUDIES				
Serum iron	Decreased	Decreased	Increased	Normal/increased
Serum ferritin	Normal/increased	Decreased	Increased	Normal/increased
Total iron binding capacity	Decreased	Increased	Normal/decreased	Normal
% Saturation	Decreased (but usually <15)	Decreased (but usually <10)	Increased (usually >75)	Normal/increased
Free erythrocyte protoporphyrin	Increased	Increased	Increased	Normal

continued

Table 2-1. Continued

Findings	Anemia of Chronic Disease	Iron Deficiency Anemia	Sideroblastic Anemia	Thalassemia
Serum soluble transferrin receptor	Normal/increased	Increased	Normal/decreased	Normal
PERIPHERAL BLOOD AND BONE MARROW FINDINGS				
Anisocytosis	No	Yes	Yes[d]	Variable
Poikilocytosis	No	Yes[e]	Yes[d]	Variable[e]
Basophilic Stippling	No	No	Yes	Variable
Stainable bone marrow iron	Increased	Decreased	Increased	Increased
Marrow sideroblasts	Decreased	Decreased	Increased	Normal

[a] Note: Bold-faced findings may be examined first to form a preliminary working diagnosis, although further studies (listed under OTHER SERUM STUDIES are often necessary to confirm the diagnosis, particularly if the clinical history is not consistent.

[b] In thalassemia minor, the microcytosis is often striking (<70 fL) and out of proportion to the mild decrease in Hb ($\cong$9–11 g/dL), unlike iron-deficiency which usually has severe decreases in Hb when the microcytosis is <70 fL.

[c] Except thalassemia major, which has an increased RDW

[d] In inherited forms

[e] Iron deficiency often causes elliptocytes, tear-drop cells, and burr cells. Thalassemia often causes target cells.

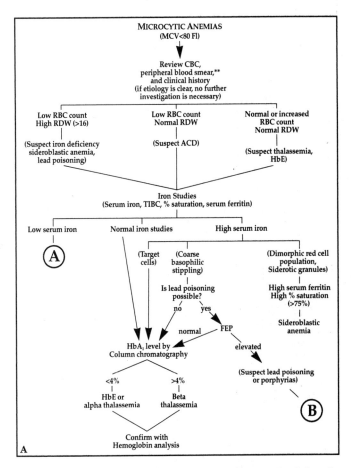

MICROCYTIC ANEMIAS
(MCV<80 Fl)

Review CBC,
peripheral blood smear,**
and clinical history
(if etiology is clear, no further
investigation is necessary)

Low RBC count	Low RBC count	Normal or increased
High RDW (>16)	Normal RDW	RBC count
		Normal RDW
(Suspect iron deficiency	(Suspect ACD)	
sideroblastic anemia,		(Suspect thalassemia,
lead poisoning)		HbE)

Iron Studies
(Serum iron, TIBC, % saturation, serum ferritin)

Low serum iron   Normal iron studies   High serum iron

Ⓐ

(Target   (Coarse   (Dimorphic red cell
cells)   basophilic   population,
             stippling)   Siderotic granules)

Is lead poisoning   High serum ferritin
possible?   High % saturation
                                            (>75%)
no   yes
                                         Sideroblastic
          normal   FEP   anemia

HbA₂ level by
Column chromatography   elevated

                              (Suspect lead poisoning
<4%   >4%   or porphyrias)

HbE or   Beta   **Ⓑ**
alpha thalassemia   thalassemia

Confirm with
Hemoglobin analysis

A

Fig. 2-4. Flow chart for microcytic anemias. ACD, anemia of chronic disease; FEP, free erythrocyte protoporphyrin; RDW, red cell distribution width; TIBC, total iron-binding capacity.

  b. Acquired. Acquired sideroblastic anemias can be primary (idiopathic) or secondary. Primary acquired sideroblastic anemias include refractory anemia with ringed sideroblasts (**RARS**), a **myelodysplastic** syndrome. Secondary acquired sideroblastic anemias can result from toxins or medications (e.g., **alcohol, lead**, cycloserine, pyrazinamide, chloramphenicol, isoniazid).
 2. Clinical findings
  a. Inherited. Pallor, splenomegaly, and anemia occur within the first few months or years of life.

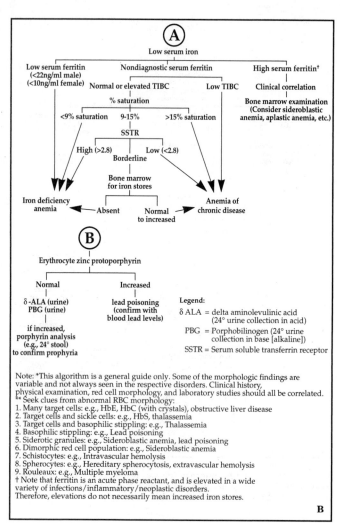

Fig. 2-4. *Continued.*

---

b. Acquired. In primary disorders (e.g., RARS), patients are typically >50 years of age. In secondary disorders, toxins or medications are often implicated and symptoms vary.

3. Laboratory findings of inherited and acquired forms. Typically, the RBC count, Hb, and MCV are decreased; however, these findings are variable (e.g., MCV in myelodysplastic syndromes tends to be increased). **Serum iron, ferritin, percent transferrin saturation, and FEP are typically increased, as is the RDW.** TIBC can be decreased or normal (Table 2-1 and Fig. 2-4).

4. Morphologic findings of inherited and acquired forms. Mixed populations of microcytic and/or hypochromic, normocytic, and occasionally even macrocytic, red cells are usually present (causing an increased RDW). **Storage iron and ringed sideroblasts are increased** in the marrow, which is often hypercellular with an erythroid predominance and signs of abnormal erythroid development (dyserythropoiesis). In RARS, the diagnostic criteria require at least 15% ringed sideroblasts in the marrow. Basophilic stippling is common, and is particularly prominent and coarse in the forms caused by lead poisoning.

D. Thalassemias and hemoglobin E. See below in hemoglobinopathy section.

E. Renal disease, when associated with hematuria and subsequent iron deficiency

F. Lead poisoning (normal reference range: children <9 µg/dL). Lead blocks several of the enzymes (e.g., δ-aminolevulinic acid dehydrogenase synthetase) necessary for the production of heme. Clinical findings include skin lesions and neurologic deficits. Laboratory findings include a microcytic hypochromic anemia, with **coarse basophilic stippling**. Morphologic features of sideroblastic anemia may also be seen. The screening test for lead is **FEP** (elevated in lead exposure, porphyrias, iron deficiency, ACD, and some sideroblastic anemias), followed by **erythrocyte zinc protoporphyrin** levels (more specific for lead exposure) and **blood lead levels** (Fig. 2-4).

G. Porphyrias. This group of at least six disorders involves defects in enzymes necessary for the production of heme. Some forms are hereditary, whereas others are acquired. The porphyrias can be grouped into **erythropoietic porphyrias** (e.g., porphyria cutanea tarda, which causes microcytic hypochromic anemia and photosensitive skin lesions) and **hepatic porphyrias** [e.g., hereditary coproporphyria, which causes hepatic dysfunction and central nervous system (CNS) defects]. Laboratory testing should include **FEP** as a screen, followed by separate 24-hour urine collections for **δ-aminolevulinic acid** (collected in acidic preservative) and **porphobilinogen** (collected in alkaline preservative). Confirmation is by a 24-hour stool specimen test for porphyrins. Specimens should be collected when the patient is symptomatic (Fig. 2-4).

V. Normocytic normochromic anemias, characterized by a normal MCV and MCHC, result from diverse causes. Some types of anemia (e.g., hemorrhage, hemolytic anemias) have normocytic normochromic mature red cells, but the increased number of responding reticulocytes (which are large cells) increases the average red cell size (MCV). (They will be discussed in the normocytic category for conceptual simplicity.) **A reticulocyte index (RI), which is essential** in evaluating normocytic anemias, allows their categorization in terms of increased red cell loss or destruction (with an increased RI) or decreased red cell production (with a decreased RI, Fig. 2-3). In some anemias of decreased red cell production, the reticulocyte count may be elevated but still relatively decreased, in that the mild elevation is not as high as would be expected of a healthy marrow responding to the given degree of anemia. Therefore, the RI is the best measure of reticulocyte response.

A. Calculating the reticulocyte index. The RI starts with the reticulocyte count and corrects it for the degree of anemia (i.e., corrects for the decreased total red cell count, and for the increasingly immature reticulocytes that are released from the marrow). The calculation is:

RI = (reticulocyte count) × (patient hematocrit/45)
    × 1/maturation factor

[The maturation factors (MF) are as follows: if the patient Hct is 45, MF = 1; if the Hct is 35, MF = 1.5; if the Hct is 25, MF = 2; if the Hct is 15, the MF is 2.5]

RI < 2 = decreased (suggesting decreased production)
RI > 2 = increased (suggesting blood loss or destruction)

B. Normocytic normochromic anemias with a decreased RI

1. Anemia of chronic disease; synonyms include "anemia of chronic inflammation" and "chronic simple anemia." ACD is the most common normocytic normochromic anemia; however, the red cells may become hypochromic and finally microcytic. ACD is associated with **chronic conditions** involving tissue injury and **inflammation**, including sarcoidosis, collagen-vascular diseases (e.g., rheumatoid arthritis, systemic lupus erythematosis), chronic infections (e.g., tuberculosis, osteomyelitis), and neoplasms (e.g., carcinoma and malignant lymphoma).

  a. Pathophysiology. ACD results from at least three defects: **lack of erythropoiesis** (caused by inhibitory cytokines such as interleukin-1 and tumor necrosis factor), lack of available iron for hemoglobin synthesis (from **trapping of iron in macrophages**), and decreased red blood cell survival (caused by cytokine-stimulated extravascular **hemolysis**). The end result is that the reticulocyte count is insufficient, although normal numbers of marrow stem cells are found.

  b. Clinical findings. ACD is usually mild to moderate and the patient's symptoms are usually attributed to the underlying disease.

  c. Laboratory findings. The RBC count, Hgb, and Hct are typically decreased. The MCV, MCH, MCHC, and RDW are usually normal. If the MCV, MCH, and MCHC are decreased, the MCHC tends to decrease before the MCV decreases, which is the opposite of what occurs in iron-deficiency anemia. **The RI is low. Serum iron, TIBC, and percent saturation are usually decreased. Serum ferritin is often increased**, but can be normal (Table 2-1 and Fig. 2-4).

  d. Morphologic findings. No specific findings are seen. RBCs appear normochromic, normocytic, or may be mildly microcytic and/or hypochromic. Usually, no significant anisopoikilocytosis, and little polychromasia (few reticulocytes) are seen. The bone marrow has adequate erythroid precursors. Iron stains show markedly **increased storage iron** (in macrophages) and **decreased sideroblastic iron** (in red cells).

e. Treatment. Treatment of the underlying disease process is the therapy of choice.

2. Chronic renal disease. The anemia associated with chronic renal disease resembles ACD.

a. Pathophysiology. The anemia of renal disease occurs primarily as a result of **decreased erythropoietin** production, and, to a lesser extent, from uremia (which damages red cells and suppresses the marrow).

b. Clinical findings. Symptoms of anemia are variable.

c. Laboratory findings. The RBC count, Hgb, and Hct are typically decreased. The MCV, MCH, MCHC, and RDW are usually normal.

d. Morphologic findings. The red cells are normocytic or normochromic. Findings include mild to moderate aniso-poikilocytosis, including **echinocytes** ("burr cells," caused by azotemia) and occasional schistocytes (particularly common in the hemolytic uremic syndrome).

e. Treatment. Treatment of the underlying disease process is the therapy of choice. Recombinant human **erythropoietin** is also frequently administered.

3. Chronic endocrine disorders. Numerous hormones are involved in erythropoiesis and may influence erythropoietic tissue function.

a. Pathophysiology. Growth hormone, thyrotropin, corticotropin, and androgens stimulate erythropoiesis, either directly or indirectly. Decreased pituitary, thyroid, adrenal, or gonadal function often results in a normocytic, normochromic anemia. However, hypothyroidism can cause a macrocytic anemia.

b. Clinical findings, typically, are related to the underlying disease state.

c. Laboratory findings. The RBC count, Hgb, and Hct are typically decreased. The MCV, MCH, MCHC, and RDW are usually normal.

d. Morphologic findings, usually, are similar to those seen with ACD.

e. Treatment: hormone replacement therapy.

4. Liver disease and alcoholism. Alcoholism is the most common cause of anemia from liver disease.

a. Pathophysiology. Anemia caused by alcoholic liver disease can have **multiple mechanisms**, including ACD (i.e., chronic hepatitis), lipid abnormalities, and nutritional deficiencies (e.g., folate, iron). **Alcohol has direct toxic effects** on bone marrow and red cells (**causing macrocytosis**), and can also cause an acquired secondary **sideroblastic anemia**.

b. Clinical findings. Symptoms depend on the severity of the liver disease and the anemia.

c. Laboratory findings. The laboratory findings depend on the dominant underlying disorder. Chronic alcoholic hepatitis causes an anemia of chronic inflammation, which is usually normocytic and normochromic. Folate deficiency as well as the direct effects of alcohol will result in a macrocytic anemia (increased MCV). Severe iron deficiency will cause a microcytic, hypochromic anemia (decreased MCV). If all occur together, the average MCV may be normal.

d.   Morphologic findings. Target cells, spherocytes, microspherocytes, and spur cells are present. In alcoholism without severe liver disease, **macrocytic** red cells are often seen. Acute massive ingestion of alcohol causes vacuolization of erythroid precursors. The marrow is often hypocellular. Chronic alcoholism increases **ringed sideroblasts** (acquired sideroblastic anemia).

e.   Treatment: withdrawal of alcohol and supplementation of any nutritional deficiencies.

5.   Aplastic anemia. This group of disorders has markedly decreased bone marrow cellularity, leading to blood cytopenias (usually pancytopenia). The disorders can involve all hematologic lineages or be restricted to red cells, and they can be hereditary or acquired.

a.   Aplastic anemias associated with pancytopenia. The most common hereditary aplastic anemia is **Fanconi's syndrome**, an autosomal recessive disease associated with pancytopenia, short stature, renal abnormalities, and skeletal abnormalities (e.g., bifid thumbs). Most cases of acquired aplastic anemia are idiopathic, and may represent immunologic attack on bone marrow stem cells. Some cases have known causes (e.g., **chemicals, drugs, viral infections, irradiation**). The anemia is normocytic/normochromic, with a **low RI** and **elevated erythropoietin** levels. The bone marrow is hypocellular, without evidence of other hematologic disease.

b.   Aplastic anemias involving only the red cell lineage (pure red cell aplasia), may be hereditary (e.g., Blackfan–Diamond disease) or acquired from toxins, neoplasms, viral infections (e.g., **parvovirus B19**), and so on.

6.   Congenital dyserythropoietic anemias (CDA). CDA is a family (three types) of hereditary abnormal red cell maturation disorders. All types show normocytic to macrocytic anemia, increased indirect bilirubin, and **megaloblastic or bizarre multinucleated red cell precursors**. One subtype of type II is hereditary erythroblast multinuclearity with positive acidified serum test (**HEMPAS**), which is distinguished from paroxysmal nocturnal hemoglobinuria by having a negative sucrose hemolysis test.

7.   Bone marrow replacement. Myelophthisis refers to the replacement of marrow space (and loss of hematopoietic capacity) by an extrinsic process. A myelophthistic (i.e., **leukoerythroblastic**) blood pattern refers to the presence of **immature myeloid cells, nucleated red cells, teardrop cells**, and occasionally schistocytes; this pattern is caused by premature release of cells from the marrow or extramedullary hematopoiesis. Anemia is usually normocytic/normochromic, and the RI can vary, depending on the amount of residual marrow capacity. Common causes include:

a.   Metastatic tumor or primary hematologic malignancies, including leukemias, lymphomas, metastastic carcinomas, or other tumors.

b. Systemic infections or inflammation, including granulomatous infections (e.g., fungal, mycobacterial), some bacterial infections [e.g., *Staphylococcus*, *Salmonella* (typhoid fever)], sarcoidosis, and so forth.

c. Fibrosis can occur as a primary disorder (myelofibrosis with myeloid metaplasia, see section VI.B. White Blood Cells) or as a response to bone marrow injury or tumor.

d. Storage disorders can occur when macrophages filled with abnormal metabolic products replace the marrow (e.g., Gaucher's disease, Niemann-Pick disease, Tay-Sachs disease).

7. Ineffective erythropoiesis. Many disorders cause abnormal red cell maturation, which then lyse within the marrow before they can enter the circulation (e.g., myelodysplasia, vitamin deficiencies). The bone **marrow is hypercellular** with increased red cell precursors, and the **RI is decreased**. Anemia is often macrocytic (see sections below), but can be normocytic or normochromic.

C. Normochromic normocytic anemias with an increased RI

1. Acute and chronic blood loss. Although the mature red cells are normocytic and normochromic, the increased numbers of reticulocytes (which are large) can cause the MCV to be increased. The problem is self-correcting if the blood loss is stopped.

2. Hemolytic anemias. The hemolytic anemias result from premature destruction of circulating red cells. They can be divided into two groups, based on the cause of the hemolysis: **intrinsic** (from abnormal red cells) and **extrinsic** (from destructive factors acting on normal red cells, Fig. 2-3). Regardless of the cause of the hemolysis, the destruction of the RBCs can occur within the circulation (**intravascular hemolysis**) or as a result of phagocytosis by macrophages within the liver, spleen, and bone marrow (**extravascular hemolysis**).

a. Commonly used tests to evaluate hemolysis. The CBC indices (normocytic, normochromic anemia with increased RDW), reticulocyte index (increased), and red cell morphology are helpful tests. The following additional laboratory studies are often useful; they can indicate the presence of hemolysis and whether it is primarily intravascular or extravascular, thus providing clues about the cause. **Extravascular hemolysis is reflected by increased indirect bilirubin, urobilinogenuria, increased lactate dehydrogenase (LDH), and microspherocytes. Intravascular hemolysis is reflected by increased free plasma hemoglobin, decreased haptoglobin, increased LDH, hemoglobinuria, hemosiderinuria, and urobilinogenuria; schistocytes** and other red cell fragments may or may not be present. Many cases of hemolytic anemia do not have purely intravascular or purely extravascular hemolysis, but instead show a **mixture of the two**, with one or the other predominating.

(1) Serum bilirubin, total and fractionated (normal reference range for adults = total: 0.3–1.0 mg/dL; direct: <0.4 mg/dL; indirect: <0.6 mg/dL). Bilirubin is the primary metabolic product of heme as it is metabolized by macrophages. Within the liver, unconjugated bilirubin (indirect bilirubin) becomes conjugated (direct bilirubin) for secretion into the intestine. **Increases** in indirect serum bilirubin support a diagnosis of hemolysis (particularly **extravascular hemolysis**).

(2)   **Plasma hemoglobin** (normal reference range: <10 mg/dL). **Increases** indicate **intravascular hemolysis**.

(3)   **Serum haptoglobin** (normal reference range: 40–180 mg/dL). Haptoglobin is an α_2 globulin protein produced by the liver that binds free hemoglobin for transport to the liver. **Absence of haptoglobin is seen with intravascular hemolysis** and liver failure. Haptoglobin, also an **acute phase reactant**, is elevated in a variety of inflammatory, infectious, and neoplastic conditions; therefore, an **elevated or normal serum haptoglobin level does not rule out hemolysis**.

(4)   **Lactic dehydrogenase** (normal reference range for adults: 90–170 U/L, but varies with method). Serum LDH increases with damage to a variety of tissues and cells, including the liver, heart, kidney, lymphocytes, and erythrocytes. **Hemolytic anemias** are one cause of elevations in LDH. LDH isoenzyme fractionation may help determine the source: LDH-1 is the isoenzyme found within erythrocytes, heart, and kidney.

(5)   **Urine hemoglobin and hemosiderin**. When the level of free hemoglobin in the blood exceeds the renal excretion threshold, hemoglobinuria results. A few days later, hemosiderin may be detectable in renal epithelial cells from the urine sediment. Hemoglobinuria or hemosiderinuria **suggests hemolysis**.

(6)   **Urine urobilinogen** (normal reference range for 2-hour test: male 0.3–2.1 mg/2 h; female 0.1–1.1 mg/2 h). Conjugated and excreted bilirubin is transformed into urobilinogen by gut bacteria. It may then be partly reabsorbed by the gut, and excreted by the kidneys. Increases in urine urobilinogen **suggest hemolysis**.

(7)   **Direct antiglobulin test (DAT; direct Coombs' test)**. The DAT detects antibodies bound to red cells *in vivo*, and detects **antibody-mediated hemolytic anemias**.

   b.   **Intrinsic hemolytic anemia**. The intrinsic hemolytic anemias result from defects inherent to the patient's RBCs. **Most intrinsic hemolytic anemias are inherited**, and normal RBCs transfused into these patients are not affected by the hemolytic process.

(1)   **Red cell membrane disorders** are caused by abnormalities in integral proteins or the cytoskeleton, and have a propensity for premature lysis. Such defects can be hereditary or acquired, and result in decreased deformability, instability, or increased sensitivity to complement.

(a)   **Hereditary red cell membrane disorders**. Most of the common RBC membrane disorders are hereditary and involve the cytoskeleton. Abnormal red cell cytoskeletons lead to the loss of membrane lipids, decreased red cell surface area, and formation of spherocytes. **Spherocytes** are poorly deformable and tend to be retained in the spleen where they are prematurely lysed (extravascular hemolysis).

(i) **Hereditary spherocytosis (HS)**

(*) **Clinical findings.** The severity of hemolysis ranges from asymptomatic to severe anemia, with improvement following splenectomy. Gallstones are seen in approximately 50% of the patients (caused by increased bilirubin).

(**) **Laboratory findings.** Spherocytes are present, and have increased osmotic fragility. The size of the spherocytes is important: **hereditary spherocytosis usually has spherocytes that are close to the normal red cell size, whereas other forms of extravascular hemolysis** (e.g., hemolytic transfusion reactions) **usually show microspherocytes.** Approximately 50% of patients will have a normal MCV and MCH, with an increased MCHC. Reticulocytes are increased and the marrow shows erythroid hyperplasia. If significant hemolysis is occurring, there will be increased unconjugated (indirect) bilirubin and LDH, decreased haptoglobin, and detectable urine urobilinogen. Measurement of cytoskeletal proteins by gel electrophoresis or radioimmunoassay is definitive but usually not required; diagnosis is made on clinical features, demonstration of spherocytes, and **increased osmotic fragility.**

(***) **Molecular pathology.** Heterogeneous molecular abnormalities exist, including deficiencies in spectrin, proteins band 3 or band 4.2, and so on. Inheritance can be autosomal dominant or recessive. The most common disorder is an **autosomal dominant spectrin** deficiency.

(ii) **Hereditary elliptocytosis (HE).** This family of disorders includes **common HE, spherocytic HE, stomatocytic HE**, and a subgroup of common HE called **hereditary pyropoikilocytosis (HPP).**

(*) **Clinical findings.** The most common disorder is common HE, which is most often seen in black and Southeast Asian populations, and is asymptomatic or has minimal hemolysis. Rare cases (particularly HPP) have severe hemolysis requiring splenectomy.

(**) **Laboratory findings.** Variable numbers of **elliptocytes** (range: 15%–100%) are present in all forms of HE. In spherocytic HE, spherocytes are also seen. In stomatocytic HE, stomatocytes are also seen, with usually no evidence of hemolysis. In HPP, **fragmented red cells, tear drop cells, and microspherocytes** are also seen, along with anemia that may be severe. Osmotic fragility is normal in most cases of common HE, and is increased in spherocytic HE and HPP. In HPP, increased **thermal instability** at 50°C leads to red cell fragmentation (whence the name "pyropoikilocytosis"). Measurement of cytoskeletal proteins by gel electrophoresis and polymerase chain reaction (PCR) testing for spectrin mutations can be done, but the diagnosis is usually made based on clinical history, CBC indices, and red cell morphology.

(***) **Molecular pathology.** Elliptocyte formation is usually caused by spectrin gene mutations leading to the impaired formation of spectrin heterodimers, and most cases are **autosomal dominant.**

c. **Acquired red cell membrane disorders. Most disorders are associated with abnormal lipid metabolism** (e.g., acanthocytosis) or with acquired hematopoietic stem cell defects [e.g., paroxysmal nocturnal hemoglobinuria (**PNH**)].

(1) **Acanthocytosis**. These abnormal red cells have **irregular, asymmetric membrane projections**, often with tiny bulbous ends. They occur in patients with abnormal lipid metabolism, which causes accumulation of nonesterified cholesterol in red cell membranes, and is followed by splenic remodeling. They are associated with **severe liver disease, abetalipoproteinemia**, some neurologic disorders, some cases of severe malnutrition, and **McLeod** or I_N blood types.

(2) **Paroxysmal nocturnal hemoglobinuria (PNH)**. This rare, acquired disorder, which is caused by a hematopoietic **stem cell mutation**, causes increased red cell **sensitivity to complement-mediated lysis**.

(a) **Pathophysiology**. Complement fixation on red cells leads to breech of the cell membrane and hemolysis. This is normally prevented by regulatory proteins [e.g., **decay accelerating factor (DAF**) and **membrane inhibitor of reactive lysis (MIRL**)] on the red cell membrane that inhibits the complement cascade. PNH has decreased phosphatidylinositolglycan-A (**PIG-A**) anchoring of DAF and MIRL, which in turn allows increased complement-mediated lysis. Because the main defect is in a stem cell, **leukocytes and platelets also may be abnormal**.

(b) **Clinical findings**. Patients with PNH are usually middle-aged or older; they have an insidious onset of anemia of variable severity. **Episodic hemolysis with hemoglobinuria** can occur, causing dark morning urine. Platelet abnormalities can cause venous thrombotic events, including mesenteric thromboses, headaches, or pulmonary embolism. Leukocyte abnormalities lead to leukopenia and increased susceptibility to infection. The disease course can be fulminant or chronic, with most patients succumbing to infection, bleeding, thrombosis, or hematopoietic malignancy (the abnormal stem cells may transform into leukemia).

(c) **Laboratory findings**. Patients have **anemia with or without leukopenia or thrombocytopenia**. Red cells may be normocytic or normochromic, or microcytic and hypochromic because of a superimposed iron deficiency (from hematuria). **Hemosiderinuria** is present, with hemoglobinuria present from time to time. Complement is normally activated by sucrose and acidification; therefore, patients with PNH have a **positive sucrose hemolysis test**. Patients also have a **positive acidified serum test (Ham's test)**, and flow cytometric demonstration of **decreased red cell expression of CD55 (DAF) and CD59 (MIRL)**, which provide definitive diagnostic evidence of PNH.

(d) **Molecular pathology**. Molecular analysis may demonstrate mutations in the PIG-A gene, but this is primarily a research tool. Cytogenetic analysis is nonspecific, but may show trisomy 9 or loss of chromosome Y.

(2) **Red cell enzyme deficiencies**. This family of hereditary disorders involves quantitative, qualitative, or both defects in enzymes of the glycolytic or hexose monophosphate shunt pathways, which results in premature lysis of red cells.

(a) **Glycolytic pathway disorders**. Red cells are dependent on glycolysis to provide **ATP** for essential cellular functions. Patients with glycolytic enzyme deficiencies show a nonspherocytic, variably severe, hemolytic anemia first seen in childhood. Patients have anemia, jaundice, gallstones, and slight to moderate splenomegaly. Aplastic crises can occur. Enzyme deficiencies include the following:

(i) **Pyruvate kinase deficiency (90% of glycolytic defects): autosomal recessive**. Qualitative fluorescent screening test is based on reduced nicotinic acid dehydrogenase (NADH) fluorescence [glycolysis causes NADH (fluorescent) to be oxidized to NAD+ (nonfluorescent) when sufficient pyruvate kinase is present]. Enzyme levels may also be quantitated.

(ii) **Other glycolytic pathway deficiencies** are identified by direct enzyme level determinations. Autosomal recessive disorders include deficiencies in **hexokinase, glucose-6-phosphate isomerase, phosphofructokinase, aldolase, diphosphoglycerate mutase,** and **triose phosphate isomerase** (which may have neurologic manifestations). **Phosphoglycerate kinase** is an X-linked disorder that may also have neurologic manifestations.

(b) **Hexose monophosphate shunt pathway disorders**. Red cells use this pathway to produce **NADPH** and **reduced glutathione** (GSH), which function to detoxify oxygen radicals. Deficiencies in this pathway leave red cells **unable to deal with oxidative stress**, leading to cellular damage and premature hemolysis.

The most common enzyme deficiency is the **X-linked glucose-6-phosphate dehydrogenase (G6PD) deficiency**, which is also the most prevalent inborn disorder of red cells. **Other hexose monophosphate shunt pathway deficiencies are rare**.

    (i)   Clinical findings. Heterozygous women may have variable penetrance because of preferential X-inactivation. Patients have episodic hemolysis following infection or ingestion of oxidant drugs, and anemia of varying degree.

    (ii)   Laboratory tests. Plasma hemoglobin levels can be increased. No distinctive red cell morphologic clues may be seen. **Heinz bodies** (particles of denatured hemoglobin and other proteins) may be demonstrated with supravital staining (e.g., new methylene blue) early in a hemolytic episode. The qualitative fluorescent screening test is most useful in men without active hemolysis (reticulocytes cause false-negative test results). Quantitative enzyme assays are more useful in patients with active hemolysis, increased reticulocytes, or in heterozygous women.

  (c)   Glutathione pathway deficiencies. These rare disorders include deficiencies of glutathione reductase, glutathione (GSH) synthase and gamma-glutamyl cysteine synthase. Episodic hemolytic anemia occurs that is similar to G6PD deficiency. GSH qualitative screening tests (by spectrophotometry) and quantitative tests are available.

(3)   Hemoglobinopathies (see later section).

  (a)   Extrinsic hemolytic anemia. The extrinsic hemolytic anemias occur as a result of **damage to the patient's normal red cells by external factors**. Extrinsic hemolytic anemias, which are **acquired**, typically are the sequelae of an underlying disease state. Transfused RBCs will undergo hemolysis similar to the patient's own RBCs.

(1)   Etiologies

  (a)   Mechanical damage. RBCs can be damaged by mechanical heart prostheses, abnormal great vessels, intense exercise ("march hemoglobinuria"), burns, fibrin strands within the microcirculation [microangiopathic hemolytic anemia (MAHA)], and so on. MAHA occurs with disseminated intravascular coagulation, hemolytic uremic syndrome, thrombotic thrombocytopenic purpura; hemolysis, elevated liver enzymes, low platelets (HELLP syndrome), and so forth.

  (b)   Damage by antibodies. Autoantibodies, alloantibodies, and drug-induced antibodies can cause both damage to RBCs and premature hemolysis. Autoantibodies can be warm reactive (IgG) or cold reactive (IgM). **Warm-reactive autoantibodies** are associated with **autoimmune diseases** (e.g., collagen-vascular diseases) and chronic disease states, or they can be idiopathic. **Cold-reactive autoantibodies** are associated with infections [e.g., *Mycoplasma pneumoniae* (anti-I), **infectious mononucleosis** (anti-i)], cold agglutinin disease, and so on. **Alloantibody-induced hemolysis occurs in hemolytic disease of the newborn and hemolytic blood transfusion reactions**.

(c) Plasma lipid abnormalities. Alterations in the lipid content of red cell membranes can result in RBC hemolysis. This is commonly seen in association with liver disease.

(d) Hypophosphatemia. Severe hypophosphatemia impedes the regeneration of ATP within red cells, leading to hemolysis.

(e) Toxins and infectious agents. Bacterial endotoxins, malaria, babesia, and some snake venoms induce RBC hemolysis.

(2) Clinical findings. Patients may complain of weakness, fatigue, and malaise; fever, jaundice, and splenomegaly may be present.

(3) Laboratory findings. The RBC count, Hgb, and Hct are decreased. The RI is increased. The WBC, serum bilirubin, plasma hemoglobin, and LDH may be increased. Serum haptoglobin is decreased. MAHA is associated with increased D-dimer levels, decreased plasma fibrinogen, and thrombocytopenia. Antibody-induced hemolytic anemia is associated with a positive Coombs' test.

(4) Morphologic findings. Spherocytes are often seen in autoantibody-induced hemolysis. Mechanical damage causes RBC fragments and schistocytes. Plasma lipid abnormalities result in target cells and acanthocytes.

VI. Hemoglobinopathies comprise a large group of hereditary disorders that are caused by globin gene mutations, which trigger either **decreased hemoglobin synthesis (quantitative disorders) or production of an abnormal hemoglobin (qualitative disorders**, Table 2-2). The quantitative disorders (e.g., thalassemias, Table 2-3) usually cause microcytic anemias.

Table 2-2. Summary of common hemoglobins (Hb)

Hemoglobin Type	Protein (Globin) Chains that Compose the Hb
Hb A	2 alpha and 2 beta
Hb A$_2$	2 alpha and 2 delta
Hb F	2 alpha and 2 gamma
Hb H	4 beta
Hb Bart's	4 gamma
Hb S	2 alpha and 2 beta$^{(6\ glutamic\ acid \rightarrow valine)}$
Hb C	2 alpha and 2 beta$^{(6\ glutamic\ acid \rightarrow lysine)}$
Hb E	2 alpha and 2 beta$^{(26\ glutamic\ acid \rightarrow lysine)}$
Hb D	2 alpha and 2 beta$^{(121\ glutamic\ acid \rightarrow glutamine)}$

Phrases in parentheses show the position of the abnormal amino acid (from the NH$_2$ terminal end), the normal amino acid, and the abnormal amino acid, respectively; for example, HbS has a valine that has replaced the normal glutamic acid at the sixth position.

Table 2-3. Summary of hemoglobin analyses in thalassemias

Condition[a]	Electrophoresis Findings
Normal newborn	Hb A ($\cong$25%), Hb F ($\cong$75%), Hb A$_2$ (1%)[b]
Normal 6 month-old	Hb A ($\cong$85%–90%), Hb F ($\cong$10%), Hb A$_2$ (2%)
Normal adult	Hb A (96%), Hb F (1%), Hb A$_2$ (3%)
Beta thalassemia	
Minor (β°/β)	Hb A ($\cong$90%), Hb A$_2$ (3%–8%), ± Hb F
Intermedia (β^+/β^+)	Hb A (50%–70%), Hb F (20%–40%), Hb A$_2$ (3%–8%),
Major (β°/β°)	No Hb A, Hb F (>90%), Hb A$_2$ (3%–8%)
Delta/beta thalassemia	
Minor ($\delta\beta^\circ/\delta\beta$)	Hb A (80%–90%), Hb F (5%–20%), Hb A$_2$ (3%)
Major ($\delta\beta^\circ/\delta\beta^\circ$)	Hb F (100%), No Hb A, No Hb A$_2$
Alpha thalassemia	
Silent carrier ($-\alpha/\alpha\alpha$)	Normal
Minor ($--/\alpha\alpha$)	Normal
Intermedia ($--/-\alpha$) (Hb H disease)	Hb A (70%–90%), Hb H (5%–30%), (Hb Barts present at birth and replaced by Hb H during first few months of life)
Major ($--/--$) (Hydrops fetalis)	Hb Barts (>80%), Hb H (10%–20%), No Hb A
Beta thalassemia/sickle-cell syndrome (β^+/S)[c]	Hb A (15%–30%), Hb S (70%–85%)
Alpha thalassemia/sickle-cell syndrome [($--/-\alpha$)/S][c]	Hb A (40%–60%), Hb S ($\cong$20%), Hb F (10%–20%)
Sickle cell	
Trait (A/S)[d]	Hb A ($\cong$60%), Hb S ($\cong$40%)
Disease (S/S)	No Hb A, Hb S (>80%), Hb F (<20%)
Hemoglobin C	
Trait (A/C)[d]	Hb A ($\cong$60%), Hb C ($\cong$40%)
Disease (C/C)	No Hb A, Hb C (>90%), Hb F (<10%)
Hemoglobin E	
Trait (A/E)[d]	Hb A ($\cong$60%), Hb E ($\cong$40%)
Disease (E/E)	No Hb A, Hb E (>90%), Hb F (<10%)

[a] Note that these conditions are examples of some possible genotypes, and that there is a wide variety of other genotypes with varying degrees of clinical severity.
[b] Note that the Hb A$_2$ gene is defective in one aspect, in that it *never* produces more than 8% of the total hemoglobin in a cell, even in disease conditions. If the electrophoretic band at the Hb A$_2$ location is >8%, *another hemoglobin* (e.g., Hb C, Hb E, Hb O) migrating to the same location must account for the band. Increases in Hb A$_2$ are of such small magnitude that quantification by special chromatography techniques is required.
[c] Double heterozygotes that have a qualitatively abnormal globin gene (Hb S, C, E) and a quantitative defect in the other beta gene (e.g., beta-thalassemia) have *more* of the qualitatively abnormal Hb (e.g., HbS) than the expected amount usually seen in the trait. If the quantitative defect is an alpha-thalassemia, the patient will have less than the expected amount of the qualitatively abnormal Hb (e.g., HbS).
[d] Hemoglobinopathy traits do not show equal amounts of each hemoglobin, because the normal gene (Hb A) usually produces more protein product than the abnormal gene (e.g., Hb S).

The qualitative disorders (e.g., sickle cell disease, HbC) usually cause normocytic anemias; the main exception is HbE, which causes a microcytic anemia.

A. Normal globin chains. Normal adult hemoglobin (**HbA**, ~96%) contains **two alpha chains and two beta chains** $\alpha_2\beta_2$, Fig. 2-1). Other minor hemoglobins found in adults are **HbA$_2$** [**two alpha and two delta** $(\alpha_2\delta_2)$; ~3% of total], and **HbF** [fetal hemoglobin: **two alpha and two gamma** $(\alpha_2\gamma_2)$; ~1% of total]. At birth, the predominant hemoglobin is HbF, which is replaced by HbA in the first year of life.

B. Laboratory analysis of hemoglobins (Hb). The following tests identify quantitative and qualitative hemoglobin abnormalities, and should be correlated with clinical data, CBC indices, and red cell morphology.

    1. Hemoglobin analysis is the **main tool** used to identify and quantify abnormal hemoglobins (Fig. 2-5).

        a. Gel electrophoresis. After cell lysis, hemoglobin is run on a **cellulose acetate** gel (pH 8.4–8.8) and on a **citrate agar** gel (pH 6.2), which separate the hemoglobins into bands based on net charge. Bands can be quantitated by densitometry. Both the alkaline and the acidic gels are needed to characterize some hemoglobins, because several different hemoglobins migrate to the same place on one or both gels.

        b. High performance liquid chromatography (HPLC). This rapid screening method detects and quantifies abnormal hemoglobins on the basis of charge, using a

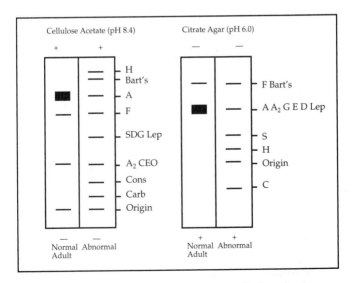

Fig. 2-5. Hemoglobin electrophoresis patterns. Carb, carbonic anhydrase; Cons, Hb constant spring; Lep, Hb lepore.

porous cation-exchange column. The method is US Food and Drug Administration-approved for preliminary identification of unusual hemoglobins (the **elution times of >700 variants** have been catalogued). Because some hemoglobins overlap, use of gel electrophoresis, solubility testing, or globin chain analysis may be additionally required for definitive diagnosis.

2.   Additional tests for detection of hemoglobin S (HbS).

   a.   Sickle test. Cells containing HbS may not appear sickled on standard blood smears. Cells can be induced to sickle when exposed to **sodium metabisulfite** before smear preparation.

   b.   Solubility test for HbS. Exposure of a red cell lysate (containing HbS) to a reducing agent causes polymerization of the HbS and an increase in **solution turbidity**.

3.   Additional tests for detection of fetal hemoglobin (HbF).

   a.   Kleihauer–Betke stain. Acid treatment of RBCs will elute HbA and precipitate HbF. Cells containing HbA will appear as ghosts, whereas cells containing **HbF will appear densely red**.

   b.   Flow cytometry. Flow cytometric methods can identify HbF by immunologic methods.

4.   Additional methods for quantification of HbA$_2$. Ion exchange chromatography (using an anion-exchange column) allows accurate quantification of HbA$_2$ (2%–3% increases are diagnostically important); gel electrophoresis is insensitive. HPLC methods can also be used to quantitate HbA$_2$.

5.   Supravital staining. HbH (seen in alpha-thalassemia) and **Heinz bodies** (seen, e.g., in G6PD) can be detected by supravital stains such as new methylene blue or brilliant cresyl blue.

6.   Globin chain analysis. Mutational analysis of globin chains can be done by Southern blotting, PCR, or other methods to provide definitive identification of a hemoglobin species (usually not required).

C.   Microcytic, hypochromic hemoglobinopathies: quantitative disorders (thalassemias) and HbE. Quantitative disorders (i.e., thalassemias) have mutations that lead to decreased or absent production of one of the globins, with a resultant overproduction of the other globins (Table 2-3). This unbalanced globin chain production leads to **decreased normal hemoglobin**, with a subsequent microcytic or hypochromic anemia. Thalassemias, which are classified by the globin chain defect, were first described in patients of Mediterranean descent ("thalassa" is Greek for "sea"). Because of a marked ineffective erythropoiesis, these patients are also susceptible to iron overload (particularly if they are transfused), and many patients have increased storage and serum iron. HbE, a qualitative hemoglobinopathy that causes a microcytic or hypochromic anemia, will be discussed later with the other qualitative hemoglobinopathies.

   1.   Alpha thalassemia. The severity of the disease depends on **how many of the four α-globin genes (αα/αα)** are defective, and whether the defect is a **partial (α^+) or a total (α^0)** deletion. The most common defects are complete deletions. When α-globin genes are deleted, red cells respond by producing excess β-globins **(HbH)** or excess γ-globins **(Hb Bart's)**, which form unstable tetramers that predispose to hemolysis. HbH and Hb Bart's can be detected by electrophoresis or HPLC, and HbH can also be detected with supravital staining. Alpha thalassemia occurs primarily in African, Mediterranean, Middle Eastern, and Southeast Asian populations: α^0 mutations (total deletions of one or more α-genes) are most common in Asian and Mediterranean populations, whereas African and Middle Eastern populations tend to have α^+ mutations (partial deletions).

   a.   Alpha thalassemia minor. One α-globin gene is affected ($-\alpha/\alpha\alpha$). These individuals are **silent carriers** with no significant anemia. The MCV is normal to slightly decreased. Small amounts of HbH (1%–2%) may be present at birth, which disappear later (Table 2-3).

   b.   Alpha thalassemia trait. Two α-globin genes are affected (α -/α- or $\alpha\alpha$/- -), giving rise to red cell microcytosis (MCV <70 fL) with **mild anemia**. Electrophoresis shows 5% to 10% HbH at birth, which disappears later.

   c.   Alpha thalassemia major (hemoglobin H disease). Three α-globin genes are affected (α -/- -), giving rise to microcytic, hypochromic anemia (MCV <70 fL), with significant ongoing hemolysis. Electrophoresis shows predominantly Hb Bart's (a tetramer of four gamma chains) at birth, with a gradual shift to **HbH** (5%–30%) over the first few months of life.

   d.   Hydrops fetalis. Four α-globin genes are affected (- -/- -), which is a lethal genetic defect. Electrophoresis shows predominantly **Hb Bart's**. The complete absence of α-globin chains in the fetus usually leads to intrauterine **death from severe hypoxia**. The hypoxia is caused by Hb Bart's high oxygen affinity (which prevents release of O_2 to the tissues), and, in turn, the hypoxia causes massive fluid accumulation. Prenatal screening may identify patients at risk and allow for in utero transfusion. This is more common in Southeast Asian and Mediterranean populations because of the predominance of the α^0 phenotype.

   2.   Beta thalassemia. One or both β-globin genes have mutations that cause partial (β^+) or total (β^0) loss of β-chain production. The number of genes affected and the type of mutation (partial or complete) will determine the disease severity (>50 different mutations have been described). Most beta-thalassemic syndromes have a significant degree of ineffective erythropoiesis, and are seen primarily in Southeast Asian, Mediterranean, Middle Eastern, African, and Indian subcontinent populations.

   a.   Beta thalassemia minor (trait). A single β-globin gene is affected (β^0/β). Decreased β-chain production leads to mild anemia (Hb 9–11 g/dL) or no anemia, normal to **increased RBC counts**, and **microcytosis** (MCV 60–70 fL). Electrophoresis shows **mild increases in HbF,**

and quantification of HbA_2 by column chromatography shows **increased HbA_2** (3%–8%).

b.   Beta thalassemia intermedia. This is most commonly caused by a **partial deletion (β^0) of both beta-genes (homozygous: β^+/β^+)**. A wide spectrum of disease is seen, with moderate to severe anemia (Hb 6–10 g/dL), growth retardation, and bony abnormalities (caused by reactive marrow hyperplasia), although this occurs later in life than with beta-thalassemia major. Electrophoresis shows **increased HbF** (20%–40%) and **increased HbA_2** (3%–8%).

c.   Beta thalassemia major (Cooley's anemia). Both β-globin genes (homozygous) have complete deletions β^0/β^0. Marked microcytic and hypochromic anemia (MCV <70 fL; Hb 2–3 g/dL) is present, with hepatosplenomegaly, bony deformities, and failure to thrive as an infant. **HbF is significantly elevated** (usually >90% of total Hb), and **HbA_2 is increased** (3%–8% of total Hb). Patients are transfusion dependent.

3.   Delta-beta thalassemia. This group of disorders involves mutations in the delta-gamma-beta globin gene cluster that affect more than one globin gene. These patients have a **lack of both β-globin and δ-globin chains ($\delta\beta$)°**, or form abnormal hemoglobin chains (Hb Lepore) with β-globins that are missing the central portion of the protein. The clinical spectrum tends to be less severe than the beta thalassemias and is dependent on the type of deletion. Most patients are heterozygotes. These disorders are found sporadically in many racial groups.

4.   Hereditary   persistence   of   fetal   hemoglobin (HPFH). This group of disorders is clinically similar to beta thalassemia, although milder. The **defective β-globin** synthesis is almost completely compensated for by production of γ-globin chains (homozygotes: 100% HbF; heterozygotes: 70% HbA and 30% HbF).

5.   Hemoglobin E: see discussion below.

D.   Normocytic, normochromic hemoglobinopathies: qualitative hemoglobin disorders. These disorders are caused by globin gene mutations that cause **structurally abnormal globins with altered function** (unlike the thalassemias, which have abnormal amounts of structurally normal globins). Many of the mutations have been designated with letters (e.g., HbS for the sickle cell disease hemoglobin, Table 2-2), but can also be designated by the mutation (e.g., HbS is $\alpha_2\beta_2^{6Glu->Val}$).

1.   Sickle cell disease (HbS) is the most common qualitative hemoglobinopathy in the world. It is due to a **β-globin chain mutation** that gives rise to HbS $\alpha_2\beta_2^{6Glu->Val}$; **valine** replaces the normal glutamic acid at the sixth amino acid position). When deoxygenated, HbS polymerizes into crystalline arrays that cause the red cell to sickle. **Sickled cells lodge in small vessels**, giving rise to vaso-occlusive events (e.g., abdominal crises, painful crises, stroke). With repeated sickling, the red cell membrane becomes progressively more abnormal in lipid content and function, leading to premature hemolysis. The heterozygous state confers some protection against malarial infection (the abnormal cells lyse before the intracellular malarial parasites can mature into infective forms). Sickle cell disease is **autosomal recessive**, and found primarily in blacks from Africa.

   a. Sickle cell trait (A/S trait: carrier state): hetero-zygous for HbS (β/S). Most patients are asymptomatic, and have normal CBC indices or a mild normocytic, nor-mochromic anemia. Red cell morphology is often normal. Hemoglobin electrophoresis shows **HbS** (~40%) and **HbA** (~60%). The solubility test and the sickling test are both positive.

   b. Sickle cell disease (S/S disease): homozygous for HbS (S/S). Patients have moderate to severe nor-mochromic, normocytic anemia (Hb 5–11 g/dL). The RI is increased, and circulating nucleated RBCs may be seen. Signs of splenectomy (Howell–Jolly bodies, anisopoikilocy-tosis) are present because of repeated splenic infarctions (**autosplenectomy**). Indirect bilirubin levels are elevated. The **solubility test and the sickle cell test are both pos-itive**, and occasional sickled cells may be present on the reg-ular blood smear. Electrophoresis shows **HbS** (>80%), **HbF** (<20%), **HbA$_2$** (3%–8% of total), and **no HbA** (Fig. 2-5).

   2. Hemoglobin C (HbC): the second most common hemoglobinopathy seen in the United States. It is caused by an autosomal recessive beta-chain mutation ($\alpha_2\beta_2^{6Glu\rightarrow Lys}$) that causes red cells to be rigid, resulting in frag-mentation and microspherocyte formation, and a decreased life span of 30 to 35 days. In patients who have had a splenec-tomy, **crystals** of HbC may be seen within red cells. HbC is found primarily in patients of West African descent, and spo-radically in other populations.

   a. Hemoglobin C trait (A/C trait): heterozygous for HbC (β/C). Patients may have mild anemia, but are usu-ally asymptomatic. Electrophoresis shows **HbA** (60%) and **HbC** (40%) (Fig. 2-5).

   b. Hemoglobin C disease (C/C disease): homozy-gous for HbC (C/C). Patients have splenomegaly and mild to moderate normocytic or normochromic anemia (Hb 8–12 g/dL). **Target cells**, spherocytes, RBC fragments, and intraerythrocytic HbC **crystals** may be seen. Dehy-dration of red cells with a hypertonic solution may accen-tuate HbC crystals in the smear. Osmotic fragility is nor-mal to decreased. Electrophoresis shows **HbC** (>90%), **HbF** (<10%), and **no HbA**.

   c. Hemoglobin C/hemoglobin S disease (S/C dis-ease): caused by heterozygous inheritance of a HbS gene and a HbC gene. Patients have moderate normocytic or nor-mochromic anemia (with increased MCHC), and spleno-megaly. **Numerous target cells**, folded red cells and occa-sional sickled cells are present. The **solubility test** and **the sickle cell test are positive**. Hemoglobin electrophoresis shows the presence of **HbS** (>40%), **HbC** (>40%), **HbF** (<10%), and **no HbA**.

3.   Hemoglobin D (HbD). Several **autosomal recessive** mutations give rise to HbD variants. HbD, which migrates on alkaline gels to the same position as HbS, has normal solubility in the solubility tests. HbD is seen in blacks and people from India (and sporadically in other races).

   a.   Hemoglobin D trait (A/D trait): heterozygous for HbD and entirely asymptomatic. Electrophoresis shows **HbD** (40%) and **HbA** (60%) (Fig. 2-5).

   b.   Hemoglobin D disease (D/D disease): homozygous for HbD, is very rare, and causes mild anemia.

4.   Hemoglobin E (HbE). This **autosomal recessive beta-chain mutation** gives rise to HbE ($\alpha_2\beta_2^{26Glu\rightarrow Lys}$). **HbE is the second most common qualitative hemoglobinopathy worldwide (after HbS), the third most common in the United States** (after HbS and HbC), and is particularly common in **Southeast Asian** populations (e.g., Thailand). HbE is unstable when subjected to oxidative stress. Red cells are **microcytic**, unlike the other qualitative hemoglobinopathies that are normocytic.

   a.   Hemoglobin E trait (A/E trait): heterozygous for HbE (β/E). Patients are asymptomatic, have no anemia, and have mildly microcytic red cells (MCV 70–80 fL). Electrophoresis shows **HbE** (40%) with **HbA** (60%) (Fig. 2-5).

   b.   Hemoglobin E disease (E/E disease): homozygous for HbE (E/E). Patients have marked microcytosis (MCV <70 fL) and hypochromia, and mild anemia (Hb > 10 g/dL). Electrophoresis demonstrates **HbE** (>90%), **HbF** (<10%), and **no HbA**.

5.   Other hemoglobinopathies are rare in comparison to HbS, HbC, HbD, and HbE. More than 700 different α- and β-globin chain abnormalities have been described that cause a variety of defects ranging from erythrocytosis to anemia, with variable clinical significance. These disorders usually require detailed globin chain analysis for definitive identification. Some hemoglobins have an **increased affinity for** O_2 **(e.g., Hb Chesapeake, Hb Rainier)**, and are associated with polycythemia (secondary to tissue hypoxia). Some hemoglobins have a **decreased affinity for** O_2 **(e.g., Hb Kansas)**. Other hemoglobins are **unstable, causing intracellular Heinz bodies to form (e.g., Hb Bart's, Hb H, Hb Torino).**

E.   Mixed hemoglobinopathies. Because of the increased frequency of thalassemic syndromes and qualitative hemoglobin mutations in the same populations, some patients have both. The most common is the **sickle-thalassemia** syndrome (HbS/beta thalassemia). These patients have fewer vaso-occlusive crises than patients with S/S disease, because of the lower hemoglobin concentration within the red cells (which decreases polymerization of HbS). Patients have splenomegaly and moderate, mildly microcytic anemia. Laboratory findings include numerous target cells in the blood smear and a positive solubility test. Electrophoresis shows **HbS** (80%) and **HbA** (20%).

VII.   Macrocytic anemias are characterized by **a MCV of >100 fL.** They are divided into **megaloblastic** and **nonmegaloblastic groups**, based on their cause and whether megaloblastic changes occur within the blood and bone marrow (Fig. 2-6).

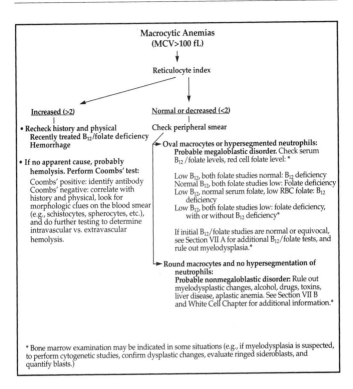

Macrocytic Anemias
(MCV>100 fL)
↓
Reticulocyte index

Increased (>2)
• Recheck history and physical
  Recently treated B_{12}/folate deficiency
  Hemorrhage

• If no apparent cause, probably
  hemolysis. **Perform Coombs' test:**
  Coombs' positive: identify antibody
  Coombs' negative: correlate with
  history and physical, look for
  morphologic clues on the blood smear
  (e.g., schistocytes, spherocytes, etc.),
  and do further testing to determine
  intravascular vs. extravascular
  hemolysis.

Normal or decreased (≤2)
Check peripheral smear

Oval macrocytes or hypersegmented neutrophils:
  Probable megaloblastic disorder. Check serum
  B_{12}/folate levels, red cell folate level: *
  Low B_{12}, both folate studies normal: B_{12} deficiency
  Normal B_{12}, both folate studies low: Folate deficiency
  Low B_{12}, normal serum folate, low RBC folate: B_{12}
    deficiency
  Low B_{12}, both folate studies low: folate deficiency,
    with or without B_{12} deficiency*

  If initial B_{12}/folate studies are normal or equivocal,
    see Section VII A for additional B_{12}/folate tests, and
    rule out myelodysplasia.*

Round macrocytes and no hypersegmentation of
  neutrophils:
  Probable nonmegaloblastic disorder: Rule out
  myelodysplastic changes, alcohol, drugs, toxins,
  liver disease, aplastic anemia. See Section VII B
  and White Cell Chapter for additional information.*

* Bone marrow examination may be indicated in some situations (e.g., if myelodysplasia is suspected,
to perform cytogenetic studies, confirm dysplastic changes, evaluate ringed sideroblasts, and
quantify blasts.)

Fig. 2-6. Flow chart for macrocytic anemias.

A. Megaloblastic anemia

1. Etiology: usually due to **deficiencies of vitamin B_{12}, folate, or both**. Both of these vitamins are involved in the conversion of homocysteine to methionine, and the synthesis of thymidine triphosphate (TTP, used for DNA synthesis). B_{12} and folate deficiencies cause **impaired DNA synthesis and delayed cell division, whereas hemoglobin synthesis proceeds normally**. This leads to large red cells with immature (finely distributed) nuclear chromatin and increased amounts of mature hemoglobinized cytoplasm (**nuclear or cytoplasmic dysynchrony**). Although B_{12} and folate deficiencies have several findings that overlap, it is nevertheless **essential to differentiate between them**. Mistakenly treating a B_{12} deficiency with large amounts of folate may partially correct some of the abnormal CBC indices (masking the lack of B_{12}), but will not **prevent the permanent neurologic damage associated with the B_{12} deficiency. Therefore, always exclude B_{12} deficiencies before starting long-term folate replacement.**

a.   **Vitamin B$_{12}$ (cobalamin) deficiency**. Vitamin B$_{12}$ is supplied in the diet by meat, eggs, and dairy products. Gastric parietal cells secrete **intrinsic factor**, which binds to B$_{12}$ and allows its absorption in the ileum. Vitamin B$_{12}$ is transported in the bloodstream by **transcobalamin II**. People normally store approximately **3 year's** worth of B$_{12}$; therefore, chronic disorders (e.g., pernicious anemia, Crohn's disease, Imerslund–Graesbeck syndrome) are the usual causes of B$_{12}$ deficiency, rather than transient dietary inadequacies. **Pernicious anemia, the most common cause of B$_{12}$ deficiency**, is characterized by gastric atrophy with associated production of autoantibodies. The autoantibodies are most commonly directed against parietal cell antigens but can also be against intrinsic factor. Dietary deficiencies, increased utilization (as in pregnancy), tapeworms (*Diphyllobothrium latum*), **intestinal (ileum) resection**, and **malabsorption** syndromes (e.g., sprue) can also result in B$_{12}$ deficiency.

b.   **Folate deficiency**. Folate in the form of methyltetrahydrofolate, the methyl group donor for the formation of methionine from homocysteine, is necessary for normal DNA synthesis. Dietary folate is supplied by leafy green vegetables and meat, and is **absorbed in the first portion** of the small intestine. People normally store only **3 month's** worth of folate. Therefore, folate deficiency most commonly results from **dietary deficiencies and transient states of increased utilization** (e.g., growth spurts, pregnancy), and less commonly from altered absorption as a result of drugs or malabsorption syndromes.

2.   **Commonly used studies to evaluate megaloblastic anemia**.

a.   **Reticulocyte index**. The RI is used to assess effective RBC production. This is normally increased after acute blood loss or hemolysis, but is decreased in cases of nutritional deficiencies, marrow aplasias or replacement, exposures to toxic agents, and so on.

b.   **Serum B$_{12}$ levels**. Serum B$_{12}$ levels below 90 pg/mL, with an associated normal folate level, indicate B$_{12}$ deficiency. **Folate deficiencies can cause artifactually decreased serum B$_{12}$ levels, which will return to normal when folate is replenished**.

c.   **Serum and RBC folate levels**. Serum folate levels below 3 ng/mL, with a normal serum B$_{12}$ level, suggest folate deficiency. **Red cell folate levels reflect chronic tissue folate status better** than serum folate levels (serum levels can change acutely after a single nutritious meal). **Vitamin B$_{12}$ deficiencies are usually associated with normal or increased serum folate levels, but can cause artifactually decreased red cell folate levels**.

d.   **Serum homocysteine. Levels of serum homocysteine increase** with B$_{12}$ or folate deficiency.

e.   **Serum bilirubin, LDH. Increases in indirect bilirubin and LDH** occur in megaloblastic anemias, because of lysis of defective RBCs within the marrow (ineffective erythropoiesis).

f. Antibodies to intrinsic factor and gastric parietal cells. The presence of antibodies against the B_{12} binding site on intrinsic factor strongly indicates pernicious anemia. Antibodies to gastric parietal cells, thyroid gland, and adrenal gland are commonly seen in patients with pernicious anemia, but they are less specific findings.

g. Urine methylmalonic acid levels are increased with B_{12} deficiency. Confirmation with other tests such as the Shilling test and serum B_{12} levels may be useful.

h. Urine formiminoglutamic acid (FIGLU) levels are increased with folate deficiency.

i. Shilling test. Tests the ability of the patient to absorb vitamin B_{12} first without, and then with, a dose of exogenous intrinsic factor. Radiolabeled B_{12} is ingested, and then a 24-hour urine sample is obtained. If >7% of the administered radioactivity is excreted in the urine, absorption is normal. **If <7% is excreted, B_{12} absorption is abnormal**. If absorption is abnormal, the test is repeated with the addition of intrinsic factor. If absorption corrects, this suggests a deficiency in endogenous intrinsic factor as is seen with pernicious anemia. If it does not correct, intestinal malabsorption is the most likely cause of the B_{12} deficiency.

j. Deoxyuridine suppression test. This test is based on the principle that B_{12} and folate are necessary to convert deoxyuridine into thymidylate, a building block for DNA synthesis. The test incubates the patient's lymphocytes with deoxyuridine and radioactive thymidine. In normal patients, the deoxyuridine is converted into thymidylate, which is then incorporated into DNA. In patients with B_{12} or folate deficiency, an alternate pathway occurs that converts the radioactive thymidine into radioactive thymidylate, which is then incorporated into the DNA and measured. In summary, **B_{12} or folate deficiency leads to the measurable incorporation of radioactive thymidylate into the DNA**.

3. Clinical findings. In both B_{12} and folate deficiencies, patients may have signs and symptoms of **anemia**, pallor, jaundice, weight loss, **glossitis**, and stomatitis. **In B_{12} deficiency, the patients may also have nervous system pathology**, such as psychological problems ("megaloblastic madness"), motor disorders, posterior column defects (e.g., paresthesias, loss of proprioception), and peripheral neuropathy.

4. Laboratory findings. The RBC count, Hct, and Hgb are decreased, with **macrocytic** red cells (MCV > 100). Thrombocytopenia and leukopenia are also common (i.e., **pancytopenia**). LDH values are often markedly elevated. In addition, depending on the cause, any of the tests described above for the workup of megaloblastic anemia may be abnormal.

5. Morphologic findings. The RBCs are characteristically large and oval (oval macrocytes), which is the most specific finding, but one that occurs late in the disorder. The **RI is decreased**. Some neutrophils contain **hyperlobated**

nuclei (look for >5% of the cells to have >5 lobes), which is one of the earliest changes. The bone marrow is hypercellular. Megaloblastic changes (e.g., **"dysynchrony"**—large nuclei with immature chromatin, and mature cytoplasm) may be seen in the erythroid, granulocytic, and megakaryocytic cell lineages. Giant metamyelocytes and large megakaryocytes are frequently encountered. Iron stores are usually increased.

B. Nonmegaloblastic macrocytic anemia

  1. Etiology

    a. Alcoholism often results in a MCV in the range of 100 to 110 fL. **Alcohol directly increases red cell size** and causes large, round red cells (in fact, the MCV has occasionally been used by corporations as a screen for alcoholism). Associated nutritional deficiencies (e.g., folate, iron) may also be present.

    b. Liver disease. Patients with cirrhosis, portal hypertension, and congestive splenomegaly commonly have a macrocytic anemia, usually caused by **increased plasma lipids** that enter the red cell membrane. The red cells are often **large and round, or target shaped**.

    c. Myelodysplastic syndromes. Macrocytic anemia (with or without pancytopenia) is seen in many myelodysplastic syndromes (MDS). Other changes of MDS can be seen in leukocytes and platelets (e.g., alterations in nuclear segmentation, cellular maturation, and cytoplasmic granulation).

    d. Drugs. Drugs that interfere with folate utilization and DNA synthesis commonly cause macrocytic anemias. Alcohol, methotrexate, trimethoprim, diphenylhydantoin, zidovudine, and several chemotherapeutic agents are well-known examples.

    e. Pregnancy can cause a slight elevation in the MCV, with or without a folate deficiency.

    f. Hypothyroidism often causes a mild normocytic to macrocytic anemia.

    g. Hemolysis. Increased reticulocyte counts associated with hemolytic anemias often result in an increased MCV (see "normocytic, normochromic anemias with increased reticulocytes"). The mature red cells are normocytic and normochromic, whereas the reticulocytes are large, round, pale blue cells (polychromasia).

  2. Clinical findings. The clinical findings are dependent on the patient's underlying disease. Many patients complain of fatigue and malaise; some are asymptomatic.

  3. Laboratory findings: macrocytic anemia, often with an increased LDH and indirect bilirubin level. The RI is decreased, except in cases caused by hemorrhage or hemolysis.

  4. Morphologic findings depend on the patient's underlying disease. Target cells are commonly seen with alcoholism and liver disease. Polychromasia is present in hemolytic anemias. The myelodysplastic syndromes may show pancytopenia, dysplastic features, and ringed sideroblasts within the marrow (see section in chapter 2.2, *White Blood Cells*).

VIII. Polycythemia

A. Definition. Polycythemia is an increase in red cell mass, and may be primary or secondary.

B. Causes

1. Primary polycythemia: erythropoietin-independent increase in red cell production (e.g., polycythemia vera; see Chapter 2.2, *White Blood Cells*). **Erythropoietin levels are low**.

2. Secondary polycythemia: erythropoietin-dependent increase in red cell production. **Erythropoietin levels are high**, and may be appropriate (responding to tissue hypoxia) or inappropriate.

a. Polycythemia as an appropriate response to tissue hypoxia resulting from smoking, high altitude acclimatization, **chronic pulmonary diseases** that cause hypoxia (e.g., chronic obstructive pulmonary disease), hypoventilation (e.g., impaired chest wall movement, sleep apnea, obesity), **cardiovascular diseases** with right-to-left shunt, abnormal hemoglobins that do not release oxygen readily (e.g., high affinity hemoglobins, methemoglobinemia) or chemical hypoxia (cobalt poisoning).

b. Inappropriate polycythemia: renal diseases leading to inappropriate release of erythropoietin (e.g., renal vascular disease, hydronephrosis, renal cysts and tumors, transplant rejection). Uterine leiomyomas, cerebellar hemangioblastomas, hepatomas, and some endocrine disorders (pheochromocytoma, adrenal cortical hyperplasia) can also cause erythrocytosis.

c. Idiopathic or essential erythrocytosis often have inappropriately high erythropoietin levels. Seen in very young patients or familial cohorts. No cause for erythrocytosis can be identified.

d. Autotransfusion (blood doping) or injection of erythropoietin. Athletes trying to increase performance may increase their red cell mass.

C. Signs and symptoms of polycythemia caused by increased red cell mass and hyperviscosity

1. CBC. Increased RBC count and hematocrit (>60%). Usually normocytic and normochromic indices, although microcytosis may be present if the iron intake is inadequate for the red cell production rate. Must exclude **relative polycythemia** (elevated hematocrit caused by fluid volume depletion, from dehydration, excess urination, or gastrointestinal water loss).

2. Blood hyperviscosity. Associated with slight increase in the incidence of strokes.

3. Clinical features. May have rubor (red "ruddy" skin). Splenomegaly should be absent. Signs of other disease (e.g., "clubbing" in pulmonary diseases) may be present.

D. Laboratory findings (Fig. 2-7)

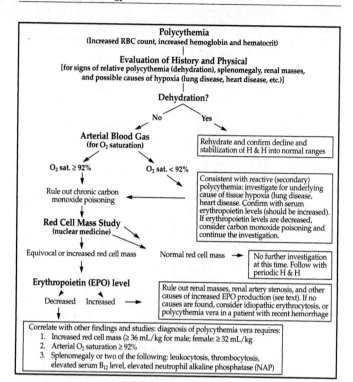

Fig. 2-7. Flow chart for polycythemia. H & H, hemoglobin and hematocrit.

White Blood Cells

Barbara J. Bain

I. Basic science review. Hematopoiesis takes place in the yolk sac (embryonic time period), then the liver and spleen (fetal time period), and finally the bone marrow (during the last third of intra-uterine development). A wide variety of tissues, regulatory factors, and stem cells are involved in hematopoiesis. Pluripotent stem cells can differentiate into lymphoid and multipotent myeloid stem cells. Multipotent myeloid stem cells can further differentiate into granulocytic, monocytic, erythrocytic, and megakaryocytic lineages. This chapter will discuss disorders of neutrophils, eosinophils, basophils, monocytes, and lymphocytes.

A. Neutrophils originate from multipotent stem cells and develop by exposure to sequential growth factors (including interleukins and colony-stimulating factors). Stages include **myeloblast, promyelocyte, myelocyte, metamyelocyte, band, and polymorphonuclear cell (PMN)**. PMNs leave the marrow, marginate along endothelial surfaces, and are attracted to sites of injury by chemotactic factors. PMNs spend 7–10 hours in the circulation. Neutrophils **phagocytize foreign materials** and **kill microbial organisms** (especially when opsonized by immunoglobulins or complement); killing mechanisms include superoxide radicals, hydrogen peroxide, and halide acids. **Primary granules contain myeloperoxidase; secondary granules are lysosomes containing lactoferrin and lysozyme**. Some storage of neutrophils occurs in the bone marrow.

B. Eosinophils follow a maturation sequence similar to neutrophils. Eosinophils have primary roles in **allergic reactions** and **reactions to parasites**. Their granules contain major basic protein and various enzymes.

C. Basophils follow a maturation sequence similar to neutrophils. Basophils have primary roles in **hypersensitivity reactions** (e.g., allergies, anaphylaxis, delayed hypersensitivity). Their granules contain histamine, slow-reacting substance of anaphylaxis, peroxidase, and so forth.

D. Monocytes originate from multipotent stem cells; stages include **monoblasts, promonocytes,** and **monocytes**. Monocytes differentiate into **macrophages**, which may be wandering (e.g., peritoneal macrophages), deposited in tissue (e.g., microglial cells), or line various spaces (e.g., alveolar macrophages, Kupffer's cells). Monocytes have important roles in **phagocytosis**, and mediate multiple **immunologic functions** (e.g., through the secretion of cytokines, interaction with T-cells).

E. Lymphocytes originate from pluripotent stem cells in the bone marrow; stages include **lymphoblasts** and **mature lymphocytes**, and they can live for **decades**. Antigen-independent development occurs in the bone marrow (**B cells**) and thymus (**T cells**). Antigen-dependent maturation then occurs in peripheral lymphoid tissues (e.g., lymph nodes, spleen, tonsils).

Lymphocytes have primary roles in the **humoral immune system** (through antibody production by B-cell–derived plasma cells) and the **cellular immune system** (T-helper and T-suppressor cells).

II. Approach to laboratory testing

 A.   Normal reference ranges. Most laboratories list normal reference ranges that represent the range of values seen in 95% of a healthy population. Therefore, by definition, **2.5% of healthy subjects will have test results above the normal range and another 2.5% will have test results below the normal range**. It is also important to realize that for many tests, **a patient's test results may fall within the normal reference range and yet still be quite abnormal compared with that specific patient's baseline values**. For example, a man with a baseline hemoglobin value of 17 g/dL could develop a chronic gastrointestinal (GI) bleed that results in a hemoglobin value of 14.5 g/dL, which is within the "normal range," but is clearly abnormal for that patient. Finally, it should be remembered that **a single "normal" test result is an isolated measurement and could represent a stable, healthy patient, or it could be part of a dramatically rising or falling trend**.

 B.   Units. Ideally, hematologic variables should be expressed in **SI units** [e.g., white blood cell (WBC) count: $10 \times 10^9/L$ (SI) = $10,000/\mu L$ (conventional)]. When interpreting cell counts, it is important **always to assess the absolute cell counts rather than the percentages**. To illustrate, a lymphocyte percentage of 95% with a neutrophil percentage of 5% could indicate either severe neutropenia with a normal lymphocyte count (e.g., agranulocytosis) or a markedly elevated lymphocyte count with a normal neutrophil count (e.g., chronic lymphocytic leukemia). The absolute numbers are calculated by multiplying the total WBC by the individual cell percentages.

III.   White blood cell morphology. Sometimes, the morphology of a blood smear suggests a hereditary or acquired disorder. Conversely, when some metabolic defects are suspected clinically, a blood smear should be examined. Common morphologic abnormalities are listed in Table 2-4.

IV.   Increased white blood cell counts. The first and most important question to answer is whether the high WBC is caused by **neutrophilia, lymphocytosis, eosinophilia,** or **significant numbers of an abnormal cell population (e.g., blasts)**. Occasionally, the WBC count may be spuriously elevated (depending on the type of analyzer) because of interference by nucleated red cells, giant or clumped platelets, or cryoglobulins; these usually show up as increased numbers of small particles at the lower end of the WBC histogram.

 A.   Neutrophilia

  1.   Causes of neutrophilia. Neutrophilia is the most common quantitative WBC abnormality, and is physiologic in the **neonatal period** and **during pregnancy**. Neutrophilia also occurs after **stress, vigorous exercise,** or **pain** (because of demargination of PMNs), with up to a doubling of the neutrophil count, but without an increase in band

(*text continues on page 102*)

Table 2-4. Morphologic variations in leukocytes in blood or bone marrow

Condition (Inheritance)	Abnormality Observed	Clinical Significance
Hereditary Pelger-Huët anomaly (AD)	Granulocyte nuclei show reduced or absent lobulation (spectacle-like: "pince-nez" nuclei)	Neutrophils are functionally normal; acquired forms may be seen in MDS and some drug reactions.
May-Hegglin anomaly (AD)	Döhle-like (but larger and more angular) inclusions in granulocytes; thrombocytopenia with giant platelets	Neutrophils are functionally normal; patients may have bleeding diathesis.
Alder-Reilly anomaly (mainly AR)	Dense azurophilic granules (lysosomes) in all white cell lineages; lysosomes contain storage material.	As an isolated anomaly has no significance, but occurs in mucopolysaccharidoses, Tay-Sachs disease and Batten-Spielmeyer-Vogt disease
Chédiak-Higashi syndrome (AR)	Large magenta and gray granules (lysosomes) in all white cell lineages; pancytopenia; primary disorder of lysosomes and melanosomes.	A serious and ultimately fatal disease characterized by partial oculocutaneous albinism, immune deficiency and recurrent infections
Myelokathexis (uncertain)	Very long filaments separating the lobes of hypersegmented neutrophils; associated neutropenia	Associated skeletal abnormalities and growth retardation
Neutrophil hypersegmentation: (AD; acquired form is more common)	Hypersegmented neutrophils	Hereditary form has no clinical significance; acquired form is most often indicative of megaloblastic erythropoiesis, but may occur in uremia and iron deficiency; >5% of cells have five lobes, or at least one cell with ≥ 6 lobes

continued

Table 2-4.   *Continued*

Condition	Abnormality Observed	Clinical Significance
Inherited increase in macropolycytes (AD)	1%–2% of neutrophils are macropolycytes	No significance; as an acquired phenomenon occurs in megaloblastic anemia and a variety of other conditions
Vacuolated lymphocytes	Vacuoles within the cytoplasm of lymphocytes	Occurs in many serious metabolic disorders including the mucopolysaccharidoses, Batten-Spielmeyer-Vogt disease, Tay-Sach's disease, Wolman's disease, I-cell disease, Jordan's anomaly, Pompe's disease and type II sialidosis
Gaucher disease (AR)[a]	Large histiocytes (macrophages) with copious amounts of weakly basophilic wrinkled "tissue-paper-like" cytoplasm	Caused by accumulation of glucocerebroside. Pseudo-Gaucher cells are seen in myeloproliferative disorders from ingested lipids
Niemann-Pick disease (AR)[a]	Histiocytes with copious amounts of foamy cytoplasm	Caused by accumulation of sphingomyelin
Sea-blue histiocytosis[a]	Histiocytes with copious amounts of deep blue cytoplasm (on WG stains); filled with ceroid or lipofuscin	Caused by accumulation of ceroid; associated with hereditary lipid storage disorders and acquired myeloproliferative disorders
Foamy macrophages[a] (hereditary or acquired disorders)	Macrophages with copious amounts of foamy cytoplasm	Niemann-Pick disease, hypercholesterolemia, hyperchylomicronemia, Wolman's disease, late-onset cholesterol ester storage disease, Fabry's disease, Batten's disease, Tangier disease

Cystine crystals within macrophages[a]	Birefringent crystals in polarized light	Cystinosis
Vacuolated hematopoietic cells and ring sideroblasts		Pearson's syndrome and other mitochondrial cytopathies; as an acquired phenomenon, may be caused by excess ethanol ingestion
Acquired		
Döhle body	Pale blue irregular cytoplasmic inclusion in neutrophils; due to RNA in ribosomes or rough endoplasmic reticulum	Commonly occurs in association with infection or inflammation, but is a feature of normal pregnancy
Toxic granules	Primary granules (with myeloperoxidase) within neutrophils	Commonly occurs in association with infection or inflammation, but is also a feature of normal pregnancy
Platelet satellitosis	Platelets surround neutrophils	EDTA artifact: causes falsely decreased platelet counts
Charcot-Leyden crystal	Sharp, blue crystals (WG stain) that represent remnants of eosinophil granules.	Associated with death of eosinophils

AD, autosomal dominant; AR, autosomal recessive; MDS, myelodysplastic syndromes; WG, Wright-Giemsa (stain).
[a] Requires tissue biopsy (e.g., bone marrow) to diagnose.

cells. Neutrophilia is expected in cases of **tissue injury, bacterial infection, inflammation,** and **in some neoplasias** (Table 2-5). If a patient fits one of these clinical circumstances, no further workup of the neutrophilia is required. However, remember that more than one process may be occurring. For example, patients on corticosteroids have neutrophilia; they may also have a bacterial infection (to which they are susceptible).

The significance of mild to moderate increases in the **band percentage** ("left shift") is controversial because of its non-specific nature and significant interobserver differences. However, a significant left shift may be particularly helpful from a diagnostic standpoint, when infection is considered in the following groups: **patients on corticosteroid therapy** and **crying newborns** (in the absence of infection, both groups normally show neutrophilia without a left shift), and in patients who are **elderly** or **receiving chemotherapy** (who have reduced abilities to produce neutrophilia, but who may respond to infection with a left shift).

2.   Morphologic variations associated with infection. When neutrophils are activated in response to bacterial infection, significant tissue damage (e.g., burns, infarction, cancer) or to severe inflammation, the neutrophils will show a **left**

Table 2-5.   Important causes of neutrophilia

Physiologic
Neonatal period
Pregnancy (third trimester), labor
Vigorous exercise[a]
Stress[a]

Pathologic
Pain[a]
Acute hemorrhage
Nausea and vomiting[a]
Infection [particularly bacterial; also viral (first 2–3 days), fungal, rickettsial]
Infarction or ischemia (e.g., myocardial infarction, pulmonary embolism, peripheral gangrene, essential hypertension, eclampsia, sickle cell crisis)
Tissue damage (e.g., trauma, surgery, burns)
Inflammation (e.g., ulcerative colitis, rheumatoid arthritis, vasculitis, thyroiditis, gout, uremia)
Diabetic ketoacidosis
Drugs [e.g., epinephrine (adrenaline)[a], corticosteroids, lithium]
Cigarette smoking
Epileptiform convulsions[a]
Splenectomy, particularly during the first few months after splenectomy
Myeloproliferative disorders and chronic myeloid leukemias

[a] The mechanism is mobilization of the marginated granulocyte pool; bands will generally not be a prominent feature.

shift, and will contain **toxic granules, Döhle bodies,** and **cytoplasmic vacuoles**. These findings also occur to a minor extent during pregnancy and the postpartum period. Neutrophil vacuolation is the most specific feature of bacterial infection (when the blood smear is prepared by finger stick and without EDTA), but can also occur as an EDTA artifact.

3. Unexplained neutrophilia. When neutrophilia is unexplained, it is necessary to **reassess the clinical history, the drug history,** and **the physical examination findings**. The blood film should then be examined for **morphologic signs of infection, inflammation,** or **for any features suggesting a hematologic neoplasm**. When the WBC and neutrophil counts are very high, myeloid leukemia may be suspected. Acute myeloid leukemia is, in fact, one of the least common causes of neutrophilia, and often causes pancytopenia. However, chronic myeloid leukemia (CML; also commonly referred to as "chronic granulocytic leukemia") causes neutrophilia, and must be differentiated from a reactive leukocytosis. **A low-grade fever, splenomegaly, basophilia, and a lack of toxic granules in the neutrophils favor CML, whereas a high-grade fever, lack of splenomegaly, and toxic granules favor a reactive neutrophilia** (Table 2-6).

B. Lymphocytosis. The first step in interpreting lymphocytosis is to **use age-specific reference ranges**, because children have much higher normal lymphocyte counts (see appendix).

1. Causes of lymphocytosis. The common causes of lymphocytosis (Table 2-7) are different in children than in adults. **In children, viral infections are the most common causes of lymphocytosis, but bacterial infections (e.g., pertussis) can also cause lymphocytosis. In adolescents, lymphocytosis is also most often caused by viral infections [particularly Epstein–Barr virus (EBV)]**, whereas bacterial infections would be unlikely. **In adult hospital patients, one of the most common causes of lymphocytosis is acute stress**, which causes a transient lymphocytosis followed within a few hours by lymphopenia. Sustained lymphocytosis in adults is often caused by a lymphoproliferative disorder.

2. Unexplained lymphocytosis. Further investigation is usually warranted, including a re-evaluation of the clinical history, a directed physical examination, and evaluation of the blood smear.

a. Clinical history. Particular attention should be paid to the likelihood of viral or other types of **infection**, any acute **severe illness** or injury, and previous **splenectomy**, all of which can cause lymphocytosis. If the patient is acutely ill, the complete blood cell (CBC) count should be repeated in 24 hours to exclude a transient, **stress-induced** lymphocytosis. **Cigarette smokers** typically have a mild lymphocytosis with cytologically normal lymphocytes. If reason is seen to suspect human immunodeficiency virus (HIV) infection, testing should be performed according to local guidelines.

(*text continues on page 106*)

Table 2-6.   Useful features in making a distinction between reactive neutrophilia and various chronic myeloid leukemias

Condition	Characteristic Features
Reactive neutrophilia (leukemoid reaction)	The white blood cell (WBC) count is rarely above $50 \times 10^9/L^a$. **Toxic granulation, neutrophil vacuolation and Döhle bodies** are present in neutrophils. Myelocytes and promyelocytes are uncommon, and blast cells are rare. The lymphocyte, basophil, and eosinophil counts are normal or reduced; lymphocytes may show reactive changes such as increased cytoplasmic basophilia. Monocytes are sometimes increased. The platelet count may be high, normal, or low; platelets are generally small. The leukocyte alkaline phosphatase **(LAP) score is increased**.
Chronic granulocytic leukemia (Philadelphia positive)	The WBC is often above $50 \times 10^9/L$. **Toxic changes in neutrophils are absent**. A characteristic "double peak" of segmented neutrophils and myelocytes is present (the spectrum looks like normal bone marrow), and a few blast cells are usually present. The **basophil count is invariably increased,** and the eosinophil count is usually increased. The lymphocyte count is normal or increased. Monocytes are increased, but not in proportion to the increase in the neutrophil count. The platelet count is usually normal or increased; platelet size is increased. The **LAP score is decreased in 95% of cases.**
Atypical chronic myeloid leukemia	**Toxic changes in neutrophils are absent**. Dysplastic features are often present. Basophilia and eosinophilia are less common than in chronic granulocytic leukemia, but monocytosis is much more common. The platelet count is less often elevated than in chronic granulocytic leukemia.
Chronic myelomonocytic leukemia	**Toxic changes in neutrophils are absent**. Dysplastic features may or may not be present. In comparison with atypical chronic myeloid leukemia, immature granulocytes are less numerous and eosinophilia

Table 2-6. *Continued*

Condition	Characteristic Features
	and basophilia are usually absent. The platelet count is usually normal or reduced, but is elevated in a minority. The **monocyte count is increased** (if using the FAB classification $> 1 \times 10^9$/L).
Eosinophilic leukemia	**Increased eosinophils** alone or increases in eosinophils plus monocytes and sometimes also neutrophils
Neutrophilic leukemia	Increased neutrophils without an increase in eosinophils or basophils, and without granulocyte precursors in the peripheral blood. In contrast to other chronic myeloid leukemias, toxic granulation may be present; some cases show dysplastic features.

[a] Reactive WBC counts $> 50 \times 10^9$/L (leukemoid reactions) can sometimes be seen in severe infections [acute (e.g., bacterial) and chronic (e.g., disseminated tuberculosis)], burns, electric shock, infarction, acute hemorrhage, metastatic carcinomas, and so on. *Transient* acute leukemia (the WBC count may be above 100×10^9/L) may occasionally occur in neonates with Down's syndrome.

Table 2-7. Important causes of lymphocytosis

Physiologic
Neonatal period, infancy, and childhood
Vigorous exercise

Pathologic
Drug and toxin reactions (e.g., sulfonamides, phenothiazines, diphenylhydantoin, lead, chlorinated solvents)
Infections: Particularly viral; also syphilis, mycoplasma, pertussis, and other bacterial infections in children
Stress-induced lymphocytosis (e.g., following myocardial infarction, cardiac arrest, severe asthma, sickle cell crisis, epileptiform convulsions)
Administration of epinephrine (adrenaline)
Immunologic disorders: Autoimmune diseases, graft rejection, dermatitis
Splenectomy
Cigarette smoking
Persistent B-cell polyclonal lymphocytosis
Lymphoid neoplasms (e.g., chronic lymphocytic leukemia and low-grade non-Hodgkin's lymphoma; rarely Hodgkin's disease).

b.   Physical examination. If the cause is still unclear, the patient should be re-examined for any **features suggesting infection** (e.g., pharyngitis, fever, or rash) or any abnormalities of lymph nodes, liver, or spleen. **When associated with infection, an enlarged liver or spleen is usually soft; lymph nodes are mobile, only moderately enlarged, and sometimes tender**. No associated organomegaly is seen in stress-induced lymphocytosis. **Lymphoproliferative disorders (e.g., chronic lymphocytic leukemia) often cause hepatomegaly, splenomegaly, or lymphadenopathy, and the organs are firm**. T-lineage lymphomas are additionally associated with skin lesions (e.g., plaques).

c.   Blood smear. Examination of the blood film is very important, and the first decision to make is whether the lymphocytes appear normal or abnormal.

   (1)   Morphologically normal cells. Pertussis (whooping cough), coxsackie viruses, some adenoviruses, some echoviruses, and some other viruses cause lymphocytosis with very little cytologic abnormalities. Hyposplenism may be suggested by the presence of Howell–Jolly bodies or Pappenheimer bodies, target cells and acanthocytes, and prominent large granular lymphocytes.

   (2)   Morphologically abnormal cells

      (a)   "Atypical" (reactive) lymphocytes. The term "atypical" is often used to refer to a type of reactive lymphocyte.

         (i)   Morphology. Atypical lymphocytes are medium to large, pleomorphic cells with irregular nuclei and **a large amount of basophilic cytoplasm**; the basophilia may be confined to the peripheral cytoplasmic edges, forming dark blue "scallops" around adjacent red cells. Some atypical lymphocytes have an immature chromatin pattern and large nucleoli, and others have prominent cytoplasmic granules.

         (ii)   Causes of atypical lymphocytes. The most common causes are viruses [particularly the EBV and cytomegalovirus (CMV)], but other viruses can also cause them). Other causes are listed in Table 2-8. Patients with numerous atypical lymphocytes should have serologic tests for heterophile antibodies; if the tests are negative, they should be repeated in 2 weeks.

      (b)   Malignant lymphocytes. Specific, **cytologic features of malignant lymphocytes are very important** in making a diagnosis of acute lymphoblastic leukemia, chronic lymphocytic leukemia, or non-Hodgkin's lymphoma (see sections on acute and chronic leukemia). This is in contrast to patients with Hodgkin's disease, who occasionally may have lymphocytosis, but the circulating lymphocytes are reactive, cytologically normal cells. If a lymphoproliferative disorder is suspected, immunophenotyping is indicated as an initial step.

**Table 2-8.   Important causes of lymphocytosis
with atypical lymphocytes**[a]

Viral infections: Primary infection with Epstein–Barr virus,
cytomegalovirus, human herpes virus 6, human immuno-
deficiency virus (HIV), hepatitis A virus, adenovirus
  Established infection by HIV or human T-cell lymphotropic virus I
  (HTLV-I)
Rickettsial infections: Tick typhus, scrub typhus, murine typhus
Parasitic infection: Toxoplasmosis, malaria, and so on
Bacterial infections: Brucellosis, tuberculosis
Stress
Hypersensitivity reactions to drugs

[a] Etiologic clues: In infectious mononucleosis, cold agglutinins may be produced
that cause red cell agglutination. Some infections can cause thrombocytopenia
in addition to lymphocytosis. In drug reactions, neutrophilia and eosinophilia
are common, and plasmacytoid lymphocytes may be present.

A rare condition, but one that is likely to cause diagnostic confusion, is persistent polyclonal B-cell lymphocytosis. This occurs mainly in middle-aged women
who are cigarette smokers. Cytologic features are very
distinctive in that binucleated and deeply lobulated
lymphocytes are present.

   C.   Eosinophilia. The common causes of eosinophilia differ
greatly in different parts of the world. **In developed countries, the most common identifiable cause is an allergic
reaction** (e.g., to environmental allergens, foods, medications);
however, it is important to realize that many, if not most, cases
of eosinophilia remain idiopathic, despite thorough workups.
In less-developed parts of the world, parasitic diseases
are responsible for most of the cases. Some of the important
causes of eosinophilia are shown in Table 2-9. Eosinophils have
a diurnal variation, with highest levels in the morning.

   1.   Clinical history. The **clinical history is of considerable importance**, and should include questions about
traveling (even in the distant past) to areas where parasites
are prevalent. A history of atopic eczema, asthma, or allergic
rhinitis should also be elicited, and the possibility of an allergic reaction to a drug should be considered.

   2.   Physical examination. Physical examination is often
noncontributory, but may disclose relevant features such
as a skin rash, lymphadenopathy (e.g., Hodgkin's disease),
hepatosplenomegaly, or signs of relevant systemic disease.

   3.   Ancillary studies. A **chest x-ray** study is indicated to
detect pulmonary infiltration (e.g., sarcoidosis, "eosinophilic
pneumonia" or Löffler's syndrome) and any mediastinal
lymphadenopathy. If the patient has a very high eosinophil
count and the eosinophils are degranulating, **electrocar-
diography** and **echocardiogaphy** are necessary to assess
any cardiac damage. Other tests are listed in Table 2-10, and
should be applied selectively based on clinical circumstances.

Table 2-9.   Important causes of eosinophilia

Neonates

Allergic reactions: e.g., allergic rhinitis, atopic eczema, urticaria, asthma, allergic bronchopulmonary aspergillosis, dermatitis, drug allergies.

Parasitic infections: e.g., hookworm, strongyloidiasis, filariasis, trichinosis, visceral larva migrans, scabies

Connective tissue disorders: Churg–Strauss variant of polyarteritis nodosa and systemic necrotizing vasculitis, systemic sclerosis, systemic lupus erythematosus, rheumatoid arthritis, and eosinophilia-myalgia syndrome following ingestion of L-tryptophan

Immune deficiency syndromes: e.g., Wiskott–Aldrich syndrome, Job's syndrome

Administration of recombinant growth factors including G-CSF, GM-CSF, and interleukins 2, 3, and 5

Acute hemorrhage or hemolysis

Leukemia: Some cases of acute lymphoblastic leukemia, certain subtypes of acute myeloid leukemia, Philadelphia-positive chronic granulocytic leukemia, eosinophilic leukemia

Lymphoma: Hodgkin's disease and non-Hodgkin's lymphoma

Carcinoma, sarcoma, malignant melanoma

Idiopathic hypereosinophilic syndrome

G-CSF, granulocyte colony-stimulating factor; GM-granulocyte-macrophage.

4.   Blood smear. The blood smear must always be examined carefully to detect any blast cells, immature granulocytes, or lymphoma cells. Degranulation of eosinophils should be noted if it is present. Observation of cytologically abnormal eosinophils is not diagnostically useful, because they can be seen in benign (e.g., secondary eosinophilia, idiopathic hypereosinophilic syndrome) or malignant conditions.

5.   Further investigation. In countries where parasitic infection is uncommon, investigation of mild unexplained eosinophilia in a healthy appearing patient rarely reveals significant pathology. At the other end of the spectrum, **patients who are unwell, who have symptoms or signs suggesting a systemic disease, or who have marked elevation of the eosinophil count clearly require study**. If the patient has marked eosinophilia with eosinophil degranulation, tissue damage from the degranulation is likely, and investigation and treatment is therefore urgent.

6.   Eosinophilic leukemia and the "idiopathic" hypereosinophilic syndrome. If no cause for secondary eosinophilia can be found, the diagnosis rests between eosinophilic leukemia and the "idiopathic" hypereosinophilic syndrome. **Significant anemia, thrombocytopenia, or hepatosplenomegaly favor a diagnosis of eosinophilic leukemia**, which is confirmed if blast cells are increased or if a clonal cytogenetic abnormality is detected. A diagnosis of the idiopathic hypereosinophilic syndrome is appropri-

Table 2-10. Investigations into the cause of eosinophilia

Clinical Suspicion	Investigation
Parasitic disease	Fecal examination, duodenal aspiration (if *Strongyloides stercoralis* is suspected), blood film examination (if filariasis is suspected), biopsy of the gastrocnemius muscle (if the patient is seriously ill and trichinosis is suspected), serologic tests for parasites
Atopy or allergy	Quantification of serum IgE, skin tests
Connective tissue disease	Autoantibody screen (antinuclear antibodies and so on)
Acute leukemia	Bone marrow aspiration, cytogenetic analysis, and immunophenotyping
Hodgkin's disease or non-Hodgkin's lymphoma	Chest x-ray, computed tomography scanning of chest and abdomen, bone marrow or lymph node biopsy
Chronic myeloid leukemia or chronic eosinophilic leukemia	Bone marrow aspiration and cytogenetic analysis
"Idiopathic" hypereosinophilic syndrome	Investigations, including bone marrow aspiration and cytogenetic analysis, to exclude eosinophilic leukemia and all probable causes of secondary eosinophilia; immunophenotypic analysis of peripheral blood lymphocytes and molecular analysis for detection of aberrant T-cell clones

ate if the **eosinophil count is above 1.5 × 10⁹/L and sustained for 6 months** (during which time no cause for a secondary eosinophilia can be found), and there is tissue damage from eosinophil degranulation. In the absence of these findings, a diagnosis of idiopathic hypereosinophilic syndrome may be tentatively made and the patients followed clinically. Some of these patients later will be shown to have eosinophilic leukemia, whereas others may have an abnormal T-cell clone (that secretes interleukin-5) and develop overt T-cell lymphoma.

D. **Monocytosis** is a **relatively nonspecific finding associated with infection, inflammation, and neoplasia, that is commonly seen in association with collagen vascular diseases and malignancies** (Table 2-11). Previously, common causes included tuberculosis and subacute bacterial endocarditis.

E. **Basophilia** is occasionally reactive (Table 2-12). It is one of the initial signs on a CBC count that **suggests that a proliferation of myeloid lineages may be malignant** (e.g., chronic myelogenous leukemia, polycythemia rubra vera).

Table 2-11.   Some causes of monocytosis

Physiologic
Neonates (first 2 weeks)
Infections (acute, chronic, and granulomatous; wide variety
  of causative agents)
Medications: (e.g., corticosteroids)
Collagen-vascular disorders
Tissue damage (e.g., trauma, infarction, radiation)
Hematologic and nonhematologic malignancies

V.   Acute leukemia. Acute nonlymphocytic leukemia
(ANLL, also called "acute myelogenous leukemia" or AML) **occurs**
most frequently in middle-aged and elderly adults, and is
often classified according to the French-American-British (FAB)
classification (Table 2-13). **Acute lymphocytic leukemia (ALL)**
occurs most frequently in children and, to a lesser extent, in
the elderly. ALL can be classified according to the FAB morphologic
classification or an immunophenotypic classification (Table 2-14).
Clues to differentiate between AML and ALL are in Table 2-15.
Figure 8 is an overview of hematologic malignancies.

   A.   Clinical history. Suspect acute leukemia in a patient who
presents with **pallor** and **purpura**, associated with nonspecific
symptoms such as **breathlessness, malaise,** and **fever**. In children, there may be bone pain. **Some patients are gravely ill**
at presentation, with sepsis and hemorrhage, whereas **others**
have only minor symptoms.

   B.   Physical examination may show bruises and petechiae,
mild hepatomegaly and splenomegaly (marked enlargement is
uncommon, except in young children), or pharyngitis with cervical lymphadenopathy. Generalized or **marked lymphade-**
nopathy is most suggestive of ALL, although it is also sometimes seen in AML with monocytic differentiation (e.g., M4 or
M5). **AML with monocytic differentiation also is associ-**
ated with gum or skin infiltration. Retinal hemorrhages or
exudates can occur in acute leukemias, and signs of hyperviscosity (e.g., venous distention and papilloedema) can occur in
those with a very high WBC count. **Prominent hemorrhagic**
manifestations (e.g., bleeding from venipuncture sites) **should**
suggest the possibility of acute hypergranular promy-
elocytic leukemia (M3), with disseminated intravascular
coagulation, and is a medical emergency.

   C.   CBC count and blood smear comprise the initial diagnostic procedure. The most common findings are **anemia,**

Table 2-12.   Some causes of basophilia

Allergic and hypersensitivity disorders
Endocrine disorders (e.g., hypothyroidism)
Some inflammatory conditions (e.g., ulcerative colitis)
Hematologic malignancies (e.g., myeloproliferative disorders,
  myelodysplastic syndromes)

Table 2-13. FAB classification of acute nonlymphocytic leukemia (ANLL)[a,b]

M0: acute myeloblastic leukemia: ≥90% of myeloid cells are blasts; ≤3% of the blasts show cytochemical staining (SB+, MPO+); identification as myeloid is by immunophenotyping. No Auer rods are present (Auer rods are abnormal, crystallized primary granules); **CG:** various abnormalities.

M1: acute myeloblastic leukemia (15%–20% of ANLL): ≥90% of myeloid cells are blasts; ≥3% of the blasts show cytochemical staining (SB+, MPO+); myeloid line can also be confirmed by immunophenotyping. Auer rods may be present. **CG** (some cases only): +8, −5, −7.

M2: acute myeloblastic leukemia (≅ 30% of ANLL): 30%–80% of the myeloid cells are blasts; at least 10% of the cells show some maturation (promyelocytes or beyond); >50% show cytochemical staining (SB+, MPO+); myeloid line can also be confirmed by immunophenotyping, if desired; may have Auer rods. **CG: t(8;21)** and other abnormalities.[c]

M3: acute promyelocytic leukemia (5%–10% of ANLL): nuclei are typically "butterfly" shaped and uniform with many primary granules (vs. monocytic leukemia in which the nuclei vary a lot); strong cytochemical staining (SB+, MPO+); **CG: t(15;17)**[d], involves gene for alpha-retinoic acid receptor (RAR); M3 micro-granular variant may not have visible granules.

M4: acute myelomonocytic leukemia (≅ 30% of ANLL): both granulocytic and monocytoid differentiation occurs; 30%–80% of the myeloid cells are myeloblasts and neutrophil precursors; promonocytes and monocytes make up >20% and <80% of the cells; **CG:** abnormalities in **11q**[e]; **inv(16)** or del(16) are seen in some cases of M4 eosinophilic variants (>5% of the myeloid cells are abnormal eosinophils).

M5: acute monocytic leukemia (≅ 10% of ANLL): **CG:** abnormal 11q including t(9;11)

　M5a: poorly differentiated (>80% of the myeloid line are monoblasts)

　M5b: well-differentiated (<80% of the myeloid line are monoblasts, and the remainder are promonocytes and monocytes).

M6: erythroleukemia (<5% of ANLL): >50% of the bone marrow is composed of red blood cell precursors, and >30% of the non-erythroid cells are blasts. Dysplastic changes are common in all of the marrow myeloid cell lines; **CG:** various abnormalities.

M7: megakaryoblastic leukemia (<5% of ANLL): highly pleomorphic circulating blasts, with abnormal megakaryocytes and fibrosis in the marrow; identified by staining for VIII-related antigen, glycoproteins Ib, IIb/IIIa (CD41); **CG:** inv(3q) or other abnormalities in 3, t(1;22); bone marrow aspirate is often a "dry tap."

CG, cytogenetics; FAB, French-American-British; MPO, myeloperoxidase; SB, Sudan Black B.

continued

Table 2-13. *Continued*

[a] To diagnose M0, M1, M2, M4, M5, and M7, blasts (excluding erythroblasts) must make up >30% of all myeloid-lineage cells in the marrow. When <30% of the myeloid line are blasts, the diagnosis will be a myelodysplastic syndrome. Myeloid-lineage cells include blasts, granulocytes (and their precursors), monocytes (and their precursors), megakaryocytes (and their precursors), and erythroid cells (and their precursors). If erythroblasts make up >50% of all nucleated cells in the marrow, and blasts (other than erythroblasts) make up >30% of all myeloid-lineage cells (other than erythroid cells), the diagnosis is M6 (erythroleukemia). The criteria for M3 are somewhat less stringent, and diagnosis is by morphologic criteria (a dominant population of promyelocytes in the bone marrow, with the characteristic t(15;17) translocation.

[b] ANLL in general may show abnormalities in chromosomes 5 (−5, 5q−), 7(−7,7q−), 8 (+8), and 21.

[c] M2 and M4 with basophilia may show t(6;9).

[d] (15;17) is present in almost all cases of M3, including M3 variant acute myeloid leukemia.

Table 2-14. Classification of acute lymphoblastic leukemia (ALL)

FAB CLASSIFICATION

L1 (85% of ALL in children): Uniformly small cells, diffuse chromatin, round nuclei, rare nucleoli, scant cytoplasm; **CG:** t(10;14), t(11;14), t(9;22); correlates with early/pre-B or T-cell ALL.

L2 (60% of ALL in adults): Heterogeneous population (cells vary markedly in size, from small to large), irregular nuclear outlines, ± large nucleoli, scant to moderate cytoplasm; correlates with early/pre-B or T-cell ALL; **CG:** as for L1.

L3 (Burkitt-like, 2% of ALL at any age): Uniformly large cells, round nuclei, large nucleoli, moderate amounts of intensely basophilic cytoplasm with vacuolization; correlates with the B ALL phenotype; **CG: t(8;14)**[a], t(8;22), t(2;8)

IMMUNOPHENOTYPIC CLASSIFICATION

Early B and common ALL: Most common type of ALL[b]; Tdt +, CD19 (pan-B)+, CALLA (CD10) ±, **CG:** t(9;22), 6q−, high hyperdiploid.

Pre-B ALL: Tdt+, CD19+, CD20+, CALLA+, cIg μ (cytoplasmic μ heavy chains); **CG:** t(1;19), t(1;11).

B ALL (Burkitt-like): Least common type; Tdt−, CD19+, CD20+, CD10−, SIg+ (surface immunoglobulin); **CG:** t(8;14)[a], t(8;22), t(2;8) (correlates with the L3 morphology).

T-cell: Second most common type of ALL; occurs in older children and adults, associated with a mediastinal mass, CNS involvement, hepatosplenomegaly, and a high WBC count; CD2 (pan-T)+, CD5+, CD7+, CD4/8 ±; **CG:** abnormalities in chromosomes 11 or 14

CG, cytogenetics; CNS, central nervous system; FAB, French-American-British; WBC, white blood cell (count).

[a] t(8;14) and other abnormalities associated with chromosome 8 are present in almost all cases of L3/B ALL.

[b] Prognostic factors: The **best prognosis** for ALL is associated with common ALL (CALLA+), hyperdiploidy (>50 chromosomes), L1 morphology, or WBC < 10 × 10⁹/L (10,000/μL). **Intermediate prognosis** is associated with pre-B ALL with hyperdiploidy (47–50) or deletions in 6q, 9p, 12p. **Poor prognosis** is associated with hypodiploidy, pre-B with Philadelphia chromosome t(9;22), t(1;19), T-cell types [t(11;14), t(8;14)], WBC > 50 × 10⁹/L, and CNS involvement. Mature B-cell ALL [Burkitt-like (with sIg), showing t(8;14), t(2;8), t(8;22)] has historically had a poor prognosis, but with modern intensive therapies these patients do quite well.

Table 2-15.   Summary of clues[a] to help differentiate acute lymphoblastic leukemia (ALL) from acute myeloblastic leukemia (AML)

Feature	ALL	AML
Age of patient	Children and some-times in the elderly	Middle-aged and older adults
Pattern of organ involvement	Common in spleen, liver, lymph nodes, CNS, and gonads	Common in spleen, liver; rare in nodes, CNS, and gonads
Cell morphology	Smudgy, fine nuclear chromatin; no nucleoli or one nucleolus; scant cytoplasm	Diffuse, fine nuclear chromatin; multiple, prominent nucleoli, moderate amounts of cytoplasm
Cytochemical stains		Myeloperoxidase +, Sudan Black B +, specific esterase (granulocytic)+ or nonspecific esterase (monocytic)+
Immuno-phenotyping	B-cell antigens; T-cell antigens Tdt + (except mature B-cell ALL)	Granulocytic/ monocytic surface antigens

CNS, central nervous system; Tdt, terminal deoxynucleotidyl transferase.
[a] In many cases, the presentation and morphology are not sufficient to make the diagnosis, and cytochemical staining and/or immunophenotyping by flow cytometry is required.

thrombocytopenia, and **leukocytosis with blast cells**; however, some patients have pancytopenia with few or no blast cells in the peripheral blood, and the pancytopenia can only be diagnosed by bone marrow examination.

D.   Further investigative tests. A hemato-oncologist should be immediately consulted if the patient appears seriously ill, is septic or hypoxic, has a reduced level of consciousness, has a very high white cell count, or exhibits petechiae or other hemorrhagic manifestations. Urgent specialist assistance is also needed if acute hypergranular promyelocytic leukemia (AML-M3), or the L3 subtype of ALL (Burkitt's lymphoma-related ALL) is suspected. The following tests will probably be needed.

1.   Bone marrow aspiration and cytogenetic analysis, possibly supplemented by molecular genetic analysis. Genetic analysis may detect specific DNA rearrangements associated with a relatively good (or particularly poor) prognosis. Cytogenetic analysis is more successful when performed on a bone marrow aspirate than on peripheral blood (even when circulating blast cells are present). Essential tests (including some of the tests listed below) should be ordered on

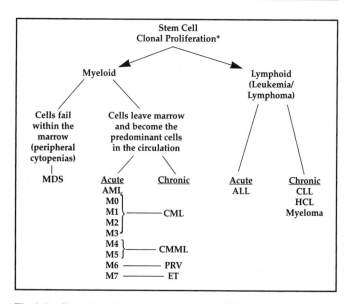

Fig. 2-8.   Overview of hematologic malignancies. ALL, acute lympho-blastic leukemia; AML, acute myeloblastic leukemia; CLL, chronic lymphocytic leukemia; CML, chronic myeloid leukemia; CMML, chronic myelomonocytic leukemia; ET, essential thrombocythemia; HCL, hairy cell leukemia; MDS, myelodysplastic syndromes; M0-7, subtypes of AML; PRV, polycythemia rubra vera. *Some neoplastic stem cells can show both myeloid and lymphoid differentiation (e.g., biphenotypic acute leukemia, chronic granulocytic leukemia).

the aspirate, to quickly obtain the information and avoid un-necessary repeat bone marrow examinations.

   2.   Cytochemical stains on peripheral blood (if numer-ous blast cells are present), or on the bone marrow aspirate, to confirm cell lineage (ALL vs. AML).

   3.   Immunophenotyping performed on the peripheral blood (if numerous blast cells are present) or on the bone mar-row aspirate

   4.   Blood group typing for possible transfusion

   5.   Chest radiography

   6.   Biochemical screening, including tests of liver and renal function and measurement of plasma uric acid

   7.   Coagulation screen, including fibrinogen assay and D-dimer

   8.   Blood cultures or other relevant cultures in febrile patients

E.   Purposes of testing. The tests listed above are intended primarily to answer three questions:

   1.   Does the patient have acute leukemia? This is usu-ally answered without difficulty by examining the blood and bone marrow aspirate smears.

2. Is the acute leukemia lymphoblastic or myeloblastic? This is sometimes answered by examining the blood and bone marrow smears, if Auer rods or other obvious granulocytic or monocytic signs of differentiation are seen. Otherwise, cytochemical stains should be carried out (Table 2-16). **Essential stains include a myeloperoxidase or Sudan black B stain (to demonstrate granulocytic or monocytic differentiation), and a nonspecific esterase stain (to demonstrate monocytic differentiation).** If an acute leukemia can be characterized as myeloid on the basis of cytology and cytochemistry, immunophenotyping is NOT necessary. However, immunophenotyping is mandatory in all cases that are not obviously myeloid. Immunophenotypic markers are not totally lineage-specific, so **a panel of markers should always be used that include B, T, nuclear terminal deoxynucleotidyl transferase (Tdt), and myeloid markers (Table 2-17). Tdt, if positive, is useful in confirming a diagnosis of acute lymphoblastic leukemia or lymphoblastic lymphoma,** rather than a lymphoma of mature B or T cells. It should be noted that small blue cell tumors of childhood sometimes masquerade as acute leukemia, and should be suspected if immunophenotypic markers for myeloid and lymphoid cells are negative.

3. Does the patient fall into a subgroup with particularly good or particularly poor prognostic features? Local protocols should be followed for detecting cytogenetic and molecular abnormalities that influence treatment choice. Good prognosis abnormalities (e.g., high hyperdiploidy in

Table 2-16. Summary of cytochemical stains used for acute leukemias

Type of Cell	Myeloperoxidase	Sudan Black B	Specific Esterase	Non Specific Esterase	Tdt
Myeloblasts	+	+	+	+/–	+/–[a]
Monoblasts	+	+	–	+++	+/–[a]
Lymphoblasts[b]	–	–	–	+/–	+++
M3 (promyelocytes)	+++	+++	+++	+/–	–
M6 (erythroblasts)[b]	–	–	–	+/–	–

Tdt, terminal deoxynucleotidyl transferase.

Myeloperoxidase stain: stains myeloperoxidase in primary granules of neutrophils and monocytes.

Sudan Black B: stains primary granules (granule membranes in neutrophils and monocytes; granule contents in neutrophils).

Specific esterase (chloroacetate esterase): stains primary granules of neutrophils.

Nonspecific esterase (α-naphthyl butyrate esterase): strongly stains monocytes, and is inhibited by fluoride pretreatment.

[a] A minority of myeloblasts and monoblasts may show some staining with Tdt.
[b] Lymphoblasts and erythroblasts also show a dense, blocky periodic acid-Schiff (PAS) staining, unlike the diffuse PAS staining of the other cells listed; lymphoblasts stain with Tdt [except the B-cell (Burkitt-like) type], whereas most myeloid cells do not. B-cell acute lymphoblastic leukemia shows pan-B immunophenotyping.

Table 2-17. Useful immunophenotypic markers in the diagnosis of acute leukemia

Marker	Interpretation
CD13, CD33, CD117, anti-myeloperoxidase	Pan-myeloid: CD117 is detectable only on immature cells, whereas the other markers will also be positive on maturing cells; antimyeloperoxidase and CD117 are the most specific markers of myeloid differentiation; other myeloid markers include CD14, CD15, CD65 and antilysozyme.
CD3	T lineage: techniques for the detection of cytoplasmic CD3 are more sensitive than techniques that detect only surface membrane CD3. CD2, CD7, and CD4 are sometimes used in immunophenotyping panels for suspected acute leukemia but are much less specific for T lineage than is CD3.
CD19, CD79a, CD22	B lineage: testing for cytoplasmic CD79a and CD22 is more sensitive than testing for surface membrane antigen; CD20 and CD24 are also immunophenotypic markers of B lineage.
CD10 (CALLA)	A subset of B-lineage ALL (early, common, and pre-B ALL).
Surface membrane immunoglobulin	Mature B-cell ALL
Antiglycophorin	Erythroid lineage
CD41, CD42, CD61	Megakaryocyte lineage
Antiterminal deoxynucleotidyl transferase (Tdt; nuclear)	Usually positive in ALL but also positive in a few cases of acute myeloid leukemia; it should be noted that in children who do not have acute lymphoblastic leukemia, up to 10% of their bone marrow cells may be positive for terminal deoxynucleotidyl transferase.

ALL, acute lymphocytic leukemia; CALLA, common ALL antigen.

childhood ALL) are an indication to use standard treatment regimens, whereas poor prognosis abnormalities (e.g., the Philadelphia chromosome) are a justification for more intensive and experimental methods of treatment. In particular, the **M3 or M3 variant subtype of AML** should be identified, because a combination of chemotherapy and differentiating therapy (**all-trans retinoic acid**) is most effective. Similarly, the confirmation of Burkitt's lymphoma-related ALL is important, because the best outcome is achieved with alternative chemotherapeutic regimens.

VI.   Chronic myeloproliferative disorders (MPD). The MPD group of malignancies involves myeloid elements that are relatively well-differentiated. The primary defect in each disorder is **a clonal multipotent stem cell, which affects all myeloid lineages (granulocytes, monocytes, erythrocytes, megakaryocytes), with one lineage usually proliferating in a dominant manner**. The disorders include chronic myeloid leukemia [the term "chronic granulocytic leukemia" (CGL) is sometimes used synonymously]; polycythemia rubra vera (PRV); essential thrombocythemia (ET); and myelofibrosis with myeloid metaplasia (MMM). **Common features of these disorders include anemia (except PRV and ET), increased white cell counts with immature neutrophils, basophilia, eosinophilia, and quantitative and qualitative platelet disorders. Hepatosplenomegaly often occurs** as the result of malignant involvement as well as extramedullary hematopoiesis, and hyperuricemia is common. The bone marrow is usually hypercellular with varying degrees of fibrosis (caused by fibroblast growth factors secreted by abnormal megakaryocytes). All of the MPD have the potential to transform into acute leukemia.

A. Chronic myeloid leukemia. When CML is suspected, two questions need to be answered:

- **Does the patient have CML or reactive leukocytosis?**
- **If the patient has CML, is it Philadelphia-positive CGL or another type of chronic myeloid leukemia?**

1. Clinical history and physical examination. Suspect CML in **young, middle-aged, or elderly patients who present with low-grade fever, weight loss, pallor, sweating, splenomegaly, and leukocytosis**. Alternate reactive causes of marked splenomegaly may be suggested by the history or physical examination (e.g., malaria, chronic liver disease). Alternative reactive causes of leukocytosis (e.g., cellulitis or osteomyelitis) may also be suggested by the history and physical examination. The physical examination findings in myelofibrosis with myeloid metaplasia are similar to those of CML, and require a bone marrow examination to differentiate between the two. Marked splenomegaly is less common in the other myeloproliferative disorders. The detection of **lymphadenopathy generally suggests a lymphoproliferative rather than a myeloproliferative disorder**, although lymphadenopathy can occur during acute (blastic) transformation of CML. Conversely, **some lymphoid leukemias** and **lymphomas** (e.g., splenic lymphoma of villous lymphocytes and hairy cell leukemia) **are characterized by splenomegaly without significant lymphadenopathy**.

2. Laboratory testing

a. CBC count and differential. If CML is suspected, the initial test is a CBC count with a differential count. The blood smear should be carefully **examined for toxic (suggesting a reactive cause) or dysplastic features (suggesting a neoplastic cause)**. Table 2-6 shows helpful features in making a distinction between reactive neutrophilia and CML. **CGL differs from AML in that CGL typically shows a wide spectrum of neutrophilic precursors (including a few blasts), unlike AML that shows two predominant populations: blasts and mature neutrophils**.

   b.   Additional tests (if CGL is still suspected)
      (1)   Bone marrow aspirate and cytogenetic analysis. In CGL, the marrow is almost **100% cellular, with a markedly increased myeloid: erythroid ratio** (almost always >10:1); cytogenetic analysis shows the **Philadelphia (Ph) chromosome** [a small chromosome 22 caused by **t(9;22)** (q34;q11)] in nucleated cells from white, red, and megakaryocytic cell lines.
      (2)   Molecular genetic analysis for detection of the *BCR-ABL* fusion gene. This should be performed in patients with the hematologic features of CGL, but in whom a Philadelphia chromosome is not detected in the cytogenetic analysis.
      (3) It should be noted that a neutrophil alkaline phosphatase score (i.e., leukocyte alkaline phosphatase score or LAP) is redundant when cytogenetic and molecular genetic analysis is available, and is potentially misleading because a normal result is obtained in 5% of patients with CGL.
   3.   Disease course. The average life expectancy, if treated by chemotherapy, is 3–4 years. Most patients have an accelerated phase followed by acute leukemia [>10% blasts in the peripheral blood: 80% of the cases show myeloblasts, whereas 20% show lymphoblasts (early B lineage)]. Some patients die from marrow fibrosis.
B.   Myelofibrosis with myeloid metaplasia [i.e., idiopathic myelofibrosis (IM)]. Idiopathic myelofibrosis is characterized by **progressive marrow fibrosis with extramedullary hematopoiesis**.
   1.   Presentation. This entity occurs in older adults, who may present with a bleeding diathesis, abdominal fullness (from splenomegaly), or have signs and symptoms of anemia.
   2.   Physical examination. Splenomegaly is always present, because of extramedullary hematopoiesis.
   3.   Laboratory studies
      a.   CBC count and peripheral smear. The CBC count shows neutrophilia with anemia and thrombocytosis, progressing to **pancytopenia**. The smear shows a **leukoerythroblastic** pattern (immature leukocytes and nucleated red cells), tear drop cells, marked anisopoikilocytosis, and giant or otherwise abnormal platelets.
      b.   Bone marrow aspirate and trephine biopsy. The aspirate is often a **dry tap**; the biopsy shows hypercellularity with increased background fibrosis, which progresses to hypocellularity with dense fibrosis. Abnormal megakaryocyte aggregates are common. No diagnostic cytogenetic abnormalities are seen, although +8, +9, and 13q– are common findings.
   4.   Disease course. The average life expectancy is 5 years, with death occurring from hemorrhage, infection, or transformation (20%) into acute leukemia.
C.   Polycythemia rubra vera and essential thrombocythemia. See later individual sections on polycythemia and thrombocytosis, respectively.

VII. Chronic lymphoproliferative disorders

A. Chronic lymphocytic leukemia (CLL) occurs in **middle-aged** or **elderly patients** (rare <40 years of age), and is the most common adult leukemia in the United States. Most (98%) of the cases are of **B-cell origin**.

1. Clinical history and physical examination. Consider CLL when elderly patients present with **generalized lymphadenopathy, hepatomegaly, and splenomegaly, with or without pallor or systemic symptoms such as fatigue and weight loss.** In this circumstance, the differential diagnosis also includes Hodgkin's and non-Hodgkin's lymphoma (viral or other infections are rarely responsible for this clinical picture). However, the most common scenario by far is for a clinician to suspect CLL when lymphocytosis is incidentally noted in a CBC count performed to investigate another disorder. The differential diagnosis then includes CLL, non-Hodgkin's lymphoma, hyposplenism, and stress-induced lymphocytosis. The differentiation between reactive and neoplastic causes of lymphocytosis has been discussed.

2. Laboratory tests. If CLL, Hodgkin's, or the leukemic phase of non-Hodgkin's lymphoma is suspected, the following tests are indicated.

a. CBC count with a differential count and a careful assessment of the cytologic features of peripheral blood cells (Table 2-18).

b. Immunophenotyping. The purpose of immunophenotyping is to establish **clonality**, and to help in the differentiation between various lymphoproliferative disorders (Table 2-18). **Neoplastic B lymphocytes**, being the progeny of a single cell, express **either kappa or lambda light chains but not both** (i.e., **light chain restriction**). **Neoplastic T cells show monoclonal T-cell receptor genes.** In reactive lymphocytosis is seen a mixture of B and T lymphocytes is seen, there is no light chain restriction, and no monoclonal T-cell receptor genes.

c. Bone marrow aspirate and trephine biopsy. A bone marrow aspirate often yields little additional information in lymphoproliferative disorders, whereas a trephine biopsy contributes to the differential diagnosis. **In CLL or prolymphocytic leukemia**, the pattern of infiltration may be interstitial, nodular, mixed, or diffuse (packed marrow pattern), but with no **paratrabecular infiltration. Paratrabecular infiltration may be seen in non-Hodgkin's lymphoma,** (particularly follicular center cell lymphoma), and nodular infiltration is uncommon, although random focal infiltration may occur.

d. Some cases will also require lymph node biopsy. A lymph node biopsy is required to diagnose Hodgkin's lymphoma, and may be useful in the diagnosis of non-Hodgkin's lymphoma (it is not always required). A lymph node biopsy is unnecessary for CLL.

e. Supplementary tests. Other tests that may be useful include **serum protein electrophoresis and quantification of immunoglobulins.** Patients with lymphoplasmacytoid lymphoma or splenic lymphoma with villous

(*text continues on page 122*)

Table 2-18.   Cytologic and immunophenotypic features of reactive and malignant lymphoproliferative disorders

Condition	Cytologic Features	Typical immunophenotypic[a] (IP) and Possible Cytogenetic (CG) Features
Reactive lymphocytosis	Heterogenous appearance, ± atypical (reactive) lymphs	**IP:** Expected normal antigens on B or T cells, without aberrant expression; polyclonal; B cells: kappa to lambda ratio ≅ 2:1; **CG:** no clonal rearrangement of T-cell receptor genes.
Chronic lymphocytic leukemia (CLL)	95% are B-cell origin; 5% are T-cell origin (worse prognosis); uniform population of small, mature lymphocytes with dense chromatin showing a mosaic ("dried cracked mud") pattern; smudge cells are typical but not pathognomonic[b]	**IP:** Weak expression of SmIg, CD5+, CD20 weak+, CD22−, CD23+, CD79a+, CD79b−, FMC7−; **CG:** +12, 13q, 14q+
Chronic lymphocytic leukemia, mixed cell type	>10% and <55% prolymphocytes, or an admixture of small, mature lymphocytes and larger cells that may have cytoplasmic basophilia or nuclear irregularity	**IP:** similar to chronic lymphocytic leukemia but sometimes have some atypical immunophenotypic features
Prolymphocytic leukemia (PLL)	>55% prolymphocytes; vast majority are B cell; medium-sized lymphocytes with chromatin that is not as condensed as in CLL, and with a large, prominent nucleolus; moderately abundant cytoplasm	**IP:** some cases have strong SmIg and are CD5−, CD20+, and FMC7+; others have an IP that is intermediate between this phenotype and that of CLL; CD22+, CD79b+; **CG:** 14q+
Hairy cell leukemia	Moderately large lymphocytes with moderately diffuse chromatin, and moderately abundant weakly basophilic, vacuolated cytoplasm; "hairs" project from the surface and keep the surrounding red blood cells at a distance	**TRAP+; IP:** CD 19+, CD20+, CD25+, CD 11c+, CD5 ±, SIg ±; **CG:** 6q−

Splenic lymphoma with villous lymphocytes	Small, mature lymphocytes that are more pleomorphic than those of CLL; some have a small nucleolus; some have cytoplasmic projections ('villi') that may be polar; some plasma cytoid differentiation	**IP:** strong SmIg and sometimes cytoplasmic expression of Ig; CD5−, CD20+, CD22+, CD23−, CD79b usually +, FMC7+; CD38 sometimes +
Lymphoplasmacytoid lymphoma	Small, mature lymphocytes; some showing plasmacytoid features such as an eccentric nucleus and cytoplasmic basophilia; rouleaux formation or red cell agglutination may occur	**IP:** strong SmIg and some cytoplasmic expression of Ig; CD5−, CD20+, CD22+, CD23−, CD79b+, FMC7+; CD38 some-times+
Follicle center cell lymphoma	Small lymphocytes with evenly condensed chromatin, angular or clefted nuclei, nucleoli, scanty cytoplasm; more pleomorphic than CLL	**IP:** SmIg strong, CD5−, CD20+, CD22+, CD23−, CD79b+, FMC7+, CD10 more often+ than in other lymphomas; **CG:** t(14;18)
Mantle cell lymphoma	Pleomorphic small and medium-sized lymphocytes, some with nucleoli, some with nuclear clefting	**IP:** SmIg strong, CD5+, CD20+, CD22+, CD23−, CD79b+, FMC7+; **CG:** t(11;14)
Sézary syndrome	Small, medium, or large lymphocytes with hyper-chromatic convoluted nuclei	**IP:** CD2+, CD3+, CD4+ (helper); CD5+, CD7+
Adult T-cell leukemia/lymphoma	Medium to large highly atypical lymphocytes with hyperchromatic nuclei, some with "flower-shaped" or convoluted nuclei	**IP:** CD2+, CD3+, CD5+, CD7+; usually CD4+ (helper), CD 25+
Large granular lympho-cyte leukemia	Medium-sized lymphocytes with plentiful weakly basophilic cytoplasm containing prominent azurophilic granules	**IP:** Various phenotypic expressions; T-cell variant: (CD2,3,5,7,8+; natural killer cell variant: (CD 2, 16, 56)+; most common is CD2+, CD3+, CD16+, CD56+

CyIg, cytoplasmic immunoglobulin; SmIg, surface membrane immunoglobulin; TRAP, tartrate-resistant acid phosphatase.

[a] Most importantly, the B-cell neoplasias will have B antigens (e.g., CD19, CD24, and CD79a) with light-chain restriction (expression of kappa or lambda, but not both). The T-cell neoplasias will have T antigens (e.g., CD3) with clonal T-cell receptor genes.

[b] Smudge cells may be prevented by mixing a drop of albumin with the blood before smearing.

lymphocytes usually have a paraprotein (i.e., monoclonal protein), whereas patients with advanced CLL tend to have hypogammaglobulinemia. A direct antiglobulin test (**Coombs' test**) is indicated for any patient whose blood smear shows spherocytes. This is most often seen in CLL, but also sometimes occurs in non-Hodgkin's lymphoma. Other useful laboratory tests include lactate dehydrogenase and tests of renal and liver function.

   f.   Cytogenetic and molecular genetic analysis on peripheral blood cells. Such tests, together with the cytologic and immunophenotypic features, can confirm a diagnosis of follicular lymphoma or mantle cell lymphoma.

   g.   Rai staging. Stage 0: absolute lymphocyte count >15,000/μL, and >40% lymphs in the marrow; stage 1: stage 0 with lymphadenopathy; stage 2: stage 0 with hepatosplenomegaly; stage 3: stage 0 with anemia; stage 4: stage 0 with thrombocytopenia.

   h.   Disease course. The average life expectancy is 10–15 years, ranging from 1–2 years for stage 4, to 15 years for stage 0. Of patients, 5% will undergo a Richter's transformation (large cell lymphoma, usually B-cell immunoblastic). Common causes of death are infection, autoimmune hemolytic anemia, and secondary malignancies.

   B.   Prolymphocytic leukemia (PLL) occurs predominantly in **middle-aged** and **elderly** individuals. Most cases (80%) are of **B-cell origin**. The **WBC count is usually markedly elevated** (>100,000/μL), and >**55% of the lymphocytes must be prolymphocytes** in order to make the diagnosis (10%–55% prolymphocytes is considered a "mixed CLL/PLL," a variant of chronic lymphocytic leukemia). **Massive splenomegaly** is common. The average length of survival is 3 years.

   C.   Hairy cell leukemia makes up <3% of leukemias, and is of **B-cell origin**; it occurs predominantly in **middle-aged men** (male:female = 4:1), **and often presents with splenomegaly**, severe monocytopenia, or pancytopenia. Bone marrow aspirates are usually **dry taps**. Trephine biopsies show **fried egg** artifacts (space around nuclei). Splenic involvement is within the **red pulp** (in contrast to most lymphoproliferative disorders that involve the white pulp). Disease course is variable, but with modern treatment is usually >10 years.

   D.   Large granular lymphocyte leukemia [a.k.a. T-gamma lymphocytosis, natural killer (NK) cell leukemia, T-cell lymphoproliferative leukemia] occur in **middle-aged** adults, **T-cell (T suppressor) or natural killer cell types**, with or without pancytopenia or decreases in individual cell lines. Neoplastic cells may be of NK- or T-lineage. Recurring bacterial infections, arthritis, and splenomegaly may be present. The disease usually has a smoldering course, except for patients with the NK type that is more aggressive.

   E.   Sézary syndrome is of T-cell (T-helper) origin, with a circulating phase of mycosis fungoides.

VIII.   Polycythemia is defined as an **increased red cell count, hemoglobin, or hematocrit**. In a patient with polycythemia, it is necessary to determine if the cause is a decrease in the plasma volume (pseudo- or **relative polycythemia**) or an increase in red cell mass (**true polycythemia**). In patients with true polycythemia, it is necessary to distinguish between **secondary polycythemia** (reacting to hypoxia) and **primary proliferative polycythemia** (i.e., PRV). A classification of the causes of relative and true polycythemia is given in Table 2-19.

A. Clinical history and physical examination. A careful history and physical examination are very important. **Dehydration and other causes of decreased plasma volume should be ruled out initially. Potential causes of tissue hypoxia should then be sought**, which would cause a reactive polycythemia (e.g., a smoking history, cyanotic heart disease, or hypoxic lung disease) and, if found, no further investigation is needed. **Renal masses**, which might represent an erythropoietin-producing tumor, should also be sought. Patients with **PRV are usually older adults** (rarely <40 years of age), and often present with **facial and conjunctival plethora, peripheral gangrene, splenomegaly, ischemic heart disease, peptic ulceration, transient ischemic attacks, and the patients may complain of itching (particularly after a hot bath).**

B. Laboratory testing. If no obvious cause of polycythemia is found, then it is essential to confirm the high hemoglobin concentration with a **repeat blood sample** taken without prolonged venous constriction. A minimal elevation of hemoglobin does not necessitate further investigation (bearing in mind that 2.5% of healthy persons will fall above the "normal" range). If the hemoglobin is significantly elevated on at least two estimates, true polycythemia is suggested, and must be investigated with **red cell mass** and **plasma volume studies** (using radioisotope dilution techniques). If the red cell mass and plasma studies are normal, no further investigation is indicated (but smokers should be advised to stop). If true polycythemia is confirmed, appropriate further investigation includes the following:

Table 2-19. Some causes of relative and true polycythemia

Relative or pseudopolycythemia
Acute: Dehydration or shock
Chronic:
  Cigarette smoking (reduced plasma volume)
  Idiopathic

True polycythemia
Living at high altitude
Cyanotic heart disease or hypoxic lung disease
Morbid obesity with hypoventilation (Pickwickian syndrome)
Sleep apnea
Cigarette smoking (increased carboxyhemoglobin)
High affinity hemoglobin (e.g., Hgb Rainier, Hgb Chesapeake)
Erythropoietin-secreting tumors (e.g., carcinoma of the kidney, hepatoma, cerebellar hemangioblastoma, uterine fibroids)
Other renal lesions including renal cysts and renal artery stenosis
Essential erythrocytosis
Polycythemia rubra vera

1. **CBC with differential count**. Most patients with PRV have a **hematocrit above 55%** (normocytic, normochromic), although **some patients may have suffered a GI blood loss** and present with a normal hematocrit (microcytic, hypochromic caused by iron deficiency). **The WBC and platelet counts are usually normal or mildly elevated, and basophilia may be present.**

2. **Serum erythropoietin assay: decreased in PRV; increased in secondary polycythemia**

3. **Ultrasound examination of the abdomen**, assessing liver, spleen, and kidneys

4. **Blood gases** (arterial O_2 saturation is usually $\geq 92\%$ in PRV, and usually $<92\%$ in secondary polycythemia caused by hypoxia).

5. **Chest x-ray study**

6. **Bone marrow aspirate and trephine biopsy** (not necessary to diagnose PRV, but may sometimes be helpful): the **marrow is hypercellular, with increased myeloid, erythroid, and megakaryocytic lines; iron stores are reduced or absent.**

7. **Other tests** that provide supportive evidence for PRV include (a) increased serum vitamin B_{12} concentration; (b) increased plasma urate concentration; (c) increased neutrophil (i.e., leukocyte) alkaline phosphatase score; and (d) abnormal cytogenetic analysis. No specific cytogenetic abnormalities are associated with PRV, but some patients have clonal abnormalities (e.g., 1q+, 20q−, +8, +9, −5).

A **diagnosis of PRV is made in cases of otherwise unexplained polycythemia, with evidence of a myeloproliferative disorder (e.g., hepatomegaly, splenomegaly, neutrophilia, basophilia, thrombocytosis, decreased serum erythropoietin concentration, high serum vitamin B_{12} concentration, high leukocyte alkaline phosphatase score, increased bone marrow cellularity, increased megakaryocytes, or a clonal cytogenetic abnormality**). In patients with true polycythemia that remains unexplained after appropriate investigation, but in whom no adequate supporting evidence is found for a diagnosis of PRV, it is appropriate to make a diagnosis of **idiopathic erythrocytosis**. On follow-up, some of these patients develop clear evidence of PRV.

C. **Disease course**. The average life expectancy is 10–15 years. A few (<10%) progress to acute leukemia; 10% progress to myelofibrosis with myeloid metaplasia ("spent phase of PRV"). Many of the disease complications are caused by hemorrhage or thrombosis.

IX. **Thrombocytosis**

A. **Causes**. The discovery of a high platelet count should lead to a review of clinical features. The cause is often readily apparent and no further investigation is indicated. **Common causes of thrombocytosis include hemorrhage, iron-deficiency, myeloproliferative disorders (e.g., PRV, CML), hyposplenia, chronic infections, chronic inflammation, and other malignancies** (e.g., lymphoma, carcinoma, see Table 2-20). Up

Table 2-20. Some causes of thrombocytosis

Surgery, trauma
Severe infection
Acute inflammation or severe chronic inflammation
Hemorrhage
Iron deficiency
Rebound after recovery from bone marrow failure (e.g., following treatment of megaloblastic anemia)
Malignancies [e.g., carcinoma, myeloproliferative disorders, myelodysplastic syndromes (a minority of cases)]
Hyposplenism
Essential thrombocythemia

to 40% of patients admitted to community hospitals with an isolated platelet count $>500 \times 10^9$ may have an occult malignancy.

B.   Essential thrombocythemia (ET)
    1.   Presentation. Essential thrombocythemia is uncommon. ET usually occurs in **older adults** (rare <40 years of age). The **platelet count is often > 1,000 × 10⁹/L (1,000,000/μL), the WBC count may be mildly increased and mild anemia may be present. Platelets are functionally abnormal, and both bleeding and thrombotic disorders occur.**
    2.   Laboratory testing. The diagnosis of ET is often made in the presymptomatic phase; it is usually discovered first in the CBC count. If essential thrombocythemia is suspected, further testing includes the following.
        a.   Review of the blood smear, looking for giant platelets, neutrophilia, or basophilia.
        b.   Bone marrow aspirate and trephine biopsy. The bone marrow is hypercellular, with aggregates of morphologically abnormal megakaryocytes (nondiagnostic).
        c.   Cytogenetic analysis (in some situations). If the basophil count is markedly elevated, cytogenetic analysis may identify a Philadelphia chromosome, in which case the patient should be managed in a manner similar to chronic granulocytic leukemia. Other patients have other clonal cytogenetic abnormalities.
    Diagnostic criteria for ET are intended to rule out other myeloproliferative disorders, and require a platelet count > 600 × 10⁹/L, hemoglobin ≤13 g/dL or normal RBC mass, stainable bone marrow iron (or failure of iron therapy), absence of Ph chromosome, absent marrow collagen fibrosis (or < 30% fibrosis with no splenomegaly and no leukoerythroblastic pattern), and no known cause for a reactive thrombocytosis. It should be noted that it may be difficult to distinguish PRV with iron deficiency from essential thrombocythemia. However, making the distinction is not important for patient management. Administering iron to the patient merely to make a diagnosis is not recommended.
    3.   Disease course. The average survival time is close to that of normal individuals; however, rarely, patients trans-

form to another form of chronic myeloproliferative disorder or acute leukemia.

X.   Chronic lymphoplasmacytic proliferations typically produce dysproteinemias, which are characterized by synthesis of **monoclonal immunoglobulins** or portions of immunoglobulins. Multiple myeloma makes up $\cong$75% of plasmacytic dysproteinemias, and is associated with the production of IgG (60% of dysproteinemias) or IgA (15% of dysproteinemias). **Waldenström's macroglobulinemia** makes up $\cong$10% to 15% of the dysproteinemias, and is associated with the production of IgM. **Light-chain disease** makes up <10% of dysproteinemias, and may be part of multiple myeloma, Waldenström's macroglobulinemia, or its own disease entity. Light-chain disease is associated with the production of light chains (kappa or lambda). When spontaneous **dimers form of two kappa chains or two lambda chains**, the result is called **"Bence Jones protein,"** and has the additional characteristic of being soluble at room temperature, precipitating at 56°C, and resolubilizing at higher temperatures. Disorders that produce only **heavy chains** (e.g., α-chain disease in Mediterranean subjects) are rare. Dysproteinemias that do not meet the diagnostic criteria for the aforementioned entities are termed **"monoclonal gammopathies of undetermined significance (MGUS),"** and occur in 2% to 3% of all people over 70 years of age. These patients should be followed clinically, as ~10% will develop multiple myeloma.

A.   Multiple myeloma (MM)

1.   Presentation. Most patients are **more than 50 years of age**. Clinical and laboratory features suggesting the possibility of multiple myeloma include **bone pain, hypercalcemia, pathologic fractures, anemia, high erythrocyte sedimentation rate (ESR), renal failure, and infection**.

2.   Laboratory testing. The appropriate initial investigation is **serum protein electrophoresis (SPE), quantification of immunoglobulins, and quantification of any paraproteins (monoclonal proteins or M-proteins)** present. **Multiple myeloma is associated with the presence of a monoclonal protein and a reduction of normal immunoglobulins**. Do not forget, some patients with multiple myeloma have neither a serum nor a urinary monoclonal protein (nonsecretory myeloma). A polyclonal increase in immunoglobulins and an increase in α_2 macroglobulin in the SPE are consistent with a benign process (e.g., infection, inflammation). If multiple myeloma is still suspected after SPE, further relevant tests include the following.

a.   A 24-hour urine collection to identify and quantify urinary light chain excretion (Bence Jones proteins).

b.   CBC count and ESR. Pancytopenia may be seen. Abnormal serum proteins cause rouleaux formation and increased ESR.

c.   Bone marrow aspiration and trephine biopsy: show increased plasma cells.

d.   Biochemical screen including creatinine, electrolytes, uric acid, calcium, liver function tests.

e. β_2-microglobulin (of prognostic significance).

f. **Measurement of plasma viscosity** (if any clinical features suggest hyperviscosity).

i. **Chest x-ray study and skeletal survey**.

Diagnostic criteria for multiple myeloma are listed in Table 2-21.

3. **Disease course and prognosis**. Average life expectancy is 2–3 years, and depends on the extent of the disease: poor prognostic features include a high tumor load (amount of M-protein, degree of anemia, lytic lesions, hypercalcemia, and β_2 microglobulin elevation), renal disease, and Bence Jones proteins in the urine (particularly lambda type).

B. **Waldenström's macroglobulinemia (WM)** is a form of lymphoma; it tends to have a slow and insidious progression; typically presents in older male patients, with signs and symptoms caused by the **intravascular accumulation of IgM**, including vascular occlusion (e.g., Raynaud's phenomenon, blurred vision, central nervous system abnormalities, cardiac ischemia), and **bleeding** (most likely because of abnormal protein-coated platelets). The laboratory workup is similar to that for multiple myeloma. The average length of survival is 5 years.

XI. Decreased cell counts and qualitative disorders of leukocytes

A. **Neutropenia, qualitative disorders of neutrophils, and pancytopenia**. It is important to **note whether the patient has isolated neutropenia or whether other lineages are also affected**. Some important causes of isolated neutropenia or pancytopenia are shown in Table 2-22. Some conditions that usually cause pancytopenia may, in some patients, cause isolated neutropenia. For example, aplastic anemia sometimes presents initially with neutropenia.

1. **Clinical history.** It is essential to **consider the ethnic origin** of the patient. The normal neutrophil range in blacks,

Table 2-21. Diagnostic criteria for multiple myeloma

More than one major criterion, **or** one major criterion and one minor criterion, **or** three minor criteria (including B1 and B2), must be present to diagnose multiple myeloma[a]

Major criteria
1. Bone marrow shows > 30% plasma cells
2. Tissue plasmacytoma
3. Monoclonal protein
   a. Serum: IgG > 3.5g/dL, IgA > 2 g/dL
   b. Urine: Bence Jones protein > 1 g/24 h

Minor criteria
1. Bone marrow shows 10%–30% plasma cells
2. Monoclonal proteins present, but less than major criteria
3. Lytic skeletal lesions
4. Reduced amounts of normal immunoglobulins: IgG < 600 mg/dL; IgA < 100 mg/dL; IgM < 50 mg/dL

[a] Modified from several sources; other diagnostic criteria schemes may be less stringent.

Table 2-22.   Some important causes of neutropenia (including rare causes)

Isolated neutropenia
Inherited
−Congenital neutropenia [e.g., Kostmann's syndrome (infantile genetic agranulocytosis; autosomal recessive)]
−Reticular dysgenesis (lymphocyte count also reduced)
−Shwachman−Diamond syndrome
−Familial benign neutropenia or familial severe neutropenia
−Myelokathexis
−Cartilage-hair hypoplasia
−X-linked agammaglobulinemia
−Cyclical neutropenia
Acquired
−Idiosyncratic reaction to drugs (e.g., sulfonamides, third and fourth generation penicillins, analgesics, anticonvulsants, antihistamines, benzodiazepines, and antithyroid drugs)
−Transient neutropenia (3–5 days) secondary to many viral infections (with more chronic decreases in some infections such as AIDS)
−Postinfection neutropenia
−Overwhelming infections (particularly in the elderly)
−Alloimmune neutropenia (in neonates)
−Autoimmune neutropenia (isolated autoimmune neutropenia or as part of collagen-vascular diseases)
−Cyclical neutropenia
−Large granular lymphocyte leukemia

Neutropenia as an aspect of pancytopenia
Inherited
−Mitochondrial cytopathies, including Pearson's syndrome
−Inherited aplastic anemia (e.g., Fanconi's anemia and dyskerotosis congenita)
−Chediak−Higashi syndrome
−Metabolic defects (e.g., oroticaciduria)
Acquired
−Decreased production
  —Predictable effect of drugs (e.g., chemotherapeutic agents, azathioprine, zidovudine)
  —Radiation
  —Acquired aplastic anemia (idiopathic or induced by a drug, toxin, or infection)
  —Megaloblastic anemia
  —Excess alcohol intake
  —Copper deficiency
  —Malignancies (e.g., acute myeloid leukemia, myelodysplastic syndromes, idiopathic myelofibrosis, bone marrow infiltration)
−Increased destruction or egress to tissues
  —Hypersplenism [including causes related to systemic lupus or rheumatoid arthritis (Felty's syndrome)]
  —Severe infection (particularly in neonates)
  —Paroxysmal nocturnal hemoglobinuria

AIDS, acquired immunodeficiency syndrome.

Yemenite Jews, and Afro-Caribbeans is lower than that of whites. Healthy blacks may have a neutrophil count of 1×10^9/L, which in a Caucasian would likely indicate significant disease. **Age is also crucial**. Neutrophil counts are high at birth and drop precipitously within a day or two. A careful history is very important regarding medications and possible exposure to toxins. Physical examination is not usually very helpful. Often, neutropenia does not require any investigation because the cause is apparent from the history. **In modern medical practice, most cases are attributable to idiosyncratic or predictable effects of prescribed drugs, or transient neutropenia caused by viral infections**.

   2. **Laboratory tests.** When the cause of the cytopenia is not apparent, investigation should start with a careful examination of the **blood smear**. Other relevant investigations can include a **bone marrow aspirate and trephine biopsy**, and an autoantibody screen.

   3. **Congenital causes of neutropenia** (Table 2-22).

     a. **Agranulocytosis of Kostmann type** is extremely rare, and severe.

     b. **Chronic benign neutropenia** may cause significant neutropenia, because of a pseudomaturational arrest at the metamyelocyte stage; anti-neutrophil antibodies are sometimes seen.

     c. **Cyclic neutropenia** involves periodic marrow failure (nadirs every 21 days) caused by a stem cell defect; it is associated with oral ulcers, skin and respiratory infections.

     d. **Fanconi's syndrome** is a chromosomal fragility syndrome that leads to aplastic anemia with pancytopenia, and is also associated with mental retardation, skeletal abnormalities (e.g., short stature, bifid thumbs), abnormal skin pigmentation, renal abnormalities, and increased risk for cancer.

     e. **Dyskeratosis congenita** is progressive marrow failure with chromosomal abnormalities; failure to thrive early in life, with dyskeratosis and poor dental or nail formation.

     f. **Myelokathexis** results from an inability to release mature PMNs from marrow; nuclei are pyknotic with thin filamentous strands between them.

   4. **Congenital qualitative defects in neutrophils**

     a. **Chediak–Higashi syndrome** is an autosomal recessive defect in chemotaxis and killing; giant lysosomes are present in neutrophils; also affects whales and mink.

     b. **Myeloperoxidase deficiency** causes clinically mild disease; it is associated with *Candida* infections.

     c. **Chronic granulomatous disease of childhood** is X-linked; a lack of oxidative "burst" limits the ability of phagocytes to kill organisms, leading to pyogenic infections and granuloma formation; is tested with nitroblue tetrazolium.

     d. **Hyperimmunoglobulin E syndrome** (Job's syndrome) is seen with high levels of IgE with decreased neutrophil functioning, recurrent infections, and "cold abscesses."

B. **Leukoerythroblastic anemia**. The term "leukoerythroblastic" refers to the presence of **granulocyte precursors and**

nucleated red blood cells in the peripheral blood. Such patients are usually anemic, and the term "leukoerythroblastic" anemia is then used. Some important causes of a leukoerythroblastic blood smear are shown in Table 2-23. Initial assessment of a leukoerythroblastic blood smear requires consideration of the clinical history, physical examination findings, and the blood smear morphology.

1.   **Clinical history**. The clinical circumstances usually indicate if the leukoerythroblastic features are the result of **acute blood loss, severe infection, shock or hypoxia, recovery from bone marrow failure, or have resulted from treatment of a severe hematinic (e.g., vitamin B_{12} or folate) deficiency**. The medical history may include a primary neoplasm that may have metastasized to the bone marrow.

2.   **Physical examination**. Three of the more significant signs to look for are splenomegaly, lymphadenopathy, and jaundice. **Splenomegaly is suggestive of idiopathic myelofibrosis, lymphoma, or other hematologic malignancy** and, at the same time, suggests that metastatic carcinoma is a very unlikely cause of the leukoerythroblastic anemia. **Lymphadenopathy suggests the possibility of bone marrow infiltration by Hodgkin's disease, non-Hodgkin's lymphoma, or other tumor. Jaundice suggests hemolysis, megaloblastic anemia, or malignant disease with hepatic as well as bone marrow infiltration.**

3.   **Blood smear**. Careful examination of a blood smear may suggest a cause of leukoerythroblastic anemia that was not apparent from the history and physical examination. **"Tear drop" poikilocytes** suggests bone marrow fibrosis, but does not permit a distinction between idiopathic myelofibrosis and fibrosis secondary to bone marrow infiltration (myelophthistic disorders). Features that suggest idiopathic myelofibrosis or another hematologic neoplasm include hypogranular or agranular neutrophils, neutrophils showing the acquired Pelger-

**Table 2-23.   Some important causes
of a leukoerythroblastic blood film**

Physiologic
−Neonatal period
Pathologic
−Shock or hypoxia
−Severe infection
−Severe hemolysis
−Severe megaloblastic anemia
−Rebound following administration of hematinic agents to a
    deficient patient (vitamins B_{12}/folate)
−Bone marrow infiltration (e.g., carcinoma or lymphoma)
−Bone marrow fibrosis, either primary (idiopathic myelofibrosis)
    or secondary
−Hematologic neoplasms (e.g., acute and chronic myeloid leukemias
    and the myelodysplastic syndromes)

Huët anomaly, bare megakaryocyte nuclei, and circulating micromegakaryocytes.

   4. Bone marrow examination. If a hematologic neoplasm or bone marrow fibrosis is suspected, bone marrow examination is indicated. If bone marrow aspiration is possible, it may be useful to use some of the aspirate for cytogenetic analysis. However, when the bone marrow is fibrotic, no aspirate can be obtained ("dry tap"). On other occasions, only blood can be aspirated ("blood tap") or the aspirate contains bone marrow cells but is very dilute. In these circumstances, a bone marrow trephine biopsy is essential for adequate assessment.

   C. Lymphopenia is a very common response to any acute illness, and slowly resolves when the underlying disease resolves. Some of the cases are readily explicable, and common causes are shown in Table 2-24. Unless a specific reason exists to suspect a congenital or acquired immune deficiency, no further investigation of lymphopenia is immediately indicated.

XII.   Myelodysplastic syndromes (MDS) are diseases resulting from **clonal hematopoietic stem cell proliferation** that differ from leukemias in two main aspects. First, **the percentage of marrow blasts in MDS is <30%,** whereas acute leukemias have >30% (the newly proposed World Health Organization classification uses a cut-off point of 20%). Second, **the proliferating cells in MDS fail within the marrow and, therefore, lead to peripheral cytopenias** rather than the increased peripheral circulating cell counts associated with leukemias.

   A. Clinical history and physical examination. Myelodysplastic syndromes usually present with abnormalities in a CBC count or blood smear in **middle-aged** or **elderly** patients, or in a patient of any age who has previously been exposed to cyto-

Table 2-24.   Causes of lymphopenia

Inherited
Reticular dysgenesis, severe combined immunodeficiency, common variable hypogammaglobulinemia, Swiss-type agammaglobulinemia, some cases of DiGeorge syndrome, ataxia telangiectasia, Wiskott–Aldrich syndrome

Acquired
Acute stress (e.g., trauma, surgery, burns, severe acute illness)
Acute infection
Some chronic infections (e.g., acquired immune deficiency syndrome, Whipple's disease)
Some chronic inflammatory disorders (e.g., systemic lupus erythematosus, sarcoidosis)
Protein-calorie malnutrition
Cushing's syndrome and corticosteroid therapy
Immunosuppressive therapy (e.g., with azathioprine, cyclosporin, or antilymphocyte globulin)
Anticancer chemotherapy or radiotherapy
Aplastic anemia
Acute and chronic renal failure
Malignancies (e.g., advanced carcinoma, Hodgkin's disease)

toxic chemotherapy or radiotherapy. The clinical history is important in eliminating causes of secondary dysplastic changes similar to those of MDS. For example, **reversible dysplastic changes can be caused by exposure to heavy metals** (e.g., lead, arsenic) or to **various drugs** (e.g., anti-cancer drugs, azathioprine, zidovudine, anti-tuberculosis drugs). **Excess alcohol** intake can cause macrocytic anemia, other cytopenias, and minor dysplastic changes. Infections, including HIV, can likewise cause cytopenia with dysplastic features. The physical examination is usually noncontributory in making the diagnosis of MDS.

B.   **Laboratory Tests**

1.   **CBC count and peripheral smear**. Peripheral blood abnormalities that raise the possibility of MDS include the following.

a.   **Unexplained anemia** (particularly when macrocytic), with or without anisopoikilocytosis, a low reticulocyte index, and nucleated red cells

b.   **Dimorphic blood film** with a major population of normochromic normocytes (or macrocytes) and a minor population of hypochromic microcytes

c.   **Pappenheimer bodies, basophilic stippling**

d.   **Unexplained thrombocytopenia**; hypogranular, giant, or vacuolated platelets

e.   **Monocytosis**, with or without neutrophilia, but without any toxic changes in neutrophils

f.   The acquired **Pelger-Huët anomaly**

g.   **Unexplained neutropenia; hypogranular or agranular white cells**

h.   Small numbers of **blast cells**

Of the abnormalities listed, those that are **most specific for MDS are the acquired Pelger-Huët anomaly and agranular neutrophils**. The observation of blast cells, with or without Auer rods, is usually indicative of MDS or acute leukemia.

2.   **Other tests**. When MDS is suspected, **it is important to exclude other possible causes** for the abnormality observed. For example, in a patient with macrocytic anemia, it is necessary to exclude vitamin B_{12} or folate deficiency, liver disease, excess alcohol intake, and hypothyroidism. Other tests that should be requested when MDS is suspected include the following.

a.   **Bone marrow aspirate and trephine biopsy**. Marrow studies usually show **hypercellularity, with dysplastic features in one or all cell lines**; erythrocyte precursors sometimes show megaloblastic features [large cells with copious, maturing cytoplasm, and nuclei that are more immature than would be expected for the degree of cytoplasmic maturation (nuclear or cytoplasmic asynchrony)]. MDS secondary to chemotherapy or radiation therapy may have a hypocellular marrow and fibrosis, along with the dysplastic cells. Myeloperoxidase stains should be performed to ensure that any Auer rods that may be present are detected.

b.   **Cytogenetic analysis** shows a variety of abnormalities, including −5, **5q−** (the most common finding), 7q−, −7 (a particularly bad prognostic sign in childhood cases of

MDS), +8, +9, inv(3), iso(17q), 20q–, and others. The prevalence of cytogenetic abnormalities increases with the severity of the MDS [e.g., more cases of refractory anemia with excess blasts in transformation (RAEB-T) show cytogenetic abnormalities than RA].

C. **Classification of MDS**. MDS are often **classified as suggested by the FAB** (French-American-British) cooperative group (Table 2-25). The diagnosis of refractory anemia can be difficult if there are neither dysplastic features nor a cytogenetic abnormality. In such circumstances, a definite diagnosis may not be possible and the patient should be kept under review. Patients with RAEB and RAEB-T should be kept under close observation because disease progression is sometimes rapid. Although the FAB group classifies RAEB-T as an MDS, it is often appropriate to treat as though the patient had AML, particularly when the patient is young with *de novo* MDS.

D. **Disease course.** The disease course is variable, with some patients ultimately transforming to acute leukemia, other patients succumbing to marrow failure (e.g., infection, bleeding), and others remaining stable for long periods of time. Approximately 15% of the patients with RA or RARS transform into AML, whereas 30% of RAEB, 40% of CMML, and almost 100% of patients with RAEB-T progress to AML. Greater numbers of chromosomal abnormalities are also associated with a greater risk of transformation into AML.

XIII. Splenomegaly

A. **Clinical history and physical examination**. The history and physical examination are of considerable importance.

Table 2-25. **The FAB classification of the myelodysplastic syndromes**

Classification (Usual Abbreviation)	Criteria
Refractory anemia (RA)	Anemia with PB blasts: $\leq 1\%$; monocytes: $\leq 1 \times 10^9$/L; BM blasts; <5%; ring sideroblasts: $\leq 15\%$
Refractory anemia with ring sideroblasts (RARS)	Anemia with PB blasts: $\leq 1\%$, monocytes: $\leq 1 \times 10^9$/L; BM blasts: <5%; ring sideroblasts: >15%
Refractory anemia with excess of blasts (RAEB)	Anemia with *either* 1%–5% PB blasts **or** 5%–20% BM blasts; monocytes: $\leq 1 \times 10^9$/L
Refractory anemia with excess of blasts in transformation (RAEB-T)	Anemia with >5% PB blasts **or** >20 but <30% BM blasts **or** Auer rods present in blasts in either PB or BM
Chronic myelomonocytic leukemia (CMML)	Monocytes: $>1 \times 10^9$/L; PB blasts: <5%; BM blasts: $\leq 20\%$

Blasts are calculated based on the nonerythroid myeloid-lineage cells.
BM, bone marrow; FAB, French-American-British; PB, peripheral blood.

The history should include the family history, travel history, and any history of recent illness. The physical examination must include a search for lymphadenopathy, jaundice, and signs of chronic liver disease. **A history of fever or travel to an area with endemic parasites (e.g., malaria), a recent illness of short duration, and a soft spleen suggest an infective cause of the splenomegaly. Liver disease suggests portal hypertension**. The presence and characteristics of the **lymphadenopathy may suggest a lymphoproliferative disease**.

   B.   Laboratory tests. Useful initial laboratory tests include the following:

   1.   CBC count and smear may suggest infectious mononucleosis, a myeloproliferative or lymphoproliferative disorder, an inherited or acquired hemolytic anemia, betathalassemia major or intermedia, hemoglobin H disease, or sickle cell disease, e.g., sickle cell/hemoglobin C disease (but, in an adult, not sickle cell anemia).

   2.   Liver function tests, serum protein electrophoresis, and quantification of immunoglobulins. Findings may suggest liver disease or a lymphoproliferative disorder.

   3.   Further testing may include an autoantibody screen, hepatitis serology, a bone marrow aspirate and trephine biopsy, a chest x-ray study, a computed tomography scan of the abdomen, and an ultrasound examination of the liver. Bone marrow biopsy may be a relatively noninvasive method to diagnose lymphoma (particularly in patients with no circulating lymphoma cells), storage diseases (e.g., Gaucher disease or Niemann–Pick disease), and light-chain associated amyloidosis (increased plasma cells and, less often, interstitial or blood vessel deposition of amyloid is present).

XIV.   Lymphadenopathy. An adequate assessment of lymphadenopathy requires a detailed history and a careful assessment of the location and characteristics of enlarged lymph nodes.

   A.   Clinical history. In addition to a general medical history, the patient should be asked about any recent **exposure to infectious mononucleosis or other acute infections, previous exposure to tuberculosis, and exposure to pets** or other animals. Risk factors for **sexually transmitted diseases** and other risk factors for HIV infection should be assessed. Residing in, or traveling to, a geographic area where **human T-lymphotropic virus-I infection or histoplasmosis** is endemic should be noted. **Smoking history, diet** (e.g., eating rare meats that might contain *Toxoplasma* organisms) and current **drug intake** should be noted (phenytoin is the drug that most often causes lymphadenopathy). The patient should be specifically interrogated for **symptoms suggesting the possibility of carcinoma, such as weight loss**, anorexia, alteration of the voice, cough, indigestion or altered bowel habit. A history of **lymphoma-related symptoms (e.g., fever, sweats, itch)** and alcohol-related pain should be sought (but note that night sweats may be caused by tuberculosis or other infections as well as lymphoma).

   B.   Physical examination. In addition to a general physical examination, specific assessment should be made of the **liver, spleen, and all lymph node areas**. In patients with cervical lymphadenopathy, the mouth, pharynx, ears, and, when appropriate, the larynx, should be examined. In those with inguinal lymphadenopathy, the genitalia and perineum should be examined.

1. **Physical characteristics of lymph nodes**. **Lymph nodes that are soft, tender, warm, and only moderately enlarged are often indicative of infection** (but can also occur in aggressive lymphomas when rapid enlargement of nodes is occurring). Firm nodes that are 0.5–1 cm in diameter (called "shotty nodes" because their size is similar to lead shot), or nodes with fluctuant areas are almost always indicative of infection (e.g., tuberculosis in the case of fluctuant nodes). In general, **lymph nodes with lymphoma or chronic lymphocytic leukemia are usually moderately or markedly enlarged, firm, and nontender. Nodes with metastatic carcinoma are often hard, and may be bound together** or bound to the overlying skin or underlying soft tissues.

2. **Location of nodes**. The site of the nodes is of some relevance. Nodes in the **anterior triangle of the neck are often indicative of metastatic carcinoma** from the head and neck. Nodes in the **posterior triangle are more likely to be the result of infection or lymphoma. Isolated supraclavicular nodes may indicate metastatic disease** from an intra-abdominal carcinoma. Enlarged **posterior occipital nodes or nodes near the elbow joint are suggestive of non-Hodgkin's lymphoma. Chronic lymphocytic leukemia or non-Hodgkin's lymphoma can cause enlarged nodes in the cervical, axillary, or inguinal regions. In Hodgkin's disease, cervical lymphadenopathy is most common, but axillary and inguinal nodes are sometimes involved.**

C. **Laboratory testing**. A CBC count and blood smear should be performed without delay in any patient with significant lymphadenopathy. Further investigations (Table 2-26) will depend on the specific clinical circumstances and on whether the CBC count and smear reveal lymphocytosis or abnormal lymphoid cells. When lymph nodes are confined to the anterior triangle of the neck, an otolaryngologist should be consulted without delay, before invasive procedures are performed. **When metastatic carcinoma is suspected, fine needle aspiration** is the appropriate initial investigation; fluctuant nodes should also be aspirated and cultured for mycobacteria and other bacteria. **When lymphoma is suspected, a lymph node biopsy must be performed**, which permits the architecture of the node to be assessed. In addition to histologic examination, supplementary tests might include culture for tuberculosis, immunophenotyping, and freezing a portion for molecular analysis, should this subsequently be required.

XV. **Lymphomas**
A. **Introduction**. A discussion of lymphomas is beyond the scope of this book; however, the following information is offered as a cursory overview. Lymphomas are malignancies of lymphocytes and other immune-related cells that originate within lymph nodes and other lymphoid tissues (e.g., spleen, bone

Table 2-26.   Tests that may be indicated in patients with lymphadenopathy

In patients with lymphocytosis or cytologically abnormal lymphocytes in the blood
Infectious mononucleosis screening test
Viral serologies: for EBV, CMV, HIV, HTLV-I
Chest x-ray
Immunophenotyping
Bone marrow aspirate and trephine biopsy
Lymph node biopsy

In patients without lymphocytosis or cytologically abnormal lymphocytes in the blood
Chest x-ray
Tuberculin skin test
Serologic tests for toxoplasmosis, histoplasmosis, cat scratch
    disease, lymphogranuloma venereum, syphilis
Serum calcium and angiotensin-converting enzyme levels
    (for sarcoidosis)
Autoantibody screen
Bone marrow aspirate and trephine biopsy
Fine needle aspirate or biopsy of lymph node

CMV, cytomegalovirus; EBV, Epstein-Barr virus; HIV, human immunodeficiency virus; HTLV-I, human T-lymphotropic Virus-I.

marrow, GI, and other mucosal surfaces). Lymphomas are generally divided into Hodgkin's disease and non-Hodgkin's lymphomas. A multitude of classifications have been used in the past, based on morphology, immunophenotyping, clinical behavior, and so on. The current classification most widely used in the United States is the Revised European American Lymphoma classification (REAL), which is based on well-defined types of lymphoma and uses specific molecular abnormalities, immunophenotyping, and so forth.

B.   Hodgkin's disease has a bimodal age distribution, with peaks at 25 years of age and at >50 years of age. Most patients present with painless enlargement of the cervical lymph nodes. Hodgkin's disease tends to involve axial nodes (e.g., cervical, mediastinal, para-aortic), spreads from one contiguous lymph node to the next, and rarely enters the blood stream. Patients may be asymptomatic (stage A) or have systemic symptoms (stage B: fevers, night sweats, weight loss). Hodgkin's disease involves large cells called Reed–Sternberg cells, in a background of reactive cells (lymphocytes, plasma cells, eosinophils, histiocytes). Reed–Sternberg cells are binucleate, with prominent nucleoli giving an "owl's eye" appearance; the cells stain with CD15 and CD30. Reed–Sternberg variants are also present in some subtypes. Hodgkin's disease is divided into the following four main groups.

1.   Lymphocyte predominant. The predilection is for males; Reed–Sternberg variants in this subtype are called L and H cells ("popcorn cells"); background cells are primarily small, mature, benign lymphocytes; L and H cells are the malignant cells, probably of B-cell origin (L and H cells stain with CD45, CD20, and EMA (epithelial membrane antigen), and are negative for CD15 or CD30, unlike the other RS cells).

2. Mixed cellularity. The predilection is for males; Reed–Sternberg cells are common.

3. Lymphocyte depleted. The predilection is for males; classic Reed–Sternberg cells are most common in this subtype.

4. Nodular sclerosing. The predilection is for females; most common subtype of Hodgkin's disease. Bands of fibrous tissue are a feature. Reed–Sternberg variants in this subtype are called "Lacunar cells," and stain with CD15 and CD30.

C. Staging is essential for prognosis and treatment selection, and may involve imaging of the liver, spleen, and abdomen; bone marrow and liver biopsies. Splenectomy is now rarely indicated. Lower stages can be successfully treated with radiation, whereas higher stages, "B" symptoms, or both require chemotherapy.

D. Non-Hodgkin's lymphomas (NHL) arise from a malignant clone in lymphoid tissues. Most NHL arise in older adults (50–60 years of age), and involve low-grade (e.g., small lymphocytic and follicular small cleaved types) or intermediate-grade (e.g., diffuse large cell) types. NHL in children tend to be high grade types (e.g., Burkitt's lymphoma, lymphoblastic lymphoma). Unlike Hodgkin's disease, the malignant cells do not necessarily spread from one node to the next contiguous node, and patients often have widespread disease when diagnosed. Extranodal involvement by B-cell NHL is common in the spleen, liver, bone marrow, and mucosal surfaces of the body, whereas T-cell NHL has a predilection for the skin.

Low-grade NHL tend to have a long, insidious course, but are generally incurable by chemotherapy. High-grade NHL are much more aggressive, but almost 50% of patients are cured by chemotherapy. The histologic and immunophenotypic classification of NHL is the most important prognostic feature. Important features include a nodular (better prognosis) versus a diffuse pattern of proliferation, small or mature cell morphology (tend to be low-grade) versus large or blastic (tend to be high grade), and immunophenotyping (B-cell NHL tend to have a better prognosis than T-cell NHL of the same general type).

A variety of cytogenetic abnormalities are present in NHL; common findings involve chromosomes 2 (kappa light chain gene), 22 (lambda light chain gene), 14 (q11: T-cell receptor gene; q32: immunoglobulin heavy chain gene), and 18 (*BCL2* oncogene).

Some types of lymphoma involve cells that are identical to the cells involved in leukemia: the lymphoma cells are first diagnosed in lymphoid tissue, whereas leukemias are first diagnosed in the blood. For example, Burkitt's lymphoma cells are identical to those in B-cell ALL type L3; lymphoblastic lymphoma cells are identical to those in T-cell, ALL, and small lymphocytic lymphoma cells are identical to those in chronic lymphocytic leukemia.

XVI. Conclusion

A. In cases of a diagnostic problem, always review the history very carefully. This is often more illuminating than a battery of laboratory tests.

B. In cases of an apparently abnormal test result, always ask:

1. Is this normal for this patient?
2. If it is abnormal, does it matter?
3. If it might matter, what should be done next?

C. Do not do any test without knowing why you are doing it, and how it will influence management of the patient.

D. Take the patient into your confidence. Tell the patient what sort of tests you are doing and why. If a test result may have a major impact on the patient's future, explain why you think it should be done and get the patient's implied consent before testing.

E. When requesting a laboratory test, accept the responsibility of checking the result and acting on it.

BIBLIOGRAPHY

Bain BJ. *Blood cells*, 3rd ed. Oxford: Blackwell Science, 2001.

Bain BJ. *Leukaemia diagnosis*, 2nd ed. Oxford: Blackwell Science, 1999.

Bain BJ. *Interactive haematology imagebank*. Oxford: Blackwell Science, 1999.

Platelets, Coagulation, and Fibrinolysis

Ann T. Moriarty

I. Platelets—basic review

A. Summary of clotting. An intravascular injury induces formation of a **platelet plug**. The **coagulation (and anticoagulation)** cascade occurs on the platelet and vascular surfaces. **Fibrinolysis** occurs after healing.

B. Formation of the platelet plug. Collagen and subendothelial von Willebrand factor (vWF) are exposed by injury. Circulating vWF then attaches to the site of injury. Circulating **platelets adhere to the vWF by glycoprotein (GP) Ib** and **GP IX** (a heterodimer). Activation of platelets then occurs, and platelet granules are released. The release of adenosine diphosphate (ADP) and thromboxane A_2 (TXA$_2$) from the platelet granules recruits additional platelets. Platelet aggregation occurs and plugs the vascular defect. **Fibrinogen binds to GPIIb/IIIa on the platelet surfaces**. The coagulation cascade can then occur on the platelet surfaces, and a thrombus is created.

C. The von Willebrand factor (vWF) is found subendothelially, on platelets, and it also circulates as a protein complex. **The protein factor VIII complex is composed of factor VIII procoagulant** (VIII:C; also called antihemophilic factor) **and vWF (VIII:R;** factor VIII:related protein). The bulk of the factor VIII complex is made up of vWF, which serves as the carrier protein for factor VIII:C.

II. Clinical findings of platelet abnormalities.

Patients with platelet abnormalities have "skin and mucosal" bleeding patterns, including petechiae, ecchymoses, epistaxis, menorrhagia, and **immediate postsurgical bleeding**. Platelet abnormalities are usually divided into **quantitative** (abnormal platelet count) and **qualitative** (abnormal platelet function) disorders. **Deep muscle, joint, intracerebral, or retroperitoneal bleeding and delayed postsurgical bleeding (1–4 hours after) are *not* characteristic of platelet abnormalities, but suggest a defect in the coagulation cascade.**

III. Laboratory evaluation of platelets

A. Platelet count. The normal reference range for platelet count is $150-400 \times 10^9$/L. The standard automated blood counter is the most **reliable *quantitative* test**.

B. Bleeding time. The normal reference range varies from laboratory to laboratory, and is usually 6–10 minutes. The test is **extremely variable** and depends on the person performing the test. The test is *always* abnormal with aspirin and platelet counts <90,000/µL, and is usually abnormal in patients with von Willebrand's disease (vWd) and vascular disorders. This test should be used to evaluate patients with a history that suggests a **qualitative** platelet bleeding disorder. The bleeding time is a crude tool and is **not a good screening test for bleeding during surgery**. It neither predicts the likelihood of bleeding nor the likelihood of not bleeding.

   C.   Aggregation studies. Performed at reference laboratories, aggregation studies are used for rare platelet disorders **to define qualitative platelet abnormalities**. These tests require a fresh, platelet-rich, turbid plasma solution, to which aggregating agents are added, including ADP, ristocetin, epinephrine, collagen, and arachidonic acid. Platelet responses are reflected by an increase in light transmission through the specimen. The response to the specific aggregating agent, as well as the portion of the response affected, help to identify the qualitative disorder.

   D.   von Willebrand assays can usually be ordered as a **panel of tests** that include platelet aggregation studies, ristocetin cofactor activity, factor VIII:Ag (representing the amount of circulating protein factor VIII complex as measured by immunologic methods), and high molecular weight multimers (HMWM) of factor VIII sodium dodecyl sulfate-polyacrylamide gel electrophoresis (SDS-PAGE).

   E.   Miscellaneous platelet tests available from reference laboratories. Among the other studies available from reference laboratories are surface receptor studies, granule contents, and adenosine triphosphate (ATP):ADP ratios.

   F.   How to predict patients who may bleed because of platelet abnormalities
      1.   History of **aspirin** or other drugs that affect platelets
      2.   History of **oozing** or blood loss with minor dental procedures, significant blood loss with menses, or **easy bruising**
      3.   **Low platelet count**
      4.   Do **not** use a bleeding time as a screen to predict bleeding.

IV.   Quantitative defects of platelet function
   A.   Measurement of the platelet count. Most reported platelet counts are derived from automated instruments that count millions of particles. A rough estimate of platelet number can be derived from a peripheral blood smear: 10–20 platelets/high power field or 1 platelet/20 red blood cells are "normal" estimates.

   B.   Types of quantitative defects (Table 2-27). Quantitative defects can be divided into production disorders, distribution disorders, and destruction disorders. An abnormal bleeding time always occurs when platelets are <90,000/μL. However, *spontaneous bleeding does not occur until platelets fall below 5,000/μL*.

   C.   Selected quantitative platelet disorders.
      1.   **Thrombotic thrombocytopenic purpura (TTP). TTP is defined by a clinical pentad of thrombocytopenia, microangiopathic hemolytic anemia, renal abnormalities, neurologic changes, and fever**. TTP often occurs after a viral prodrome. Some forms of TTP have a multimeric vWF/factor VIII processing defect: **unusually large vWF bind to the fibrinogen-binding sites (GP IIb/IIIa) on circulating platelets, causing circulating microthrombi** (and thereby consuming platelets). The thrombi can hemolyze red cells through shearing by fibrin strands (this process is

Table 2-27. Quantitative platelet disorders

Platelet production disorders

Congenital	Fanconi's anemia, TAR syndrome, May–Hegglin anomaly, Wiskott-Aldrich syndrome, Bernard–Soulier syndrome
Acquired	Alcohol, B_{12}/folate deficiency, drugs (including chemotherapy), aplastic anemia (e.g., from radiation, toxins, viral infections), granulomatous inflammation (e.g., TB), autoimmune disease, myelodysplasia, paroxysmal nocturnal hemoglobinuria, myelophthistic disorders (e.g., metastatic carcinoma, sarcoidosis), hematologic malignancies (e.g., leukemia/lymphoma, idiopathic myelofibrosis)

Platelet distribution disorders

Pooling	Hypersplenism, hypothermia, vascular
Dilution	Massive transfusion[a]

Platelet destruction disorders

Coagulative consumption	DIC, urosepsis, snake venom, crush injury
Isolated consumption	TTP, HUS, HELLP
Immune destruction	ITP, HIT, isoimmune neonatal purpura, post-transfusion purpura, drugs, collagen-vascular disease, infections (e.g., HIV), neoplasia

DIC, disseminated intravascular coagulation; HELLP, hemolytic anemia/elevated liver enzymes/low platelets; HIT, heparin-induced thrombocytopenia; HIV, human immunodeficiency virus; HUS, hemolytic uremic syndrome; ITP, immune thrombocytopenic purpura; TAR, thrombocytopenia with absent radii; TB, tuberculosis; TTP, thrombotic thrombocytopenic purpura.
[a] Dilutional effects, in general, are perhaps the most common cause of thrombocytopenia in a community hospital.

called "microangiopathic hemolysis"), causing the red cell fragmentation (schistocytes) noted on peripheral smears. Other causes of TTP have included, for example, collagen-vascular diseases, multiple myeloma, metastatic carcinoma, pregnancy, and various drugs. **Plasma exchange** is the treatment of choice. **Platelet transfusions are contraindicated**.

2. **Hemolytic uremic syndrome (HUS)**. HUS is similar to TTP, but demonstrates **less pronounced neurologic sequelae and more pronounced renal symptoms**. HUS has been associated with *Escherichia coli* **O157:H7** (often in poorly cooked hamburger), *Shigella dysenteriae*, pregnancy, cancer, drugs (e.g., mitomycin C), and so on. **Dialysis** may be necessary.

3. **HELLP (*h*emolysis, *e*levated *l*iver enzymes, *l*ow *p*latelets) syndrome** is an obstetric disease similar to TTP.

It is associated **with pregnancy or delivery** (a significant number of cases arise 24–48 hours after delivery), and produces a **microangiopathic hemolysis**. The most common presenting symptom is abdominal **right upper quadrant pain**. Complications from HELLP include hepatic rupture, blindness, disseminated intravascular coagulopathy (DIC), and seizures.

   4. Immune thrombocytopenic purpura (ITP). ITP occurs in children and adults. **Children usually have the acute form** of ITP (80%–90% of the cases are acute), whereas **adults have the chronic form** (99.9% of the adult cases are chronic).

   a. Acute ITP is associated with a preceding **viral infection**; it has an abrupt onset, lasts approximately **4 weeks**, does not usually require therapy, and is associated with **full recovery**.

   b. Chronic ITP is rarely associated with viral infections; it has an **insidious onset**, lasts for **years**, often requires **steroids or splenectomy** or both as treatment, and **rarely resolves** completely.

   ITP occurs when IgG (e.g., platelet-associated immunoglobulin: **PAIgG**) attaches to the fibrinogen-binding sites (anti-GPIIb/IIIa) or vWF binding sites (anti-GPIb/IX) on platelets, leading to splenic destruction of platelets without splenomegaly. No morphologic abnormalities are noted on the smear and no routine laboratory tests identify this disorder. Paradoxically, these patients **do not readily bleed**.

   5. Neonatal isoimmune thrombocytopenic purpura. This disorder is analogous to Rh disease of the newborn, and occurs in 1:3000 births. The platelet alloantigen HPA-1a (**PLA-1**) is inherited from the father, and **evokes a maternal antibody response**, which crosses the placenta and destroys the fetal platelets. If therapy is necessary, **maternal platelets can be given** to the neonate (the maternal platelets lack the offending HPA-1a).

   6. Heparin-induced thrombocytopenia (HIT). HIT is a complication of heparin therapy. The most serious form of HIT is caused by an **antibody directed at the heparin platelet factor 4 (PF4) complex**. It occurs most commonly in association with unfractionated heparins. The diagnosis rests primarily in the clinical picture. Few reliable (and available) tests exist to confirm the diagnosis, although platelet aggregation studies (using heparin) may offer supportive evidence.

   a. Type 1 HIT occurs in the **first several days** after instituting heparin therapy; it causes **mild thrombocytopenia** (counts usually remain >100,000/µL), is often **not associated with antibodies**, may resolve without discontinuing heparin, and patients are usually **asymptomatic**.

   b. Type 2 HIT occurs **5–15 days** after the start of heparin (or can occur immediately if the patient has been previously sensitized); it can cause moderately **severe thrombocytopenia** (<100,000/µL) and a paradoxical risk for thrombosis (venous or arterial) in sites that were not originally indicated for anticoagulation. **Heparin must be immediately stopped** for type 2 HIT, and an alternative anticoagulant must be used. **Coumadin may worsen thrombosis**, and recombinant **hirudin** may be the drug of choice.

7. **Drug-induced thrombocytopenia**. A large (almost endless) number of agents have been reported to cause thrombocytopenia.

a. **Agents that cause general marrow aplasia**: radiation, benzene, chemotherapeutic agents [e.g., sulfur and nitrogen mustard agents (busulfan, cyclophosphamide), antimetabolites (e.g., methotrexate, cytosine arabinoside)], colchicine, some antibiotics (e.g., adriamycin, daunorubicin), and so forth.

b. **Agents that selectively suppress platelet production**: ethanol, estrogens, chlorothiazides, and so forth.

c. **Agents that selectively destroy platelets through immune mechanisms**: acetaminophen, cephalothin, diazepam, phenytoin, heparin, methicillin, methyl-DOPA, penicillins, rifampin, sulfisoxazole, and others.

d. **Agents with unknown mechanisms**: allopurinol, ampicillin, aspirin, carbemazepine, chlorpheniramine, cimetidine, codeine, desipramine, digoxin, erythromycin, gentamicin, imipramine, insecticides, isoniazid, lidocaine, minoxidil, nitrofurantoin, nitroglycerine, phenobarbital, phenytoin, prednisone, procainamide, promethazine, sulfamethoxazole, tetracycline, turpentine, vinyl chloride, and so on.

8. **Thrombocytosis**. Thrombocytosis is a quantitative disorder that **can cause bleeding or thrombotic complications** depending on whether the platelets maintain their ability to function. Platelets tend to act like acute phase reactants, and can be elevated in any condition associated with inflammation. **Reactive states rarely cause clinical signs** (although platelet counts can rise above 1 million/μL) (Table 2-28). Essential or **neoplastic thrombocytoses are often associated with dysfunctional platelets**.

V. **Qualitative abnormalities of platelet function**. Qualitative platelet disorders, which may or may not be associated with a normal platelet count, include connective tissue disorders, adhesion disorders, platelet-platelet interaction disorders, and disorders of platelet granules.

Table 2-28. Common causes of thrombocytosis

Reactive	Essential
Iron deficiency	Essential thrombocytosis
Recent hemorrhage	Polycythemia rubra vera
Inflammation	Chronic myelocytic leukemia
Neoplasia (e.g., carcinoma)	Myelodysplasia (RARS)
Splenectomy	AML-M7 with inv(3)
Drugs	

AML, acute myeloblastic leukemia; RARS, refractory anemia with ringed sideroblasts.

A. Connective tissue disorders may interfere with the exposure or adherence of vWF to the subendothelial connective tissue. Inherited disorders include Ehlers–Danlos syndrome and hereditary hemorrhagic telangiectasia. Acquired disorders include amyloidosis, scurvy, and anorexia.

B. Adhesion disorders. Normal platelet aggregation requires adequate amounts of functional vWF, which binds subendothelial proteins to GPIb/IX on platelet surfaces.

  1. Hereditary adhesion disorders

    a. Bernard–Soulier disease: a severe, rare, autosomal recessive disorder in which the **platelets lack the GPIb/IX that normally binds vWF**; it is also associated with thrombocytopenia. **Giant platelets** can be seen on peripheral blood smears. The platelets have an **impaired response** to ristocetin in platelet aggregation studies. Paradoxically, the tendency to bleed resolves somewhat over the patient's lifetime.

    b. von Willebrand's disease is the **most common congenital bleeding disorder**. Many types of vWD are seen. **Most are associated with an abnormality in vWF, and most have *normal* platelets** (Table 2-29). The clinical presentation is variable and many people with vWD are relatively asymptomatic. VWF also serves as the carrier protein for factor VIII:C; therefore, the **factor VIII: Ag level** (which is the quantity of VIII:C as measured by immunologic methods) **is usually decreased, along with vWF**. However, remember that factor VIII:Ag is an acute phase reactant. During pregnancy, healing, or inflammation, VIII:Ag levels often rise to normal levels in patients with vWD.

      (1) vWD, type I: the "classic" and **most common form** of vWD; it is autosomal dominant and associated with an **absolute decrease** in vWF and an absolute decrease in factor VIII coagulant activity (VIII:C). Laurell rocket electrophoresis was the classic method for detecting a decrease in vWF antigen. **Ristocetin cofactor activity is decreased** (reflecting a decreased amount of vWF to interact with platelets).

      (2) vWD, type IIA: autosomal dominant; **high-molecular weight multimers (HMWM) are absent in plasma and platelets** (VIII:Ag is also dysfunctional). **Ristocetin cofactor activity is absent**. In platelet aggregation studies, **no response to ristocetin** occurs.

      (3) vWD, type IIB: autosomal dominant; HMWM is absent in plasma, because **all HMWM binds to platelets**. A mild decrease is seen in ristocetin cofactor activity in the plasma. In platelet aggregation studies, a **hypersensitive response to ristocetin** occurs (increased aggregation because of the increased binding of vWF to platelets). **Desmopressin analogues (DDAVP) are contraindicated** in these patients, because they cause the release of more vWF and subsequent thrombosis to occur.

      (4) vWD, type III: autosomal recessive; **vWF:Ag is absent** and **ristocetin cofactor activity is absent. Factor VIII:C is severely decreased** (1–5 U/dL).

Table 2-29. Laboratory differentiation of von Willebrand's disease types

Laboratory Test	Type I	Type IIA	Type IIB	Type III
Platelet count	Normal	Normal	Normal	Normal
Bleeding time	Normal to increased	Increased	Increased	Increased
Factor VIII: C (plasma level)	Decreased	Normal or mildly decreased	Normal or mildly decreased	Severely decreased
vWF (plasma level)	Decreased	Mildly decreased	Mildly decreased	Severely decreased
Ristocetin cofactor activity	Decreased	Severely decreased	Normal to decreased	Severely decreased
Platelet aggregation with ristocetin	Normal to decreased	Severely decreased	Increased	Severely decreased

vWF, von Willebrand factor.

   2. Acquired adhesion disorders: uremia and various medications.
C. **Platelet-platelet interaction disorders**
   1. **Hereditary platelet-platelet interaction disorders**
      a. **Glanzman's thrombasthenia** is an extremely rare, autosomal recessive disorder in which the **platelets lack GPIIb/IIIa**; therefore, **no fibrinogen bridging occurs**. Patients present with moderate bleeding and normal platelet morphology. Also seen is an associated decrease of platelet antigen PLA-1. The platelet aggregations are "opposite" those of vWD, as they **aggregate *only* with ristocetin**.
      b. **Hereditary fibrinogen disorders**: afibrinogenemia, hypofibrinogenemia, dysfibrinogenemia, for example.
   2. **Acquired platelet-platelet interaction disorders**: fibrin degradation (split) products (e.g., DIC), paraproteins (e.g., from multiple myeloma), various medications.
D. **Disorders of platelet granules and granule release. Two types of platelet granules are seen. Dense body granules** contain ADP, ATP, seratonin, and calcium. **Alpha granules** contain proteins of adhesion (e.g., fibrinogen, vWF), coagulation (e.g., HMWK, factor V), and growth (e.g., platelet-derived growth factor, transforming-growth factor). **Arachidonic acid metabolism** is intimately associated with granule function.
   1. **Dense body disorders.** Hereditary dense body disorders are listed in Table 2-30. Acquired dense body disorders can be associated with autoimmune disorders (e.g., systemic lupus erythematosis, immune thrombocytopenic purpura, various myeloproliferative malignancies, and some leukemias.

Table 2-30. Hereditary disorders of platelet dense body granules

Inherited Syndrome	Clinical Findings	Platelet Tests
Hermansky–Pudlak	Albinism, ceroid deposition in the reticuloendothelial system.	
Chédiak–Higashi	Partial albinism, increased pyogenic infections	Prolonged bleeding times, ↓ADP, ↓ Seratonin, ↓Ca^{++}, ↑ATP:ADP
Wiskott–Aldrich	Eczema, thrombocytopenia, increased serum IgM levels	
Thrombocytopenia with absent radii	Cardiac and skeletal abnormalities, increased bleeding times	

ADP, adenosine diphosphate; ATP, adenosine triphosphate; IgM, immunoglobulin M.

  2.   Alpha granule disorders. Alpha granule disorders are listed in Table 2-31. Acquired alpha granule disorders include cardiopulmonary by-pass surgeries.

  3.   Arachidonic acid is metabolized to TXA_2 by cyclo-oxygenase in the dense tubular system of platelets. TXA_2 is a potent platelet "recruiter." Aspirin, myelodysplasia, and drugs interfere with the cyclo-oxygenase pathway. An inherited cyclo-oxygenase deficiency also exists (the so-called "aspirin-like" defect), and may be diagnosed with platelet aggregation studies.

  E.   Drug-related platelet dysfunction. Many drugs have been found to inhibit platelet function. Aspirin, ticlopidine, and **clopidogrel (Plavix; ADP-binding inhibitor)** are the most important drugs that actually cause clinical bleeding. A partial list of other drugs that affect platelet function to a lesser extent include nonsteroidal anti-inflammatory drugs (NSAIDS; reversible effects that last only as long as the drug is present), anti-biotics (penicillins, cephalosporins, nitrofurantoin, miconazole), heparin, tissue plasminogen activator (TPA), cardiovascular drugs (nitroglycerin, propranolol, sodium nitroprusside, verapamil, diltiazem, nifedipine), chemotherapeutic drugs (daunorubicin, mithramycin), psychotropic drugs (amitryptyline, haloperidol, chlorpromazine), and antihistamines.

VI.   Coagulation

  A.   Overview. Platelets provide fibrinogen, close contact factors, and a phospholipid surface upon which coagulation factors (and circulating fibrinogen) can aggregate. Activation of proteases (e.g., coagulation factors) occurs on platelet surfaces, which then cleave fibrinogen into fibrin, and finally cross links the fibrin. The coagulation system is a **cascade**, in that factors are activated in sequential fashion with amplification. The system is divided into an intrinsic and an extrinsic pathway that meet in a common pathway (Fig. 2-9). The **intrinsic pathway** occurs within the circulation, is initiated by denuded endothelial surfaces or negatively charged substances, and is evaluated by the activated partial thromboplastin time (**aPTT**). The initial components of the intrinsic pathway are called "contact factors," and include high molecular weight kininogen (HMWK) and prekallikrein. The **extrinsic pathway** occurs in extravascular sites, is initiated by tissue factor (a transmembrane glycoprotein), and is evaluated by the prothrombin time (**PT**). Key facts regarding coagulation factors include the following.

  1.   Vitamin K is essential for post-translational carboxylation of factors **II, VII, IX, and X.**

  2.   Factor VIII is the only factor *not* produced in the liver.

  3.   Many of coagulation factors are decreased at birth (and do not reach adult levels for several months), and the aPTT and PT tests cannot be used in newborns.

  4.   Fibrinogen or platelets are at normal levels at birth, and factor VIII:C and VIII:Ag are elevated at birth.

  5.   Factor VIII: Ag and fibrinogen—acute phase reactants—are elevated in any condition associated with inflammation.

Table 2-31. Disorders of platelet alpha granules

Syndrome	Granule Content	Clinical Findings	Laboratory Findings
Gray platelet	Adhesion proteins: fibrinogen, fibronectin, vWF, thrombospondin Coagulation proteins: V, HMWK, fibrinogen Growth modulators: PDGF, CTAF, PF4, TGF, thrombospondin	Thrombocytopenia Normal bleeding time Few symptoms	↓ PF4, normal bleeding time, large gray platelets, ↓platelet aggregation with all agents ↓ PDGF
Extracorporeal circulation			

CTAF, connective tissue-activating factor; HMWK, high molecular weight kininogen; PDGF, platelet-derived growth factor; PF4, platelet factor 4; TGF, transforming growth factor; V, factor V; vWF, von Willebrand factor.

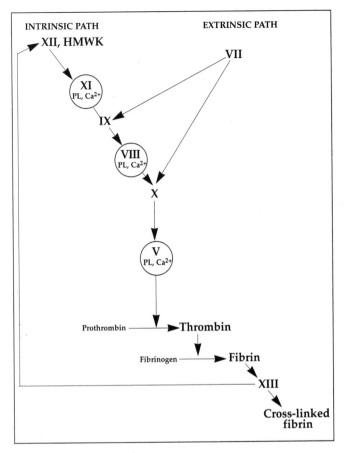

Fig. 2-9. The coagulation pathway. Circle, aggregate of phospholipid, coagulation factors, and platelets; HMWK, high molecular
weight kininogen; PL, phospholipid.

 6. Most significant coagulopathies can be detected by a good
medical history. If a factor deficiency or hepatic-associated
coagulopathy is present, surgical-associated bleeding usually
requires **fresh frozen plasma** or **factor administration**.
B. **Laboratory evaluation of coagulation**
 1. **Activated partial thromboplastin time**
  a. **Used to monitor the intrinsic pathway, to monitor unfractionated heparin therapy, and to detect
factor deficiencies.**
  b. **Evaluates all coagulation factors except VII
and XIII.**

c. **Important collection principles**. Draw in a 3.2% buffered citrated tube with a 9:1 blood:citrate ratio (citrate binds calcium and, thus, prevents coagulation. Do *not* overfill or underfill!). Draw through a peripheral site or a well-flushed line. Draw last if a series of tests are being collected.

d. **Principle of the aPTT**. The citrated blood is mixed with a negatively charged activator, a partial thromboplastin as a phospholipid source, and Ca^{++} (to replenish the Ca^{++} bound by the citrate). The time the specimen takes to form a clot is then measured.

e. **The aPTT is prolonged with factor deficiencies, factor inhibitors, heparin, or lupus anticoagulants.**

f. **If the effects of unfractionated heparin need to be reversed (e.g., postcardiac surgery), protamine sulfate can be given** (0.5 mg for every 100 units of heparin given during the last hour); the activated clotting time (ACT) is the test that is usually used to monitor these changes.

2. **Prothrombin time**

a. **Used to monitor the extrinsic pathway, to monitor warfarin therapy, and to detect a factor VII deficiency.**

b. **The PT is prolonged in the setting of vitamin K deficiency** (e.g., because of diet, changes in bowel flora caused by antibiotics, intestinal malabsorption) or liver disease, before the aPTT becomes prolonged.

c. **The PT does not detect deficiencies in factors XII, XI, IX, VIII, or XIII**.

d. The collection principles for the PT are the same as for the aPTT (see above).

e. **Principle of the PT**. The citrated blood is mixed with tissue factor and Ca^{++} (to replenish the Ca^{++} bound by the citrate). The time the specimen takes to form a clot is then measured.

f. The **International Normalized Ratio** [INR = (PT patient/mean normal PT)[ISI]]; ISI (International sensitivity index) is a measure of the sensitivity of the specific tissue factor used in the test, as compared with a World Health Organization standard (normal British brain tissue factor).

g. **Warfarin effects can be reversed in several ways**. If the INR is very high or if immediate reversal is desired, use **fresh frozen plasma**. If the INR is moderately high, **vitamin K** can be administered (which takes several hours to work). If the INR is mildly elevated, **warfarin can be simply stopped**.

3. **Thrombin clotting time (TCT)**

a. **The TCT only detects the activity of fibrinogen**.

b. **Principle of the test**. Citrated blood is mixed with thrombin and Ca^{++}, and the time it takes for the specimen to clot is measured.

c. **The TCT is prolonged with heparin, fibrin split products, dysfibrinogenemia, hypofibrinogenemia, afibrinogenemia, and thrombolytic agents.**

4. Factor assays are based on dilutions of an assayed standard; the aPTT is used for the standard curve. Patients and controls are compared with the dilutional standard aPTT curve.

5. The 5M urea clot dissolution method is the only way to detect factor XIII, which is the factor that cross links fibrin. The test detects severe deficiencies (<1 U/dL) in factor XIII by measuring the time it takes for a clot to dissolve in urea. A severe factor XIII deficiency will cause the clot to dissolve faster than 24 hours (because the uncross-linked fibrin is easier to dissolve).

6. What to do when the PT or aPTT is prolonged. The PT and aPTT are poor screening tests. **They should be obtained only in the face of a significant history pointing to liver disease, coagulopathy, or anticoagulant therapy**. If an aPTT or a PT is abnormal, but there is no history of bleeding, consider the following:

    a. Was the citrated tube underfilled?

    b. Was the citrate concentration 3.2%? (Some tubes are still available with 3.8% sodium citrate.)

    c. Was the specimen contaminated with an anticoagulant such as heparin or coumadin? (For example, is the patient taking either drug, or was the specimen drawn through a heparin-contaminated line?)

    d. Are there fibrin splits present? [Obtain fibrin split products (FSP) or D-dimer tests if suspected.]

    e. A factor deficiency, a factor inhibitor, or a lupus-like anticoagulant may be present (see Fig. 2-10 for the appropriate workup).

C. Monitoring oral anticoagulants

    1. Use blood collection tubes with 3.2% citrate, and analyze the specimen within 24 hours.

    2. Laboratories should use thromboplastin with an ISI of 0.9–1.7; different instruments can affect the ISI.

    3. The PT can be affected by heparin. If heparin contamination is suspected, a TCT is usually performed. If the TCT is prolonged, heparin contamination is assumed, and the sample should be redrawn.

    4. Lupus anticoagulants can alter PT and INR during dosing.

    5. During the initial phase, the PT should be evaluated every 2 days, noting an increase in the PT until the INR is stable. Thereafter, the frequency of monitoring should be tailored to the individual, but is often obtained once a month.

    6. The INR can only be used for monitoring patients with STABLE oral anticoagulation. INR therapeutic goals include the following:

        a. Prophylaxis = 1.3

        b. All other indications except cardiac = 2.0–3.0

        c. Cardiac (e.g., mechanical heart valve prophylaxis) = 2.5–3.5

VII. Factor deficiencies

  A. General facts

    1. All factor deficiencies will give a prolonged aPTT except VII and XIII.

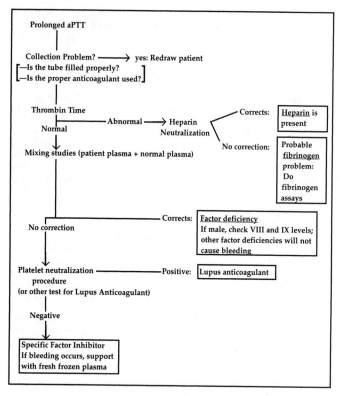

Fig. 2-10.   Evaluation of an isolated prolonged APTT.

    2. When factor deficiencies need to be treated, they should be treated with **specific factor replacements** where possible, and only **when undergoing surgery or actively bleeding**.

    3. **Cryoprecipitate and fresh frozen plasma are "emergency" replacements** for factor-deficient patients when specific factors are unavailable.

B.   Hemophilia A (factor VIII deficiency). Hemophilia A is the most common congenital coagulation factor deficiency (remember that vWD is the most common congenital bleeding disorder overall).

    1. **X-linked recessive** and, therefore, found in **males**.

    2. Associated with **large hemorrhages** into joint, body cavity, intracranial and intramuscular sites; and with **postsurgical bleeding that is delayed** (1–4 hours after surgery) (Table 2-32).

    3. **Variable clinical severity** based on factor VIII levels (normal = 100 U/dL). (See page 154.)

**Table 2-32. Common causes
of bleeding with laboratory results**

Test Results			
Platelet Count	aPTT	PT	Common Causes of Bleeding
N	↑	↑	Coumadin, heparin, ↓vitamin K (e.g., 2° diet, malabsorption, gallbladder disease), liver disease, acute DIC
N	↑	N	Heparin, factors VIII, IX, or XI deficiencies/inhibitors, lupus anti-coagulant, vWD[a]
N	N	↑	Early coumadin, factor VII deficiency/inhibitor, early vitamin K deficiency, early liver disease
N	N	N	Chronic (compensated) DIC, vWD[a], qualitative platelet disorders (e.g., aspirin, ticlopidine, uremia), factor XIII deficiency, tPA, PAI deficiency, fibrinogen disorders (e.g., dysfibrinogenemia), vascular disorders (malformations, vasculitis, scurvy), localized lesions (e.g., colonic carcinoma, endometrial polyps/atrophy)
↓	↑	↑	Acute DIC, HIT, liver disease (especially if hypersplenism is present), some cases of TTP/HUS/HELLP[b]
↓	N	N	Disorders of platelet production/distribution/destruction (see Table 2.27), hemodilution
↑	N	N	Primary hematologic proliferative disorders (e.g., CML, PRV, ET)

N, normal; ↓, decreased; ↑, increased. aPTT, activated partial thromboplastin time; CML, chronic myelogenous leukemia; DIC, disseminated intravascular coagulation; ET, essential thrombocythemia; HELLP, hemolysis/elevated liver enzymes/low platelets syndrome; HIT, heparin-induced thrombocytopenia; HUS, hemolytic uremic syndrome; PAI, plasminogen activator inhibitor; PRV, polycythemia rubra vera; PT, prothrombin time; tPA, tissue plasminogen activator; TTP, thrombotic thrombocytopenic purpura; vWD, von Willebrand's disease.

[a] A minority of the cases of vWD are associated with a prolonged aPTT, because of a concomitant decrease in factor VIII:C (which must be decreased below 45% of normal before the aPTT will be affected). Most cases of vWD have a normal aPTT. Keep in mind that the factor VIII:C level, as an acute phase reactant, may be increased in inflammatory states.

[b] TTP/HUS/HELLP are usually associated with thrombocytopenia and normal aPTT/PT; however, some cases may show prolonged aPTT/PT.

    a. <1 U/dL = severe
    b. 1–5 U/dL = moderate
    c. 5–10 U/dL = mild

    4. **Antibodies (inhibitors)** occur in 11% to 15% of severe hemophiliacs. Anamnestic responses occur (exposure to small amounts of factor VIII will cause large rises in detectable antibody in someone who has been previously sensitized). Antibodies are time- and temperature-dependent, and are measured in **Bethesda units**: ability of the patient's plasma to inactivate 50% of factor VIII activity of normal plasma after 2 hours of incubation at 37°C.

    5. **Treat with factor VIII concentrates** (see *Blood Component Therapy* chapter for calculations).

C. Hemophilia B (factor IX deficiency: "Christmas' disease")

    1. **X-linked recessive** and, therefore, found in **males**.

    2. Associated with **large hemorrhages into joint, body cavity, intracranial and intramuscular sites**; and with **postsurgical bleeding that is delayed** (1–4 hours after surgery).

    3. **Antibodies (inhibitors)** occur in 3% of all hemophilia B patients and 7% to 10% of patients with severe disease. The antibodies are immediate-acting antibodies. Titers fall after exposure.

    4. Patients with **nephrotic syndrome** may develop an acquired factor IX deficiency.

    5. Treat with factor IX concentrates (see *Blood Component Therapy* chapter for calculations).

D. "Contact factor" deficiencies: factor XII ("Hageman Factor"), HMW kininogen, prekallikrein

    1. **Autosomal recessive;** occurs in men and women, children of consanguineous relationships, and isolated gene pools.

    2. **Does not cause clinical bleeding** (Mr. Hageman died of a pulmonary embolus, not from bleeding).

E. Factor XI deficiency

    1. **Autosomal recessive**; Ashkenazi Jewish descent (4.3% gene frequency)

    2. Presentation: **mild bleeding at worst** (20%)

F. Factor VII deficiency

    1. **Autosomal recessive**

    2. **Associated with large hemorrhages into joint, body cavity, intracranial and intramuscular sites**; and with **postsurgical bleeding that is delayed** (1–4 hours after surgery). Spontaneous bleeding does not occur until factor VII levels are <3 U/dL.

    3. **PT is prolonged with a normal Russell viper venom study.**

G. Factor X deficiency

    1. **Autosomal recessive**

    2. Variety of presentations; <15% with the disease will bleed.

    3. **PT and aPTT are increased; TCT is normal.**

    4. Patients with amyloidosis may develop acquired X deficiency.

H. Factor V deficiency (also called "parahemophilia")

    1. Occurs in 1 of 1×10^6 people.

2. Is associated with bruising and soft tissue hemorrhage.

3. **PT, aPTT, and bleeding time are prolonged (platelets too are missing factor V); TCT is normal.**

I. **Factor II (prothrombin) deficiency**

1. **Autosomal recessive;** extremely **rare**

2. Absolute decreases are hypoprothrombinemia; dysfunctional proteins are also seen and are "dysprothrombinemias."

3. **PT and PTT are prolonged**

J. **Factor XIII deficiency**

1. **Autosomal recessive**

2. Presents at birth with **umbilical stump bleeding**; also associated with intracranial hemorrhage, soft tissue hemorrhage, recurrent spontaneous abortions, delayed bleeding, and poor wound healing.

3. PT and aPTT are normal; **5M urea test is abnormal** [dissolves clot in <24 hours (when factor XIII is <1 U/dL)].

K. **Fibrinogen deficiency**

1. **Afibrinogenemia**: autosomal recessive; presents with **severe hemorrhage**.

2. **Hypofibrinogenemia**: autosomal dominant; presents with **moderate bleeding**; the functional levels of fibrinogen are equal to the quantities measured by immunologic assay.

3. **Dysfibrinogenemia**: autosomal dominant; **asymptomatic**; the functional levels of fibrinogen are less than the quantities measured by immunologic assay (there is enough fibrin, but it has **abnormal function**).

VIII. **Natural anticoagulants and thrombophilia**

A. **General review. Local anticoagulation occurs in the intact blood vessel**. If anticoagulation did not occur, clot propagation would continue unchecked throughout the body. The main anticoagulants are protein C, protein S, and antithrombin III (ATIII) (Fig. 2-11).

1. **Protein C**: a vitamin K-dependent serine protease, synthesized by the liver, with plasma levels of 3–5 mg/L. During normal clot formation, **thrombomodulin** (in intact endothelium) binds thrombin, and the complex **activates protein C**. Protein C promotes anticoagulation by **cleaving factors Va and VIIIa**.

2. **Protein S**: a vitamin-K dependent cofactor (not a serine protease), synthesized by the liver, megakaryocytes, and endothelial cells, with plasma levels of 20–25 mg/L. Of protein S, 60% is normally bound by C4b-binding protein; the unbound "free" portion is the active portion. Protein S **helps bind activated protein C to phospholipid**.

3. **Antithrombin III** is a serine protease inhibitor, synthesized by the liver, with normal plasma levels of 140 mg/mL. During normal clot formation, ATIII is activated by heparin-like glycosaminoglycans on endothelial cells, and binds to (thus inhibiting) 75% of the thrombin (**heparin** enhances this reaction 2,000×, thereby preventing coagulation). ATIII also inhibits factors Xa, IXa, XIa, and XIIa.

Disorders in the natural anticoagulant system result in thrombosis. Thrombus formation is caused by three events: changes in blood flow through a vessel (i.e., hemostasis), vessel wall changes, or a hypercoagulable state. **Blood flow and**

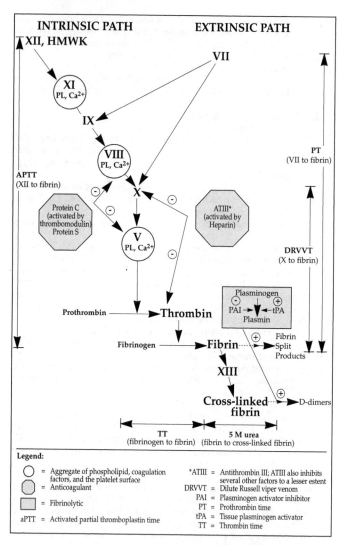

Fig. 2-11. Coagulation tests, anticoagulation, and fibrinolysis.

vessel wall changes are most often the source of thrombi (see risk factors below); hereditary defects in anticoagulants are comparatively rare. **The most common hereditary anticoagulation defect by far is activated protein C resistance, followed by a deficiency of protein C.**

B.   Risk factors for thrombosis. Surgery, trauma, malignancy, sepsis, immobility, obesity, congestive heart failure, oral contraceptives or estrogens, atherosclerosis, smoking, hypertension, diabetes, nephrotic syndrome, and family history are risk factors for thrombosis.

C.   Specific hereditary defects in anticoagulants (thrombophilia or hereditary hypercoagulability)

　1.   Protein C deficiency

　　a.   Protein C deficiency makes up **2% to 5% of all hereditary hypercoagulability cases**, and 15% of young adults with thrombosis. Homozygosity results in death during infancy (e.g., "purpura fulminans").

　　b.   The clinical sign of protein C deficiency is **coumadin-induced skin necrosis**. In normal individuals, a transient hypercoagulable state exists during loading doses of coumadin (because coumadin causes protein C to decrease before the coagulation factors such as X are decreased); this hypercoagulable state is exacerbated in patients with protein C deficiency.

　　c.   Two types of protein C deficiency are seen.

　　　(1)   Type I: Low levels of normal protein

　　　(2)   Type II: Abnormal functioning of protein C

　　d.   Treat with **heparin**; proceed with warfarin slowly.

　2.   Protein S deficiency

　　a.   Protein S deficiency is involved in **10% of the cases** of young patients (<45 years of age) with unexplained thrombosis.

　　b.   Treat with **heparin**; maintain with warfarin.

　3.   Activated protein C resistance

　　a.   Caused by a **genetic factor V alteration** (base pair substitution), which produces "factor V Leiden." **Factor V Leiden resists activated protein C (APC) degradation** and, hence, can lead to thrombus formation. The risk for thrombosis is increased any time in life.

　　b.   Of the normal population, 6% have factor V Leiden (which may make it **the most common genetic disease**). Of patients with deep venous thrombosis (DVT), 40% have factor V Leiden.

　　c.   Laboratory tests for diagnosis.

　　　(1)   APC ratio: (aPTT with APC)/aPTT

　　　Normal APC ratio = 2–3; <2 is suggestive of APC resistance

　　　(2)   Polymerase chain reaction (PCR) (factor V mutation test)

　4.   Antithrombin III (ATIII) deficiency: ATIII deficiency is **autosomal dominant** (1/2,000), and is characterized by thrombosis in unusual sites (e.g., mesenteric veins), and usually has an onset in the late teens.

D.   What to do when a patient has a suspected hyper-coagulopathy (thrombophilia)

1.   Most instances are *not* caused by inherited abnormalities of anticoagulation.

2.   Make sure to treat the thrombus with appropriate anti-coagulation, acutely and chronically.

3.   Make sure patients "at risk" have appropriate prophy-laxis for surgery or immobility.

4.   *Do not evaluate a patient for inherited thrombosis in the face of a recent thrombus* (altered levels of proteins result from recent thrombosis and therapy).

5.   When the patient is stable, order the following tests (and **be sure to tell the laboratory what chronic anti-coagulant the patient in taking**): Activated protein C resistance (factor V Leiden), protein C, protein S, ATIII, lupus anti-coagulant.

IX.   Lupuslike anticoagulants (LLA)

A.   General review. Lupuslike anticoagulants are *not usually* associated with Lupus, and do *not* cause bleeding. LLA are antibodies directed toward phospholipid (PL). Phos-pholipid is essential for the aPTT reaction, and the LLA anti-bodies inhibit the limited amount of phospholipid that is present in the aPTT test, whereas the amount of phospholipid *in vivo* is almost limitless. Therefore, LLA cause a prolongation of aPTT or aPTT-based tests such as factor assays (whence the term "anticoagulant"). LLA can also prolong the PT and PT-based tests such as the dilute Russell viper venom time (DRVVT). However, LLA paradoxically *cause thrombosis* in patients.

B.   Presentation. It is estimated that LAA cause **6% to 8% of thrombi** in patients who are otherwise healthy.

C.   Disease association. Lupuslike anticoagulants are **seen in a variety of illnesses**, including autoimmune dis-orders, viral infections, acquired immunodeficiency syndrome (AIDS) and human immunodeficiency virus (HIV) infections; malignancies; drugs of all classes; and so on. In addition, 5% to 10% of patients with systemic lupus erythematosis (SLE) have lupuslike anticoagulants.

D.   Anticardiolipin syndrome. Lupuslike anticoagulants may be associated with the anticardiolipin syndrome, which involves antibodies directed toward cardiolipin phospho-lipids. **Thromboses occurs in 23% to 58% of the patients** with the anticardiolipin syndrome, which is also associated with recurrent fetal loss and thrombocytopenia.

E.   Laboratory tests for LLA are based on limiting the amount of phospholipid in the test system.

1.   Dilute Russell Viper Venom Test (DRVVT). The phospholipid in the test is diluted to produce a normal clot-ting time of 23–27 seconds. The DRVVT is prolonged in the presence of antiphospholipid antibodies (such as LLA and anti-cardiolipin antibodies), and the prolongation is cor-rected by the addition of platelets (which provide extra phos-pholipid). The DRVVT is the **most sensitive of the tests for LLA**.

2. Kaolin clotting time (KCT). Kaolin is sensitive to the LLA, and therefore the KCT is **prolonged in the presence of LLA**.

3. Anticardiolipin antibodies are obtained if the anti-cardiolipin syndrome is suspected. In general, when interpreting the significance of anticardiolipin antibodies (and other antiphospholipid antibodies such as antiphosphatidylserine), **the clinical significance of an antiphospholipid antibody is greater when the antibody is IgG rather than IgM, when the antibody titer is high, and when the antibody titer remains elevated for a prolonged period of time** (e.g., >2 months).

F. Treatment. The LLA often resolves when the underlying condition is resolved. Treatment is not indicated except with a history of thrombosis. The anticardiolipin syndrome with thrombosis requires long-term anticoagulation.

X. Fibrinolysis

A. General review. Plasminogen is adsorbed onto fibrin polymers within the clot. **Plasminogen activator** (from surrounding endothelial cells) then "activates" the plasminogen into **plasmin, which lyses fibrin into fibrin split products. When plasmin lyses cross-linked fibrin, the results are D-dimers** (Fig. 2-11). **Alpha-$_2$-antiplasmin inactivates plasmin,** and a deficiency in alpha-$_2$-antiplasmin leads to bleeding.

B. Tests of fibrinolysis

1. Fibrinogen: both the quantity (with immunologic tests) and functional ability of fibrinogen can be measured.

2. Euglobulin clot lysis: plasminogen, tPA, and fibrinogen are precipitated with acetic acid, allowed to clot, and the dissolution time is recorded (2–4 hours); this test measures the level of **plasminogen activator**.

3. Fibrin split (degradation) products/D-dimers: antibody directed at FSP/D/E is adsorbed onto an indicator, and the patient sample is added. If FSP/D-dimers are present, clumping occurs. Serial dilutions allow **quantitation of the FSP/D-dimers**.

C. Fibrinolytic disorders

1. Disseminated intravascular coagulation. A variety of underlying disorders cause the release of tissue factors, resulting in coagulation and fibrinolysis.

a. Acute (uncompensated) DIC: factors are consumed faster than they are replenished. Occurs with sepsis, trauma, burns, shock, obstetric emergencies (e.g., amniotic fluid embolism, eclampsia, HELLP syndrome), acute promyelocytic leukemia (FAB-M3), and so forth. Laboratory findings include the following:

(1) Thrombocytopenia

(2) Microangiopathic hemolytic anemia (e.g., schistocytes); findings variable

(3) Decreased fibrinogen (for *that* patient: remember that fibrinogen is an acute phase reactant. It can be very elevated because of tissue injury and then start to decrease because of consumption), and **decreased factor VIII.**

      (4)   **Elevated PT, aPTT, TCT, fibrinopeptide A, and FSP/D-dimer; positive protamine sulfate test**
   b.   **Chronic (compensated DIC): factor consumption is compensated** (or overcompensated) by replenishment of factors. Occurs in various malignancies (e.g., pancreatic, gastric, lung, breast, leukemia), myeloproliferative disorders, paroxysmal nocturnal hemoglobinuria, obstetric disorders, and so forth (Fig. 2-12). Laboratory findings include:

      (1)   **Normal platelet count**
      (2)   **Normal PT, aPTT** and **fibrinogen**
      (3)   **TCT may be normal or elevated; elevated fibrinopeptide A and FSP/D-dimer; positive protamine sulfate test**

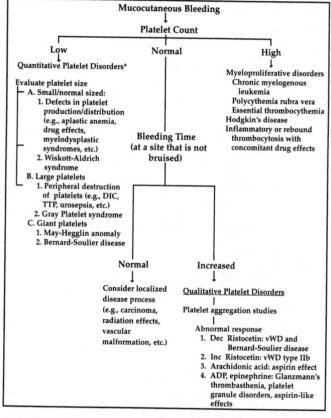

Fig. 2-12.   Evaluation of suspected platelet disorders. DIC, disseminated intravascular coagulation; TTP, thrombotic thrombocytopenic purpura; Dec, decreased platelet aggregation with the listed agent; Inc, increased platelet aggregation with the listed agent; vWD, von Willebrand's disease. *Some of these disorders have a qualitative defect as well.

2. **Systemic fibrinolysis**. A variety of disorders cause **degradation of uncross-linked fibrin**, such as liver disease, plasminogen activators (e.g., tPA), thrombolytic therapy such as streptokinase and urokinase. Laboratory findings include
   a. **Normal platelet count**
   b. **Decreased fibrinogen**
   c. **Increased FSP**
   d. **Normal (or slightly increased) D-dimer and fibrinopeptide A**
   e. **Elevated factor VIII (factor VIII is an acute phase reactant and will be elevated in various inflammatory conditions, including liver disease).**
   f. **Decreased euglobulin clot lysis**

BIBLIOGRAPHY

Brandt JT, McLendon WW, eds. College of American Pathologists Conference XXXI on Laboratory Monitoring of Anticoagulant Therapy. *Arch Pathol Lab Med* 1998;122:765–816.

Miller JL. Blood coagulation and fibrinolysis. In: Henry JB. *Clinical diagnosis and management by laboratory methods*, 19th ed. Philadelphia: WB Saunders, 1996:719–747.

Miller JL. Blood platelets. In: Henry JB. *Clinical diagnosis and management by laboratory methods*, 19th ed. Philadelphia: WB Saunders, 1996:701–719.

3

Microbiology

Microbiologic Diagnosis: Clinical and Laboratory Differentiation

James C. Overall, Jr.

I. Introduction

A. Frequency of infectious diseases. In the office or outpatient setting, infectious disease is one of the most common problems (e.g., 60%–85% of all emergent and walk-in visits to a pediatric practice). Infectious disease is also one of the most common problems encountered in the hospital setting, either as the admitting diagnosis or as a complication during admission.

B. Importance of specific microbiologic diagnosis. Making a specific microbiologic diagnosis is important for the following reasons.

1. **Proof of a particular microorganism enables specific antimicrobial therapy**.

2. **Some infectious disease clinical syndromes** (e.g., pneumonia, diarrhea, sepsis syndrome) **are caused by a variety of different microorganisms** (bacteria, viruses, fungi, parasites), and each may require a different antimicrobial agent. In a seriously ill patient, several antimicrobials may be initiated to "cover all the bases."

3. **Initial empiric broad spectrum therapy can be switched to specific targeted treatment**, thereby reducing expense, adverse effects, and pressure on emergence of antibiotic-resistant organisms (e.g., penicillin-resistant pneumococcus).

4. **Initial antimicrobial therapy may be discontinued** if a microorganism is identified that does not respond to antibiotics [e.g., demonstration of enterovirus in the cerebrospinal fluid (CSF) of a patient with partially treated meningitis]. This can also enable shortened hospitalization, reduced adverse effects, and decreased hospital costs.

5. **A treatable microbial cause may be found that was not initially treated**. For example, herpes simplex virus (HSV) may be found in a neonate or in a patient with stomatitis; influenza may be diagnosed in a patient with pneumonia and underlying cardiopulmonary disease; amebiasis may be discovered in a patient with bloody diarrhea.

II. Approach to microbiologic diagnosis: important points to consider

A. Some infectious disease syndromes can be diagnosed on clinical features alone and/or are clearly bacterial or viral. These may not require special efforts to define the cause. **Common bacterial syndromes include otitis media, cellulitis, skin abscess, and sinusitis. Viral syndromes include measles, varicella and herpes zoster, roseola** (human herpesvirus types 6 and 7), **erythema infectiosum** (parvovirus), **herpangina** and **hand-foot-mouth syndrome** (coxsackie A viruses), **croup**, and **bronchiolitis**.

B. Obtain all specimens. Before antimicrobial therapy is begun, it is important to obtain the most likely causative agents. In addition to common bacteria and fungi, think also about viruses and parasites. Specimens often forgotten include saving an acute phase serum for later serologic tests; and saving an initial CSF to test for bacterial antigens, HSV, and enteroviruses [by polymerase chain reaction (PCR)], if initial Gram's stains and cultures are negative.

C. Indicate body site source. It is **critical to indicate** on the laboratory test request slip **the body site source** of the specimen (e.g., swab of vesicle, eye, or cervix), and the presumed or **suspected diagnosis** (e.g., varicella, conjunctivitis, or cervicitis). With this information, microbiology personnel may suggest additional important diagnostic tests at the outset that can provide answers more quickly and positively influence patient management.

D. Important specimens. Those obtained during surgery or by bronchoalveolar lavage, for example, **may require special transport** conditions or follow particular **protocols in the laboratory**. Check with procedures at your institution.

E. Gram's stain and other rapid tests in the laboratory may provide information quickly that can assist decisions about initial patient management.

F. Requirements for some specimens or suspected organisms

    1. Special transport media. For example, stool for any *Enterobacteriaceae*, stool for ova and parasites; and specimens for anaerobes, *Neisseria gonorrhoeae*, or *Bordetella pertussis*.

    2. Special culture media in the laboratory. For example, *B. pertussis, N. gonorrhoeae, Franciscella tularensis, Yersinia pestis, Mycobacterium* species, *Enterohemorrhagic Escherichia coli, Mycoplasma* species, *Corynebacterium diphtheriae*.

    3. Advance notification of the laboratory because of infectious hazard to microbiology personnel, such as *M. tuberculosis, F. tularensis, Y. pestis*.

G. Common causes for false-negative results

    1. Delayed collection of specimen when the infectious agent is no longer present, or has been suppressed by therapy.

    2. Inadequate or poor specimen

        a. Pus instead of mucosal cells in an epithelial lesion

        b. Nasopharyngeal (NP) swab instead of NP aspirate in respiratory infection

        c. Sputum instead of tracheal aspirate in a freshly intubated, critically ill patient; **or instead of a bronchoalveolar lavage** in an immunocompromised patient with pneumonia

        d. Wrong kind of swab for the particular organism or specimen type

        e. Improper transport (e.g., inappropriate delay, wrong temperature)

H. For optimal microbiologic results in unusual or complex situations, contact laboratory personnel before obtaining specimens. Often, microbiology personnel can suggest additional organisms to consider, or remind physicians of one of the items in II.B–G.

III. Tables of common infectious disease syndromes (Tables 3-1 through 3-10). Physicians see patients with infectious disease clinical syndromes. The purpose of the tables below is to list the common clinical syndromes, the usual organisms in order of frequency for each syndrome, the epidemiologic and clinical features associated with each organism or group of organisms, and the preferred specimen and diagnostic test for each organism or group of organisms. The tables are arranged in an anatomic fashion (head to toe). The features listed are those which help differentiate among the causative agents for a given clinical syndrome, rather than describing similarities. This will enable the physician to consider the most likely causative agent in each syndrome and pursue the microbiologic diagnosis accordingly. For more details on a particular microorganism, consult the appropriate subsequent chapter.

Note: For each of the clinical syndrome tables, only the most common causative agents are listed. Additional microorganisms (*text continues on page 182*)

Table 3-1. Encephalitis

Etiology	Features Suggesting Etiology	Recommended Specimen; Preferred Diagnostic Test
HSV	Nonseasonal Focal neurologic findings: clinical and/or neuroradiologic	CSF; PCR for HSV genome
Arboviruses: St. Louis encephalitis, California equine encephalitis, others	Summer season, mosquito exposure More diffuse neurologic findings Geographic influence on particular virus	Serum; antibody titer rise (results in a delay in diagnosis) CSF for PCR for conserved portion of genome—available through state health laboratories
CMV; *Toxoplasma gondii*	Immunocompromised host (e.g., AIDS).	CSF; PCR for CMV and for *T. gondii* genomes
HIV	AIDS patient Different neurologic syndromes: meningitis early, encephalopathy with dementia late; also myelopathy and peripheral neuropathy	CSF; PCR for HIV genome

AIDS, acquired immunodeficiency syndrome; CMV, cytomegalovirus; CSF, cerebrospinal fluid; HIV, human immunodeficiency virus; HSV, herpes simplex virus; PCR, polymerase chain reaction

Table 3-2.   Features supporting viral rather than partially treated bacterial meningitis

Epidemiologic or clinical features
Enterovirus season: summer, fall
Enterovirus-compatible disease in the community, particularly in a close contact
Enteroviruslike rash in the patient
Decrease in severity of headache and clinical improvement after lumbar puncture (LP)
Absence of other infections that suggest bacterial disease: otitis media, lobar pneumonia

Initial cerebrospinal fluid (CSF) findings
Lymphocyte predominance in the differential count
Normal CSF sugar in relation to blood sugar
Normal CSF lactate and C-reactive protein (CRP)
Presence of atypical lymphocytes on a cytospin smear of CSF cells
Low levels of CSF tumor necrosis factor (TNF) or interleukin-6 (IL-6)
Negative bacterial antigen detection tests on CSF (perform only if gram stains and culture are negative and if the information is medically important)

If the initial CSF demonstrates neutrophil predominance, repeat LP in 24 to 48 hours
Shift to lymphocyte predominance in viral meningitis
Neutrophil predominance persists in treated bacterial meningitis

Table 3-3.   Conjunctivitis

Age or Patient Group	Etiology	Features Suggesting Etiology	Recommended Specimen and Preferred Diagnostic Test
Neonate, young infant	*Neisseria gonorrhoeae*	Onset within 3–5 days after birth Usually bilateral Gram-negative intracellular diplococci on Gram's stain	Swab of eyelid mucosa—use swab with the transport media kit; culture directly on Thayer Martin media at bedside; molecular tests also available.
Neonate, young infant	*Chlamydia trachomatis*	Onset 5–12 days after birth Usually unilateral	Transport media swab of eyelid mucosa for cell culture; molecular tests also available.

Table 3-3. *Continued*

Age or Patient Group	Etiology	Features Suggesting Etiology	Recommended Specimen and Preferred Diagnostic Test
Older infant, child	*Haemophilus influenzae* type b	Associated otitis media	Culturette swab of eyelid mucosa for culture.
Older infant, child, adult	Adenovirus	Usually bilateral, with lymphoid follicles in palpebral conjunctivae late in course; URI symptoms, cervical lymphadenopathy	Transport media swab of eyelid mucosa for cell culture.
Adult	Bacteria: *Streptococcus pneumoniae, Staphylococcus aureus,* others	Usually bilateral, with mucopurulent discharge	Culturette swab of eyelid mucosa for culture.
Any age	Herpes simplex virus	Usually unilateral, with vesicles on eyelid	Transport media swab of eyelid mucosa for cell culture; DFA stain of cells is rapid and reasonably accurate; molecular tests also available.

DFA, direct fluorescent antibody stain of cells; URI, upper respiratory infection.

Table 3-4. Pharyngitis, stomatitis

Clinical Syndrome	Etiology	Features Suggesting Etiology	Recommended Specimen, Preferred Diagnostic Test
Pharyngitis	Group A beta strep-tococcus (GABS)	Winter, spring season School-aged child Exposure to GABS in close contact Headache, abdominal pain, nausea No common cold symptoms Scarlet fever rash	Culturette throat swab for culture; antigen detection is slightly less sensitive and specific than culture.
Pharyngitis	Epstein–Barr virus (EBV)	Older school-aged child, adolescent Hepatosplenomegaly Rash with ampicillin Lymphocytosis, atypical lymphocytes Moderately elevated liver enzymes	Serum; Mono Spot test in patients >5 years of age; in young children, EBV IgM antibody present.

Pharyngitis	Adenovirus	Associated common cold symptoms Conjunctivitis	Throat swab, respiratory specimen, or eye mucosa swab for cell culture.
Pharyngitis	Coxsackie A viruses (Herpangina)	Summer, fall season Preschool-aged child Ulcers on tonsils, soft palate	Throat swab, respiratory specimen; cell culture is insensitive; do PCR for enteroviruses, if medically important.
Stomatitis	Coxsackie A viruses (Hand-foot-mouth syndrome)	Summer, fall season School-aged child Ulcers on buccal mucosa, tongue, pharynx; vesicles on palms, soles	Throat swab, respiratory specimen; cell culture is insensitive; do PCR for enteroviruses, if medically important.
Gingivo stomatitis	Herpes simplex virus (HSV)	Usually infant, toddler Ulcers on lips, gingiva, buccal mucosa, tongue Vesicles on skin around lips	Swab of ulcers, vesicles for cell culture in shell vial; antigen detection tests are less sensitive/specific.

PCR, polymerase chain reaction.

Table 3-5.   Bronchitis, bronchiolitis

Clinical Syndrome	Etiology	Features Suggesting Etiology	Recommended Specimen, Preferred Diagnostic Test
Bronchitis	Respiratory viruses, esp. respiratory syncytial virus (RSV), influenza (FLU), paraFLU, adenoviruses	Fall, winter season Common cold symptoms	Respiratory specimen[a] for cell culture; antigen detection for RSV is good, but less sensitive for the other viruses. Multiplex PCR for RSV, FLU, and paraFLU will be available in the future.
Bronchitis	*Mycoplasma pneumoniae*	Nonseasonal School-aged child Sore throat preceding cough	Respiratory specimen[a] PCR available in referral laboratories. Use only in hospitalized patients.
Bronchitis	*Bordetella pertussis*	Underimmunized or not immunized for pertussis Paroxysmal cough Lymphocytosis	Respiratory specimen[a]; PCR for *B. pertussis* genome; DFA and culture insensitive
Bronchiolitis	Respiratory viruses: RSV, FLU	Infant, toddler Expiratory wheeze Air trapping on chest x-ray	Respiratory specimen[a] Same tests as for viruses in bronchitis

DFA, direct fluorescent antibody; PCR, polymerase chain reaction.
[a] Preferred respiratory specimen: nasopharyngeal aspirate, tracheal aspirate immediately following initial intubation, bronchoalveolar lavage.

Table 3-6. Pneumonia

Age or Patient Group	Etiology	Features Suggesting Etiology	Recommended Specimen Preferred Diagnostic Test
Young infant	*Chlamydia trachomatis, Ureaplasma urealyticum,* Cytomegalovirus (CMV)	Afebrile, slowly progressive course Infiltrate on x-ray is diffuse, with air trapping	[a]Respiratory specimen, transport in M4 viral transport media[b] PCR for *C. trachomatis* Culture for *U. urealyticum,* CMV.
Infant, toddler, school-aged child, adult	Respiratory viruses: RSV, FLU, paraFLU, adeno-viruses	Fall, winter season Infiltrate on x-ray is diffuse or perihilar, nonconsolidating	[a]Respiratory specimen Tests are the same as for bronchitis, viruses
Infant, toddler, school-aged child, adult	Bacteria: *Streptococcus pneumoniae, Haemophilus influenzae, Staphylococcus aureus,* Group A beta strepto-coccus, other	Neutrophilic leukocytosis Infiltrate on x-ray is focal or localized, consolidating Pleural effusion	[a]Respiratory specimen Culture
School-aged child, young adult	*Mycoplasma pneumoniae*	Nonseasonal Atypical pneumonia syndrome Infiltrate on x-ray is nonconsolidating	[a]Respiratory specimen PCR available in referral laboratories; use only in hospitalized patients IgM antibody positive late in course
School-aged child, young adult	*Chlamydia pneumoniae*	Same as for *M. pneumoniae*	[a]Respiratory specimen Culture on special media IgM antibody titers

continued

Table 3-6.   Continued

Age or Patient Group	Etiology	Features Suggesting Etiology	Recommended Specimen Preferred Diagnostic Test
School-aged child, young adult	*Pseudomonas aeruginosa, Pseudomonas cepacia*	Cystic fibrosis	[a]Respiratory specimen Culture
School-aged child, adult	Enterobacteriaceae, *Legionella* sp.	Nosocomial acquired Infiltrate on x-ray is localized, consolidating	[a]Respiratory specimen Culture for Enterobacteriaceae DFA for *Legionella* sp.
School-aged child, adult	*Pneumocystis carinii* cytomegalovirus (CMV)	Immunocompromised patient Infiltrate on x-ray is diffuse	[a]Respiratory specimen DFA for *P. carinii.* Culture for CMV
School-aged child, adult	Mixed anaerobic bacteria	Aspiration	Lower respiratory tract specimen collected under anaerobic conditions for anaerobic culture—**not** sputum or bronchial lavage.

Note: There are many other less common causes of pneumonia: additional bacteria and viruses, fungi, rickettsia, mycobacteria, parasites. Consult clinical microbiology or infectious disease sources for more information.
DFA, direct fluorescent antibody; PCR, polymerase chain reaction.
[a] Preferred respiratory specimen: nasopharyngeal aspirate, tracheal aspirate immediately following initial intubation, bronchoalveolar lavage.
[b] M4 media for transport of viruses, *Chlamydia* sp., *Mycoplasma* sp.

Table 3-7. Hepatitis

Etiology	Features Suggesting Etiology	Recommended Specimen, Preferred Diagnostic Test
Hepatitis A virus (HAV)	Fecal oral spread, food/water borne High risk groups: family contacts, custodial care or correctional institutions, summer camps, child care centers, homosexual contacts Acute hepatitis (usually subclinical in children), no chronic disease	Serum Acute disease: anti-HAV IgM present Immunity: anti-HAV total (IgG) present, anti-HAV IgM absent
Hepatitis B virus (HBV)	Spread by blood exposure, sexual contact, transplacental transmission High risk groups: Asian and African populations; IV drug abusers, homosexual men, newborns of carrier mothers, multiple transfused patients, family intimate contacts. Acute disease infrequent; chronic carriage in 5%–10% of children and adults, 10%–90% of perinatally infected neonates	Serum Acute disease: HB surface antigen (HBsAg) and anti-HBc IgM present. Chronic carrier: HBsAg present, but anti-HBc IgM absent. Qualitative PCR for HBV genome available. Quantitative HBV DNA by RNA probe available.

continued

Table 3-7. *Continued*

Etiology	Features Suggesting Etiology	Recommended Specimen, Preferred Diagnostic Test
Hepatitis C virus (HCV)	Spread by blood exposure, organ transplantation; less often by sexual contact. High risk groups: IV drug abusers, African populations. Acute disease rare, chronic carriage in 70%–80%.	Serum Anti-HCV antibody by ELISA, confirmatory antibody by recombinant immunoblot assay (RIBA). Qualitative PCR for HCV genome available. Quantitative HCV RNA by PCR available.
Hepatitis D virus (HDV)	Can infect only patient with current acute or chronic HBV infection. High risk groups: endemic areas (south Italy, South America, Middle East, parts of Africa), homosexual men. Disease: can make HBV disease worse.	Serum Anti-HDV total (IgG) antibody present. Anti-HDV IgM antibody and HDV antigen tests available in referral laboratories.

ELISA, enzyme-linked immunosorbent assay; IV, intravenous; PCR, polymerase chain reaction.

Table 3-8. Gastrointestinal tract infections[a]

Clinical Syndrome	Etiology	Features Suggesting Etiology	Recommended Specimen Preferred Diagnostic Test
Watery diarrhea	Enterotoxigenic bacteria: *Escherichia coli*, others	Travel associated	Commercial assay for enterotoxigenic *E. coli* (ETEC) is not available.
Watery diarrhea	Protozoa: *Giardia lamblia*, others	Travel, contaminated water supply. Child care center attendance. Diarrhea can be chronic	Fresh stool for ova and parasite microscopy. *G. lamblia* rapid antigen detection test
Watery diarrhea	Preformed enterotoxins: *Staphylococcus aureus*, *Bacillus cereus*, *Clostridium perfringens*	Food-borne poisoning. Vomiting and/or diarrhea	Commercial assays for preformed toxins are not available.
Bloody diarrhea, dysentery syndrome, blood and mucus in stool	*Shigella* sp, *Salmonella* sp, Enteroinvasive and enterohemorrhagic *E. coli*, *Campylobacter* sp, *Entamoeba histolytica*, others	Travel. Fever, abdominal cramps. Fecal neutrophils present	Fresh stool. Stool culture first, follow with additional confirmatory tests. *Campylobacter* sp.—special media required. *E. histolytica*—microscopy, antigen detection. Serum antibody for amebic liver abscess

continued

Table 3-8.   *Continued*

Clinical Syndrome	Etiology	Features Suggesting Etiology	Recommended Specimen Preferred Diagnostic Test
Gastroenteritis	Enteric viruses: rotaviruses, calicivirus, astroviruses, enteric adenoviruses	Vomiting followed by watery diarrhea Fecal leukocytes variable	Fresh stool Rotavirus, enteric adeno antigen detection tests Electron microscopy for other viruses
Antibiotic-associated colitis	*Clostridium difficile*	Watery diarrhea Fecal neutrophils Pseudomembranes in colon	Fresh stool Culture, confirm by cell culture cytotoxin assay

[a] Evaluation of the etiology of GI tract infection is complex because of the large number of causative agents, and the variety of laboratory tests. In addition to the features listed above, etiology is influenced by factors such as age of patient, transmission from contaminated food or water, prior antimicrobial therapy, immunocompromised host, and nosocomial acquisition. Consult clinical microbiology or infectious disease sources for more information.

Table 3-9. Vaginitis, urethritis, genital vesicles or ulcers

Clinical Syndrome	Etiology	Features Suggesting Etiology	Recommended Specimen, Preferred Diagnostic Test
Urethritis	*Neisseria gonorrhoeae*	Abrupt onset after exposure Mucopurulent discharge Gram-negative intracellular diplococci on stain	Urethral swab Preferably inoculate on special media at bedside. If not, use GC transport media, and then culture on special media.
Urethritis	*Chlamydia trachomatis*	Gradual onset after exposure Thin mucoid discharge	Urethral swab, first portion of voided urine PCR for *C. trachomatis* genome Also, culture/ DNA probe, but less sensitive
Cervicitis	*Neisseria gonorrhoeae*	Mucopurulent discharge May have associated pelvic inflammatory disease	Endocervical swab, first portion of voided urine Tests same as for urethritis
Cervicitis	*Chlamydia trachomatis*	Mucopurulent discharge Cervical ectopy with edema Easily induced endocervical bleeding	Same as for cervicitis
Genital ulcers, vesicles	Herpes simplex virus (HSV)	Several ulcers and/or vesicles in primary disease, few vesicles in recurrent disease Painful, regional nodes	Swab from viral transport media kit Cell culture in shell vial Antigen detection tests are less sensitive

continued

Table 3-9.   *Continued*

Clinical Syndrome	Etiology	Features Suggesting Etiology	Recommended Specimen, Preferred Diagnostic Test
Genital ulcer	*Treponema pallidum*	Usually single ulcer, painless Slower onset than HSV	Serum for VDRL, confirmatory anti-IgM antibody Scraping from base of ulcer for darkfield microscopy, rapid transport to laboratory required

HSV, herpes simplex virus; PCR, polymerase chain reaction.

Table 3-10.   Molecular methods—when is it the preferred diagnostic test?

Clinical Syndrome	Etiology	Recommended Specimen, Preferred Diagnostic Test
Aseptic (viral) Meningitis	Enteroviruses	CSF PCR for enteroviruses
Encephalitis	HSV, Arboviruses	CSF PCR for HSV genome PCR for conserved portion of arbovirus genome available through state health laboratories
Encephalitis in immunocompromised (e.g., AIDS)	*Toxoplasma gondii,* CMV, VZV	CSF PCR for *T. gondii,* CMV, and VZV genomes
CNS syndromes of Lyme disease	*Borrelia burgdorferi*	CSF PCR for *B. burgdorferi genome*
CNS syndromes of infectious mononucleosis	EBV	CSF PCR for EBV genome
HIV infection—diagnosis in neonates or in adults before antibody development	HIV	[a]Plasma Qualitative PCR for HIV genome

Table 3-10. *Continued*

Clinical Syndrome	Etiology	Recommended Specimen, Preferred Diagnostic Test
Chlamydia urethritis, cervicitis	*Chlamydia trachomatis*	Swabs of urethra or cervix, first portion of voided urine from male or female PCR or LCR or SDA or TMA
Tuberculosis	*Mycobacterium tuberculosis*	Respiratory specimen, smear positive or smear negative PCR or TMA for *M. tuberculosis* genome
Pertussis	*Bordetella pertussis*	[b]Respiratory specimen PCR for *B. pertussis* genome
Pneumonia in hospitalized and/or immunocompromised patient	*Mycoplasma pneumoniae, Legionella pneumophila,* Respiratory viruses	[b]Respiratory specimen PCR for *M. pneumoniae* genome DFA for *L. pneumophila* Multiplex PCR for respiratory viruses will be available in future
Pneumonia in hospitalized, immunocompromised patient	*Legionella pneumophila*	[b]Respiratory specimen PCR
Pneumonia in hospitalized, immunocompromised patients (AIDS, transplant recipient)	Respiratory syncytial, influenza, and para-influenza viruses	[b]Respiratory specimen Multiplex PCR available in future
Quantitative viremia in immunocompromised patient (AIDS, transplant recipient)	CMV	Peripheral WBC (collect in EDTA purple top tube) Antigenemia (FA stain of cells) Molecular tests available
Quantitative viremia in hepatitis—to monitor therapy	Hepatitis B virus	Serum RNA probe hybrid capture chemiluminescence assay, others available

continued

Table 3-10.   *Continued*

Clinical Syndrome	Etiology	Recommended Specimen, Preferred Diagnostic Test
Quantitative viremia in hepatitis—to monitor therapy	HCV	[a]Plasma Automated quantitative PCR, other methods available
Quantitative viremia in AIDS—to monitor therapy	HIV	[a]Plasma Automated quantitative PCR, other methods available
Hepatitis C genotyping—to determine prognosis, response to therapy	HCV	[a]Plasma DNA sequencing of amplified PCR product

AIDS, acquired immunodeficiency virus; CMV, cytomegalovirus; CSF, cerebrospinal fluid; EBV, Epstein-Barr virus; HCV, hepatitis C virus; HIV, human immunodeficiency virus; HSV, herpes simplex virus; PCR, polymerase chain reaction; VZV, varicella zoster virus; WBC, white blood cell.

  Molecular methods have become the diagnostic technique of choice for selected situations, as indicated in the Table above. These methods include polymerase chain reaction (PCR), ligase chain reaction (LCR), strand displacement assay (SDA), and transcription-mediated amplification (TMA). Some of these tests may be available in regional medical centers, but many will require sendout to a regional or national referral laboratory.

[a] Plasma = use EDTA purple top tube.
[b] Preferred respiratory specimen: nasopharyngeal aspirate, tracheal aspirate immediately following initial intubation, bronchoalveolar lavage.

can be causative; consult clinical microbiology or infectious disease sources for more information.

BIBLIOGRAPHY

Carroll KC, Overall JC Jr. Diagnostic virology. In: McClatchey KD, ed. *Clinical laboratory medicine*, 2nd ed. Baltimore: Williams & Wilkins (*in press*). Also see other chapters on microbiology diagnosis in same textbook.

Christenson JC, Overall JC Jr. Proper use of the clinical microbiology laboratory. *Pediatr Rev* 1995;16:62–68.

Overall JC Jr. Is it bacterial or viral? Laboratory differentiation. *Pediatr Rev* 1993;14:251–261.

Long SL, Pickering LK, Prober CG. *Principles and practice of pediatric infectious diseases*. New York: Churchill Livingstone, 1997. Several chapters on gastrointestinal tract infections and intoxications and other infectious diseases.

Mandell GL, Bennett JE, Dolin R. *Principles and practice of infectious diseases*, 4th ed. New York: Churchill Livingstone, 1995. Several chapters on gastrointestinal tract infections, pneumonia, and other infectious diseases.

Bacteria

Richard B. Thomson, Jr.

I. Bacterial classification and biology

A. Taxonomic classification. Bacteria are classified according to **phenotypic** (antigens, biochemical reactivity) and **genotypic** (nucleic acid structure) characteristics. Large **families** of bacteria, such as the *Enterobacteriaceae*, are divided into closely related groups called **genera**. Genera are further divided into **species** and species **into biochemical, serological, or molecular types or variants** (i.e., biovars, serovars, and genovars). For example, the genus *Salmonella* has one species, *S. enterica*, and nearly 2,000 serovar (serotypes). *Salmonella enterica* serovar enteritidis is the most common serotype of *Salmonella* detected in the United States.

B. Bacterial structure

1. **Prokaryote cell.** Bacteria have a single **circular chromosome**, a cytoplasmic membrane consisting of a **lipid bilayer** and a rigid **cell wall**. Bacteria can have an outer membrane, a capsule, and extra-chromosomal circular **plasmid** DNA. Bacteria are hosts for lysogenic and lytic **bacteriophage** (viruses that attack bacteria).

2. **Gram-positive bacteria** are characterized by a thick, rigid cell wall consisting of **peptidoglycan**.

3. **Gram-negative bacteria** are characterized by a thin peptidoglycan layer and a thick outer lipopolysaccharide membrane containing lipid A (**endotoxin**).

C. Bacterial metabolism

1. **Aerobic** bacteria grow in the presence, but not in the absence, of oxygen.

2. **Anaerobic** bacteria grow in the absence, but not in the presence, of oxygen.

3. **Facultative** bacteria grow in both the presence and absence of oxygen.

4. **Microaerophilic** bacteria grow best in reduced (compared with ambient) concentrations of oxygen.

5. **Capnophilic** bacteria require increased concentrations of carbon dioxide (compared with ambient) to grow.

6. **Aerotolerant** bacteria are anaerobic bacteria that survive temporary exposure to oxygen.

D. Bacterial growth phases

1. The **lag phase** occurs before cell division while cells accumulate nutrient and precursor molecules.

2. **Exponential growth phase or logarithmic (log) phase** is characterized by rapid cell growth and division.

3. **Stationary phase** involves cessation of cell division following the log phase. Cell growth has exhausted nutrients and precursors. Bacterial cells lose viability over time.

E. Exchange of genetic material among bacteria. Bacteria adapt to environmental changes by acquiring genetic material from other bacteria.

1. **Conjugation**: the direct exchange of genes (DNA) through a connecting pilus or intercellular bridge.

2. **Transduction**: the exchange of genes during infection by bacteriophage.

3. **Transformation**: the uptake of DNA from the environment, after the DNA has been released from other bacteria undergoing lysis.

F. **Virulence and pathogenic mechanisms. Virulence is a measure of a microorganism's ability to cause disease** (pathology). Some bacteria are pathogenic in all human hosts (*Mycobacterium tuberculosis*), whereas others are pathogenic in compromised hosts (*Pseudomonas aeruginosa*). Bacterial pathogenic mechanisms include the following.

1. **Attachment** is required by most bacteria before causing disease (e.g., *Streptococcus pyogenes* that cause pharyngitis and *Escherichia coli* that cause enteritis).

2. **Inhibition of phagocytosis and intracellular killing**. Pneumococcal capsules inhibit phagocytosis of the bacterial cell before homologous antibody production. *Legionella pneumophilia* resists intracellular killing by macrophages, and continues to grow within phagosomes.

3. **Avoidance of immune mechanisms**. *Neisseria gonorrhoeae* avoids immune recognition by altering proteins of attachment pili.

4. **Invasion and dissemination**. *Salmonella* species invade by penetrating epithelial cell layers to reach the basement membrane. Subsequent dissemination requires avoiding immune, lymphatic, and phagocytic killing mechanisms.

5. **Toxin production. The most virulent human pathogens produce exotoxins (toxins)**. Diphtheria, botulinal, tetanus, and toxic shock toxins are examples.

6. **Autoimmune immunopathologic reaction**. Postinfectious immunopathologic lesions (e.g., rheumatic heart disease caused by *S. pyogenes*) result from cross-reacting antibodies that damage human tissue.

7. **Synergistic infection**. Infection and overwhelming disease by multiple bacteria, each one of which is relatively nonpathogenic by itself, is characteristic of synergistic necrotizing cellulitis. Mixtures of anaerobes and enteric gram-negative bacilli are responsible.

G. **Normal flora**. Skin and mucous membranes are normally and continuously colonized by bacteria that can reach concentrations as high as 10^{11}/mL bacteria in the colon. **Infections adjacent to surfaces colonized by normal flora are caused commonly by endogenous flora**. Aspiration pneumonia caused by oral anaerobes and intra-abdominal abscess caused by intestinal anaerobic and facultative flora are examples.

II. **Methods used to detect bacteria**

A. **Specimen collection**. Material for the detection of bacteria causing infection must be representative of a specific pathologic site and free of contaminating normal flora. **Tissue biopsy, needle and syringe aspiration** of fluid, pus and mucous membrane secretions with or without **irrigation, blood, urine, stool**, and **sputum** are the most useful specimens for bacterial culture.

1. Specimen collection from superficial wounds and from the respiratory, urinary, and gastrointestinal tracts (Table 3-11). **Expectorated sputum, endotracheal tube aspirates**, and secretions collected during **bronchoscopy** represent increasingly more invasive respiratory tract specimen collection methods, with a concomitant reduction in contamination and improvement in pathogen recovery. **Midstream urine** is more likely to be contaminated than urine collected by in-and-out catheterization. Urine collected by **suprapubic aspiration** and during **cystoscopy** should be sterile in the absence of pathology. **Stool**, rather than material collected on a rectal swab, is required for the detection of gastrointestinal pathogens.

2. Blood cultures. Collection of blood for culture requires strict adherence to antisepsis, volume, and number of cultures. Venipuncture site disinfection with an iodine-containing (iodine tincture or povidone-iodine) or alcoholic chlorhexidine antiseptic is required before blood culture sampling. No more than 3% of adult blood cultures should be contaminated if proper antisepsis is used. Adult blood cultures may be ordered "stat" or "routine" (Table 3-12). **Stat** cultures should be collected immediately before starting or changing antimicrobial therapy. **Routine** cultures, if anti-microbials will not be started immediately, can be collected over a 12–24 hour period to document a continuous bacteremia.

Blood volumes collected from pediatric patients vary according to patient weight; volumes should increase as the children grow (Table 3-13).

B. Specimen transport

    1. Transport media

        a. Oxygen-free for anaerobes: nitrogen or carbon dioxide atmosphere with moist, reduced medium.

        b. Stuart's or Aimes' for aerobic and facultative bacteria: maintains viability while limiting growth; usually contained in a swab-carrying device.

        c. Carbon dioxide (3%–5%) for *N. gonorrhoeae*

        d. Charcoal in medium to absorb toxic substances

        e. Boric acid solution for urine to stabilize colony counts

        f. Cary–Blair for stool to prevent acidification of specimen

    2. Transport temperature. Refrigeration or on ice for times up to 12 hours. Cerebrospinal fluid (CSF), synovial fluid specimens, and specimens thought to contain gonococci, meningococci, or anaerobes should be held at room temperature. Freezing and longer transport times (>12 hours) are not recommended.

C. Specimen processing by organ system or specimen source

    1. Blood. Twenty milliliters of blood (or the full volume when <20 mL is collected from pediatric patients) is divided evenly between aerobic and anaerobic culture broth. In some clinical settings, aerobic plus anaerobic broth media are not as useful as two aerobic broth culture bottles. The recommended volume of blood (20 mL per culture) is always necessary regardless of media used. In pediatric patients, or the

Table 3-11. Specimen collection from superficial wounds and from the respiratory, urinary, and gastrointestinal tracts

Site	Specimen	
	Appropriate	Inappropriate
Superficial wound	Aspirations of pus or local irrigation fluid (non-bacteriostatic saline); swab of purulence originating from beneath the dermis	Swab of surface material or specimen contaminated with surface material; irrigation with saline containing preservative
Lower respiratory tract	Freshly expectorated mucus and inflammatory cells (pus)—sputum	Saliva, oropharyngeal secretions, sinus drainage from nasopharynx
Nasal sinus	Secretions collected by direct sinus aspirate, or washes, curetting and biopsy material collected during endoscopy; freshly "blown" pus into clean tissue from infected sinuses	Nasal or nasopharyngeal swab, nasopharyngeal secretions, sputum, and saliva
Urinary tract	Midstream urine; urine collected by "straight" catheterization; urine collected by suprapubic aspiration; urine collected during cystoscopy or other surgical procedure	Urine from foley catheter collection bag
Gastrointestinal tract	Freshly passed stool; washes/feces collected during endoscopy	Rectal swab; specimen for bacterial culture if diarrhea developed after patient has been hospitalized for ≥ 3 days

Table 3-12. Blood collection for adult bacterial culture

Type of Culture	When Ordered	Number of Cultures	Volume of Blood/Culture
Adult-Stat	Acute febrile episode; anti-microbials are to be started immediately	2	20 mL each culture
Adult-Routine	Nonacute disease; antimicrobials will not be immediately started or changed	2–3	20 mL each culture

occasional adult, where total blood volume is less than the minimum required per bottle (usually, 3–5 mL), inoculate the entire volume into the aerobic bottle. Blood culture media is incubated for a total of 5–7 days before a final negative (no growth) report is recorded.

   2. Central nervous system. CSF Gram's stains should always be examined as quickly as possible. If >2 mL of CSF are received, cytocentrifuge for smear and pellet of cells and bacteria (centrifuge at $1,000 \times g$ for 10 minutes) should be inoculated to culture media. Brain tissue should be minced and ground gently before culture.

   3. Eye. Corneal scrapings should be inoculated directly to culture media and a smear prepared in the clinic or at bedside, because of the small amount of material collected. Each scraping is rubbed onto the agar surface in a different area. The plates should not be cross streaked by the laboratory. Contaminants are those bacteria that grow away from the inoculated spots. Other specimens (e.g., vitreous fluid, aspirates, tissue) should be processed as usual.

   4. Gastrointestinal tract. Patients who have been in the hospital for >3 days, and who did not have diarrhea at the time of admission, are extremely unlikely

Table 3-13. Blood collection for pediatric bacterial culture

Patient Weight	Number of Cultures	Volume of Blood/Culture
<18 lbs	1–2	1 mL
18–30 lbs	2	3 mL
30–60 lbs	2	5 mL
60–90 lbs	2	10 mL
90–120 lbs	2	15 mL
>120 lbs	2	20 mL

to have bacterial (other than *Clostridium difficile*) or parasitic (protozoan) gastrointestinal disease. Bacterial culture for usual pathogens and examination for parasites should not be performed. *C. difficile* toxin assay or parasite examination for helminths, if epidemiologically justified, are appropriate tests.

   5.   Genital tract. Endocervical and urethral specimens are appropriate for *N. gonorrhoeae* or *Chlamydia trachomatis* culture. A swab of the vaginal wall and a rectal swab are needed to screen for group B streptococcal carriers. Vaginal secretions are required for the diagnosis of vaginitis (*Candida* or *Trichomonas*) and bacterial vaginosis. The Gram's stained smear is used to detect patients with bacterial vaginosis (reduced lactobacillus, clue cells, anaerobic morphologies); culture is not necessary.

   6.   Respiratory tract. Sputum and endotracheal aspirates are screened for squamous epithelial cells. Elevated numbers (>10 per 10× microscope objective field) suggest specimens should not be cultured because of gross oropharyngeal contamination. Endotracheal aspirates are screened for bacteria in the Gram's stain. No bacteria seen suggests specimens should not be cultured because the results will not be helpful. Bronchoalveolar lavage (BAL) fluid should be cultured quantitatively using dilutions or a calibrated loop. The BAL smear should be screened for intra- and extracellular bacteria.

   7.   Skin. Swab specimens should be discouraged. Fluid is used to prepare a smear and is divided evenly among culture media.

   8.   Tissue. Smears of tissue should be prepared from a freshly cut surface that is rolled or gently pressed against the slide (impression smear). Tissue is minced and gently ground before inoculation to agar media.

   9.   Urinary tract. Smears of urine for Gram's staining are prepared using cytocentrifugation (sensitivity as low as 1,000/mL bacteria) or no centrifugation (sensitive to 10,000/mL bacteria). Two bacteria per average 100× microscope objective field (unspun urine) correlate to counts of 100,000/mL bacteria of urine. Quantitative culture of urine is performed using a calibrated loop.

D.   Direct detection in clinical specimens without culture

   1.   Stains. Smears of fluids are prepared using cytocentrifugation. Smears of tissue are made by blotting or rolling the freshly cut surface on a slide. Smears of pus and mucus are made by pressing the specimen between two slides, creating a monolayer of material. Gram's stains are used to differentiate gram-positive and gram-negative bacteria (Table 3-14). Methylene blue stains all cells blue. The Quellung reaction is used with methylene blue to identify encapsulated bacteria. The fluorochrome acridine orange, a nucleic acid intercalating agent, stains all bacteria.

   2.   Antigen detection. Direct and indirect fluorescent antibody stains, conventional (tube or microtiter tray), membrane (reaction membrane within a disposable handheld

Table 3-14. Interpretation of Gram-stained smears

Morphology Observed	Interpretation
Gram-positive cocci—clusters	Staphylococci
Gram-positive cocci—chains	Streptococci
Gram-positive diplococci	*Streptococcus pneumoniae*
Gram-negative diplococci	*Neisseria* and *Moraxella*
Gram-negative coccobacilli	*Haemophilus*
Gram-positive bacillus—diphtheroid	*Corynebacterium* and *Propionibacterium*
Gram-positive bacillus—boxcar	*Clostridium* and *Bacillus*
Gram-positive bacillus—branching	*Actinomyces* and *Nocardia*
Gram-positive bacillus—other	*Listeria* and *Lactobacillus*
Gram-negative bacillus	Enteric and *Pseudomonas*-like Gram-negative bacilli
Yeast cells	Yeast [e.g., *Candida* (*Torulopsis*)] and *Cryptococcus*
Yeast cells with pseudohyphae	*Candida*
Septate hyphae	Mold (e.g., *Aspergillus*)

chamber) enzyme immunoassays, and latex agglutination are used to detect bacterial antigens in patient specimens.

3. Nucleic acid detection. Nucleic acid probes are used to identify bacterial DNA or RNA that is specific for a microorganism in a patient specimen. Low copy numbers of nucleic acid sequences to be detected in a specimen can be amplified by the polymerase chain reaction (PCR), or related techniques such as the ligase chain reaction, to increase the sensitivity of the probe.

E. Culture

1. Plating. Inoculate the specimen to ¼ of the agar plate. Streak specimen into four quadrants to dilute bacteria and inhibitory substances. Quantitate bacterial growth as 1+ through 4+ by reporting the highest quadrant of growth (quadrants 1 through 4).

2. Incubation. Usual incubation is in 3% to 5% CO_2, 35°C to 37°C.

3. Media. Selective and differential media used, depending on pathogens suspected (Table 3-15).

III. Important bacteria, useful characteristics for identification, and selected disease associations

A. Gram-positive cocci occurring in chains, pairs, or clusters

1. Staphylococci: catalase-positive, gram-positive cocci that occur in clusters. Staphylococci account for >75% of suppurative diseases seen clinically. Many species exist; only those important in human disease are listed.

a. Coagulase-positive staphylococci: *Staphylococcus aureus* causes **invasive infections** (e.g., carbuncles, impetigo, wound infections, pneumonia, endocarditis) and diseases related to **staphyloccal toxins** [e.g.,

Table 3-15. Bacterial culture media

Medium	Use
Sheep blood agar	Hemolytic reactions (alpha, beta, non-hemolytic)
Chocolate agar	Fastidious bacteria (esp. *Haemophilus*)
CIN agar	Selective for *Yersinia* in stool
CNA agar	Selective for Gram-positive bacteria
EMB agar	Selective and differential for Gram-negative bacteria
GN broth	Enrichment for *Salmonella* and *Shigella* in stool
Hektoen enteric agar	Selective and differential for *Salmonella* and *Shigella*
MacConkey agar	Selective and differential for Gram-negative bacteria
Martin–Lewis agar	Selective for *Neisseria gonorrhoeae*
New York City agar	Selective for *N. gonorrhoeae*
Phenylethyl alcohol agar	Selective for *Gram-positive bacteria*
Regan–Lowe agar	Selective for *Bordetella pertussis* and *B. parapertussis*
Salmonella–Shigella agar	Selective and differential for *Salmonella* and *Shigella*
Selenite enrichment broth	Enrichment for *Salmonella* and *Shigella* in stool
TCBS agar	Selective and differential for vibrios in stool
Thayer–Martin medium	Selective for *N. gonorrhoeae* and *meningitidis*
Thioglycollate broth	All purpose broth for aerobes and anaerobes
Tryptic soy broth	All purpose broth for aerobes
XLD agar	Selective and differential for *Salmonella* and *Shigella*

food poisoning, toxic shock syndrome, toxic epidermal necrolysis (scalded baby syndrome)].
  b. Coagulase-negative staphylococci (CNS)
    (1) *S. epidermidis*. Novobiocin sensitive; **a common skin commensal** that can cause infections in, for example, immunocompromised hosts, in patients with **artificial heart valves** or **indwelling catheters**, intravenous drug users.
    (2) *S. saprophyticus*. Novobiocin resistant; a cause of **urinary tract infections** (UTI) in young women.
    (3) Others: *S. haemolyticus, S. hominis, S. capitis, S. schleiferi, S. warneri, S. lugdunensis*
  2. Streptococci-Enterococci-Abiotropha. Catalase-negative, gram-positive cocci that occur in pairs and chains.

a. Beta-hemolytic streptococci: detection of cell wall antigens by latex agglutination is used to identify groups.

(1) Group A (*S. pyogenes*). L-pyrrolidonyl-z-naphthylamdide (PYR) positive, bacitracin sensitive; causes pharyngitis ("strep throat"), impetigo, erysipelas, nephritis, scarlet fever, rheumatic fever, and so on.

(2) Group B (*S. agalactiae*). CAMP positive, bacitracin resistant; causes, for example, neonatal sepsis, meningitis, pneumonia, UTI.

(3) Others. Group C, group G, and group F

b. Group D streptococci: bile-esculin positive

(1) Enterococci (*Enterococcus faecalis* and *E. faecium*). Growth in 6.5% salt, PYR-positive; causes UTI, endocarditis, and so forth.

(2) *S. bovis*. No growth in 6.5% salt, PYR negative; small association with colon cancer.

c. Pneumococci (*S. pneumoniae*): bile-soluble (sensitive), optochin-sensitive, >80 capsular serotypes; the most common cause of lobar and bronchopneumonia; also a common cause of adult meningitis and pediatric otitis media.

d. Viridans group streptococci ("oral streptococci"): bile-esculin negative, bile-insoluble (resistant), optochin-resistant. These include the *S. anginosus* (milleri) group (small association with occult abscesses), *S. mitis* group, *S. mutans* group (causes most dental caries), and *S. salivarius* group; all these organisms can cause endocarditis.

e. *Abiotropha* (nutritionally variant streptococci): only grow near other bacteria, especially staphylococci, that provide missing nutrients ("satellite" growth) or on supplemented media, such as chocolate agar.

(1) *A. defectiva*: ONPG positive

(2) *A. adiacens*: ONPG negative

B. Gram-negative cocci. Occur in the Gram's stain as single or paired cells. When paired, the adjacent sides are flattened (gram-negative diplococci).

1. *Neisseria and Moraxella*. Oxidase-positive, gram-negative diplococci

a. *Neiserria gonorrhoeae*: uses glucose; causes, for example, urethritis, proctitis, pharyngitis, neonatal conjunctivitis, sepsis, Fitz-Hugh-Curtis syndrome, arthritis.

b. *Neisseria meningitidis*: uses glucose and maltose; causes sepsis, epidemic meningitis.

c. Other *Neisseria* species: many nonpathogenic species exist.

d. *Moraxella catarrhalis*: tributyrin or DNAase positive; causes otitis media in children and lower respiratory tract disease in adults with underlying lung disease.

C. Gram-positive bacilli. Includes diphtheroid, boxcar, branching, and straight- or regular-shaped bacilli.

1. *Corynebacterium* species. Gram-positive diphtheroid morphology, catalase-positive.

a. *Corynebacterium diphtheriae*: Elek test for toxicogenic strains; causes diphtheria, infections associated with insect bites, and so on.

b. *C. jeikeium*: resistant to many antimicrobials.

    c. **C. urealyticum**: rapidly urea-positive; causes urinary tract infection in adults with underlying uropathology.

  2. **Lactobacillus species**. Catalase-negative; normal oral and vaginal flora, can cause endocarditis.

  3. **Bacillus species**. Gram-positive boxcar morphology, catalase-positive, endospores

    a. **Bacillus anthracis**. Medusa head colony, non-hemolytic, nonmotile; causes anthrax [cutaneous, pulmonary (Woolsorter's disease), and gastrointestinal forms].

    b. **B. cereus**: beta-hemolytic, motile; causes food-poisoning (e.g., rice).

  4. **Listeria monocytogenes**. Beta-hemolytic, catalase-positive, motile; causes sepsis or meningitis in newborns or the immunocompromised.

  5. **Erysipelothrix rhusiopathiae**. Alpha-hemolytic, catalase-negative, H_2S-positive; causes skin infections in fisherman, veterinarians, and so forth.

  6. **Arcanobacterium hemolyticum**. Beta-hemolytic, catalase-negative; causes pharyngitis in young adults.

D. **Gram-negative bacilli—"fermenters"**
Fermenters of glucose; other carbohydrates may or may not be fermented.

  1. **Glucose-fermenters that are oxidase-negative.**

    a. **Enterobacteriaceae (enteric bacilli): nitrate positive**

      (1) **Lactose-fermenting colonies on differential media**

        (a) **E. coli**. Indole-positive; causes UTI, neonatal infections, enteritis, wound infections, sepsis, pneumonia, nosocomial infections, abscesses, hemolytic uremic syndrome (*E. coli* O157:H7), and so on.

        (b) **Klebsiella pneumoniae**. Mucoid colony; causes UTI, wound infections, sepsis, pneumonia, nosocomial infections, abscesses, meningitis, endocarditis, and so forth.

      (2) **Nonlactose-fermenting colonies on differential media**

        (a) **Proteus mirabilis**. Swarming colony on blood agar; causes UTI, pneumonia, wound infections, sepsis.

        (b) **Morganella morganii**. Causes disease similar to *Proteus*.

        (c) **Providencia species**. Causes disease similar to *Proteus* (especially nosocomial infections in nursing homes).

        (d) **Salmonella enterica**. H_2S-positive, nearly 2,000 serovars; causes typhoid fever, invasive enteritis, sepsis, osteomyelitis, food poisoning.

        (e) **Shigella species**. Nonmotile; includes *Shigella boydii* (serogroup C), *S. dysenteriae* (serogroup A), *S. flexneri* (serogroup B), and *S. sonnei* (serogroup D); causes, for example, food poisoning (watery diarrhea), invasive enteritis.

        (f) **Yersinia enterocolitica**. Causes food poisoning, invasive enterocolitis, and so on.

   (3)   Lactose or nonlactose fermenting colonies on differential media
      (a)   *Citrobacter* species. Includes *Citrobacter freundii* and *C. koseri* (formerly *diversus*); causes nosocomial UTI.
      (b)   *Enterobacter* species; includes *Enterobacter cloacae* and *E. aerogenes*; causes nosocomial UTI.
      (c)   *Serratia* species. Causes, for example, nosocomial UTI, sepsis (may be fatal in neonates, immunocompromised, or elderly patients).
      (d)   *S. marcescens*
2.   **Glucose-fermenters that are oxidase-positive**
   a.   **Vibrio-Aeromonas-Pleisomonas**
      (1)   *Vibrio* species. Halophilic (grow in 6% salt).
         (a)   *Vibrio cholera*. Sucrose-positive; causes cholera.
         (b)   *V. parahaemolyticus*. Sucrose-negative; causes self-limited enteritis associated with poorly cooked fish.
         (c)   Others include *V. vulnificus*
      (2)   *Aeromonas hydrophila*. Not halophilic, other related species
      (3)   *Pleisomonas* species. Not halophilic
E.   **Gram-negative bacilli–"nonfermenters." Although glucose is not fermented it can be oxidized, or it may not be utilized at all.**
   1.   **Glucose nonfermenters that are oxidase-negative**
      a.   ***Acinetobacter baumannii***: glucose-oxidizer; low-grade opportunistic infections
      b.   ***A. lwoffi***: glucose-nonoxidizer
      c.   ***Stenotrophomonas maltophilia***: rapid maltose-oxidizer, glucose oxidizer
   2.   **Glucose nonfermenters that are oxidase-positive**
      a.   ***Pseudomonas aeruginosa***: fluorescent pigment, blue-green pigment (pyocyanin), fruity odor, growth at 42°C; causes pneumonia (very common in cystic fibrosis patients), wound and burn infections, catheter-induced UTI, skin infections, otitis, and conjunctivitis (in extended contact lens wearers).
      b.   ***P. fluorescens*** and ***P. putida***: fluorescent pigment, no growth at 42°C
      c.   ***Burkholderia cepacia***: dry, yellow colony on iron-containing media
      d.   ***Alkaligenes* species**: sweet odor
F.   **Gram-negative bacilli–"fastidious."** Gram-negative bacilli that do not grow, or grow very poorly, on selective media for gram-negatives (e.g., MacConkey and EMB agars). Some fastidious gram-negative bacilli require special media or incubation conditions.
   1.   ***Haemophilus* species. Require growth factor X, growth factor Y or X and V for growth; grow on chocolate agar**
      a.   ***Haemophilus influenzae***: require X and V, serotypes A–F; causes meningitis, buccal cellulitis, and septic arthritis in infants; the most common cause of bacterial conjunctivitis (*H. influenzae* subgroup aegyptius: "pink-eye") and bacterial epiglottitis; also causes pneumonia and osteomyelitis.

    b. *H. parainfluenzae*: requires V
    c. *H. aphrophilus*: dry adherent colony, no X or V requirement
    d. *H. ducreyi*: requires X; causes chancroid
  2. **HACEK group: oral flora bacteria**, grow on blood and/or chocolate agars. Includes *Haemophilus aphrophilus*, *Actinobacillus actinomycetemcomitans*, *Cardiobacterium hominis*, *Eikenella corrodens*, *Kingella kingii*; causes endocarditis after dental manipulation.
  3. *Bordetella pertussis*. Detect or confirm growth with FA stain; causes "whooping cough."
  4. *Pasteurella multocida*. Skin infections associated with cat or dog bites.
  5. *Brucella* species. Many are rapidly urea positive, small gram-negative coccobacilli; cause brucellosis (undulant fever).
  6. *Campylobacter* species. Small, curved gram-negative bacilli; cause enteritis.
    a. *C. jejuni*: microaerophilic, growth at 42°C
    b. *C. coli*: microaerophilic, growth at 42°C
    c. *C. fetus*: no growth at 42°C
  7. *Capnocytophaga* species. Fusiform cell morphology, require CO_2.
  8. *Francisella tularensis*. Requires cysteine for growth; small gram-negative coccobacillus; causes tularemia (associated with handling animal carcasses, particularly rabbits).
  9. *Helicobacter pylori*. Small curved gram-negative bacilli, strongly urea positive; associated with almost 100% of duodenal ulcers and 70% of gastric ulcers.
  10. *Legionella* species. More than 30 species; require cysteine for growth; includes *L. pneumophila*, which has >12 serogroups; serogroup 1 is most common in humans; causes pneumonia (Legionnaires' disease) and Pontiac fever.
G. **Bacteria without cell walls**
  1. *Mycoplasma* and *Ureaplasma*. Cell membrane only, osmotically fragile
    a. *M. pneumoniae*: fried egg colony, resistant to thalium acetate; causes "walking pneumonia" (may cause one half of all nonviral community-acquired pneumonias)
    b. *M. hominis*: occasionally grows on blood agar; a common cause of postpartum sepsis; also causes wound infections
    c. *U. urealyticum*: rapid urea hydrolysis in broth; causes acute urethritis in women, neonatal pneumonia, and chorioamnionitis
H. **Uncultivable or very difficult to cultivate bacteria.** The following bacteria have not yet been cultivated or do not reliably grow on artificial media, or are strictly intracellular and require cell culture or animal inoculation for growth.
  1. *Afipia* species. Cause rare disorders clinically similar to cat-scratch disease.
  2. *Bartonella* species. Freshly prepared blood agar for growth; *B. henselae* causes cat-scratch disease. *B. quintana* causes quintana fever ("trench fever"; sometimes seen in homeless alcoholics). *B. henselae* and *B. quintana* both cause

bacillary angiomatosis in immunosuppressed patients (e.g., those with the acquired immunodeficiency syndrome).
   3. *Chlamydia* **species. Intracellular pathogens**
      a. *C. trachomatis*: giemsa or fluorescent antibody (FA) stains, enzyme immunoassay, cell culture, PCR
         (1) Serovars A–C cause conjunctivitis ("trachoma"; the most common cause of blindness in some parts of the world)
         (2) Serovars D–M cause urethritis, epididymitis, endometritis, salpingitis, neonatal conjunctivitis and pneumonitis.
         (3) Serovars L1-3 cause lymphogranuloma venereum
      b. *C. pneumoniae*. Cell culture and PCR; a common cause of respiratory disease in young adults and the elderly
      c. *C. psittaci*: cell culture; causes psittacosis (e.g., pneumonia, sepsis, associated with bird-handlers)
   4. *Coxiella burnetii* causes Q-fever.
   5. *Ehrlichia* **species**. Intracellular bacteria, arthropod vector; cause ehrlichiosis (similar to Rocky Mountain spotted fever, but without the rash)
   6. *Rickettsia* **species**. Intracellular bacteria, arthropod vector; cause Rocky Mountain spotted fever (*R. rickettsii*), "epidemic" typhus (*R. prowazekii*), "scrub" typhus (*R. tsutsugamushi*), and so on.
   7. Spirochetes. Motile, loose to tight spirals
      a. *Borrelia burgdorferi*: cultivated with difficulty on special media; causes Lyme disease
      b. *B. recurrentis*: motile with loose spirals, cultivated with difficulty on special media; causes relapsing fever
      c. *Leptospira* **species**: darkfield microscopy, spirals with hooked ends; can be cultivated in broth medium; causes leptospirosis
      d. *Treponema pallidum*: darkfield microscopy, tight spirals; causes syphilis
   8. *Tropherema whippelii*. Periodic acid-Schiff-positive bacilli in macrophages; causes Whipple's disease
I. Anaerobic bacteria. Grow only in the absence of oxygen. Most clinically significant anaerobes withstand short (up to 1 hour) exposure to oxygen, remaining viable when returned to anaerobic conditions. Occasional "anaerobes" grow showing small (pinpoint) colonies in aerobic (3%–5% CO_2) incubation (e.g., *P. acnes* and *C. tertium*).
   1. Anaerobic gram-negative bacilli
      a. *Bacteroides fragilis* **group**: bile resistant, resistant to kanamycin, vancomycin, and colistin; includes *B. fragilis*, *B. thetaiotaomicron*, *B. vulgatus*, *B. distasonis*, *B. ovatus*, and *B. uniformis*; cause abscesses (e.g., abdominal, from perforated viscera), particularly when associated with bowel flora, bacteremia, pelvic inflammatory disease, necrotizing fasciitis, and so forth.
      b. *Bacteroides* **species, not** *B. fragilis* **grosup**: *B. ureolyticus* is usually bile sensitive; causes abscesses in association with facultative bacteria and other anaerobes, within and adjacent to the respiratory, gastrointestinal, and genital tracts.

    c. *Bilophila wadsworthia*: bile resistant but sensitive to kanamycin, and colistin; resistant to vancomycin

    d. *Porphyromonas* **species**: asaccharolytic, bile sensitive, black colonies; cause, for example, abscesses in perioral locations and in the brain, aspiration pneumonia, infections associated with human bites.

    e. *Prevotella* **species**: saccharolytic, bile sensitive, black colonies; cause diseases similar to *Porphyromonas* (see above).

    f. *Fusobacterium* **species**: fusiform or long filamentous bacilli; include *F. nucleatum*, *F. mortiferum*, and *F. necrophorum*; common in the oral cavity; can cause infection in surrounding sites, aspiration pneumonia, Lemierre's disease (caused by *F. nucleatum*), and so forth.

2. **Anaerobic gram-positive bacilli that do not form endospores**

    a. *Actinomyces israelii*: branching, knotted filaments; cause, for example, soft tissue infections near the oral cavity, pulmonary disease, endometritis.

    b. *Propionibacterium acnes*: anaerobic "diphtheroid" (microscopic morphology shows clubbing, Chinese lettering, and palisading); causes infections in prosthetic joints, endocarditis, and so forth.

    c. *Eubacterium* **species**

    d. *Lactobacillus* species: anaerobic strains

    e. *Bifidobacterium* species: rudimentary branching "bifids"

3. **Anaerobic gram-positive bacilli that do form endospores**. *Clostridium* species: boxcar shaped bacilli in Gram's stain

    a. *C. perfringens*: double zone of hemolysis on blood agar; causes "gas gangrene," cellulitis, abscesses, sepsis.

    b. *C. botulinum*: toxin ingested; causes botulism

    c. *C. difficile*: enterotoxin A and cytotoxin B; causes antibiotic associated and pseudomembranous colitis

    d. *C. septicum*: causes gas gangrene

    e. *C. tetani*: toxin produced in wounds; causes tetanus

4. **Anaerobic cocci**. Chains and clusters; causes abscess in association with other facultative bacteria and anaerobes, within and adjacent to the genital tract, and so on.

    a. *Veillonella* **species**: gram-negative cocci, resistant to vancomycin; causes eye infections, endometritis.

    b. *Peptostreptococcus* **species**: gram-positive cocci, susceptible to vancomycin; causes brain abscesses, aspiration pneumonia, wound infections, endometritis, and so forth.

IV. **Interpretation of culture results**

  A. **Blood specimens. Single blood cultures positive with a coagulase-negative staphylococcus, *Bacillus* species, *Corynebacterium* species, *Propionibacterium* species, nonpathogenic *Neisseria* species or a viridans group streptococcus are contaminants in most cases**. Multiple positive blood cultures, especially if collected at different times from peripheral venipunctures (not through indwelling lines), of these usual contaminants may be "significant" pathogens.

Significant implies the bacteria are involved in a pathologic progress. **The single most useful finding, which helps differentiate "significant" from "insignificant" isolates of coagulase-negative staphylococci, is whether multiple isolates are clonal** (i.e., the strains from all positive cultures are identical). Multiple blood cultures positive for coagulase-negative staphylococci have a higher likelihood of being "significant" if all strains are identical or clonal. **Usual blood stream pathogens (e.g., *E. coli*, *S. aureus*, *S. pneumoniae*) are considered "significant" whether they are detected in one or multiple blood cultures**. Single blood cultures positive for viridans group streptococci from neutropenic patients with mucositis are likely to be "significant."

  B.   Intraabdominal specimens collected during surgery. Peritonitis and intraabdominal abscess caused by intestinal bacteria entering the peritoneum are caused by usual **colonic flora**, including anaerobes, *Enterobacteriaceae* and enterococci. Culture is necessary to determine if unexpected pathogens are involved (e.g., yeasts, *S. aureus*, *P. aeruginosa*) or unusually resistant bacteria (vancomycin-resistant enterococci).

  C.   Intravascular catheter specimens. Infected intravascular catheters are a source of bacteremia and widespread dissemination of bacteria. Catheters are cultured to determine the source of bacteremia and to provide infection control data. A catheter that is removed can be cultured by rolling on an agar plate, or by sonication and quantitative culturing of the sonicate. Roll culture of the intravascular or intradermal portion should result in >**15** colonies, and quantitative culture of the sonicate should result in >**1,000** colonies if the catheter is a potential source of a bacteremia.

  D.   Gastrointestinal tract specimens. Potential bacterial pathogens detected by culture include *Salmonella enterica*, *Shigella* species, *Campylobacter* species, *Aeromonas* species; *Pleisomonas* species, *Vibrio* species, *Yersinia enterocolitica*, and *E. coli* O157:H7. *Clostridium difficile* disease is detected by toxin testing. *Helicobacter pylori* is detected by culture or histologic examination of gastric biopsy tissue, presence of urease in tissue (CLO-test), stool antigen test, or urea breath test.

  E.   Presumably sterile sites, including body fluids and deep wounds. Bacteria should not grow from these specimens unless an infectious process is present. Contaminants occasionally grow and are recognized by their identity (coagulase-negative staphylococci, corynebacteria, propionibacteria, and other bacteria of low pathogenicity) and quantity (usually one colony on a single plate). It is common for infected sterile sites to be identified by a Gram's-stained smear containing polymorphonuclear leukocytes and bacteria.

  F.   Respiratory tract specimens. All lower respiratory tract specimens that pass through the oropharynx are expected to be contaminated with normal oral flora, including those collected during bronchoscopy. Sputum specimens containing **<10 squamous epithelial cells per 10× microscope objective** lens field are unlikely to be grossly contaminated with oral bacteria and should be cultured. Predominant bacterial morphologies of usual pathogens in Gram's-stained smears, in conjunction with polymorphonuclear leukocytes, which grow as predominant isolates in culture, have the greatest chance of being significant pathogens in patients with appropriate clinical findings. Potential pathogens in less than predominant quantity may be significant if they are found within leukocytes (intracellular bacteria) in the stained smear. Endotracheal tube (ETT) secretions collected from intubated patients should not be cultured if grossly contaminated with oropharyngeal contents as indicated by >10 squamous epithelial cells per 10× microscopic field. In addition, **ETT specimens do not need culturing if bacteria are not seen in the direct Gram's stain**. Quantitative culture of BAL or protected brushing specimens collected during bronchoscopy can identify potential pathogens based on the number of bacteria that grow. In general, **>10,000/mL bacteria in culture of BAL fluid and >1,000/mL bacteria in culture of brushing specimens** increase the chance that an isolate is involved in a pathogenic process.

G. **Superficial wounds**. Culture results of wounds sampled by **collecting material from an exposed surface are not helpful. Debrided material, subcutaneous material collected by aspiration, and expressed pus should contain bacteria** and inflammatory cells in the Gram's stain that match the predominant bacteria detected by culture.

H. **Throat or pharyngeal specimens**. The pharyngeal pathogens include *S. pyogenes, Arcanobacterium hemolyticum* and *C. diphtheriae*. Beta-hemolytic streptococci groups C and G are considered by some to be pathogens. Other bacteria detected by usual or routine bacterial culture methods represent normal oropharyngeal flora.

I. **Urine specimens**. Any number of bacteria detected in urine collected during cystoscopy, by suprapubic aspiration or by in-and-out catheterization can be significant. **Urine collected from patients with indwelling urinary catheters will always contain bacteria** and should not be cultured unless the patient is septic and the urinary tract is a potential source of the bacteremia, in which case all bacteria need to be identified. Midstream urine should be interpreted as listed in Table 3-16.

Table 3-16. Interpretation of midstream urine cultures

Urine Specimen	Likely to be Significant	Not Likely to be Significant
Midstream, female with cystitis	>10^2 CFU/mL if leukocyte esterase is positive	Quantity of potential pathogen ≤ contaminating flora
Midstream, female with pyelonephritis	>10^5 CFU/mL, leukocyte esterase usually positive	Quantity of potential pathogen ≤ contaminating flora
Midstream, patient with asymptomatic bacteriuria	>10^5 CFU/mL, leukocyte esterase positive or negative	<10^5 CFU/mL, quantity of potential pathogen ≤ contaminating flora
Midstream, male with UTI	>10^3 CFU/mL, leukocyte esterase positive	<10^3 CFU/mL, quantity of potential pathogen ≤ contaminating flora

CFU, colony-forming unit; UTI, urinary tract infection.

BIBLIOGRAPHY

Doern G. Detection of selected fastidious bacteria. *Clin Infect Dis* 2000; 30:166–173.

Fan K, Morris A, Reller B. Application of rejection criteria for stool cultures for bacterial enteric pathogens. *J Clin Microbiol* 1993; 31:2233–2235.

Fredricks DN, Relman DA. Application of polymerase chain reaction to the diagnosis of infectious diseases. *Clin Infect Dis* 1999;29: 475–488.

Hooton T, Stamm W. Diagnosis and treatment of uncomplicated urinary tract infection. *Infect Dis Clin North Am* 1997;11:551–581.

Jousimies-Sommer H, Summanen P. Microbiology terminology update: clinically significant anaerobic gram-positive and gram-negative bacteria (excluding spirochetes). *Clin Infect Dis* 1999;29(4):724–727.

Morris AJ, Smith LK, Mirrett S, Reller LB. Cost and time savings following introduction of rejection criteria for clinical specimens. *J Clin Microbiol* 1996;34:355–357.

Peterson LR, Thomson RB Jr. Use of the clinical microbiology laboratory for the diagnosis and management of infectious diseases related to the oral cavity. *Infect Dis Clin North Am* 1999;13(4):775–795.

Reimer L, Carrol K. Role of the microbiology laboratory in the diagnosis of lower respiratory tract infections. *Clin Infect Dis* 1998;26: 742–748.

Reimer L, Wilson M, Weinstein P. Update on detection of bacteremia and fungemia. *Clin Microbiol Rev* 1997;10:444–465.

Thomson RB, Peterson LR. Role of the clinical microbiology laboratory in the diagnosis of infections. In: Noskin GA, ed. *Management of infectious complications in cancer patients*. Boston: Klower Academic Publishers, 1998:143–165.

Wilson ML. General principles of specimen collection and transport. *Clin Infect Dis* 1996;22:766–777.

Woods GL, Walker DH. Detection of infection or infectious agents by use of cytologic and histologic stains. *Clin Microbiol Rev* 1996;9:382–404.

Antimicrobial Testing

Richard B. Thomson, Jr.

I. **Antimicrobials**. Common antimicrobials tested by the laboratory can be classified according to their chemical structure or their mechanism of action.

   A. **Classification based on chemical structure, with some important uses** (Table 3-17)

     1. **Beta-lactams**. A four-sided beta-lactam ring is part of their chemical structure. Common examples include the following

       a. **Penicillins**

         (1) **First generation** (naturally occurring): penicillin; good for streptococci and beta-lactamase negative anaerobes

         (2) **Second generation** (antistaphylococcal, penicillinase stable): methicillin, nafcillin, oxacillin; good for methicillin-susceptible staphylococci

         (3) **Third generation** (aminopenicillins): ampicillin, amoxicillin; use similar to penicillin, plus good for some enterococci; *Escherichia coli*; *Proteus* spp. and *Haemophilus influenzae*

         (4) **Fourth generation** (carboxypenicillins): carbenicillin, ticarcillin; use similar to penicillin plus for *Enterobacteriaceae* and some *Pseudomonas aeruginosa*

         (5) **Fifth generation** (ureidopenicillins): piperacillin; use similar to fourth generation penicillins plus more *P. aeruginosa* activity

       b. **Cephems (cephalosporins)**

         (1) **First generation**: cephalothin, cefazolin; good for streptococci, methicillin-susceptible staphylococci, and some *E. coli*; *Proteus* and *Klebsiella* spp.

         (2) **Second generation**: cefoxitin, cefuroxime, cefamandole; use similar to first generation plus better for *Enterobacteriaceae*, anaerobes (cefoxitin), and pneumococcus (cefuroxime).

         (3) **Third generation**: ceftazidime, ceftriaxone, cefotaxime; same as second generation plus better for *Enterobacteriaceae*, *P. aeruginosa* (ceftazidime), and streptococci or haemophilus (ceftriaxone, cefotaxime).

         (4) **Fourth generation**: cefepime; use similar to third generation plus better for *Enterobacteriaceae,* and *P. aeruginosa*

       c. **Monobactams**: aztreonam; good for aerobic and facultative gram-negative bacilli only.

       d. **Carbapenems**: imipenem, meropenem; very broad activity. Good for most bacterial groups except *S. maltophilia*, methicillin-resistant staphylococci, and *Enterococcus faecium*.

(*text continues on page 206*)

Table 3-17.   Overview of antimicrobial therapy

Microorganisms Groups	Penicillin 1st Generation—Penicillin	Penicillin 2nd Generation—Antistaphylococcal	Penicillin 3rd Generation—Aminopenicillins	Penicillin 4th Generation—Carboxypenicillins	Penicillin 5th Generation—Ureidopenicillins	Cephem 1st Generation (e.g., Cefazolin)	Cephem 2nd Generation (e.g., Cefuroxime)	Cephem 3rd Generation (e.g., Ceftriaxone)	Cephem 4th Generation (e.g., Cefepime)	Monobactams	Carbapenems	Beta-Lactamase Inhibitors	Aminoglycosides	Glycopeptides	Lincosamides	Macrolides	Quinolones/Fluoroquinolones	Rifamycins/Ansamycins	Folate Pathway Inhibitors	Tetracyclines	Chloramphenicol	Linezolid (Oxazolidones)	Metronidazole (Nitroimidazoles)	Nitrofurantoin	Quinupristin/Dalfopristin (Streptogramins)
Gram-positive cocci																									
–Staphylococci		‡				+			+			+		‡	+		+					+			+
–Beta-hemolytic streptococci	‡		‡		+	+		+				+		+	+	+	+					+			+
–Enterococci			‡		+								s	+								+		u	+

–Pneumococci	++		++		+	+		++				+		+	+	++	++		+	+					
–Viridans group streptococci	++		++		+			++						+											
Gram-negative cocci																									
–*Neisseria gonorrhoeae*	+		+					++									++								
–*N. meningitidis*	++		++					++											+	+					
–*Moraxella catarrhalis*								+				++				++	+		++	+					
Gram-positive bacilli																									
–Corynebacterium	++		++											++	+	+									
–Lactobacillus																									
–Bacillus	++										+			++	+	+	+			+					
–*Listeria monocytogenes*	+		++													+			++						
–*Erysipelothrix rhusiopathiae*	++		++					++																	
–*Arcanobacterium haemolyticum*	++															++									
Gram-negative bacilli																									
–Enteric bacilli			+	+	++	+	+	++	++	++	++	+	++				++		+						
–Vibrio/aeromonas							+	+	+		+		+				++		+	+				u	
–Nonfermentative Gram-negative bacilli					++			++	++	++	+	++	++				++								
Fastidious Gram-negative bacilli																									

continued

Table 3-17. Continued

Microorganisms Groups	Penicillins: 1st Generation—Penicillin	Penicillins: 2nd Generation—Antistaphylococcal	Penicillins: 3rd Generation—Aminopenicillins	Penicillins: 4th Generation—Carboxypenicillins	Penicillins: 5th Generation—Ureidopenicillins	Cephems: 1st Generation (e.g., Cefazolin)	Cephems: 2nd Generation (e.g., Cefuroxime)	Cephems: 3rd Generation (e.g., Ceftriaxone)	Cephems: 4th Generation (e.g., Cefepime)	Monobactams	Carbapenems	Beta-Lactamase Inhibitors	Aminoglycosides	Glycopeptides	Lincosamides	Macrolides	Quinolones/Fluoroquinolones	Rifamycins/Ansamycins	Folate Pathway Inhibitors	Tetracyclines	Chloramphenicol	Linezolid (Oxazolidones)	Metronidazole (Nitroimidazoles)	Nitrofurantoin	Quinupristin/Dalfopristin (Streptogramins)
Haemophilus influenzae			+					‡			+	‡				+	‡		+						
HACEK			‡				+	‡					‡												
Bordetella pertussis																‡			‡						
Pasteurella multocida	‡		‡				+	+				+				+	+		+	+					
Brucella spp.													‡				+	+	+	‡					

Table (rotated; column headers appear on the facing page and are not visible on this page). Row labels (organism groups) from top to bottom:

- *Campylobacter jejuni/coli*
- *Helicobacter pylori*
- *Legionella pneumophila*
- Cell wall deficient bacteria
- –*Mycoplasma*/*Ureaplasma*
- Noncultivatable or very difficult to cultivate bacteria
- –*Bartonella*
- –*Chlamydia*
- –*Coxiella burnetii*
- –*Ehrlichia*
- –*Rickettsia*
- –*Borrelia*
- –*Leptospira*
- Anaerobic bacteria
- –Anaerobic Gram-negative bacilli
- –Anaerobic Gram-positive bacilli
- –Anaerobic cocci

Usual antimicrobial therapies matching groups of microorganisms and antimicrobial families. ++, usual first line therapy; +, alternate or second line therapy; HACEK = Haemophilus aphrophilus, Actinobacillus actinomycetemcomitans, Cardiobacterium hominis, Eikenella corrodens, Kingella Kingii; s, second drug used for synergy; u, therapy for urinary tract only.
Most therapies require *in vitro* testing to confirm activity.

  e. **Beta-lactamase inhibitors**: clavulanic acid, sulbactam, tazobactam. Common combinations include amoxicillin/clavulanate, ticarcillin/clavulanate, ampicillin/sulbactam, and piperacillin/tazobactam; good for most streptococci and enterococci, some facultative gram-negative bacilli, and most anaerobes.

 2. **Aminoglycosides**: gentamicin, tobramycin, amikacin; good for aerobic and facultative gram-negative bacilli.

 3. **Glycopeptides**: vancomycin, teicoplanin; good for most gram-positive aerobic, and facultative and anaerobic bacteria.

 4. **Lincosamides**: clindamycin; good for streptococci, staphylococci, and anaerobes.

 5. **Macrolides**: erythromycin, clarithromycin, azithromycin; good for streptococci, *Moraxella catarrhalis*, *Legionella* spp., *Chlamydia* spp., and *Bordetella pertussis*.

 6. **Quinolones and fluoroquinolones**: good for facultative gram-negative bacilli and pneumococci; fair for streptococci; some are fair for anaerobes.

  a. **Quinolones**: naladixic acid

  b. **Fluoroquinolone**: norfloxacin, ciprofloxacin, levofloxacin, moxifloxacin, gatifloxacin

 7. **Rifamycins and ansamycins**: rifampin; good for *Mycobacterium tuberculosis*. Not used alone (as single drug therapy) for treatment of any infection.

 8. **Folate pathway inhibitors**: trimethoprim–sulfamethoxazole, sulfonamides; good for facultative gram-negative bacilli.

 9. **Tetracyclines**: tetracycline, doxycycline, minocycline; good for facultative gram-negative bacilli.

 10. **Miscellaneous**

  a. **Chloramphenicol**: good for streptococci; meningococci and *H. influenzae*, especially in central nervous system disease, and facultative gram-negative bacilli.

  b. **Linezolid** (oxazolidones): good for vancomycin-resistant enterococci.

  c. **Metronidazole** (nitroimidazoles): excellent for anaerobes.

  d. **Nitrofurantoin**: good for gram-negative bacilli and enterococci causing urinary tract infections.

  e. **Quinupristin and dalfopristin** (streptogramins): good for methicillin-resistant staphylococci and vancomycin-resistant *E. faecium*.

B. **Classification based on mechanisms of action**

 1. **Drugs that interfere with cell wall synthesis**: beta-lactams and glycopeptides

 2. **Drugs that interfere with protein synthesis**: aminoglycosides, chloramphenicol, lincosamides, macrolides, streptogramins, oxazolidones, and tetracyclines

 3. **Drugs that affect DNA**

  a. Drugs that affect DNA synthesis: quinolones/fluoroquinolones

  b. Drugs that cause DNA strand breakage: nitroimidazoles

 4. **Drugs that affect RNA synthesis**: rifamycins

5. Folate pathway inhibitors: sulfonamides–sulfonamide combinations

II. In vitro antimicrobial testing. In vitro antimicrobial susceptibility tests are used to help predict whether a specific antimicrobial will eradicate a pathogen from an infected site. Laboratories perform in vitro tests when they isolate a likely pathogen that has an unpredictable antimicrobial profile and proved methods exist that determine susceptibility and resistance. Consensus methods used to test antimicrobial susceptibility are published by the National Committee for Clinical Laboratory Standards (NCCLS), Wayne, PA.

A. Minimum inhibitory concentration (MIC). The lowest concentration of antimicrobial that inhibits growth of a bacterium.

B. Breakpoint. The concentration of antimicrobial that is used to differentiate "susceptible" from "resistant." In theory, the breakpoint is the concentration of antimicrobial **achieved at the site of infection** after normal dosing.

C. Interpretation. The term "susceptible" implies that the concentration of antimicrobial at the site of infection will exceed the MIC of the offending pathogen following normal drug dosing. Growth of microorganisms will be inhibited. The term **"resistant"** implies that **the concentration of antimicrobial at the site of infection will be lower than the MIC** and inhibition of growth is not likely to occur. The term **"intermediate"** means **that the concentration of antimicrobial and MIC are approximately equal** at the site of infection and, unless higher than normal doses are used or the antimicrobial is concentrated at the infected site (e.g., urine), a different drug should be selected to which the organism is susceptible.

D. Methods used to determine MICs

1. Broth dilution testing. Twofold dilutions of antimicrobial are prepared in standard broth (e.g., Mueller–Hinton broth). A standard inoculum of strain to be tested is added to each antimicrobial dilution so that the final concentration of bacteria in the tube or well is 5×10^5/mL. The broth is incubated overnight at 35°C, and then read as "growth" (turbidity) or "no growth" (visually clear). **Macrobroth dilution** methods are performed in standard test tubes. **Microbroth dilution** methods are performed in microtiter trays. The final report includes the **MIC value** and the interpretation as either **susceptible, intermediate, or resistant.**

2. Agar dilution. Dilutions of the antimicrobial are prepared in agar plates. Each plate contains a different concentration. Approximately 35 different bacterial strains are tested per plate. Each strain is inoculated to a spot (10^4 bacteria per spot), and then read as growth or no growth for each strain. This was originally considered to be the "gold standard" for MIC testing, but is currently performed in reference laboratories only.

3. E-test. Paper strips are used with an antimicrobial gradient applied to one side. Antimicrobial concentrations are printed along the length of the strip from high to low. A standard inoculum of the strain to be tested (i.e., turbidity equivalent to **0.5 McFarland standard**) is applied to a

Mueller–Hinton agar medium. E-test strips are then applied to the freshly inoculated medium. After overnight incubation, an inhibitory ellipse occurs around the end of the strip with the higher concentration of antimicrobial. Bacterial growth intersects the paper strip where antimicrobial concentration approximates MIC. The final report includes the **MIC value** along with the interpretation as either **susceptible, intermediate, or resistant.**

   4.   Disk diffusion testing. Agar disk diffusion (a.k.a. the Kirby–Bauer test) is a MIC test on the surface of an agar plate. High potency disks containing the antimicrobials to be tested are placed on the surface of a Mueller–Hinton agar plate that has been inoculated with a "lawn" of bacteria (0.5 McFarland suspension). The antimicrobial diffuses into and across the agar surface, creating a concentration gradient that mimics the dilutions one uses in the broth dilution procedure, with a high concentration near the disk and a low concentration far from the disk. Bacteria grow toward the disk until they reach their MIC, forming a circular zone of inhibited growth around the disk. Statistical analysis has been used to determine the MIC and breakpoint zone diameter equivalents for disk diffusion with most antimicrobial and organism combinations. Results of disk testing are reported as **susceptible**, **intermediate**, or **resistant** without including the approximated MIC equivalent.

   5.   Semiautomated methods. Semiautomated instruments that perform MIC tests include the Microscan Walkaway (Dade MicroScan, Inc., West Sacramento, CA) and the Vitek (bioMerieux, Inc., Hazelwood, MO). The Walkaway instrument incubates and reads turbidity in conventional broth microdilution trays. The Vitek incubates and reads light scattering in nonconventional cards containing antimicrobial-filled microchambers. A semiautomated instrument for the performance of disk diffusion testing is the BIOMIC Video System (Giles Scientific, Inc., Santa Barbara, CA). Images of disk diffusion plates and software containing NCCLS breakpoint data are used to rapidly determine zone diameters and **susceptible**, **intermediate**, or **resistant** interpretations.

E.   Special conditions needed for testing fastidious bacteria. Bacteria that do not grow in Mueller–Hinton broth for MIC testing or on Mueller–Hinton agar for disk testing (within 24 hours in an ambient 35°C incubator) require special testing conditions. Fastidious bacteria include the following.

   1.   Anaerobes. Because of discrepancies between broth and agar dilution MIC results, testing is not routinely recommended. **Published antibiogram data should be used to select empiric therapy**. Testing in rare circumstances can be performed using the E-test.

   2.   *H. influenzae*. Use *Haemophilus* **Test Medium** (HTM), 35°C, ambient air, and 20- to 24-hour incubation.

   3.   *Neisseria gonorrhoeae*. Use **GC agar base** with 1% defined growth supplement, 35°C, 5% CO_2, and 20- to 24-hour incubation.

4. Streptococci (including beta-hemolytic, viridans group, and pneumococci). Use **Mueller–Hinton broth with lysed horse blood**, 35°C, ambient air, and 20- to 24-hour incubation.

5. Oxacillin screen for penicillin-resistant pneumo-cocci. A 1-µg oxacillin disk is used to screen for penicillin non-susceptible pneumococci. **Zone sizes of ≥20 mm indicate penicillin susceptibility** (MIC ≤0.06). Penicillin MICs should be determined for isolates with zone sizes of ≤19 mm, because pneumococci with zones ≤19 mm may be resistant (MIC ≥2 µg/mL), intermediate (MIC 0.12–1.0 µg/mL), or occasionally susceptible.

F. Testing for difficult-to-detect resistance. Many bacteria acquire or develop resistance to antimicrobials that is not readily detected by standard MIC or disk diffusion methods. Supplemental testing is needed to confirm *in vitro* susceptibility as determined by usual methods (Table 3-18). For example, beta-lactamase testing is performed using the chromogenic cephalosporin method, referred to as the "nitrocefin test." Nitrocefin is a colorless or faint yellow cephalosporin antimicrobial that is hydrolyzed rapidly by most beta-lactamases. The hydrolysis product is pink. The bacterium to be tested is applied to a paper disk containing nitrocefin. A pink color developing within minutes (positive test) indicates a beta-lactamase producing bacterium.

G. Antimicrobial assays are used to measure the concentration of antimicrobials in blood or other body fluid (Table 3-19). Assays document compliance with a prescribed regimen, ensure adequate therapeutic concentrations, and document that concentrations are not at toxic levels. Assays of aminoglycoside and vancomycin concentrations are used most commonly. Levels of antimicrobials are commonly monitored after the third dose (steady-state achieved). Regimens and frequency of testing varies with patient condition and disease state. Use of assays can be minimized in most patients with normal renal formation.

H. Synergy testing. Synergy occurs when the combined effect of two antimicrobials is greater than if the effects of each used alone were to be added together. Testing to document synergy is necessary on a routine basis when treating **endocarditis caused by enterococci**. The combination of a cell wall active antimicrobial (usually ampicillin or vancomycin) and an aminoglycoside (usually gentamicin) will be synergistic if the enterococcus is susceptible to the cell wall agent and is unable to inactive the aminoglycoside with aminoglycoside-inactivating enzymes. A test for aminoglycoside-inactivating enzymes is performed with a one-tube MIC test (500 µg/mL). Enterococci susceptible to this concentration will be killed by combination therapy. Enterococci resistant to 500 µg/mL will be inhibited by the cell wall drug but not killed by the combination (no synergy).

III. Reporting results

A. Laboratory reports indicate MIC values and susceptible (S), intermediate (I), or resistant (R) interpretations if MIC testing is performed, or "S," "I," or "R" if disk diffusion

Table 3-18.   Supplemental testing needed to confirm in vitro susceptibility

Bacteria	Antimicrobial	Supplemental Test	Resistance Mechanism
Staphylococcus aureus			
All staphylococci	Penicillin	Beta-lactamase assay	Beta-lactamase production
	Methicillin and related drugs	MEC-A gene analysis, or agar and broth dilution testing with increased concentrations of NaCl	Altered penicillin binding
	Vancomycin	Broth or agar dilution MIC; disk diffusion not recommended	Altered cell wall morphology which consumes excess drug
Enterococci	Vancomycin	Broth or agar dilution MIC; disk diffusion not recommended	Altered cell wall structure which reduces binding of drug
Escherichia coli/Klebsiella	Cephalosporins	Review overall antimicrobial pattern Ceftazidime or another extended spectrum cephalosporin is tested with and without clavulanate	Extended-spectrum beta-lactamase production
Haemophilus influenzae	Ampicillin	Beta-lactamase assay	Beta-lactamase production
Moraxella catarrhalis	Ampicillin	Beta-lactamase assay	Beta-lactamase production
Neisseria gonorrhoeae	Penicillin	Beta-lactamase assay	Beta-lactamase production

MIC, minimum inhibitory concentration.

**Table 3-19. Collection of specimens and interpretation
of results for aminoglycoside and vancomycin assays**

Antimicrobial	Timing of Blood Specimen	Interpretation
Vancomycin	Peak level (60 min after end of infusion)	25–40 µg/mL
	Trough level (before next dose)	5–15 µg/mL
	Random level (anytime)	Redose if <5–15 µg/mL
Gentamicin or Tobramycin	Peak level: conventional dosing (30 min after end of infusion)	4–8 µg/mL
	Trough level: conventional dosing (before next dose or 18 h after every 24-h dose)	<2 µg/mL
	Peak level: synergy dosing[a] (30 min after end of infusion)	3–5 µg/mL
	Trough level: synergy dosing (before next dose)	<1 µg/mL
	Random level (anytime)	Redose if <2 µg/mL
Amikacin	Peak level: conventional dosing (30 min after end of infusion)	15–30 µg/mL
	Trough level: conventional dosing (before next dose)	<10 µg/mL
	Random level (anytime)	Redose if <10 µg/mL

[a] Synergy dosing refers to lower doses used to treat enterococci in combination with a second antimicrobial.

testing is used. The best antimicrobial to use is not necessarily the one with the lowest MIC, because all drugs do not have the same breakpoint (serum level differentiating S from R). In addition, most antimicrobials that test as susceptible do not show improved effectiveness as the MIC drops. **The MIC value is most helpful when selecting therapy for infections in areas of the body where drug concentrations differ from usual serum levels** (e.g., the central nervous system).

B. Antibiograms are compilations of antibiotic testing results over a defined period of time. A common antibiogram lists the percentage of bacteria susceptible to a battery of antimicrobials routinely reported for all common isolates during the past year. Antibiograms are used to assess the overall activity of antimicrobials against the community's pathogens. **Every hospital or community has a different bacterial flora** and, consequently, will have different percentages in their antibiogram. **The most important use of antibiograms is to help determine empiric therapy regimens for the hospital or community.**

BIBLIOGRAPHY

Cockerill FR. Genetic methods for assessing antimicrobial resistance. *Antimicrob Agents Chemother* 1999;43(2):199–212.

Gold HS, Moellering R. Antimicrobial-drug resistance. *N Engl J Med* 1996;19:1445–1453.

Jorgensen H. Selection criteria for an antimicrobial susceptibility testing system. *J Clin Microbiol* 1993;Nov:2841–2844.

Jorgensen H, Ferraro M. Antimicrobial susceptibility testing: general principles and contemporary practices. *Clin Infect Dis* 1998;26: 973–980.

Jorgensen JH. Laboratory issues in the detection and reporting of antibacterial resistance. *Infect Dis Clin North Am* 1997;11(4):785–802.

Kiska D. In vitro testing of antimicrobial agents. *Seminars in Pediatric Infectious Diseases* 1998;Oct:281–291.

Murray B. Antibiotic resistance. *Advances in internal medicine*. St. Louis: Mosby-Year Book, 1997:42.

Sahm D. Emerging trends in antimicrobial resistance: a laboratory perspective. *Antimicrobial resistance: a crisis in health care*. New York: Plenum Publishing, 1995.

3.4

Mycobacteria

Elmer W. Koneman

I.   **Introduction. Mycobacteria are aerobic, slow-grow-ing, weakly Gram-positive, acid-fast, non–spore-forming, slightly curved or straight bacilli** that are closely related to the genera *Corynebacterium* and *Nocardia*. Mycobacteria have cell walls with a **high lipid content** that retain carbol-fuchsin dye despite decolorization attempts with acid (whence, acid-fast).

Mycobacterium tuberculosis **and** *M. bovis*, **which cause tuberculosis, are transmitted by the inhalation of infected droplets** (*M. tuberculosis*) **or by ingestion of milk from in-fected cows** (*M. bovis*). Disseminated tuberculosis can involve almost any organ of the body [e.g., the lungs, cervical lymph nodes (**scrofula**), meninges (**tuberculous meningitis**), spinal vertebra (**Pott's disease**), gastrointestinal tract, kidneys, adrenals, male and female genital systems]. Risk factors include malnourishment, close human-to-human contacts in crowded living environments, intravenous (IV) drug use, pre-existent pulmonary pathology, and immunodeficiencies [e.g., acquired immunodeficiency syndrome (**AIDS**), immunosuppression, chronic debilitating diseases]. Since the 1980s, the world-wide incidence of tuberculosis has **steadily increased** (in part, because of AIDS), and **multidrug-resistant strains** have emerged. Patients with AIDS tend to have particularly aggressive disease with accelerated rates of bacterial repli-cation, and the high concentrations of the organism increase the likelihood of transmitting the infection.

The incidence of *M. avium/intracellulare* **(MAI)**, which is common in patients with **AIDS**, has particularly increased. *M. lep-rae*, **the cause of leprosy**, is uncommon in the United States, but is historically important. Mycobacteria can be highly communica-ble, and are arguably **one of the world's leading infectious causes of death**.

II.   **Pathophysiology**. Pathogenic mycobacteria cause tissue damage by "hiding" within macrophages and inciting delayed-type, cell-mediated hypersensitivity reactions (**type IV hyper-sensitivity**). Virulence factors in the mycobacterial cell walls include the toxic glycolipids called **cord factor and sulfatides**. Histologically, *M. tuberculosis* causes **caseating granulomas** with Langhans' type multinucleated giant cells, whereas MAI usually shows large, **foamy macrophages** (foamy, because of the intracellular MAI organisms) within the lamina propria of the gastrointestinal tract or in the reticuloendothelial system.

III.   **Specimen collection**

A.   **Sputum. Early-morning** specimens are collected on **three to five successive mornings**.

B.   **Urine. First-of-the-morning, clean-catch** specimens are collected on **three** successive mornings.

C.   **Stool**. Stool is collected in a **clean** (not necessarily sterile) container with a lid.

D.   Blood. Lysis centrifugation blood culture system (Isolator™) is used.

IV.   Specimen preparation. Specimens must be prepared and decontaminated to prevent bacterial overgrowth. A common decontaminant is **NaOH** (4%), which kills bacteria but not mycobacteria (because of the lipid content of the cell walls), with *N*-acetyl-*L*-cysteine (NALC), which lyses mucin within which mycobacterial cells may be trapped. Direct smears are then performed for acid-fast staining, and culture media are inoculated.

V.   Culture media. The classic media are **Löwenstein–Jensen** (LJ, egg-based) and **Middlebrook 7H10** (agar-based). Because of increased sensitivity of recovery and shortened colony growth times, **broth culture** (e.g., **Bactec 12B**) is the medium currently preferred. The use of automated instruments and p-nitroacetylamino-hydroxypropiophenone (NAP) in broth cultures has dramatically improved detection and shortened the time for diagnosis.

VI.   Additional tests for mycobacteria. Additional tests for the diagnosis of tuberculosis include purified protein derivative (**PPD**) skin testing, direct smears for **acid-fast stains**, and **polymerase chain reaction (PCR)/DNA** probes. The nucleic acid probes are very sensitive (>95%), specific (≥99%), rapid (same-day culture confirmation), and cost competitive.

VII.   Stains

   A.   Classic acid-fast stains. Ziehl-Neelsen ("hot" stain; uses heat to effect cell wall penetration of the dye); **Kinyoun** ("cold" stain: uses phenol to effect penetration); both use carbol-fuchsin (red), with methylene blue counterstain and acid alcohol as a decolorizer. **Fite** stains are used to detect *M. leprae*.

   B.   Fluorescent. Auramine and **auramine-rhodamine** require a fluorescent microscope, but allow rapid screening using 10× or 20× objectives instead of 40× that must be used when examining the acid-fast stains.

VIII.   Biochemical tests. Several biochemical tests can be used for species identification. Most are performed at specialized centers. Tests include niacin accumulation, nitrate reduction, iron uptake, Tween 80 hydrolysis, growth inhibition by thiophene-2-carboxylic hydrazide, growth on MacConkey agar, and the synthesis of arylsulfatase, catalase, pyrazinamidase, and urease. Most laboratories use nucleic acid probe assays to confirm *M. tuberculosis*, and **MAI**.

IX.   Susceptibility testing. *Mycobacterium tuberculosis* isolates are **resistant to at least one drug in 10% to 20% of the cases** (in some locations higher). Use of broth cultures is recommended for susceptibility testing. If >1% of bacilli in an isolate show *in vitro* resistance to a drug, that drug will not be useful clinically. Susceptibility testing of MAI isolates require special interpretative criteria. In general, MAI is resistant to isoniazid and pyrazinamide.

X.   Classification with clinical syndromes and key characteristics. *Mycobacterium* species are generally divided (with a few exceptions) according to the **Runyon** classification system. Mycobacterium species are divided into the *M. tuberculosis* **complex** (consisting of *M. tuberculosis*, *M. bovis*, *M. ulcerans*, and

M. africanum, all of which probably represent a single species), and **mycobacteria other than** *M. tuberculosis* (MOTT). MOTT are then **further classified into four groups**, based on pigment production and growth rate: (a) photochromogens, (b) the scotochromogens, (c) the nonchromogens, and (d) the rapid growers.

A. **Mycobacterium tuberculosis complex**

1. *M. tuberculosis* causes **tuberculosis (TB)**. The classic **primary infection** results in a residual calcified lung nodule and hilar lymphadenopathy (**Ghon complex**). **Secondary infections** (or disease reactivation) typically cause **cavitary, caseating granulomas** in the lung apices. Hematologic spread to any organ of the body (**miliary TB**) can occur in primary or secondary infections, and is particularly common in patients with AIDS. Key characteristics include the following.

a. Optimal growth temperature: 37°C

b. Growth time: **7 days** (broth culture) or **2–4 weeks** (LJ culture)

c. Pigmentation: none (**buff colored**)

d. Biochemical reactions: **niacin accumulation positive, nitrate reduction positive, catalase negative**

e. Serpentine arrangement of cells (**cording factor**)

f. Failure to grow in NAP

g. Cells are **red, thin, curved, and beaded**

2. *M. bovis* causes **gastrointestinal tuberculosis** (with spread to other organs); it commonly infects **cattle, dogs, cats** (causes up to 40% of tuberculosis in cattle or in dairy industry regions such as Scotland and Czechoslavakia). Urine isolates may be recovered in patients who have received bacillus Calmette–Guérin (BCG)—lavage (which contain attenuated strains of *M. bovis*) for treatment of transitional cell carcinoma; the BCG stimulates an immune response that destroys the carcinoma cells.

3. *M. ulcerans* causes painless, shallow, nonhealing **skin ulcers (Barnsdale ulcer)**; it is more common in Africa, Mexico, Australia.

B. **MOTT groups**

1. **Group I. Photochromogens (produce pigment when grown in the light)**

a. *M. marinum*: **skin infections** (painful, red-blue, subcutaneous nodules) from exposure to contaminated salt or fresh water (**swimming pool granuloma**) or inadequately chlorinated fresh water. Skin lesions that appear in tropical fish aquarium owners or salt-water fishermen are examples.

b. *M. kansasii*: **pulmonary disease**, not communicable (transmitted by contaminated dust).

c. *M. simiae*: a rare isolate causing pulmonary disease.

2. **Group II: Scotochromogens (produce pigment when grown in the light *or* grown in the dark)**

a. *M. gordonae*: (**tap-water bacillus**); a **common contaminant** (usually not pathogenic, but rare cases of infection have been recorded).

b. *M. flavescens*: **contaminant** (usually not pathogenic)

   c.   *M. xenopi* causes pulmonary disease (particularly in immunosuppressed patients), from contaminated hot and cold tap water, more common in Europe and North America (second most common nontuberculous mycobacterium cultured in the province of Ontario). Recovery is optimum at 42°C.

   d.   *M. scrofulaceum* causes unilateral cervical lymphadenitis involving nodes high in the neck (frequently draining to skin surface) in children (**2–4 years of age**) and teenagers (**16–18 years of age**), probably related to **teething** or eruption of molars.

   e.   *M. szulgai*: very rare isolate causing pulmonary disease.

   3.   Group III: Nonchromogens (do not produce pigment in either the light or the dark)

   a.   *M. avium-M. intracellulare* causes gastrointestinal disease (from contaminated food or water or from disseminated pulmonary infections) and **pulmonary disease** (from inhaled droplets). MAI usually occurs in association with immunodeficiency. MAI is the most common mycobacterial infection in patients with **AIDS**; usually occurs late in the AIDS disease course; presents with low-grade fever, weakness, and weight loss; and is often disseminated throughout the reticuloendothelial system. Pulmonary lesions tend to be necrotizing rather than granulomatous. Gastro-intestinal infections show **foamy histiocytes** in the lamina propria (resembling Whipple's disease). Blood cultures are often positive. Note that most isolates from patients with AIDS are unusual in that they *do* produce pigment.

   b.   *M. malmoense* causes pulmonary disease in middle-aged men with chronic lung disease; more common in Europe and the United States; cultures require **8–12 weeks** to grow (often cultures are destroyed before these colonies are visible and, therefore, infections are underdiagnosed).

   4.   Group IV: The rapid growers (form visible colonies within 7 days)

   a.   *M. fortuitum/chelonei* complex causes **skin infections** (draining abscesses) and pulmonary disease from surgical contamination, needle-sticks, trauma, and so on; disseminated in immunosuppressed patients.

C.   Miscellaneous

   1.   *M. paratuberculosis*: recovered from some patients with Crohn's disease, but evidence of a causal relationship is unclear.

   2.   *M. hemophilum* requires hemoglobin for growth. Risk factors include AIDS, renal dialysis, steroid therapy.

   3.   *M. thermoresistible* grow at 52°C. Minimal virulence.

   4.   *M. genavense*: patients with AIDS; grows only in broth, 165 rRNA gene assay necessary to establish an identification.

3.5

Viruses

Diane S. Leland

I. Introduction. The contemporary virus laboratory provides a broad range of services—timely, cost-effective, diagnostic information important in patient management and therapy. This is of increasing significance now that antivirals are available for the treatment of many viral infections. Viral infections that were previously diagnosed strictly on clinical grounds are now seen in partially immunized or immunocompromised individuals in whom classic signs and symptoms are absent or atypical; laboratory confirmation of these infections is essential for accurate diagnosis. **This chapter describes two approaches for viral disease diagnosis: direct detection of viral antigens or nucleic acids and virus isolation. Common viruses and their syndromes are also discussed**. Detection of viral antibodies is described in chapter 3.9, *Infectious Serology*.

II. Direct detection of viral antigens or nucleic acids. In viral antigen detection, known antiviral antibodies are used in the test system, and binding of this antibody to the target viral antigen identifies the viral antigen in the sample. In nucleic acid detection, labeled segments of viral nucleic acids (probes) hybridize to complementary sequences within the nucleic acid of viruses in the patient's sample. The hybridization process can be carried out in a solid or liquid environment, involving amplification of the target viral nucleic acid or of the signal associated with the bound probe. **Isolation (culture) of the virus is not required for the direct detection of viral antigens or nucleic acids**.

   A. Advantages of direct detection. Direct detection provides rapid results (1–6 hours), good specificity, and no dependence on viral proliferation.

   B. Disadvantages of direct detection. Most viral antigen detection methods have lower sensitivity than virus isolation methods, which can result in false-negative findings. Nucleic acid detection methods have very high sensitivity, which sometimes results in false-positive or positive findings because of a latent virus not involved with disease production. Direct detection also lacks a viral isolate for use if additional subtyping or susceptibility testing is required, and each assay is specific for only a single virus—in contrast to viral culturing in which many viruses may be detected.

   C. Immunofluorescence (IF) in viral antigen detection

      1. Specimen collection. The patient's sample must contain intact infected cells and should be collected in exactly the same manner as a sample for viral culturing, placed in transport medium, and transported to the laboratory (Table 3-20, Table 3-21). In the laboratory, the cells in the sample can be concentrated through centrifugation of the transport medium, and the cell pellet is used to prepare small antigen smears.

(text continues on page 221)

Table 3-20.   Selection of specimens for isolation of viruses in standard cell cultures

Clinical Syndromes: Related Viruses	Clinical Specimens for Virus Isolation: Target Virus[a, b]
Respiratory tract infection: Adeno, CMV, entero, HSV, influenza, mumps, parainfluenza, RSV	**Blood:** CMV **Throat, N/P swab:** All **Sputum:** All except mumps **Urine:** Adeno?, CMV, mumps **Stool/rectal:** Entero **BAL:** CMV, influenza, parainfluenza
Exanthem: Entero, HSV, measles, rubella, VZV	**Blood:** Measles, VZV? **Throat, N/P swab:** All except HSV, VZV? **Vesicle, lesion:** Entero, HSV, VZV **Urine:** Measles?, rubella? **Stool/rectal:** Entero **CSF:** Rubella? Serologic testing is useful for measles and rubella.
Gastroenteritis: Entero, rotavirus, adeno (types 40–41), Norwalk	**Throat, stool/rectal** for entero The other viruses (which cause most of the cases of gastroenteritis) are unculturable; use direct antigen detection or electron microscopy for unculturable viruses.

Febrile illnesses: Tick, dengue, and yellow fevers.

CNS infection: Entero, HSV, measles, mumps, rubella, rabies, arthropod-borne encephalitis viruses.

These viruses are unculturable[c]; use serology.
Blood: measles
Throat, N/P swab: Entero, HSV?, mumps
Vesicle, lesion: HSV
Urine: Mumps
Stool/rectal: Entero
CSF: Entero, HSV, measles, mumps
Brain: Entero, HSV.
Rabies and arthropod-borne encephalitis viruses (e.g., western equine, eastern equine, St. Louis, and California encephalitis) are unculturable[c], and serologic testing is useful for these viruses and for rubella.

Congenital: CMV, entero, HSV, rubella, VZV

Blood: CMV
Throat, N/P swab: All
Vesicle, lesion: HSV, VZV
Urine: CMV, HSV?, rubella?
Stool/rectal: entero
CSF: HSV?, rubella?
Rubella is best confirmed by IgM serology.

Mononucleosis syndrome: CMV, EBV, and hepatitis viruses A, B, and C.

Blood, throat, N/P swab, urine for CMV.
The other viruses are unculturable[c]; use serology.

Adeno, adenovirus; BAL, bronchoalveolar lavage; CMV, cytomegalovirus; CNS, central nervous system; CSF, cerebrospinal fluid; EBV, Epstein-Barr virus; entero, enteroviruses (polio, coxsackie, echoviruses); HSV, herpes simplex virus; RSV, respiratory syncytial virus; VZV, varicella zoster virus.
[a] Question marks following any term indicate questionable usefulness or association.
[b] In all syndromes, appropriate biopsy or autopsy tissue may be helpful.
[c] Unculturable refers to standard cell cultures and vials. Some of these viruses can be isolated in specialized cell cultures not available in most virology laboratories.

Table 3-21.   Collection of specimens for viral culture

Autopsy tissue: Collect samples as soon as possible after death. Place cubes of 1 cm³ or less in VTM[a]. *Do not place tissue in formalin.*

Biopsy tissue: Remove tissue surgically from the site of infection. Place intact specimen in VTM. *Do not place tissue in formalin.*

Blood (anticoagulated): Collect whole blood in heparin, EDTA, or ACD. Sample should arrive in the laboratory within 2 hours of collection.

Eye exudate: Remove exudate or pus with a sterile swab and discard. Rub corneal or conjunctival ulcers with a sterile swab moistened with sterile saline. Place swab in VTM[b].

Genital, cervical: Sample lesions of the external genitalia as any other lesion (see lesions, ulcers, and vesicles). Collect cervical specimens after the cervix has been cleared of mucus and pus. Swab any lesions; if no lesions are present, insert the swab 1 cm into the cervical canal and rotate it. Place swab in VTM[b].

Lesions, ulcers, and vesicles: Collect specimens within 3 days of eruption. Aspirate vesicle fluid with a syringe with a 26 or 27 gauge needle. Place aspirated fluid in VTM. Rub lesion, ulcer, or opened vesicle with a swab, being sure to obtain cells from the base of the lesion or active edge (rather than necrotic center) of the ulcer. Place swab in VTM[b].

Nasal swab: Sample turbinates, not anterior nares. Insert dry cotton swab gently into nose. Leave the swab in the nose for a few seconds so that secretions can be absorbed. Sample both nasal passages. Place swabs in VTM[b].

Rectal swab: Insert dry cotton swab 4–6 cm into the anal orifice and rotate it against the mucosa. Place swab in VTM[b].

Spinal fluid: Collect at least 1.0 mL of CSF; 2–3 mL is preferred. Collect in a sterile screw-capped container. *Do not place fluid in VTM.* Refrigerate during transport to laboratory.

Sputum: Collect expectorated sputum in a sterile screw-capped container.

Stool: Collect a 2–4 g specimen in a sterile container.

Throat swab: Vigorously rub the posterior pharyngeal wall and posterior nasal passages with a dry cotton swab. Place swab in VTM[b].

Urine: Collect 10–50 mL of freshly voided urine in a sterile container. Refrigerate during transport to laboratory. *Do not freeze.*

Washings (throat nasal): Infuse 10–15 mL of sterile physiologic saline into nasal passages. Use suction device to collect washings. Place washings in a sterile, screw-capped container.

---

[a] VTM, viral transport medium. Many types of viral transport media are available commercially. Most contain a balanced salt solution; gelatin, albumin, or fetal bovine serum; antibiotics; and a color indicator.

[b] Break off swab above tip by pressing it against the inside of the transport medium tube.

2. IF principles. All results are viewed with a fluorescence microscope to evaluate quantity and distribution of fluorescence.

    a. Direct. Fluorescein-labeled monoclonal antibodies are applied to the smear of patient cells.

    b. Indirect. Unlabeled monoclonal antibodies (e.g., mouse antibodies) are applied to the smear of patient cells, followed by fluorescein-labeled, antispecies anti-bodies (e.g., anti-mouse antibodies).

3. Applications of IF in viral antigen detection (Table 3-22)

D. Enzyme immunoassay (EIA) in viral antigen detection

    1. Specimen collection. For most EIAs, specimens collected for virus isolation are satisfactory. EIAs have the capacity to detect viral antigens that are free in solution, so intact infected cells are not essential.

    2. EIA principle. A solid phase surface (wall of a microwell, the surface of a plastic bead, or a membrane contained in a plastic cassette) coated with antiviral antibodies is used. When the sample is exposed to the solid phase, the antiviral antibodies bind any viral antigen present in the sample, and subsequent assay steps result in a color change to signal that the viral antigen has been detected. Most EIAs require approximately 2–4 hours to complete, but some cassette-type EIAs require only 15–20 minutes.

    3. Applications of EIA in viral antigen detection (Table 3-22)

E. Molecular techniques (viral nucleic acid detection)

    1. Specimen collection. Samples are collected as for traditional cell culture. Anticoagulated peripheral blood may also be used for many determinations.

    2. Principles of molecular assays

      a. Signal amplification

        (1) *In situ* **probes**: nucleic acid probes are applied directly to tissue section.

        (2) Hybrid capture: RNA probes hybridize to viral DNA to make DNA:RNA hybrids, which are then detected.

        (3) Branched chain DNA (bDNA): virus-specific "extender" probes hybridize to the viral target. bDNA containing numerous branched chains then binds to the probes; bound bDNA is then detected.

      b. Target amplification

        (1) Polymerase chain reaction (PCR). Viral nucleic acid is multiplied through repetitive cycles that create new copies of the viral nucleic acid, which are then identified.

        (2) Many other target amplification methods (**NASBA, LCR**) are now available; each is unique, but all multiply the viral DNA before detection.

    3. Applications of molecular assays (Table 3-22)

III. Virus isolation (traditional cell cultures, shell vials, engineered cell lines). Isolation of viruses in cell cultures depends on the viability of the virus, which must infect living cells and produce cellular changes (cytopathogenic

(*text continues on page 224*)

Table 3-22. Direct detection (IF, EIA, and molecular techniques) and isolation of viruses

Virus	IF	EIA/Other	Molecular	Culture
Adenovirus	Detects group antigens in samples from respiratory tract and eyes	Not available for culturable adenoviruses; use for nonculturable, enteric strains (40,41)	Not routinely available	SCC (7–10d), SV
CMV	Antigenemia (peripheral blood only)	Not available	**Nonamplified:** hybrid capture, bDNA (peripheral blood only) **Amplified** (PCR, others): all specimen types	SCC (14–21d), SV
EBV	Not available	Not available	**Nonamplified:** *In situ* probes for paraffinized tissues **Amplified:** (PCR, others): all specimen types	No SCC
Enterovirus	Not available	Not available	**Amplified** (PCR, others): all specimen types; especially useful for spinal fluids	SCC (2–4d), SV
HSV	Detects group or type antigens in genital, oral, and skin lesion samples	EIA for group antigens from genital, oral, or skin lesion samples Agglutination for group antigens	**Amplified** (PCR, others): all specimen types; especially useful for spinal fluids	SCC (1–2d), SV, ELVIS

Virus				
Hep A, B, C, D, others	Not available	Hepatitis B antigens in peripheral blood	**Nonamplified:** hybrid capture and bDNA for hepatitis B in peripheral blood **Amplified** (PCR, others): hepatitis B and hepatitis C for diagnosis and quantitation	No SCC
HIV-1	Not available	HIV-1 antigens in peripheral blood	**Amplified** (PCR, others): diagnosis and quantitation	No SCC
Influenza A, B	Detects group antigens in respiratory samples	EIA for group A in respiratory samples and for group A and B in some combination assays	Not routinely available	SCC (7–10d), SV
Parainfluenza 1,2,3,4	Detects group antigens in respiratory samples	Not available	Not routinely available	SCC (7–10d), SV
Rotavirus	Not available	EIA and agglutination in fecal samples	Not routinely available	No SCC
RSV	Detects antigen in respiratory samples	EIA for antigen in respiratory samples	Not routinely available	SCC (7–10d), SV
Rubella	Not available	Not available	Not routinely available	SCC difficult
VZV	Detects antigen in samples from lesions	Not available	Not routinely available	SCC (7–10d), SV

bDNA, branched chain DNA method for nucleic acid detection; CMV, cytomegalovirus; d, days; EIA, enzyme immunoassay; EBV, Epstein–Barr virus; ELVIS, enzyme-linked virus inducible (culture) system; Hep, hepatitis virus; HIV, human immunodeficiency virus; HSV, herpes simplex virus; IF, immunofluorescence; PCR, polymerase chain reaction; RSV, respiratory syncytial virus; SCC, standard cell culture; SV, shell vial culture; VZV, varicella zoster virus.

effect-CPE) or otherwise alter the cells as evidence of their replication. Virus isolation can be accomplished in several different formats, although the principles of specimen collection are generally the same regardless of the format.

A.   **Specimen collection. Virus shedding is greatest during the acute stage** of illness. The chance of **viral recovery is best during the first 3 days after disease onset** and is greatly reduced with many viruses beyond 5 days. The selection of the specimen is based on the site of infection, clinical syndrome, or the virus suspected (Table 3-20), and collection varies according to specimen source (Table 3-21). Swabs are used for collection of many types of samples. **Swab tips made of rayon, Dacron, cotton, or polyester are acceptable for use**, whereas calcium alginate-tipped swabs are toxic for herpes simplex virus (HSV) and should not be used. Specimens should be sent to the laboratory immediately. If the specimen cannot be sent immediately, but will be received in the laboratory within 3–5 days after collection, it should be refrigerated at 2°C to 8°C. Specimens that will not be received by the laboratory for more than 3–5 days after collection should be frozen at –70°C or colder. Freezing has been shown to decrease the infectivity of some viruses, and, if the suspected virus is respiratory syncytial virus (RSV) or cytomegalovirus (CMV), **do not freeze the specimen**; store at 2°C to 8°C and send to the laboratory as soon as possible. **Make sure that the suspected virus(es) is clearly identified for each specimen**.

B.   **Viral isolation methodologies**

1.   **Traditional cell cultures. Patient samples are inoculated into test tubes that contain a monolayer of adherent cells. Cells generally are one of three types**: (a) primary cell lines that do not replicate (e.g., **primary monkey kidney**); (b) cell lines that undergo a finite number of divisions (e.g., **human diploid fibroblasts** from newborn foreskin); and (c) cell lines that divide indefinitely [e.g., **HEp-2** (human laryngeal epidermoid carcinoma)]. Different viruses grow best in different types of cell lines, and **determining the cell line in which they grow offers helpful diagnostic information**. Following incubation of cell culture tubes in rotating racks at 37°C, visible **viral cytopathic effects** [CPE: e.g., vacuoles, syncytia (large multinucleated cell masses), swelling, shrinking, loss of adherence, granulation] may offer diagnostic clues, but **follow-up testing is required** to confirm the viral identification. Viruses that are commonly isolated in standard cultures include adenovirus, CMV, many of the enteroviruses (coxsackie B, echovirus, and poliovirus); HSV types 1 and 2; influenza A and B; measles; mumps; parainfluenza types 1, 2, 3, and 4; RSV; and varicella zoster. **Hemadsorption** (adherence of erythrocytes to virus-infected monolayers) can be used to detect some viruses that produce CPE slowly or not at all.

2.   **Shell vial cultures. This system uses centrifugation-enhanced inoculation of cell monolayers grown on coverslips contained in 1-dram shell vials**. After a short incubation period (usually 24–48 hours), an antigen or nucleic acid detection method is performed on the cells in the mono-

layer to detect viral proliferation. The shell vial system has been especially important in detection of CMV, which often requires 7–21 days to produce characteristic CPE in traditional cell cultures. Other viruses sometimes isolated in the shell vial system include HSV and respiratory viruses (adenovirus; influenza A and B; parainfluenza 1, 2, and 3; and RSV).

3. Genetically engineered cell lines. An *Escherichia coli LacZ* gene can be inserted behind an inducible HSV-1 promoter in a line of baby hamster kidney cells, resulting in a cell line that will express detectable β-galactosidase only after infection with HSV. This system, named "enzyme-linked virus inducible system" (**ELVIS**), is sensitive for HSV isolation and is used in many laboratories.

IV. Antivirals. Many antivirals are currently available or nearing approval (Table 3-23). **Because these are virus-specific, rather than broad spectrum such as many antibiotics, definitive viral identification is often required** before initiating therapy with any of these agents.

V. Viruses and their syndromes. Viruses are structures containing **DNA** or **RNA**, with an **outer capsid** made up of capsomeres. The shape of most capsids is either **helical** or **icosahedral**. Some viruses have an additional **outer lipid bilayer envelope** that coats the capsid; it is obtained from the host cell's own cell membrane. Enveloped viruses also have viral-encoded glycoproteins on the envelope surface. A **virus replicates by attaching to receptors** on living cell surfaces (which determine the type of cell or organ that the virus can infect), then **penetrating** the cell wall, followed by an uncoating of the virus' genetic material. The genetic material **utilizes some of the cell's enzymatic functions to replicate itself** and produce viral proteins (usually divided into "early" and "late" proteins). The new viral genetic material and proteins are then assembled into new viruses (**"virions"**). **Enveloped viruses are released from the host cell by budding** (which does not kill the cell), whereas **nonenveloped viruses are released by lysis** of the host cell (which kills the cell). Viruses vary in size from 20 nm (e.g., parvoviruses) to 400 nm (e.g., poxviruses).

Viruses can be transmitted to humans in various ways, including direct contact [e.g., hand-mouth, hand-eye (e.g., common cold viruses), mouth-mouth (e.g., Epstein–Barr virus)], **sexual contact** (e.g., human immunodeficiency virus; HIV), **respiratory droplets** (e.g., influenza), **fecal-oral route** (e.g., rotavirus), **contaminated blood** (e.g., hepatitis C), from **infected animals** (e.g., rabies), or from **infected arthropods** (e.g., western equine encephalitis). **After the initial entry of the virus, a generalized viremic stage often occurs, followed by deposition in a final target tissue** for which the virus has a predisposition (e.g., the brain, kidneys). Most DNA viruses have a latent stage that can persist indefinitely in the patient (except for parvovirus B19, which causes transient infections). **RNA viruses have various life spans** within patients, with many lasting for a small finite time period. **Some viruses are oncogenic**, and are associated with specific malignancies (Table 3-24).

The main **DNA viruses** include adenoviruses, hepadnaviruses, herpesviruses, papovaviruses, parvoviruses, and poxviruses. The

Table 3-23. Antivirals

Virus	Antiviral Generic Name (Trade Name)[a]
CMV	Ganciclovir (Cytovene), Cidofovir (Vistide), Foscarnet (Foscavir)
EBV	Some HSV and VZV antivirals may have some clinical effect
Enterovirus	Pleconaril[b]
HSV	Acyclovir (Zovirax), Valacyclovir (Valtrex), Famciclovir (Famvir), Vidarabine (Vira-A), Idoxuridine (Herplex Liquifilm, Stoxil), Trifluridine (Viroptic), Foscarnet (Foscavir)
Hepatitis B	Interferon alfa 2a (Roferon), Lamivudine, also known as 3TC (Epivir HBV), Famciclovir (Famvir), Lobucavir[b], Adefovir dipivoxil (Preveon)[b]
Hepatitis C	Interferon alfa 2b (Viraferon), Interferon in combination with Ribavirin (Virazole)
HIV	Dideoxynucleoside analogues: Zidovudine AZT (Retrovir), Didanosine (Videx), Zalcitabine (Hivid), Stavudine (Zerit), Lamivudine (Epivir) Protease inhibitors: Saquinavir (Invirase), Indinavir (Crixivan), Ritonavir (Norvir), Nelfinavir (Viracept) Nonnucleoside reverse transcriptase inhibitors: Nevirapine (Viramune), Delavirdine (Rescriptor), Efavirenz (Sustiva)
Influenza A	Amantadine (Symmetrel), Rimantadine (Flumadine), Zanamivir (Relenza)
Influenza B	Zanamivir (Relenza)
Rhinovirus	Pleconaril[b]
RSV	Ribavirin (Virazole)
VZV	Acyclovir (Zovirax), Valacyclovir (Valtrex), Famciclovir (Famvir), Vidarabine (Vira-A), Idoxuridine (Herplex Liquifilm, Stoxil), Trifluridine (Viroptic)

CMV, cytomegalovirus; EBV, Epstein-Barr virus; HIV, human immunodeficiency virus; HSV, herpes simplex virus; RSV, respiratory syncytial virus; VZV, varicella-zoster virus.

[a] At this writing, no antivirals are marketed for adenovirus, hepatitis A, parainfluenza viruses, rotavirus, or rubella.

[b] In clinical trials at this writing.

Table 3-24.   Viruses and their relationship to malignancy

Virus	Malignancy
Epstein–Barr virus	Burkitt's lymphoma Nasopharyngeal carcinoma B-cell lymphomas in immuno- suppressed patients
Hepatitis B virus	Hepatocellular carcinoma
Human T-cell lymphotrophic virus-1 (HTLV-I)	Adult T-cell lymphoma/leukemia
Human papillomavirus	Carcinoma (uterine cervical carcinoma)

main **RNA viruses** include bunyaviruses, coronaviruses, ortho-myxoviruses, paramyxoviruses, picornaviruses, retroviruses, rhab-doviruses, and togaviruses.

The most common viruses detected by community laboratories **in children include RSV, rotavirus, enteroviruses, and parainfluenza viruses**. The most common viruses detected **in youth and adults include Epstein–Barr virus, herpes simplex viruses, and CMV**. Table 3-25 provides brief descriptions of the most significant viruses that infect humans.

(*text continues on page 236*)

Table 3-25.   Significant human viral pathogens

ADENOVIRUS

General: A family of viruses (>40 serotypes), 80 nm in size, double-stranded DNA, icosahedral, no envelope; "adeno," from Gr. meaning "gland," referring to upper respiratory infections of "glands" such as tonsils and adenoids.

Disease association: Transmitted by fecal-oral, respiratory, and direct contact (e.g., conjunctivitis) routes. Causes upper and lower respiratory tract infections, ocular infections, gastroenteritis (e.g., types 40 and 41), cystitis, serious disseminated disease in transplant recipients or other immunosuppressed patients. Some types (e.g., 4 and 7) may cause epidemics in groups with close contact (e.g., dorm students or military personnel). Adenovirus remains latent within lymphoid tissues.

Laboratory diagnosis: Most strains isolated in standard cell cultures, with IF used for antigen detection. Enteric adenoviruses (types 40 and 41) are nonculturable in standard cell lines, and EIA is used for antigen detection. Antibodies detected by complement fixation for determining seroconversion and monitoring changes in antibody titers.

Specimens: Samples from upper and lower respiratory sites for virus isolation or antigen detection. Viruses may also be isolated from conjunctiva, feces, or urine. Submit clotted blood for antibody detection.

continued

Table 3-25.   *Continued*

ARBOVIRUSES

General: A group of viruses that are transmitted by arthropod vectors ("arbo," from "*ar*thropod-*bo*rne"). These viruses include members of the flavivirus, togavirus, bunyavirus (from African bunyamwera virus), rhabdovirus, arenavirus, and reovirus families.

Disease association: Transmitted by arthropods (e.g., mosquitoes); cause a spectrum of disease, from asymptomatic infections to meningitis/encephalitis (e.g., eastern equine, western equine, Venezuelan, St. Louis, and California), yellow fever, dengue, and so on.

Laboratory diagnosis: Antibody detection by indirect fluorescence for determining seroconversion and monitoring changes in antibody titers.

CORONAVIRUS

General: 80–150 nm, single-stranded RNA, helical shape, enveloped; "corona" from Gr. meaning "crown," referring to the crown of projections on the viral surface seen with EM.

Disease association: Common cold

Laboratory diagnosis: Cannot be isolated in standard cell culture; antigen and antibody detection are not available. Diagnosis is made on clinical grounds alone.

COXSACKIEVIRUSES (SEE ENTEROVIRUSES)

CYTOMEGALOVIRUS (CMV)

General: A member of the herpes family, 150 nm, double-stranded DNA, icosahedral, enveloped.

Disease association: CMV can be transmitted by respiratory secretions or saliva, organ transplants, blood transfusions (CMV is carried by the white cells), contaminated breast milk, and transplacentally. In immunocompetent individuals, most infections are subclinical or insignificant, although an infectious mononucleosis-like syndrome is seen in teenagers and young adults (CMV is the most common cause of heterophile-negative infectious mononucleosis). The virus establishes latency in all patients. Primary infections in seronegative pregnant females can produce congenital infections that result in a variety of symptoms. In immunocompromised individuals (especially bone marrow transplant recipients), serious and often fatal pneumonia is seen.

Laboratory diagnosis: Isolated in standard cell cultures and shell vials. Antigen detection by IF in peripheral blood samples ("antigenemia" assay); not routinely productive in other types of samples. Detection of antibodies by many methods (passive latex agglutination, EIA, IF) for determining immune status, detecting seroconversion, and monitoring changes in antibody level. Nucleic acid detection (by signal and target amplification methods) available for various specimen types. Histologically, infected cells are quite enlarged (whence the name "cytomegalo")

Specimens: Urine and peripheral blood are the two samples that yield virus most frequently in culture. In infected, immunocompromised patients, bronchoalveolar lavage as well as lung and other appropriate biopsy samples are most useful. Anticoagulated

Table 3-25. *Continued*

peripheral blood is used for antigenemia assays. Submit clotted blood for antibody detection and EDTA plasma for molecular diagnostics. Nucleic acid detection can be performed on various specimen types including biopsy tissue, amniotic fluid, CSF, urine, and sputum.

ECHOVIRUSES (SEE ENTEROVIRUSES)

ENTEROVIRUSES

General: Members of the picornavirus family ["pico"(small) + "RNA"], 25 nm, single-stranded RNA, icosahedral, no envelope; includes the following viruses:

–1. Poliovirus (from Gr. meaning "gray", referring to CNS gray matter infections)

–2. Coxsackieviruses (named for Coxsackie, NY, where it was discovered)

–3. Echoviruses (from *enteric cytopathic human orphan*: initially, the isolated virus was not thought to "belong" to any specific disease association)

–4. Enteroviruses (including hepatitis A virus, which is enterovirus 72).

Disease association: transmitted by fecal-oral route; causes polio (poliovirus), herpangina and hand-foot-mouth disease (coxsackie A), myocarditis (coxsackie B), hemorrhagic conjunctivitis (enterovirus 70), meningitis (enteroviruses), hepatitis (enterovirus 72), and summer/early fall influenza (most viruses in this family).

Laboratory diagnosis: polio: cultures and serology; coxsackie and enteroviruses: culture

EPSTEIN-BARR VIRUS (EBV)

General: Named after a physician and a virologist; a member of the herpes family, 100 nm, double-stranded DNA, icosahedral, enveloped.

Disease association: transmitted by saliva. Produces classic EBV infectious mononucleosis in otherwise healthy adolescents and young adults. Subclinical infections are common in children. The virus establishes latency after primary infection and may reactivate when the host is stressed or immunocompromised. EBV also causes oral hairy leukoplakia and is associated with Burkitt's lymphoma, nasopharyngeal carcinoma, and B-cell lymphomas in immunocompromised patients.

Laboratory diagnosis: Cannot be isolated in standard cell cultures, and antigen detection assays are not available. Heterophile antibodies detected in 80%–90% of classic EBV infectious mononucleosis. Several methods (EIA, IF) are used to detect and identify a variety of EBV-related antibodies (e.g., VCA, EA, EBNA, discussed in detail in the chapter *Infectious Serology*) for determining antibody status and in detecting seroconversion and monitoring changes in antibody level. This is especially important in heterophile-negative infectious mononucleosis and in EBV-related syndromes such as nasopharyngeal carcinoma and Burkitt's lymphoma. Molecular assays may detect EBV DNA in clinical samples.

continued

Table 3-25.   *Continued*

Specimens: Submit clotted blood for antibody detection and EDTA plasma for molecular assays. Biopsy tissue can be used in molecular assays.

HANTAVIRUS

General: also called **sin nombre virus** (literally "without name"), member of the Bunyavirus family, 100 nm, single-stranded RNA, spherical shape, enveloped.

Disease association: Transmitted by contact with infected animal feces; causes influenza like illness, which may progress to respiratory failure. In the United States, cases have been reported in many states west of the Mississippi River. Contact reference laboratories for suspected cases.

HEPATITIS A VIRUS (ENTEROVIRUS TYPE 72)

General: A member of the picornavirus family, 25 nm, single-stranded RNA, icosahedral, no envelope.

Disease association: Transmitted by fecal-oral route. Causes classic "infectious" acute hepatitis. No carrier state.

Laboratory diagnosis: Cannot be isolated in standard cell cultures, and antigen detection not available routinely. Detection of IgM and total (IgM and IgG) antibodies widely available by EIA.

Specimens: Submit clotted blood for antibody detection.

HEPATITIS B VIRUS (HBV)

General: A member of the hepadnavirus family ["hepadnavirus" from "Hepa"(liver) + "DNA"], 40 nm, double-stranded DNA, globoid or elongated shape. "Dane particle" is a synonym for the entire HBV virion. "Australia antigen" is a synonym for the HBV surface antigen.

Disease association: Transmitted by direct person contact (e.g., sexual activity), intravenous (IV) drug use, contaminated blood products, and so on. Causes classic "serum" hepatitis. Of infections, 90% are acute and self-limited (two thirds of these cases are asymptomatic), 1% of the infections are fulminant (sometimes requiring liver transplant), and 9% of the infections are chronic. Chronic infections can be asymptomatic (carrier states), or can cause chronic hepatitis, cirrhosis, or hepatocellular carcinoma. Infections in children are associated with a higher likelihood of chronicity than in adults.

Laboratory diagnosis: Cannot be isolated in standard cell cultures. Detection of HBV surface antigen and HBV e antigen by EIA. Detection of several HBV-related antibodies (HBV core total—IgG and IgM, HBV core IgM, HBV e antibody, HBV surface antibody) by EIA (see *Infectious Serology* chapter). Molecular diagnostics used to detect viral nucleic acids.

Specimens: Submit clotted blood for use in antigen, antibody, and nucleic acid detection assays. EDTA plasma can also be used for most of these assays.

HEPATITIS C VIRUS (HCV)

General: A member of the flavivirus family ("flavi" from L. meaning "yellow", referring to the yellow fever virus in this family), 50 nm, single-stranded RNA, enveloped. It is found world-wide, with a high prevalence in the Mediterranean, Africa, and the Orient.

Table 3-25. *Continued*

Disease association: Transmitted by sexual contact, IV drug use, and particularly through contaminated blood products (causes 90% of the transfusion-related cases of hepatitis). Causes "non-A, non-B" hepatitis. Of the acute infections, 75% are asymptomatic; >50% of the infections become chronic, and 50% of the chronic infections lead to cirrhosis. HCV is also associated with hepatocellular carcinoma.

Laboratory diagnosis: Cannot be isolated in standard cell cultures, and antigen detection not available routinely. Total antibody IgM and IgG detected by EIA. Identity of antibodies confirmed by immunoblotting (recombinant immunoblot assay—RIBA). Molecular methods for viral nucleic acid detection are available (e.g., cDNA-PCR).

Specimens: Submit clotted blood for antibody and nucleic acid detection. EDTA plasma can be used for most of these assays.

HEPATITIS D VIRUS (HDV)

General: A defective RNA virus that needs the hepatitis B virus to complete its replication.

Disease association: Transmitted by direct contact (see hepatitis B), and infects only in the presence of active HBV.

Laboratory diagnosis: Cannot be isolated in standard cell cultures, and antigen detection not available routinely. Total antibody IgM and IgG detected by EIA.

Specimens: Submit clotted blood for antibody detection.

HEPATITIS E VIRUS

General: Most likely a member of the calicivirus family ("calici" from L. meaning "little cup," referring to the tiny cups seen on the viral surface by EM), 33 nm, single-stranded RNA, icosahedral, no envelope.

Disease association: transmitted by fecal-oral route. Causes hepatitis that is particularly dangerous to pregnant women (20% mortality). Occurs in Asia, north and west Africa, and Mexico.

Laboratory diagnosis: Cannot be isolated in standard cell cultures, and no reagents available commercially in the United States for detection of antigens or antibodies. Consult reference laboratory.

HERPES SIMPLEX VIRUSES (HSV) (TYPES 1 AND 2)

General: 100 nm, double-stranded DNA, icosahedral, enveloped; "herpes" from Gr. meaning "to creep," referring to spreading skin lesions.

Disease association: HSV types 1 and 2 produce recurrent lesions in oral (80% from HSV-1) and genital (80% from HSV-2) areas, as well as pharyngitis (HSV-1), conjunctivitis (HSV-1), encephalitis (HSV-1), and skin infections (HSV-1 and -2, "Whitlow"). The virus establishes latency within nerve cells after primary infection and may reactivate when the host is stressed. Congenital infections (HSV-2) may occur in infants born to mothers who have genital herpes.

Laboratory diagnosis: Isolated in standard cell cultures. Antigen detected by IF or EIA. Antibodies detected by many methods (e.g., IF, EIA) for determining antibody status, detecting seroconversion, and monitoring changes in antibody level.

continued

Table 3-25. *Continued*

Specimens: For virus isolation and antigen detection, submit swabs from lesions or other infected sites. Submit clotted blood for antibody detection.

HERPES VIRUSES (PARTICULARLY TYPES 6, 7, AND 8)
General: 100 nm, double-stranded DNA, icosahedral, enveloped. There are eight types of viruses in the human herpes family, including HSV types 1 and 2, Epstein–Barr virus, cytomegalovirus, varicella zoster virus, human herpes virus (HHV) types 6, 7, and 8; see individual viruses for more information.

Disease association: HHV-6 causes roseola (exanthem subitum). HHV-7 causes a few cases of roseola and a CMV-like infection in bone marrow transplant patients. HHV-8 is associated with all forms of Kaposi's sarcoma, and with some cases of primary effusion lymphomas (nonsolid lymphomas) as well as multicentric Castleton's disease. For other herpes viruses, see under individual name.

Laboratory diagnosis: Serology (e.g., EIA).

Specimens: Submit clotted blood for antibody detection.

HUMAN IMMUNODEFICIENY VIRUS-1,2 (HIV), AND HUMAN T-CELL LYMPHOTROPHIC VIRUS 1,2 (HTLV)
General: Members of the retrovirus family, 100 nm, single-stranded RNA, icosahedral, enveloped. Viruses contain reverse transcriptase, which makes DNA from RNA (whence the name "retro").

Disease association: Transmitted by sexual contact, IV drug use, contaminated blood products, contaminated breast milk, and transplacentally. HIV-1 and HIV-2 infect T lymphocytes (T-helper cells) and monocytes. Monocytes are the probable reservoir of the virus within the body. HIV-1 and HIV-2 infection results in acquired immunodeficiency syndrome (AIDS), which starts as an acute self-limited illness (e.g., sore throat, myalgias), includes a chronic phase with progressive viral replication and lymphadenopathy, and reaches a crisis phase represented by breakdown of the immune system, decreased CD4 cell counts, and opportunistic infections. Opportunistic infections include *Pneumocystis carinii, Candida, Mycobacterium avium-intracellulare, Cryptococcus, Toxoplasma*, herpes simplex, cryptosporidium, and so on. Malignancies (e.g., Kaposi's sarcoma, non-Hodgkin's lymphomas) are also likely to occur.

HTLV 1,2 are transmitted primarily in contaminated blood products, and the prevalence is relatively high in the Orient and Caribbean: HTLV 1,2 causes adult T-cell leukemia-lymphoma and HTLV-1–associated myelopathy (also known as tropical spastic paraparesis).

Laboratory diagnosis: Viruses cannot be isolated in standard cell cultures. HIV-1 antigen detection by EIA (positive after 35 days of infection). Antigen detection not widely available for other viruses. Antibody detection for all viruses, with EIA used extensively for screening, and immunoblotting (Western blotting) used for confirmation. For HIV-1, diagnosis requires two of the following three bands on immunoblotting: p24, gp41, gp120/160. Nucleic acid detection (e.g., PCR, turns positive after 20 days of infection) for confirmation of active infection and for quantitation of viral load. Ancillary tests include CD4 (T-helper) lymphocyte

Table 3-25. *Continued*

counts (decreased in AIDS), with a reversal of the CD4/CD8 ratio (the ratio becomes <1).

Specimens: Submit clotted blood for antigen, antibody, and nucleic acid detection. EDTA plasma may be acceptable for many assays.

INFLUENZA A AND B VIRUSES

General: Members of the orthomyxovirus family, 100 nm, single-stranded *segmented* RNA, helical shape, enveloped; "orthomyxo" from "ortho" (Gr. meaning "true") and "myxo" (Gr. meaning "mucous"; referring to the "true influenza viruses"). Viruses are categorized according to hemagglutinin and neuraminidase viral-related surface antigens. Viruses infect humans and animals. Mutations in influenza A generally originate in the Far East, where humans live in close proximity with infected animals. Antigenic "drift" (from minor genetic mutations) causes new yearly seasonal (winter/spring) infections. Antigenic "shifts" (which occur only in influenza A, are major changes in the viral genome, probably because of reassortment of the genetic segments with similar animal influenza viruses) cause world-wide pandemics every few decades.

Disease association: Influenza A causes upper and lower respiratory infections (including serious acute pneumonia), influenza (headache, myalgias, fatigue), and croup. Influenza B causes mild forms of influenza and gastroenteritis.

Laboratory diagnosis of influenza A and B (Influenza C does not cause significant human infection, and is not routinely tested): Isolation of most strains in standard cell cultures. IF or EIA for detection of antigen. Antibody detection (group antibodies, not strain specific) by complement fixation for determining seroconversion and in monitoring antibody titers.

Specimens: Samples from upper and lower respiratory sites for virus isolation or for viral antigen detection. Submit clotted blood for antibody detection.

MEASLES VIRUS (SEE PARAMYXOVIRUSES)

MUMPS VIRUS (SEE PARAMYXOVIRUSES)

NORWALK VIRUS

General: Possibly, a calicivirus, 25 nm, single-stranded RNA, icosahedral, no envelope; named for Norwalk, Ohio, where the first outbreak was documented.

Disease association: Sporadic, abrupt gastroenteritis in older children and adults, usually associated with contaminated food and water.

Laboratory diagnosis: Diagnostic assays are not widely available, with diagnosis usually depending on visualization of the viral particles in feces by electron microscopy. Consult reference laboratory.

PAPOVAVIRUSES (PAPILLOMAVIRUS, POLYOMAVIRUS)

General: This family of viruses is 50 nm, double-stranded DNA, icosahedral, no envelope; "Papova" stands for *pa*pillomavirus, *po*lyomavirus, *va*cuolating (the viruses cause perinuclear vacuolization).

continued

Table 3-25.   *Continued*

Disease association:

Human papillomaviruses (HPV): Cause various warts [e.g., verruca plantaris (type 1), verruca vulgaris (type 2), condyloma acuminatum and laryngeal papillomas (types 6 and 11), cervical and laryngeal dysplasia/carcinoma (types 16, 18, 31, 33), and dermatologic anomalies.]

Polyoma viruses: JC type causes progressive multifocal leukoencephalopathy; BK type causes hemorrhagic cystitis.

Laboratory diagnosis: Cannot be isolated in standard cell cultures. Antigen detection not widely available. Antibody detection not available. Diagnosis usually rests on clinical evaluation and histologic confirmation. Molecular techniques can identify viral nucleic acids.

Specimens: Contact reference or research laboratory to determine acceptable samples.

PARAINFLUENZA VIRUSES (SEE PARAMYXOVIRUSES)

PARAMYXOVIRUSES

General: This family of viruses includes parainfluenza, measles, mumps, and respiratory syncytial, 150–300 nm, single-stranded, nonsegmented RNA, helical, enveloped; "paramyxo" (from Gr. "para") meaning "similar to" (and "myxo" meaning "mucous"), referring to viruses that are similar to the true influenza viruses.

Disease Association:

–**Parainfluenza types 1, 2, 3, 4:** Transmitted by respiratory route; cause epidemics of upper and lower respiratory tract infections in the fall and spring (including pneumonia), and croup.

–**Measles virus:** Transmitted by respiratory route; causes measles in the winter and spring, atypical measles (in individuals vaccinated with killed measles viruses as children) and subacute sclerosing panencephalitis (SSPE).

–**Mumps:** Transmitted by respiratory route; causes mumps (parotitis) in the winter and spring, aseptic meningitis, nephritis, orchitis, otitis, and so on.

–**Respiratory syncytial virus:** (RSV) see separate category below.

Laboratory diagnosis: Virus isolation in standard cell cultures. Antigen detection by IF for parainfluenzas. Type-specific antibodies for parainfluenza are detected by complement fixation (used for determining seroconversion and monitoring changes in antibody levels). Measles antibodies are detected by EIA. Mumps antibodies are detected by IF or EIA.

Specimens: Samples from upper and lower respiratory sites for virus isolation and viral antigen detection. Submit clotted blood for antibody detection.

PARVOVIRUS

General: 20 nm, single-stranded DNA, icosahedral, no envelope; "parvo" from L. meaning "small."

Disease association: Parvovirus B19 infects nucleated red cell precursors in the bone marrow. Parvovirus B19 has been implicated as the agent of fifth disease (erythema infectiosum) in children, in aplastic crisis in patients with chronic hemolytic disorders (e.g., sickle cell disease, thalassemia), and in hydrops fetalis.

Table 3-25. *Continued*

Laboratory diagnosis: Cannot be isolated in standard cell cultures. Antigen detection is not available. Antibody testing is available in reference laboratories. Molecular diagnostic techniques may be used to detect parvovirus B19 DNA

Specimens: Submit clotted blood for antibody detection. Contact reference laboratory to identify proper specimens for molecular assays.

POXVIRUSES (VARIOLA, MOLLUSCUM CONTAGIOSUM, ETC.)

General: Large 200–400 nm, double-stranded DNA, enveloped; "pox" from Anglo-Saxon meaning "spot."

Disease association: All poxviruses cause skin lesions. Variola virus produces classic smallpox. This virus is now reported by the World Health Organization to be eradicated from the planet. *Molluscum contagiosum* produces skin or genital lesions. Vaccinia virus is the vaccine virus used formerly in smallpox vaccine.

Laboratory diagnosis: No testing available in routine clinical laboratories

RABIES VIRUS

General: "Rabies" from L. meaning "to rage," a member of the rhabdovirus family, 180 nm long, single-stranded RNA, bullet-shaped, enveloped; "rhabdo" from Gr. meaning "rod-shaped."

Disease association: Causes rabies.

Laboratory diagnosis: Histology with direct immuno-fluorescence, serology.

RESPIRATORY SYNCYTIAL VIRUS (RSV)

General: A member of the paramyxovirus; single-stranded nonsegmented RNA, helical, enveloped.

Disease association: Transmitted by respiratory route or by direct contact (hand). Most common cause of seasonal (winter) severe respiratory problems in infants and young children.

Laboratory diagnosis: Virus isolation in standard cell cultures (infected cells form a giant syncytium, whence the virus name). Antigen detection by IF or EIA. Antibody detection by many methods (complement fixation, IF) for detecting seroconversion and monitoring changes in antibody level.

Specimens: Samples from upper and lower respiratory sites for virus isolation and viral antigen detection. Submit clotted blood for antibody detection.

RHINOVIRUS

General: "Rhino" from Gr. meaning "nose," a member of the picornavirus family, 25 nm, RNA, icosahedral, no envelope; >100 serotypes.

Disease association: Transmitted by respiratory secretions. Causes the common cold. Laboratory diagnosis is usually not necessary.

ROTAVIRUS

General: "Rota" from L. meaning wheel, referring to the virus' appearance under EM; a member of the reovirus family, 70 nm, double-stranded, segmented RNA, icosahedral, no envelope.

continued

Table 3-25. *Continued*

Disease association: Transmitted by fecal-oral route or by contact with contaminated surfaces; causes seasonal (winter/spring) gastroenteritis in infants (6 months to 2 years of age).

Laboratory diagnosis: Antigen detection by several methods (e.g., EIA, latex agglutination).

RUBELLA VIRUS

General: "Rubella" from L. meaning "red" referring to the skin rash, member of the togavirus family, 60 nm, single-stranded RNA, icosahedral, enveloped; "toga" refers to the envelope that "cloaks" the virus.

Disease association: Transmitted by respiratory route and transplacentally; causes rubella (German measles); congenital rubella is particularly serious.

Laboratory diagnosis: Viral isolation in cell cultures is difficult. Antibody detection by hemagglutination inhibition and EIA for detecting seroconversion and monitoring changes in antibody level.

VARICELLA-ZOSTER VIRUS (VZV)

General: "Varicella" from L. for the "pox disease"; "zoster" from Gr. meaning "girdle", referring to the rash; a member of the herpes family, 100 nm, double-stranded DNA, icosahedral, enveloped.

Disease association: Transmitted by respiratory secretions; VZV causes chickenpox. The virus remains latent in the dorsal root ganglia. Reactivation is called shingles.

Laboratory diagnosis: Isolated in standard cell cultures. Antigen detected by IF. Antibodies detected by many methods (passive latex agglutination, EIA, IF).

Specimens: For virus isolation and viral antigen detection, scrapings or swab samples collected from lesions should be submitted. Submit clotted blood for antibody detection.

CNS, central nervous system; CSF, cerebrospinal fluid; EIA, enzyme immunoassay; EM, electron microscopy; Gr., Greek; IF, immunofluorescence; L., Latin; PCR, polymerase chain reaction.

BIBLIOGRAPHY

Leland DS. *Clinical virology*. Philadelphia: WB Saunders, 1996.

Lennette EH, Lennette DA, Lennette ET. *Diagnostic procedures for viral, rickettsial, and chlamydial infections*, 7th ed. Washington, DC: American Public Health Association, 1995.

Lennette EH, Smith TF. *Laboratory diagnosis of viral infections*, 3rd ed. New York: Marcel Dekker, 1999.

Mycology

Elmer W. Koneman

I. Introduction

Fungi are eukaryotic cells with the morphologic forms of either molds or yeasts. Molds are hyphal (filamentous) structures, whereas **yeasts are spherical**. Hyphae may or may not have septa (**septate or aseptate**), and may be **clear (hyaline) or dark (dematiaceous)**. Fungi reproduce **sexually or asexually**, and are often categorized according to the morphologic and biochemical characteristics of their yeast, mold, and reproductive structure (spore) forms. Although thousands of different fungi exist in nature, only a few have yet caused infections in humans.

II. Definitions

A. **Yeasts are spherical** fungal cells that reproduce **asexually by budding** (forming blastoconidia).

B. **Molds** are synonymous with **"mycelium."** They are long, **filamentous** fungal cells (hyphae) that reproduce either **sexually or asexually**.

C. **Mycelium** is a "mat" of **hyphae growing together**.

D. **Reproductive structures (spores)** can be formed asexually or sexually.

    1. **Asexual spores** (also called **conidia**, which means "dust") can be large (**macroconidia**) or small (**microconidia**), and formed from vegetative or aerial hyphae.

        a. **Vegetative production**: conidia arising from hyphal or yeast forms that are submerged beneath the substrate

            (1) **Arthroconidia**: formed by the fragmentation of parent hyphae

            (2) **Blastoconidia**: formed by budding of parent yeast cells

            (3) **Chlamydoconidia**: thick-walled, resilient structures formed from parent hyphae

        b. **Aerial production**: conidia arising from specialized structures extending above the substrate called **"fruiting bodies"**

    2. **Sexual spores**: rarely seen in clinical isolates, they include ascospores, basidiospores, and zygospores

E. **Dimorphic**: fungi that grow as molds (hyphae) at ambient temperature, and as yeasts at body temperature

III. Collection

A. **Blood.** After decontamination of the skin (as for bacterial blood cultures), blood is collected into special fungal culture media containers (e.g., BACT-i-FLASK).

B. **Urine.** The first early morning void into a sterile container is the one most useful.

C. **Cerebrospinal fluid (CSF).** Samples are obtained via a spinal tap. Sterile containers with CSF (same as for bacterial culture) are appropriate.

D. **Sputum.** Respiratory samples should be obtained by induction, bronchoscopy, or alveolar lavage.

   E. Skin, hair, and nails. Decontamination of the skin (using
70% alcohol swabs) is important before obtaining scrapings;
scrapings should be performed at the edge of skin lesions, using
the side of a scalpel blade or the edge of a glass microscopic slide.
Plucked hair should be placed in a clean container. Nails should
be sampled by scraping the soft material underneath the nail
plate, not the outer surface of the nail.
   F. Wounds and deeper tissues. Swab specimens are not
recommended (superficial specimens often miss the deeper fungal organisms, and are heavily contaminated). Deep scrapings,
aspirates, or biopsy material are best. Place biopsies in sterile,
saline-soaked gauze; do not place in formalin.

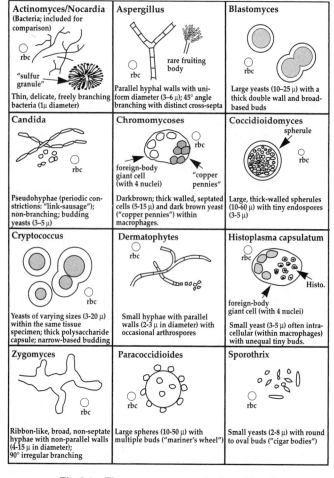

Actinomyces/Nocardia (Bacteria; included for comparison)	Aspergillus	Blastomyces
Thin, delicate, freely branching bacteria (1μ diameter)	Parallel hyphal walls with uniform diameter (3–6 μ); 45° angle branching with distinct cross-septa	Large yeasts (10–25 μ) with a thick double wall and broad-based buds
Candida	**Chromomycoses**	**Coccidioidomyces**
Pseudohyphae (periodic constrictions: "link-sausage"); non-branching; budding yeasts (3–5 μ)	Darkbrown; thick walled, septated cells (5-15 μ) and dark brown yeast ("copper pennies") within macrophages.	Large, thick-walled spherules (10–60 μ) with tiny endospores (3-5 μ)
Cryptococcus	**Dermatophytes**	**Histoplasma capsulatum**
Yeasts of varying sizes (3-20 μ) within the same tissue specimen; thick polysaccharide capsule; narrow-based budding	Small hyphae with parallel walls (2-3 μ in diameter) with occasional arthrospores	Small yeast (3-5 μ) often intracellular (within macrophages) with unequal tiny buds.
Zygomyces	**Paracoccidioides**	**Sporothrix**
Ribbon-like, broad, non-septate hyphae with non-parallel walls (4-15 μ in diameter); 90° irregular branching	Large spheres (10-50 μ) with multiple buds ("mariner's wheel")	Small yeasts (2-8 μ) with round to oval buds ("cigar bodies")

Fig. 3-1.   Tissue appearances of selected fungi.

G.   Vagina. Swabs are appropriate. Keep moist with saline or place in an appropriate transport container.

IV.   Media

Physicians should indicate on the request slip a suspected diagnosis when submitting clinical samples, so that laboratory personnel can select appropriate media and incubation conditions. Two general types of media (nonselective and selective) are required to ensure recovery of all significant fungi.

   A.   Nonselective media. Allow growth of virtually all fungal species.

   1.   Inhibitory mold agar (or SABHI agar): recommended

   2.   Sabouraud dextrose agar (SDA): not recommended as a primary isolation medium except for cutaneous or vaginal cultures.

   B.   Selective media. Prevent the overgrowth of rapidly growing fungi, allowing slowly growing fungi to be recovered.

   1.   Sabouraud's dextrose agar (SDA) with cycloheximide and chloramphenicol (SDA with C&C); particularly useful for cutaneous cultures.

   2.   Brain-heart infusion media (BHI) with antibiotics and antifungal agents prevents the overgrowth of bacteria and rapidly growing fungal contaminants.

V.   Methods of microscopic examination

   A.   Direct examination

   1.   KOH (potassium hydroxide): put specimen (skin, nail scraping, mucosal swab) on glass slide, add one drop of 10%–20% KOH, gently warm, coverslip, wait 10 minutes, examine under microscope.

   2.   Phase-contrast microscopy: quick, no need for direct stains, and good visualization.

   3.   India ink: primarily of historical interest; centrifuge CSF, place one drop of sediment on a glass slide, and add one drop of India ink; examine for *Cryptococcus neoformans*. Antigen detection methods have largely replaced the India ink method.

   B.   Lactophenol cotton blue. Yeasts and hyphae are stained a delicate blue color that is useful for morphologic evaluation. It is used with **tease mounts** and **scotch tape mounts** (the sticky tape surface is touched to the culture media surface, fungal elements adhere to the tape, and are then stained and examined).

   C.   Calcofluor white. A whiting agent and mordant used in the textile industry, calcofluor white binds to the cellulose and chitin in the fungal cell walls, and fluoresces under ultraviolet light. It is particularly helpful when viewing skin scrapings for dermatophytic hyphae.

   D.   Tissue sections: Periodic Acid-Schiff (PAS) and **Gamori's Methenamine Silver** (GMS) (See Fig. 3-1 for description of morphology)

VI.   General features of fungal infections

   A.   Predisposing conditions. Some conditions predispose individuals to fungal infections, including **immunosuppression** [e.g., acquired immunodeficiency syndrome (**AIDS**), organ transplant patients]; leukopenia; underlying malignancies (particularly hematopoietic); **debilitating or metabolic disorders** (e.g., **diabetes**, systemic lupus, hemochromatosis, dysgammaglobulinemia); **alcohol** or intravenous (IV) drug use; a history of **recent** travel to places where fungal infections are endemic; a history of **recent antibiotic or immunosuppressive therapy**; or a history of activities that involve **close contact with soil, vegetation, or animals**.

  B. **Presenting signs and symptoms (S&S)**

    1. **General**. S&S are often vague and nonspecific, including low-grade fever, night sweats, weight loss, and easy fatigability.

    2. **Organ-specific**

        a. **Pulmonary**: chronic cough with or without chest pain, progressive dyspnea, hemoptysis; chest x-ray showing nonresolving pulmonary infiltrates, finely nodular fibrosis, or focal abscesses.

        b. **Skin and mucous membranes**: nonhealing ulcers of the skin, oral cavity, pharynx, intestines, or genital tracts (bacterial infections rarely result in chronic, nonhealing ulcers); **thrushlike** mucosal exudates; chronic draining sinus tracts, particularly if granules are present; verrucous, scaling, or marginated pruritic skin lesions; cracking nails; alopecia.

        c. **Eyes**: unresolving conjunctivitis, particularly following trauma.

        d. **Sinuses and soft tissue**: chronic sinusitis or periorbital swelling.

        e. **Central nervous system**: abrupt or insidious symptoms, including headaches that are progressively more frequent and more severe, vomiting, vertigo, seizures, and decreased levels of consciousness.

    3. **Laboratory studies that may lead to the suspicion of fungal disease**: persistent mild elevations in the leukocyte count, with increased monocytes, eosinophils, or both; increased erythrocyte sedimentation rate; and elevated levels of serum enzymes or gamma globulin.

VII. **Superficial mycoses** infect the superficial aspects of the skin (stratum corneum) and hair.

  A. **Common disorders**

    1. **Tinea versicolor** ("tinea" is Latin for "worm"): caused by *Malassezia furfur*; usually asymptomatic; forms scaly skin lesions on the upper torso of **various colors** (pale gray to red-brown). *M. furfur* is a lipophilic yeast that requires fatty acids for growth, and tends to proliferate when personal hygiene is poor and sebum builds up on the skin; skin infections also occur at venipuncure sites in neonates receiving parenteral feedings (which are rich in lipids).

    2. **Tinea nigra**: caused by *Exophiala werneckii*; forms tan to **black skin macules** on the palms and soles of the feet.

    3. **Piedra (or "white piedra")**: caused by *Trichosporon beigelii*, forms soft, **white to tan lesions** on hair of scalp, beard, axilla, and groin.

    4. **Black piedra**: caused by *Piedraia hortae*, which forms **hard brown-black nodules** on scalp hair.

  B. **Diagnosis**: skin scrapings, culture

VIII. **Cutaneous mycoses**. Usually caused by **dermatophytes**, including *Trichophyton* species (*T. rubrum*, *T. mentagrophytes*,

T. tonsurans, T. verrucosum), **Epidermophyton floccosum**, and **Microsporum** species (*M. canis, M. gypseum*). These infections involve the skin, nails, and hair, and are commonly called "ringworm" or "tinea." Most dermatophytes are ubiquitous and infect a variety of animals as well as humans. Transmission can be from **direct contact** with an infected human or animal, or contact with contaminated surfaces (e.g., communal shower stalls, barber shop clippers). Rarely, dermatophytes may cause systemic infections in immunocompromised patients.

   A.   Common disorders. Named according to the region of the body that is involved, and include the following.

   1.   Tinea capitis: circular, bald patches on the scalp, with broken hair shafts

   2.   Tinea barbae: erythematous lesions in the bearded areas

   3.   Tinea corporis: known to laymen as "ringworm": pruritic, circular, scaly skin lesions on the trunk, with an advancing erythematous border

   4.   Tinea cruris: "jock itch," pruritic, erythematous, scaly lesions in the groin

   5.   Tinea pedis: "athlete's foot," pruritic vesicles in the toe webs

   6.   Onychomycosis: thick, yellow, malformed nails

   B.   Diagnosis. Skin or nail scrapings (taken from the edge of the advancing lesion) with KOH (look for slender hyphae that tend to break up into arthroconidia; Fig. 3-1), culture, fluorescent lamp (for *Microsporum* species).

IX.   Subcutaneous mycoses. In general, these organisms are found in **soil or in decaying vegetation**. Infections require **direct inoculation** into subcutaneous tissues, usually by trauma involving sharp, rotting vegetative material, and cause chronic granulomatous infections.

   A.   Sporotrichosis

   1.   *Sporothrix schenckii* is found on plants or decaying wood worldwide (in the United States, most cases are in the Midwest). The usual route of entry is a **skin puncture by a spore-contaminated thorn or piece of straw ("rose gardener's disease")**; it can also grow under old bricks or lumber, and may enter through cracks in the skin.

   2.   Causes local **pustule or abscess** at the site of puncture, with subsequent spread along lymphatics, with a linear pattern of **skin ulcerations**; disseminated disease (e.g., osteomyelitis, synovitis, and myositis) can occur by hematogenous spread.

   3.   Not communicable

   4.   Histology. Organisms are rare: **small (2–8 μm), round to oval budding yeasts ("cigar bodies")**

   5.   Culture

      a.   Colonies: ivory to black, wrinkled

      b.   Micro: delicate (1–2 μm in diameter) hyphae with microconidia (3–6 μm) diagnostically arranged like daisyheads

   6.   Diagnosis: history, culture, serology (Ab titers ≥1:80 strongly suggest active infection).

B.   Chromomycosis (literally "colored fungus")

   1.   Tropical infection caused by **black molds** (dematiaceous fungi) found in soil and plant material. The usual route of entry is through skin trauma in people who walk barefoot; progressive disease can occur in individuals who do not have access to prompt treatment.

   2.   Common causative organisms include *Phialophora verrucosa*, *Fonsecaea pedrosi*, and *Cladosporium carrionii*.

   3.   Causes focally necrotic, verrucoid, **cauliflowerlike** masses of the skin at the site of inoculation. Infection may spread along lymphatics (usually around the **dorsum of the feet** and the lower legs).

   4.   Not communicable

   5.   Histology: In a background of abscesses, granulomas, and pseudoepitheliomatous hyperplasia: dark-brown, septate hyphae, and (more importantly) **yellow-brown yeasts in clusters (called "Medlar bodies" or "copper pennies")** that aggregate within macrophages or multinucleated giant cells.

   6.   Culture

   a.   Colonies: small, slow-growing colonies that are brown-black and hairy, velvety-green and mattlike, or leathery.

   b.   Micro

   (1)   *P. verrucosa*: dark, septate hyphae with urn-shaped phialides and clusters of conidia at the tip.

   (2)   *F. pedrosi*: dark, septate hyphae with conidia that arise from short dentricles attached laterally to the sides of conidiogenous cells.

   (3)   *C. carrionii*: dark, septate hyphae with elliptical conidia in long chains.

   7.   Diagnosis: by culture, histology

C.   Mycetoma (literally "fungal growth"), or "maduromycosis"

   1.   Localized lesions caused by **soil molds and some bacteria** (e.g., *Actinomyces*, *Nocardia*, *Streptomyces* spp.). The usual route of entry is through **skin trauma**; the term "mycetoma" refers to severe, deeply penetrating subcutaneous infections, primarily of the **hands and feet**, in which the parts are markedly swollen.

   2.   Common causative organisms include *Pseudallescheria boydii* **(United States) and** *Madurella* **species** (**Africa**, whence the name "madura foot"). Other species include *Exophiala jeanselmei* and *Wangiella dermatitidis*.

   3.   Causes markedly **swollen lesions with deeply penetrating sinuses**. The sinuses drain purulent material to the skin surface, contain fungal **granules that vary in color** (white, gray, brown, or yellow ["sulfur granules"]), depending on the specific fungus species involved.

   4.   Not communicable

   5.   Histology: In a background of abscesses, necrosis, granulation tissue, and fibrosis: granules composed of fungal organisms are embedded in a pink matrix (antibodies).

   6.   Culture: *Scedosporium apiospermum* (asexual) or *Pseudallescheria boydii* (sexual)

a. Colonies: house-mouse gray, silky surface with tiny water droplets on surface

b. Micro: lemon-shaped, singly derived conidia (4–9 µm) (asexual) and large baglike structures filled with sexually derived "ascospores"

7. Diagnosis: by culture, histology

X. Systemic (deep) mycoses. These infections are caused by **virulent soil fungi** that are dimorphic [they grow as yeasts in tissues (at 37°C) and grow as molds (hyphae) in soil or laboratory cultures (at 25°C to 30°C)]. The mold forms are the infective forms, and the usual route of entry is by **inhalation of spores or through injection by trauma**, after which the fungi convert *in vivo* to the virulent yeast forms, which can spread to any organ. **Most infections are asymptomatic, although the organisms can cause disease (usually systemic) in healthy individuals.** These fungi can be **cultured** (exercise extreme caution if coccidioidomycosis is suspected), **and exoantigen or nucleic acid probe tests** can then be performed on isolated colonies to identify the specific fungus.

A. Blastomycosis

1. *Blastomyces dermatitidis* **is a dimorphic** fungus found in **soil and decaying wood in the Mississippi, St. Lawrence, and Ohio River valleys** (primarily Kentucky, Arkansas, Mississippi, North Carolina, Tennessee, Louisiana, Illinois, and Wisconsin). **Dogs** are often infected, as they "root around" in the soil. Also called **"North American Blastomycosis,"** but it also occurs in Central America and Africa.

2. Most infections occur after **inhalation of the spores (conidia)**; the fungi require exacting environmental conditions to sporulate (e.g., moisture, pH) and these conditions are met when soil is plowed or disturbed, buried logs are dislodged, and so forth. Infections can take several forms.

a. Primary pulmonary blastomycosis: ranges from asymptomatic to pneumonia.

b. Primary cutaneous blastomycosis: (Gilchrist's disease, caused by direct inoculation through trauma): spreading, ulcerating, wartlike lesions on unclothed areas of skin. However, most skin infections are actually the result of disseminated disease.

c. Disseminated blastomycosis usually arises from pulmonary blastomycosis, and commonly involves the **skin, bone (ribs or vertebrae), liver, spleen, and male reproductive** system (testes, epididymis, and prostate).

3. Noncommunicable

4. Histology: Organisms are **large, round yeasts (10–15 µm) with a doubly refractile cell wall and a single broad-based bud**. The background is usually ulcerative with microabscesses (in skin lesions), or granulomatous. Organisms may be seen in the **base of the ulcers within multinucleated foreign-body giant cells.**

5. Culture

a. Colonies: at 30°C, grows slowly as a white to brown mold, with delicate or hairlike mycelia. At 37°C grows as a smooth, off-white, yeastlike colony.

   b.   Micro: delicate, branching, clear (hyaline) hyphae (1–2 μm in diameter), with small, round conidia (1–4 μm) borne singly on thin conidiophores (like "lollipops").
   6.   **Diagnosis**: history, histology, culture; serum Ab titers 1:32 or greater are usually diagnostic.
B. Histoplasmosis
   1.   *Histoplasma capsulatum* is a dimorphic fungus found in the **soil of the Ohio, Missouri, and Mississippi River valleys**, particularly in areas where **bird or bat feces** are concentrated [e.g., chicken coups, caves (whence "cave fever")]. Most infections occur from **inhalation of the spores (conidia)**.
   2.   **Most acute infections are asymptomatic**, or cause mild **flulike** symptoms. Older lesions form laminated, **calcified granulomas ("histoplasmomas") in the lungs**. Some infections become systemic (particularly in the very young, very old, or immunosuppressed), involving the **reticuloendothelial system** (liver, spleen, bone marrow, and lymphoid tissues), or almost any other organ (e.g., severe pneumonia, potentially fatal infections in the adrenal glands).
   3.   **Noncommunicable**
   4.   **Histology: necrotizing** granulomas with **2–4 μm, oval yeasts inside macrophages** (sometimes with a single bud held by a delicate filament). The yeasts have a **clear area around them, simulating a capsule**, whence the name "capsulatum."
   5.   **Culture**
   a.   Colonies: at 30°C, slow-growing white or beige, delicate hairlike colonies. At 37°C the colonies are smooth, entire, yellow-white, and yeastlike.
   b.   Micro: small, oval microconidia (2–4 μm) are seen early in culture; large, spiked, thick-walled, spherical macroconidia (10–20 μm) develop later.
   6.   **Diagnosis**: history, tissue biopsies; complement fixation titers: 1:32 or greater are usually diagnostic (but beware of cross reactions with aspergillosis, blastomycosis, coccidiodomycosis); immunodiffusion tests: simultaneous appearance of H and M bands indicate active infection.
C. Coccidioidomycosis
   1.   *Coccidioides immitis* **is a dimorphic** fungus that grows beneath the hot **desert sands of the southwestern United States** and Mexico. **Arthroconidia** are carried by desert winds and, if inhaled, can cause a variety of illnesses.
   2.   **Clinical syndromes**
   a.   **Primary pulmonary coccidioidomycosis**: most individuals are **asymptomatic (60%)**, with the remainder exhibiting **flulike** symptoms (fever, cough, malaise, and myalgias) called "San Juaquin Valley fever," or simply "**valley fever**." Of those affected, 2% develop solid radiographic "**coin lesions**" or cavitary lesions.
   b.   **Primary cutaneous coccidioidomycosis**: caused by direct cutaneous inoculation, and often presents as **erythema multiforme and erythema nodosum**.
   c.   **Disseminated coccidioidomycosis**: usually arises from pulmonary infections and spreads to the **spleen, liver,**

adrenal glands, brain, and bones [particularly in some ethnic groups (i.e., **blacks, Hispanics**), in **AIDS patients,** or during **pregnancy**].

3. **Not communicable** from person to person, but exercise extreme caution when dealing with suspected cultures, as the spores are highly infectious.

4. **Histology: thick-walled spherule (up to 60 μm) with multiple endospores inside**.

5. **Culture**
    a. Colonies: white or beige, cottony or delicate cob-web colony at 30°C; a yeast form is not recovered at 37°C.
    b. Micro: hyaline hyphae that break up into alternate staining arthroconidia

6. **Diagnosis**: history, histology, complement fixation titers 1:16 or greater usually indicate active disease (but be aware of cross reactions to histoplasmosis), and may be negative in patients with acute infections or with solitary pulmonary lesions; nucleic acid probe assays are available for culture confirmation.

D. **Paracoccidioidomycosis**
    1. *Paracoccidioides brasiliensis* **is a dimorphic** fungus that grows in **soil and decaying vegetation**, and is the most common cause of systemic fungal infections in South America (particularly Venezuela, Brazil, and Colombia); also called **"South American Blastomycosis."**
    2. Most infections occur by **inhalation of the spores**. Infections can be asymptomatic or they can spread to other organs, particularly the **reticuloendothelial system** (e.g., liver, spleen, lymphoid tissues), skin, and mucous membranes.
    3. Causes **ulceration of the skin (perioral) or mucous membranes (nasal, oral cavities, anorectal mucosa)**, and necrotizing granulomas in the organs listed above.
    4. **Noncommunicable**
    5. **Histology**: necrotizing granulomas and organisms that are **large (10–20 μm), thick-walled, spherical yeasts with multiple buds around the circumference ("mariner's wheel")**. The organisms tend to aggregate **inside multinucleated foreign-body type giant cells**.
    6. **Culture**: delicate, septate, hyphal structures (2–3 μm in diameter) with tear-shaped conidia (like "lollipops").
    7. **Diagnosis**: histology; culture

XI. **Opportunistic mycoses**. These organisms **infect patients who are immunocompromised** because of AIDS, lymphoproliferative malignancies, hereditary immunodeficiencies, chemotherapy, high dose steroids or other immunosuppressive agents, diabetes with acidosis, and so on. Patients with **chronic indwelling catheters** are also at higher risk for fungemias. Some organisms come from the normal flora of the body, or from exogenous sources, particularly as inhaled spores, or when spores come in contact with wounds and burns.

A. **Candida**
    1. *Candida* species are **oval, budding yeasts (3 × 6 μm)** that are part of the **commensal flora** of the upper respiratory tract, the gastrointestinal tract, and the vagina. *Candida* species cause infection in association with **immuno-**

suppression (e.g., AIDS, chronic debilitating diseases, chemotherapy) **or suppression of normal bacterial flora** (e.g., pregnancy, diabetes, prolonged use of broad spectrum antibiotics).

   2.   The most common species causing infection is *Candida albicans*. Other species such as *C. tropicalis*, *C. parapsilosis*, and *Torulopsis glabrata*, rarely, are involved.

   3.   **Common infections**

   a.   **Mucous membranes**: mouth (**thrush**), esophagus, and **vagina**; causing redness, edema, and white patches

   b.   **Skin** (in warm, moist areas such as inframammary folds and the groin areas)

   c.   **Nails** (mimics onychomycosis and can cause paronychia)

   d.   **Fungemia** with involvement of deep organs of the body (e.g., lungs, kidneys, prosthetic or previously **damaged heart valves**); endocarditis can occur in patients with **indwelling catheters** or in those who engage in **IV drug use; peritonitis** can occur with ambulatory peritoneal dialysis.

   e.   **Chronic mucocutaneous candidiasis** can occur in patients with **hereditary cellular immunodeficiency.**

   4.   **Noncommunicable**

   5.   **Histology: oval, budding yeasts (3 × 6 μm) with a tendency to form elongated cells that resemble hyphae (pseudohyphae).** The ends of the cells are connected, giving an appearance of septa, but differ from the appearance of true hyphae in that the ends of the elongated cells are constricted where they join.

   6.   **Culture**

   a.   Colonies: white to ivory-colored, soft, smooth, pasty colonies with a yeast odor

   b.   Micro: oval, budding yeasts (3–6 μm) and blastoconidia forming clusters along pseudohyphae when observed in cornmeal agar preparations. *C. albicans*, unlike the other species, forms **germ tubes** within 2 hours after innoculation in human or rabbit serum.

   7.   **Diagnosis**: history and physical examination, biopsy, culture

B.   Cryptococcosis

   1.   *Cryptococcus neoformans* **is a soil yeast** that is **ubiquitous** in nature, particularly in soil with an alkaline pH and a high nitrogen content (e.g., such as soil contaminated with **bird feces (pigeon, chicken, turkey)**.

   2.   Most infections occur after the **spores are inhaled** (e.g., while cleaning chicken coups or excavating buildings where pigeons have perched). **Most infections are asymptomatic. Serious infections can arise from inhalation of large numbers of yeasts or in immunocompromised hosts who may have a reactivation of latent disease.**

   3.   Causes slowly developing, **chronic meningitis** (CSF has high opening pressure, high protein, low or normal glucose) that is invariably **fatal if untreated**; skin, lungs (pneumonia), kidneys (possibly because of the altered pH), and other organs may also be affected.

4. **Noncommunicable**
5. **Histology: yeast forms (round or oval), irregular in size between 4–12 μm, with narrow-based buds and widely separated by capsular material**
6. **Culture**
   a. Colonies: shiny, mucoid (from polysaccharide capsule material), cream-colored colonies that grow well at 37°C (unlike nonpathogenic *Cryptococcus* species)
   b. Micro: round or oval yeast forms (4–12 μm) that are irregular in size, with narrow-based buds (hairlike strands connect them), surrounded by a thick polysaccharide capsule
7. **Diagnosis**: history, India ink, **CSF antigen detection**, culture

C. **Aspergillosis**
1. Aspergillosis is caused by a group of *Aspergillus* species (of 700 species, *A. fumigatus*, *A. flavus*, *A. niger*, **and *A. terreus* cause 98% of human infections**) that are **ubiquitous** in nature, and found on decaying plant materials. They may **colonize breaks in the skin** surface (e.g., wounds, burns), or **can be inhaled**.
2. Persons at risk include those with some forms of **immunodeficiencies** (e.g., chronic granulomatous disease), or with **pulmonary anatomic abnormalities.**
3. Clinical syndromes: causes skin and pulmonary infections
   a. **Skin infections** occur after colonization of burns, wounds, corneal abrasions, or external ear canal (otitis externa, **"swimmer's ear" caused by *A. niger*** contamination of a cerumen plug).
   b. **Pulmonary**: three main forms
      (1) **Fungus ball**. Aspergillus grows in a tangled mass of hyphae in a preexisting lung cavity and usually does not invade the tissue.
      (2) **Allergic bronchopulmonary aspergillosis**. An *Aspergillus* species with low propensity for tissue invasion; it is associated with asthma, high levels of eosinophils and IgE, and Charcot–Leyden crystals.
      (3) **Invasive aspergillosis**. *Aspergillus* species invade deeply into lung tissues and cause hemoptosis, pneumonia, and dissemination to other body organs. Deep invasion usually occurs only in the immunosuppressed.
4. **Noncommunicable**
5. **Histology: slender (4–6 μm in diameter), hyaline septate hyphae with parallel walls, that branch at 45-degree angles**. To diagnose an infection (and not just colonization), **active invasion of blood vessel walls** or lung parenchyma must be seen.
6. **Culture**
   a. Colonies: rapidly growing colonies mature in 3–5 days. Colonies are cottony or granular with a distinct outer margin. *A. fumigatus*: green-gray, *A. flavus*: yellow, *A. niger*: black, and *A. terreus*: brown.
   b. Micro: uniform, slender (4–6 μm in diameter), clear, septate hyphae with parallel walls, and swollen vesicles with radiating chains of conidia

7. **Diagnosis**: radiographic, biopsy, culture
8. Fungal organisms that may also mimic the clinical syndromes of *Aspergillus* species include *Fusarium*, *Curvularia*, and *Pseudallescheria* (scedosporium).

D. **Zygomycosis** (commonly called **"mucormycosis"**)
1. The *Zygomycetes* are a **family of opportunistic fungi that includes *Mucor* spp., *Rhizopus* spp., *Absidia* spp., *Syncephalastrum* spp., *Circinella* spp., and *Cunninghamella* spp.**; they are **widely distributed in soil, dung, and vegetable matter**. Although the term "mucormycosis" is often used as a synonym for these infections, *Rhizopus* spp. is more commonly recovered from clinical specimens than the other species.
2. Most infections occur in **debilitated or immunocompromised hosts** (e.g., diabetics particularly with ketoacidosis, burns, lymphoproliferative malignancies, chemotherapy), and involve the **paranasal sinuses, lungs, gastrointestinal tract, and skin. IV drug use** is also a risk factor (particularly for *Cunninghamella elegans*), as is **iron overload** (e.g., in hemodialysis patients receiving deferoxamine), because iron enhances fungal growth.
3. The organisms have a propensity to **invade blood vessels**, causing subsequent **thromboses** and necrosis of surrounding tissues. The most common forms of serious infection include **pneumonia, meningitis, and disseminated disease.**
4. **Noncommunicable**
5. **Histology: wide, irregular, ribbonlike, aseptate hyphae with nonparallel walls that branch at wide angles (e.g., 90 degrees); often in a purulent background**
6. **Culture**
a. Colonies: rapidly growing (2–3 days) gray-white to gray-brown, cottony colonies without a distinctive border ("lidlifters")
b. Micro: broad, ribbonlike, aseptate hyphae with saclike sporangia and rootlike structures called rhizoids (except *Mucor* spp. which lacks rhizoids)
7. **Diagnosis**: culture, histology
E. *Pneumocystis carinii*
1. *Pneumocystis carinii* is a **common fungus** found in a variety of animals, including **rats and dogs**. It is extremely common (almost universal) in humans, being **acquired during childhood by inhalation of the cysts** from household pets or other people. **Almost all infections are asymptomatic.**
2. *P. carinii* can cause a potentially **lethal pneumonitis**, particularly in the very young, the very old, and in **immunocompromised** patients (e.g., AIDS, bone marrow transplant patients, congenital immunodeficiencies). It causes more than 50% of AIDS-related deaths.
3. **Histology**: biopsies or bronchoalveolar lavage specimens are stained **with Gomori's methenamine silver**. In a **"frothy"** background, the organisms are in groups of **eight pear-shaped sporozoites (1–3 μm each), all within a 8–10 μm cyst**. The silver highlights the cysts. PAS and modified trichrome stains highlight the individual sporozoites.

4. Diagnosis: histology, cytology
XII. Less common fungal infections (grouped by hyphal and conidial characteristics)
A. Hyalohyphomycosis. Literally, "clear hyphae," the most common clinical syndromes are **mycetoma, onychomycosis, and mycotic keratitis**. Diagnosis is by culture and histology. These organisms are ubiquitous in nature; to make a definitive diagnosis (and to rule out environment contamination), the same species must be recovered from at least two separately collected samples from the same body site. Colonies vary in color from white to yellow, green or green-gray. Organisms are grouped by the pattern of their conidia.
   1. Fungi with conidia in chains: *Penicillium* spp., *Paecilomyces* spp., *Scopulariopsis* spp.
   2. Fungi with conidia in clusters: *Acremonium* spp., *Fusarium* spp., *Trichoderma* spp.
   3. Fungi with single conidia: *Scedosporium* spp., *Chrysosoprium* spp., *Sepedonium* spp., *Beauveria* spp.
B. Phaeohyphomyces. Literally, "dark hyphae," the clinical infections include **mycotic keratitis, superficial (tinea nigra, black piedra), cutaneous (onychomycosis), and subcutaneous and deep-systemic infections**. Diagnosis is by culture and histology. These organisms are ubiquitous in nature; to make a definitive diagnosis (and to rule out environment contamination), the same species must be recovered from at least two separately collected samples from the same body site. Histologic evidence of hyphal tissue invasion is also supportive of a true infection. Colonies have a **dark-gray to jet black color on their reverse side** (bottom side, from pigmentation of the vegetative hyphae). Organisms are grouped by the appearance of their conidia.
   1. Fungi with microconidia that have transverse and longitudinal septa: *Alternaria* spp., *Ulocladium* spp., *Stemphilium* spp., *Epicoccum* spp.
   2. Fungi with microconidia that have transverse septa only: *Bipolaris* spp., *Drechslera* spp., *Exserohilum* spp., *Curvularia* spp.
C. *Torulopsis glabrata*. A common cause of urinary tract infections, *Torulopsis glabrata* is cultured in cornmeal agar, where it shows small, uniform-sized, spherical yeast cells in tight clusters (unlike *Candida* species, no pseudohyphae are present).
D. *Malassezia furfur*. A yeast that grows well in association with lipids, *Malassezia furfur* is a potential cause of fungemia in patients with long-term indwelling catheters who receive parenteral nutrition (high in lipids). Microscopically, skin scrapings show clusters of thick round yeasts and hyphae are mixed together ("spaghetti and meatballs"). Culture media must be overlaid with virgin olive oil in order to recover the yeast form.
E. *Actinomyces, Streptomyces,* and *Nocardia* spp. are bacteria that cause subcutaneous (actinomycotic mycetomas) and opportunistic infections clinically similar to fungal infections. Microscopically, **freely branching filamentous structures (1 µm in diameter)** are present, sometimes with clubbed ends. *Actinomyces* spp. tend to form radiating "sunbursts" of organisms as seen in tissue sections. *Nocardia* spp. are partially acid-fast.

Parasitology

Steven L. Jones

I. Introduction. Parasites are organisms that live within a host at some expense to the host. Human parasitic infections are common, involving literally billions of people worldwide. Risk factors include living in (or visiting) areas that are endemic for the organism, poor hygiene or sanitation, inadequately washed or cooked foods, and contaminated water. Many parasitic diseases have a long latent period before symptoms arise, and **careful patient histories are therefore essential**.

II. Sample collection and examination

A. Stool should be collected in a clean container, without urine. **Three stool specimens taken 48 hours apart** are the minimal standard. If the stool is not able to be examined within 1 hour, add fixative [polyvinyl alcohol (**PVA**) or 10% formalin]. **Examine stool grossly** (for adult worms, proglottids, and so on) and prepare fresh, warm, **wet mounts** to identify trophozoites (use the last part of the passed stool and add a drop of saline to it). Then **concentrate the specimen** by using the Ritchie formalin-ether sedimentation or the zinc sulfate flotation methods, and prepare trichrome, iron hematoxylin, or iodine stained slides. Always use an ocular micrometer when examining the slides, and examine several organisms to establish an average organism size.

B. Blood. Whole blood should be mixed with EDTA (except for suspected malaria–use finger stick). Thick smears (for screening) and thin smears (for speciation) should be prepared and stained with Giemsa stains. Pay particular attention to the edge of the smear. **Serum** is collected for serology (see *Infectious Serology* chapter).

C. Surgical biopsies (e.g., of muscle, liver, skin), **lumbar punctures** (for cerebrospinal fluid, stained with Giemsa), and **urine** collection (centrifuged for sediment and stained with trichrome) may be helpful in identifying certain parasites (Table 3-26).

III. Clinical signs and symptoms. Signs and symptoms depend on which organ is affected by the parasite (Table 3-26). **Systemic signs and symptoms** (e.g., lassitude, weight loss, generalized urticarial skin rashes) **can occur in a variety of parasitic infections. Blood eosinophilia** is a common finding, and generally is proportional to the invasiveness of the parasite. Eosinophils may also be increased in sputum, stool, and body cavity fluids, depending on the organism.

IV. Protozoa, which are **single-celled, eukaryotic animals** that feed by engulfing particles, are classified in part based on their means of locomotion (Fig. 3-2). **Amoebae** (*Sarcodina*) move by pseudopodia, **ciliates** (*Ciliophora*) move by cilia, **flagellates** (*Mastigophora*) move by flagella, and coccidia (*Sporozoa*) lack the locomotive abilities of the other groups.

(*text continues on page 258*)

Table 3-26. Common signs, symptoms, and organisms associated with parasitic involvement of various organs[a]

Organ	Signs and Symptoms	Common Organisms
Gastrointestinal Tract (including mesentery)	Diarrhea and/or abdominal pain (which may be dull or cramping)	**Protozoa** (*Entamoeba histolytica, Balantidium coli, Giardia lamblia, Dientamoeba fragilis, Cryptosporidium, Sarcocystis, Isospora, Microsporidia, Blastocystis hominis*)
		Nematodes [*Ascaris lumbricoides, Trichuris trichiura, Enterobius vermicularis,* Hookworms (*Necator americanus, Ancylostoma duodenale*), *Strongyloides stercoralis*], *Trichinella spiralis, Anisakis*
		Cestodes (*Diphyllobothrium latum, Taenia solium* and *saginata, Dipylidium caninum, Hymenolepis nana* and *diminuta*)
		Trematodes (*Schistosoma mansoni* and *japonicum, Fasciola hepatica, Fasciolopsis buski, Clonorchis sinensis*)
	Rectal prolapse	*Trichuris trichiura*
	Megaesophagus, megacolon	*Trypanosoma cruzi*
	Bowel obstruction	*Ascaris lumbricoides, Fasciolopsis buski*
	Anal itching	*Enterobius vermicularis*
	Microcytic anemia	Hookworms (*Necator americanus, Ancylostoma duodenale*)
	Megaloblastic anemia	*Diphyllobothrium latum*

continued

Table 3-26.   *Continued*

Organ	Signs and Symptoms	Common Organisms
Hepatobiliary Tract and Spleen	Jaundice, hepatosplenomegaly, or hepatitis	**Protozoa** [*Entamoeba histolytica* (metastatic abscess), *Plasmodia, Babesia, Leishmania donovani, Trypanosoma cruzi, Toxoplasma gondii*] **Nematode** [*Ascaris lumbricoides* (if the worms migrate into the biliary tract), *Toxocara canis* and *cati* (visceral larva migrans)] **Cestodes** [*Taenia solium* (cysticercosis), *Echinococcus* (hydatid disease)] **Trematodes** [*Fasciola hepatica* (in bile ducts), *Fasciolopsis buski, Schistosoma mansoni* and *japonicum, Clonorchis sinensis* (in bile ducts)]
	Portal hypertension	*Schistosoma japonicum*
	Cystic lesions	**Protozoa** [*Entamoeba histolytica* (metastatic abscess)] **Cestodes** [*Echinococcus* (hydatid disease), *Taenia solium* (cysticercosis)]
Central nervous system	Headache, vomiting, seizures meningoencephalitis, and so on	**Protozoa** (*Naegleria fowleri, Acanthamoeba castellani, Entamoeba histolytica, Plasmodium falciparum, Toxoplasma gondii, Trypanosoma* sp.) **Nematodes** [*Toxocara canis* and *cati* (visceral larva migrans), *Trichinella spiralis*] **Cestodes** [*Taenia solium* (cysticercosis), *Echinococcus* sp. (hydatid disease)]

Site	Finding	Organisms
	Cyst/abscess	**Protozoa** (*Entamoeba histolytica*) **Cestodes** [*Taenia solium* (cysticercosis), *Echinococcus* sp. (hydatid disease)] **Trematodes** (*Paragonimus westermani*)
	Insidious decrease in level of consciousness	*Trypanosoma b. gambiense*
	Stillbirths, failure to progress, learning disabilities	*Toxoplasma gondii*
	Infarctions	*Plasmodium falciparum*
	Blindness	*Toxoplasma gondii* (retinochoroiditis), *Toxocara canis* and *cati* (visceral larva migrans), *Taenia solium* (cysticercosis), *Onchocerca volvulus*
Eye	Corneal ulceration	*Acanthamoeba castellani*
	Periorbital edema	*Trypanosoma cruzi, Trichinella spiralis*
Lung	Cough[b], hemoptysis (variable), chest pain (variable), pneumonitis, and so on	**Protozoa** [*Entamoeba histolytica* (usually extending from liver abscess), *Plasmodia* spp., *Toxoplasma gondii*] **Larval nematodes** [*Ascaris lumbricoides*, hookworms (*Necator americanus, Ancylostoma duodenale*), *Strongyloides stercoralis, Toxocara cani* and *cati* (visceral larva migrans)] **Filarial nematodes** (*Dirofilaria immitis, Wuchereria bancrofti, Brugia malayi*) **Cestodes** [*Echinococcus* sp. (hydatid disease)] **Trematodes** (*Paragonimus westermani, Schistosoma haematobium*)

continued

Table 3-26.   Continued

Organ	Signs and Symptoms	Common Organisms
Heart	Cardiomyopathy, cardiomyositis, and so on	**Protozoa** [*Trypanosoma cruzi, Toxoplasma gondii, Sarcocystis, Plasmodium falciparum* (in capillaries with or without infarction)] **Nematodes** (*Trichinella spiralis*)
Genitourinary tract	Vaginal itching, malodorous discharge	*Trichomonas vaginalis* (may also cause dysuria if organisms migrate into urethra), *Enterobius vermicularis* (if worms migrate into vagina)
	Hematuria, suprapubic pain, increased frequency of urination	*Schistosoma haematobium*
	Squamous cell carcinoma of the urinary bladder	*Schistosoma haematobium*
	Renal infarction	*Plasmodium falciparum*
Muscle and connective tissues	Myalgias, and so on	**Protozoa** (*Toxoplasma gondii, Sarcocystis, Leishmania donovani, Trypanosoma cruzi*) **Nematodes** [*Trichinella spiralis, Toxocara canis and cati* (visceral larva migrans)] **Cestodes** [*Taenia solium* (cysticercosis)]
Skin and subcutaneous tissues	Subcutaneous nodules/eruptions	**Protozoa** [*Trypanosoma* sp. *Leishmania* sp. (e.g., *L. mexicana, L. tropica, L. major, L. braziliensis*)] **Nematodes** [*Ancylostoma braziliense* or *caninum* (cutaneous larva migrans), hookworms (*Necator americanus, Ancylostoma duodenale*)]

System	S&S	Parasites
	Pruritis	**Filarial nematodes** (*Onchocerca volvulus, Loa loa, Wuchereria bancrofti, Brugia malayi, Dracunculus medinensis*) **Nematodes** [*Enterobius vermicularis* (anal pruritis), hookworms (*Necator americanus, Ancylostoma duodenale*; at time of entry), *Strongyloides* (at time of entry)] **Filarial nematodes** (*Onchocerca volvulus*) **Trematodes** [*Schistosoma* sp. (at time of entry)]
Blood	Fever, chills, sweats, weight loss (many other S&S may occur such as diarrhea, pneumonitis, and so on)	**Protozoa** [*Plasmodia* sp. (e.g., *P. falciparum*), *Babesia microti*, *Leishmania* sp. (e.g., *L. donovani*; diarrhea is common), *Trypanosoma* sp.] **Microfilariae**
	Anemia	**Protozoa** [*Plasmodia* sp. (e.g., *P. falciparum*), *Babesia microti, Leishmania donovani*]; also see under gastro-intestinal section above for hookworms (*Necator americanus, Ancylostoma duodenale*) and *Diphyllobothrium latum*
Lymph nodes	Lymphadenopathy	**Protozoa** [*Toxoplasma gondii, Leishmania* sp. (e.g., *L. donovani*), *Trypanosoma* sp. (e.g., *T. cruzi*)] **Filarial nematodes** [*Wuchereria bancrofti* (also causes scrotal swelling), *Brugia malayi*]

S&S, signs and symptoms.

[a] Systemic signs and symptoms (such as lassitude, weight loss, generalized urticarial skin rashes, blood eosinophilia, etc.) may occur in a variety of parasitic infections.

[b] Symptoms occur from parasites that reside in the lungs or that have transient migrations (e.g., intestinal nematode larvae) through the lungs.

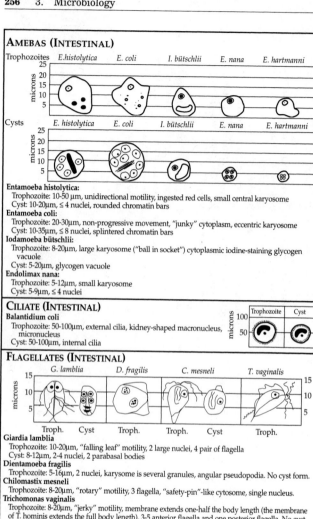

AMEBAS (INTESTINAL)

Trophozoites *E.histolytica*   *E. coli*   *I. bütschlii*   *E. nana*   *E. hartmanni*

Cysts *E. histolytica*   *E. coli*   *I. bütschlii*   *E. nana*   *E. hartmanni*

Entamoeba histolytica:
 Trophozoite: 10-50 μm, unidirectional motility, ingested red cells, small central karyosome
 Cyst: 10-20μm, ≤ 4 nuclei, rounded chromatin bars
Entamoeba coli:
 Trophozoite: 20-30μm, non-progressive movement, "junky" cytoplasm, eccentric karyosome
 Cyst: 10-35μm, ≤ 8 nuclei, splintered chromatin bars
Iodamoeba bütschlii:
 Trophozoite: 8-20μm, large karyosome ("ball in socket") cytoplasmic iodine-staining glycogen
  vacuole
 Cyst: 5-20μm, glycogen vacuole
Endolimax nana:
 Trophozoite: 5-12μm, small karyosome
 Cyst: 5-9μm, ≤ 4 nuclei

CILIATE (INTESTINAL)
Balantidium coli
 Trophozoite: 50-100μm, external cilia, kidney-shaped macronucleus,
  micronucleus
 Cyst: 50-100μm, internal cilia

Trophozoite | Cyst

FLAGELLATES (INTESTINAL)

G. lamblia   *D. fragilis*   *C. mesneli*   *T. vaginalis*

Troph. Cyst   Troph.   Troph. Cyst   Troph.

Giardia lamblia
 Trophozoite: 10-20μm, "falling leaf" motility, 2 large nuclei, 4 pair of flagella
 Cyst: 8-12μm, 2-4 nuclei, 2 parabasal bodies
Dientamoeba fragilis
 Trophozoite: 5-16μm, 2 nuclei, karysome is several granules, angular pseudopodia. No cyst form.
Chilomastix mesneli
 Trophozoite: 8-20μm, "rotary" motility, 3 flagella, "safety-pin"-like cytosome, single nucleus.
Trichomonas vaginalis
 Trophozoite: 8-20μm, "jerky" motility, membrane extends one-half the body length (the membrane
  of T. hominis extends the full body length), 3-5 anterior flagella and one posterior flagella. No cyst
  form.

A

Fig. 3-2. Common protozoa morphology.

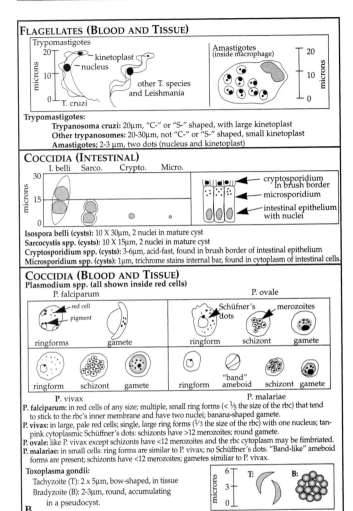

FLAGELLATES (BLOOD AND TISSUE)

Trypomastigotes:
 Trypanosoma cruzi: 20μm, "C-" or "S-" shaped, with large kinetoplast
 Other trypanosomes: 20-30μm, not "C-" or "S-" shaped, small kinetoplast
 Amastigotes; 2-3 μm, two dots (nucleus and kinetoplast)

COCCIDIA (INTESTINAL)

Isospora belli (cysts): 10 X 30μm, 2 nuclei in mature cyst
Sarcocystis spp. (cysts): 10 X 15μm, 2 nuclei in mature cyst
Cryptosporidium spp. (cysts): 3-6μm, acid-fast, found in brush border of intestinal epithelium
Microsporidium spp. (cysts): 1μm, trichrome stains internal bar, found in cytoplasm of intestinal cells.

COCCIDIA (BLOOD AND TISSUE)
Plasmodium spp. (all shown inside red cells)

P. falciparum: in red cells of any size; multiple, small ring forms (< ⅕ the size of the rbc) that tend to stick to the rbc's inner membrane and have two nuclei; banana-shaped gamete.
P. vivax: in large, pale red cells; single, large ring forms (⅓ the size of the rbc) with one nucleus; tan-pink cytoplasmic Schüffner's dots: schizonts have >12 merozoites; round gamete.
P. ovale: like P. vivax except schizonts have <12 merozoites and the rbc cytoplasm may be fimbriated.
P. malariae: in small cells; ring forms are similar to P. vivax; no Schüffner's dots. "Band-like" ameboid forms are present; schizonts have <12 merozoites; gametes similiar to P. vivax.

Toxoplasma gondii:
 Tachyzoite (T): 2 x 5μm, bow-shaped, in tissue
 Bradyzoite (B): 2-3μm, round, accumulating
   in a pseudocyst.

B

Fig. 3-2. *Continued*

A. Amoebae (from Greek "to change") are single-celled animals that move by extending cytoplasmic protrusions called **pseudopodia**. Generally, each species has two forms, a trophozoite form (from Latin, "to nourish," that represents the motile, feeding stage) and a cyst form (the nonmotile, resting stage that is resistant to environmental effects).

1. **Pathogenic intestinal amoebae**

   a. *Entamoeba histolytica*: (from "histo" [tissue], and "lysis" [destruction]). This amoeba causes **amebiasis**, and resides in the large intestine. It is transmitted by the **ingestion of cysts** (fecal-oral route or by cyst-contaminated fruits and vegetables).

   (1) **Clinical syndromes** include intestinal and disseminated disease.

   (a) **Intestinal**. Many patients are asymptomatic. Virulent strains cause **amoebic dysentery**: diarrhea with cramping, abdominal pain.

   (b) **Disseminated**. Hematogenous spread can cause **"anchovy pastelike" abscesses in the liver** (most common), spleen, lung, or brain.

   (2) **Diagnosis**: finding **motile trophozoites in fresh, warm stool, or trophozoites or cysts in fixed stool** specimens (Table 3-27, Fig. 3-2). Watery diarrhea suggests active disease (trophozoites), whereas formed stools suggest quiescent disease (cysts). Trophozoites may

Table 3-27. Guide for identifying intestinal amebae

Identifying trophozoites:

If the trophozoites move in one direction and have invisible nuclei in fresh saline mounts, with cytoplasm containing erythrocytes but no bacteria, the organism is *E. histolytica*.

If the trophozoites do not move in one direction, have occasional visible nuclei in fresh saline mounts, and have "junky" cytoplasm (granular, with bacteria but no erythrocytes), the organism is *E. coli*.

If more than half the trophozoites have 2 nuclei, the organism is *Dientamoeba fragilis*.

Small trophozoites (<12 μ) include *Endolimax nana* (large karyosome), *Entamoeba hartmanni* (small karyosome), and *Iodamoeba bütschlii* (large iodine-staining glycogen vacuole).

Macrophages *don't move* in fresh saline mounts, and contain erythrocytes *and* bacteria.

Identifying cysts:

Cysts, as they mature, develop more nuclei. For speciation, look on the slide for the cysts with the largest numbers of nuclei (mature cysts).

Large (>10μm) cysts are either *E. histolytica* (4 nuclei, small karyosomes, rounded chromatoidal bars) or *E. coli* (8 nuclei, small karyosomes, and splintered chromatoidal bars).

Small (<10μm) cysts are either *E. nana* (4 nuclei, large karyosomes), *E. hartmanni* (4 nuclei, small karyosomes), *or I. bütschlii* (1–2 nuclei, large iodine-staining glycogen vacuole).

form **flask-shaped necrotic ulcers** (the amoebae can spread through the submucosa but cannot cross the muscularis propria, except in immunosuppressed patients). Trophozoites are found at the edges of ulcers or abscesses, with few inflammatory cells. **Serologic tests** (e.g., indirect hemagglutination) may be helpful, especially for **metastatic infections**.

    2. **Nonpathogenic intestinal amoebae**: *Entamoeba coli*, *Iodamoeba bütschlii*, *Endolimax nana*, and *Entamoeba hartmanni*. The finding of nonpathogenic amoebae in a patient with diarrhea **should not end the search for pathogenic amoebae**, as both may be transferred together in similar ways.

    3. **Free-living pathogenic soil amoebas**

        a. *Acanthamoeba castellani*: causes **keratitis** (or less commonly, meningitis) after ocular trauma, from contaminated contact lenses, or through airborne cysts.

        b. *Naegleria fowleri*: causes **meningoencephalitis** in children or young adults; caused by swimming in freshwater ponds. Organisms pass through the cribriform plate into the brain.

           (1) **Diagnosis. Trophozoites** have a large distinct nucleus (but with a much smaller nuclear to cytoplasmic ratio than macrophages) and mitochondria, and **cysts** have a single nucleus without glycogen vacuoles or chromatoidal bars.

B. **Flagellates (mastigophora)** are single-celled animals with a whiplike **flagella**. **Axostyles** (central, stiff rods) and **kinetoplasts** (cytoplasmic organelles) control the flagella. Most flagellates have trophozoite (motile, feeding stage) and cyst forms (nonmotile, resting stage).

    1. **Pathogenic intestinal flagellates**

        a. *Giardia lamblia*: causes **giardiasis**, the most common diarrheal disease transmitted by **contaminated water** in the United States (chlorine does not kill it). *Giardia* occurs worldwide and is the only human protozoa that resides in the **duodenum**. It is transmitted through streams and domestic water supplies contaminated with cysts from human or wildlife feces, fecal-oral routes in child day-care centers, oral-anal sex, and so on. Symptoms include mild to severe **diarrhea**, cramping, and malabsorption. Diagnosis is made by identifying **trophozoites or cysts in stool and in surgical biopsies** (red "kite-shaped" intraluminal organisms). **Serologic tests** [e.g., enzyme-linked immunosorbent assay (ELISA)] may be helpful.

        b. *Dientamoeba fragilis*: causes abdominal pain and **diarrhea**, and has a **high association with** *Enterobius vermicularis* (pinworm) infections. Diagnosis is made by identifying **trophozoites in stool**. No cyst form exists.

    2. *Trichomonas vaginalis*: causes **sexually transmitted genitourinary infections**. Signs and symptoms include **vaginal pruritis**, **"strawberry-red" mucosa**, and **frothy exudates**. Diagnosis is made by identifying trophozoites in the vaginal discharge mixed with a drop of normal saline.

    3. **Nonpathogenic gastrointestinal flagellates include** *Chilomastix mesnili* and *Trichomonas hominis*.

4. **Pathogenic blood and tissue flagellates**
   a. *Trypanosoma*: causes trypanosomiasis (e.g., African sleeping sickness, Chagas' disease). ***Trypanosoma* and *Leishmania*** (see below) **both have identical developmental stages, each with a central nucleus and a kinetoplast**. The stages seen in human hosts depend on the individual species:

   - **Amastigote**: 2–3 μm, intracellular, sporelike stage seen in tissues (*T. cruzi* and *Leishmania*)
   - **Promastigote and epimastigote**: intermediate partially developed stages (*T. cruzi*)
   - **Trypomastigote**: 30 μm, elongated, with an undulating membrane and flagella, found in blood or cerebrospinal fluid (CSF) (in **all *Trypanosoma*, but not in *Leishmania***)

     (1) **Clinical syndromes**
        (a) **African trypanosomes**: cause a highly lethal **meningoencephalitis**, transmitted by **tsetse flies**. Trypomastigotes reside in the blood and CSF. Amastigote forms are not present in humans.
           (i) *T. brucei gambiense:* **Western Africa**; causes **"African sleeping sickness"** (indolent progression from somnolence to stupor and death)
           (ii) *T. brucei rhodesiense*: **Eastern Africa** (Lake Tanganyika); more aggressive than *T. brucei gambiense*
        (b) **American trypanosomiasis**: refers to *T. cruzi*, which causes **Chagas' disease**. It is found in Central and South America (10% of the people in some areas are infected). It is transmitted by the Reduviid "**kissing bug**," which bites the skin and then defecates. Victims rub the contaminated feces into the bite wound. **Romaña's sign** is unilateral eyelid swelling from a bug bite near the eye. Clinical syndromes include **cardiomyopathy** and gastrointestinal structural disorders (e.g., megaesophagus and **megacolon**). *T. rangeli* is found in people in Central and South America, but does not cause clinical disease, and organisms are only rarely seen in the blood.
     (2) **Morphology**: *T. cruzi* has a **C- or S-shaped** trypomastigote with a **large** kinetoplast. African trypanosomes and *T. rangeli* trypomastigotes are not C- or S-shaped, and have small kinetoplasts.
     (3) **Diagnosis: amastigote stage and intermediate stages of *T. cruzi* are seen within cardiac muscle** and other tissues. Trypomastigotes of all trypanosome species are seen in warm, fresh **blood smears**, and in **CSF smears in African trypanosomiasis. ELISA, indirect hemagglutination, complement fixation (Machado test)**, and **DNA probes** are available for *T. cruzi*. Xenodiagnosis for suspected *T. cruzi* can be performed when other tests are negative (clean triatomine bugs feed on the patient and the bug feces are later examined for trypanosomes).

b. *Leishmania* species: cause **Leishmaniasis**, which occurs in many parts of the world, and can involve the skin, subcutaneous tissues, or deep organs. Transmitted by **sandflies**. Amastigote accumulations are seen within macrophages. **Trypomastigote stages do not occur in humans.**

    (1) **Clinical syndromes.**

      (a) **Old World cutaneous leishmaniasis** ("Baghdad boil," "Oriental sore"): Southern Europe, Middle East, and Africa. *L. tropica* and *L. major* cause self-limited ulcers; *L. aethiopica* is more aggressive.

      (b) **Old World visceral leishmaniasis: ["Kala-Azar,"** "Dum Dum fever" (from the city near Calcutta)] caused by *L. donovani* complex. Transmitted by **sandflies.** May be asymptomatic or cause a fatal, disseminated involvement of the **reticuloendothelial** system (e.g., lymph nodes, spleen, bone marrow). Fevers are often "double quotidian"(two spikes per day). Onset may be up to 1 year after the sandfly bite.

      (c) **New World cutaneous leishmaniasis**: Central and South America. *L. mexicana* **("Chiclero ulcer")** causes self-limited ulcers (e.g., on the ears of forest workers harvesting gum for "Chiclets"). *L. peruviana* ("Uta") is more aggressive.

      (d) **New World mucocutaneous leishmaniasis** ("Espundia"): *L. braziliensis* causes **disfiguring erosion of the nasal septum** ("tapir nose"), with fungating masses in the oropharynx that have reportedly caused death by suffocation.

    (2) **Diagnosis: amastigotes** (see under *Trypanosoma*) **are seen within phagocytic cells in biopsies**. Amastigotes are 2–3 μm, with **two dots (a nucleus and a kinetoplast)**, versus the fungus *Histoplasma capsulatum* which only has one dot (a nucleus). **Serologic tests are available** (immunofluorescence, ELISA), and Montenegro skin tests are sometimes used in South America.

C. **Ciliates (ciliophora)** are single-celled animals that **move by cilia** (motile, hairlike cell projections). Ciliates have a **macronucleus** and **several micronuclei**. The only pathogenic human ciliate is *Balantidium coli*, the largest human intestinal protozoa, which commonly infects hogs. Most cases are asymptomatic, but occasionally **diarrhea** alternating with constipation occurs.

D. **Coccidia (sporozoa)** are single-celled animals that **lack the means of locomotion** found in other protozoa, and have a life cycle that alternates between sexual stages (**sporogony**) and asexual stages (**schizogony**). **Definitive** hosts are hosts in which sexual reproduction occurs (fusion of gametes to form oocysts and sporocysts), whereas **intermediate** hosts allow only asexual reproduction (nuclear fission to form schizonts).

    1. **Pathogenic intestinal coccidia**

      a. *Sarcocystis species*: oocysts are ingested by herbivores (intermediate hosts), become sarcocysts within muscle, and are then ingested by definitive hosts (carnivores), where they sexually reproduce in the intestines. **Humans may be intermediate hosts** (from eating contaminated vegetation) or **definitive hosts** (from eating poorly cooked beef or lamb). Symptoms include **myalgia** (in intermediate hosts) or **diarrhea** (in definitive hosts). Diagnosis is made by **serology** (e.g., complement fixation) or **tissue biopsy**.

  b.   *Isospora belli*: an intestinal protozoa that causes coccidiosis. Symptoms include self-limited **diarrhea**, which can become severe in immunocompromised hosts [always check patients for the human immunodeficiency virus (**HIV**) infection]. Diagnosis is made by identifying cysts in the stool.

  c.   *Cryptosporidium parvum*: a common infection of cattle, rodents, and fowl; transmitted to humans by **fecal-contaminated food or water** (chlorine does not kill it). Symptoms include abdominal pain and diarrhea (which can be severe in the immunocompromised). Diagnosis is made by finding **acid-fast oocysts in stool**, or identifying the 2–6 μm **organisms in the brush border** of ileal mucosal biopsies. Serologic tests (e.g., indirect immunofluorescence, ELISA) are used as epidemiologic tools.

  d.   *Microsporidia*: 1 μm; trichrome stains highlight a central bar across the organism.

  e.   *Blastocystis hominis*: has an uncertain classification (amoebae vs. coccidia); whether it is truly a pathogen is unclear; the organism is spherical, with irregular sizes (5–20 μm).

2.   Pathogenic blood coccidia

  a.   *Plasmodium* **species**: cause **malaria**, one of the most common protozoal diseases in the world (killing 1–2 million people per year). It is transmitted by the blood-sucking *Anopheles* **mosquito** (its definitive host), by transfusions, or transplacentally. Plasmodia are intracellular parasites, with an **erythrocyte cycle** and an **extra-erythrocyte cycle** (in the liver). Mosquitoes inject **sporozoites**, which divide asexually in the liver into **schizonts** (filled with merozoites). **Merozoites** then infect red blood cells and become **trophozoites** (the feeding stage, with a ringlike shape followed by an amoeboid shape). Then, they again divide into merozoites, which can infect other red blood cells (RBCs) or become **gametes** to be ingested by mosquitoes.

    Signs and symptoms include **splenomegaly**; periodic **shaking chills** ("rigors") as RBCs rupture, followed by **spiking fevers** (as merozoites penetrate other RBCs); sweats; anorexia; and joint pain. Leukopenia and normocytic anemia may also be present.

    P. falciparum (≈45%) and *P. vivax* (≈45%) **are the most common** species in the tropics (and in the United States). *P. malariae* (<5%) is also found in the tropics, but is much less common. *P. ovale* (<5%) is basically restricted to western Africa.

    (1)   *P. falciparum* ("malignant tertian malaria" with fevers every 48 hours) is the **most dangerous**

species, and infects RBCs of all stages of maturation. Usually, **only the ring forms and the gametes are seen in smears**; the presence of amoeboid forms suggests other species. Acute **intravascular hemolysis** causes hemoglobinuria ("blackwater fever"). Infected RBCs develop "sticky knobs" causing cell sludging and **infarctions of the brain, kidneys**, and so forth. Without treatment, patients die or are spontaneously cured within 1 year (no relapses). Hemoglobinopathies (e.g., sickle cell disease, thalassemia) provide some protection because the already abnormal RBCs rupture before the merozoites inside can mature.

    (2) *P. vivax* (**"benign tertian malaria"** with fevers every 48 hours) infects young RBCs (large and pale). Relapses can occur for up to 5 years. Blacks with **Duffy blood group** (a- b-) are somewhat resistant.

    (3) *P. ovale* (**"benign tertian malaria"** with fevers every 48 hours) infects young RBCs (large and pale); cytoplasm is **fimbriated**. Untreated, relapses can occur for up to 5 years.

    (4) *P. malariae* (**"benign quartan malaria"** with fevers every 72 hours) infects older (small) RBCs. Low-grade cryptic infections (recrudescences) can last for up to 40 years.

    (5) **Diagnosis**: thick (for screening) and thin (for species identification) blood smears with Giemsa stain. **First, *P. falciparum* should be looked for by identifying the ring forms or the banana-shaped gametes. Next, *P. vivax* should be looked for by identifying the ring forms, Schüffner dots, and appropriate schizonts.** *P. ovale* is restricted to a small geographic area. *P. malariae* is often diagnosed by exclusion. Immunoassays are available and may be helpful.

    b. *Babesia microti*: coccidial infection of cattle and deer, endemic to Massachusetts (e.g., **Martha's vineyard, Nantucket Island**); transmitted by ticks (*Ixodes dammini*); causes fevers, sweats, headache, arthralgia, and myalgia. Organisms look **identical to the ring forms of *P. falciparum* except for a lack of pigment**, and occasionally four ring forms attach to each other and create a "Maltese cross." Diagnosis is made by identifying **ring forms on blood smears** and by **serology** (e.g., indirect immunofluorescence).

3. *Toxoplasma gondii*: causes **toxoplasmosis**

    a. **Life cycle and transmission**. The definitive host is the cat, who releases oocysts into the feces, which then **require 48 hours to become infectious**. Oocysts are ingested by animals and become **tachyzoites**, which are the rapidly reproducing, feeding forms that attack nucleated cells throughout the body. They may encyst, particularly in the brain and eye, as **bradyzoites** (dormant organisms).

    b. **Morphology**

        (1) **Tachyzoites**: 5 μm × 2 μm, **bow- or crescent-shaped**, in tissues

        (2) **Bradyzoites: 2–3 μm, round**; aggregate within 10–50 μm **pseudocysts**

c.   Clinical syndromes

(1)   Congenital: disseminated with multiple organ involvement, particularly the **central nervous system (CNS)** and the **eye** (stillbirths, brain calcifications, convulsions, blindness)

(2)   Acquired: pregnant women are especially susceptible. Infections may be mild (chronic weakness with headaches), or may cause chorioretinitis, meningoencephalitis, cardiomyositis, and so on. In the acquired immunodeficiency syndrome (AIDS), quiescent infections can become fulminant.

d.   Diagnosis: ELISA serologic tests (IgG and IgM) are the recommended tests of choice. Positive IgM titers represent active infection (including congenital infection in neonates). The **Sabin–Feldman dye test** is the reference serologic test, but is available in only a few laboratories, and is rarely used.

V.   Helminths are worms, and include **Nematodes** (roundworms with a central body cavity) and **Platyhelminths** (flatworms with no true central body cavity). Platyhelminths include **Cestodes** (tapeworms) and **Trematodes** (flukes; Fig. 3-3). Helminth infections affect 1–2 billion people worldwide (particularly infections by *Ascaris lumbricoides*, hookworms, *Enterobius vermicularis*, and filarial worms). Transmission is often through a **fecal to oral** route; therefore, poor hygiene and poor sanitation are high risk factors.

A.   Nematodes (roundworms) have **cylindrical bodies**, an outer acellular **cuticle**, and a central digestive system. Females are typically larger than males. Their life cycles include eggs, one or more larval stages, and an adult stage. Definitive hosts have adult worms; intermediate hosts have larvae only.

1.   Pathogenic intestinal nematodes. Most of the intestinal roundworms infect humans through **fecal-contaminated soil or food. Pinworms are an exception** because they can be transmitted directly from anal skin (by scratching) to the hands of other children, making them common urban infections. *E. vermicularis* **and** *T. trichiura* **remain in the gastrointestinal tracts of their human hosts, whereas the other intestinal roundworms migrate through the lungs**, and may cause **Löeffler's syndrome** (transient lesions on chest x-ray film with blood eosinophilia). Some worms have a life span of several months (e.g., *E. vermicularis*), whereas others can live for >30 years (e.g., *Strongyloides*).

a.   *Ascaris lumbricoides* (giant roundworm): worldwide distribution; **one of the most common human intestinal roundworms in the world**.

(1)   Transmission and life cycle. Humans ingest eggs in fecal-contaminated food. Eggs release larvae, which invade the intestinal lymphovascular system and are carried to the lungs. There, they are coughed up, swallowed, and become adults that reside in the cecum.

(2)   Clinical syndromes: asymptomatic or **abdominal pain and diarrhea, Löeffler's syndrome**. Worms migrating into the bile ducts can cause **hepatitis, pancreatitis, or cholecystitis**.

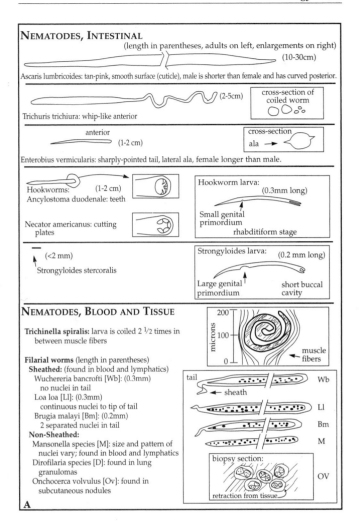

NEMATODES, INTESTINAL

(length in parentheses, adults on left, enlargements on right)

(10-30cm)

Ascaris lumbricoides: tan-pink, smooth surface (cuticle), male is shorter than female and has curved posterior.

(2-5cm)

cross-section of coiled worm

Trichuris trichiura: whip-like anterior

anterior

(1-2 cm)

cross-section

ala →

Enterobius vermicularis: sharply-pointed tail, lateral ala, female longer than male.

Hookworms: (1-2 cm)
Ancylostoma duodenale: teeth

Necator americanus: cutting plates

Hookworm larva: (0.3mm long)

Small genital primordium
rhabditiform stage

(<2 mm)

Strongyloides stercoralis

Strongyloides larva: (0.2 mm long)

Large genital primordium
short buccal cavity

NEMATODES, BLOOD AND TISSUE

Trichinella spiralis: larva is coiled 2 ½ times in between muscle fibers

Filarial worms (length in parentheses)
  Sheathed: (found in blood and lymphatics)
    Wuchereria bancrofti [Wb]: (0.3mm)
      no nuclei in tail
    Loa loa [Ll]: (0.3mm)
      continuous nuclei to tip of tail
    Brugia malayi [Bm]: (0.2mm)
      2 separated nuclei in tail
  Non-Sheathed:
    Mansonella species [M]: size and pattern of nuclei vary; found in blood and lymphatics
    Dirofilaria species [D]: found in lung granulomas
    Onchocerca volvulus [Ov]: found in subcutaneous nodules

200
microns
100
0

muscle fibers

tail   Wb
← sheath
Ll
Bm
M

biopsy section:

OV

retraction from tissue

A

Fig. 3-3. Common helminth morphology.

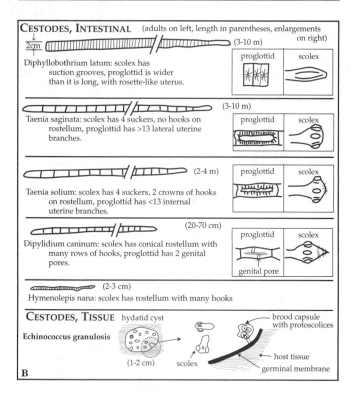

CESTODES, INTESTINAL (adults on left, length in parentheses, enlargements on right)

Diphyllobothrium latum: scolex has suction grooves, proglottid is wider than it is long, with rosette-like uterus. (3-10 m)

Taenia saginata: scolex has 4 suckers, no hooks on rostellum, proglottid has >13 lateral uterine branches. (3-10 m)

Taenia solium: scolex has 4 suckers, 2 crowns of hooks on rostellum, proglottid has <13 internal uterine branches. (2-4 m)

Dipylidium caninum: scolex has conical rostellum with many rows of hooks, proglottid has 2 genital pores. (20-70 cm)

Hymenolepis nana: scolex has rostellum with many hooks (2-3 cm)

CESTODES, TISSUE hydatid cyst

Echinococcus granulosus

(1-2 cm) scolex

brood capsule with protoscolices

host tissue

germinal membrane

B

Fig. 3-3. *Continued*

(3) **Diagnosis: adult worms/eggs in stool** [stool samples from outhouses may contain common earthworms (dark brown-purple and segmented vs. the pale, tan-pink, smooth *Ascaris lumbricoides*)].

b. ***Trichuris trichiura* (whipworm)**: worldwide distribution (tropics/subtropics)

(1) **Transmission and life cycle. Humans ingest eggs** in fecal-contaminated food. The eggs mature into adult worms that reside in the large intestine for up to a decade.

(2) **Clinical syndromes**: asymptomatic or **abdominal pain with diarrhea**. Adult worms secrete a neurotoxin which may cause **rectal prolapse** in children.

(3) **Diagnosis: adult worms or eggs in stool**

c. ***Enterobius vermicularis* (pinworm)**: worldwide distribution; **the most common intestinal roundworm in children living in urban societies.**

(1) **Transmission and life cycle**. Humans ingest eggs from **contaminated fingers** (due to scratching or handling soiled clothing). The eggs mature into adult

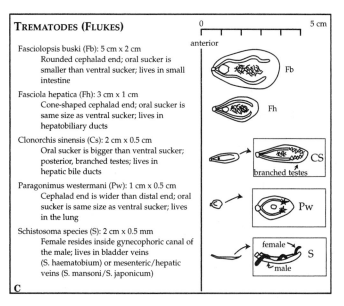

TREMATODES (FLUKES)

Fasciolopsis buski (Fb): 5 cm x 2 cm
    Rounded cephalad end; oral sucker is smaller than ventral sucker; lives in small intestine

Fasciola hepatica (Fh): 3 cm x 1 cm
    Cone-shaped cephalad end; oral sucker is same size as ventral sucker; lives in hepatobiliary ducts

Clonorchis sinensis (Cs): 2 cm x 0.5 cm
    Oral sucker is bigger than ventral sucker; posterior, branched testes; lives in hepatic bile ducts

Paragonimus westermani (Pw): 1 cm x 0.5 cm
    Cephalad end is wider than distal end; oral sucker is same size as ventral sucker; lives in the lung

Schistosoma species (S): 2 cm x 0.5 mm
    Female resides inside gynecophoric canal of the male; lives in bladder veins (S. haematobium) or mesenteric/hepatic veins (S. mansoni/S. japonicum)

0   5 cm

anterior

C

Fig. 3-3. *Continued*

worms that reside in the cecum and **migrate at night to the anal area to lay eggs**. Self-reinfection may occur.

(2) **Clinical syndromes**: intense **perianal itching**, abdominal pain

(3) **Diagnosis: cellophane tape** method to collect eggs from the perianal skin. Eggs are not usually identified in the stool.

d. **Hookworms**: *Necator americanus* (**New World hookworm**) and *Ancylostoma duodenale* (**Old World hookworm**): worldwide distribution, including the tropics and North America (*N. americanus*) and other temperate zones (*A. duodenale*, which is not endemic to the United States).

(1) **Transmission and life cycle**. Infections are common in fields fertilized with human feces ("night soil"). Eggs deposited in soil develop into **rhabdidiform** larvae and then **filariform** larvae. Filariform larvae **directly penetrate human skin**, are carried by the lymphovascular system into the lungs, and are then coughed up and swallowed. They then mature into adults that firmly attach to the small intestine mucosa (hence, are not usually found in the stool) and suck blood from small mucosal vessels. They can live up to 20 years.

(2) **Clinical syndromes**: skin infections where the larvae penetrate (**ground itch**), **Löeffler's syndrome, abdominal pain with nausea and diarrhea, and**

HELMINTH EGGS

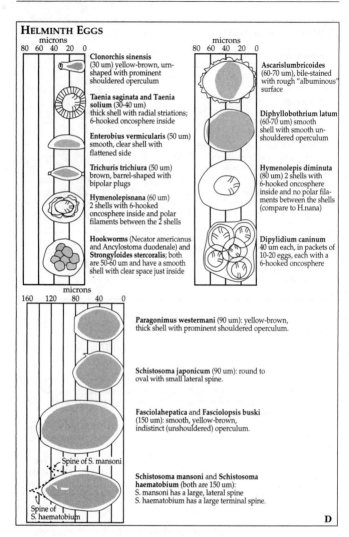

microns
80 60 40 20 0

Clonorchis sinensis
(30 um) yellow-brown, urn-shaped with prominent shouldered operculum

Taenia saginata and Taenia solium (30-40 um)
thick shell with radial striations; 6-hooked oncosphere inside

Enterobius vermicularis (50 um)
smooth, clear shell with flattened side

Trichuris trichiura (50 um)
brown, barrel-shaped with bipolar plugs

Hymenolepisnana (60 um)
2 shells with 6-hooked oncosphere inside and polar filaments between the 2 shells

Hookworms (Necator americanus and Ancylostoma duodenale) and **Strongyloides stercoralis**; both are 50-60 um and have a smooth shell with clear space just inside

microns
80 60 40 20 0

Ascarislumbricoides
(60-70 um), bile-stained with rough "albuminous" surface

Diphyllobothrium latum
(60-70 um) smooth shell with smooth un-shouldered operculum

Hymenolepis diminuta
(80 um) 2 shells with 6-hooked oncosphere inside and no polar filaments between the shells (compare to H.nana)

Dipylidium caninum
40 um each, in packets of 10-20 eggs, each with a 6-hooked oncosphere

microns
160 120 80 40 0

Paragonimus westermani (90 um): yellow-brown, thick shell with prominent shouldered operculum.

Schistosoma japonicum (90 um): round to oval with small lateral spine.

Fasciolahepatica and **Fasciolopsis buski** (150 um): smooth, yellow-brown, indistinct (unshouldered) operculum.

Spine of S. mansoni

Schistosoma mansoni and **Schistosoma haematobium** (both are 150 um):
S. mansoni has a large, lateral spine
S. haematobium has a large terminal spine.

Spine of S. haematobium

D

Fig. 3-3. *Continued*

iron-deficiency anemia caused by intestinal blood loss. Each hookworm can cause 0.2 mL/d of blood loss.

    (3)   **Diagnosis: eggs in stool** (larvae are generally not seen because the eggs require more time than the eggs of *Strongyloides stercoralis* to develop into larvae); adult worms in intestinal biopsies.

    e.   *Strongyloides stercoralis* (**threadworm**): worldwide distribution (tropic and subtropic), southern United States.

    (1)   **Transmission and life cycle**: similar to hookworms

    (2)   **Clinical syndromes**: similar to hookworms, except no blood loss. Eggs (released by adults) can develop into filariform larvae before exiting with the stool, and may reinvade the mucosa ("auto-reinfection"). **Auto-reinfection can be fatal**, particularly in the immuno-suppressed.

    (3)   **Diagnosis: larvae or eggs in stool specimens**; adult worms in intestinal biopsies; serology

    f.   **Other miscellaneous intestinal nematodes**: *Trichostrongylus* **spp**.: gastrointestinal nematode, similar to hookworms; endemic to Europe and Russia; transmitted by contaminated food. *Capillaria philippinensis*: nematode; causes abdominal symptoms; endemic to the Philippines; transmitted by eating poorly cooked fish. *Angiostrongylus cantonensis* (rat lung nematode): can cause meningoencephalitis in humans; endemic to Southeast Asia; transmitted by eating poorly cooked shrimp or snails. *Anisakis* **spp**.: gastrointestinal nematode; endemic to Japan, California, Hawaii; transmitted by eating poorly cooked salt-water fish.

2. Pathogenic tissue nematodes

    a.   **Filarial worms**. These roundworms have threadlike adult forms, and prelarval stages called "microfilaria." Microfilaria have rounded anterior ends and pointed tails, and some species have **sheaths** (empty membranes that are egg-shell remnants). Microfilaria are transmitted by **mosquitoes and flies. Diagnosis is made by identification of the microfilaria in blood or skin** (adults generally are in deep tissues). Serologic tests (e.g., indirect hemagglutination, ELISA, indirect immunofluorescence) may be helpful.

    (1)   **Sheathed microfilaria**

        (a)   *Wuchereria bancrofti*: the **most common** filarial infection; 270 μm long, **no nuclei in tail**; nocturnal activity (collect diagnostic blood from 2–4 AM); transmitted by *Anopheles mosquito*; endemic to tropical and subtropical areas. Larvae migrate through the lymphatics where they mature into adults, and cause fever, headache, and obstructive lymphadenopathy (**"elephantiasis"** and **hydroceles** of the groin).

        (b)   *Brugia malayi*: 200 μm long, **two separated nuclei in tail**; no set schedule of activity; transmitted by the *Anopheles* mosquito; endemic to the Orient. Clinical syndromes are similar to *W. bancrofti*.

        (c)   *Loa loa* (**African eyeworm**): 270 μm long, **nuclei form a continuous row to the tip of the tail**; diurnal activity (collect blood at noon); transmitted by

deer fly (*Chrysops*); endemic to tropical Africa. Microfilaria migrate through the subcutaneous and subconjunctival tissues, causing subcutaneous swellings (**"calibar"**) and **conjunctivitis**. Diagnosis is made by blood smears and skin biopsies.

(2)   Nonsheathed microfilaria

  (a)   *Mansonella* species: usually nonpathogenic; pattern of nuclei varies; endemic to Argentina and the Caribbean; reside in peritoneal cavities and blood.

  (b)   *Onchocerca volvulus*: no nuclei in tail; transmitted by **buffalo or black flies** (*Simulium*); endemic to Africa and Central and South America. Microfilaria migrate through the subcutaneous tissues and cause **loss of skin elasticity ("hanging groin")** and **"river blindness."** Diagnosis is made by **skin biopsies**.

  (c)   *Dirofilaria immitis* (dog heart worm): transmitted by **mosquitoes**; endemic to India, Southeast Asia. In humans (accidental hosts), the microfilaria travel to the **lungs**, die, and form **granulomas** ("coin lesions" on chest x-ray film). Definitive diagnosis is made by **lung biopsy**.

b.   *Trichinella spiralis*

  (1)   Transmission and life cycle. Humans eat undercooked pork or bear contaminated with encysted larvae. The larvae mature into adults, burrow into the intestine, and deposit new larvae in the lymphatics. The larvae migrate **into active, striated muscles** (e.g., diaphragm, intercostal, jaw, extraocular, calf) where they encyst.

  (2)   Clinical syndromes: causes **"trichinosis."** Early symptoms include abdominal pain, headache, and diarrhea. Later, **muscle or joint pain and periorbital edema** may develop. Death can occur from diaphragmatic exhaustion.

  (3)   Diagnosis: extreme peripheral blood eosinophilia (50%–80% of white cells). **Muscle fiber biopsies show larva with 2½ spirals**. Use regular paraffin sections, "tease" preparations or "compressed" preparations. **Serologic tests** (e.g., ELISA, immunofluorescence, Bentonite flocculation) are useful.

c.   *Toxocara canis* (dog roundworm) and *Toxocara cati* (cat roundworm): cause visceral larva migrans. *T. canis* and *T. cati* are nonhuman nematodes (dog and cat ascaris) with a worldwide distribution.

  (1)   Transmission and life cycle (in humans as accidental hosts). Humans ingest ova from infected dog or cat feces, which then develop into larvae within the intestines. The larvae migrate aimlessly into the **liver, eyes, CNS, lung, heart**, for example, where they can live for years.

  (2)   Morphology. Tissue biopsies show **granulomatous inflammation** and nematode larvae.

  (3)   Clinical syndromes: usually involve small children, causing, for example, fever, failure to thrive, hepatomegaly, CNS symptoms, and eye disorders.

(4) **Diagnosis: open biopsy** of liver or lung; **serologic tests** (e.g., ELISA) are useful.

d. *Dracunculus medinensis* (**guinea worm**): endemic to Africa, the Middle East, Asia

(1) **Transmission and life cycle**: larvae are ingested by **water fleas**, which are then **ingested by humans in contaminated water**. The larvae migrate to subcutaneous tissues (usually lower legs), and mature into adults within a **skin papule**.

(2) **Morphology**: adult females are up to 1M in length (males are 4 cm); cause one form of "**cutaneous larva migrans.**"

e. *Ancylostoma braziliense* and *Ancylostoma caninum* (**dog hookworms**): worldwide distribution; transmitted by walking barefoot in soil contaminated with dog or cat feces. The **larvae directly penetrate the skin**, migrate through the subcutaneous tissues (**"cutaneous larva migrans"**), and die within days.

B. **Platyhelminthes (flatworms)** include the **Cestodes (tapeworms)** and the **Trematodes (flukes)**. These multicellular organisms have a **flat, symmetric body**, and most are **hermaphroditic** (having both male and female sexual organs).

1. **Pathogenic intestinal cestodes (tapeworms).** Tapeworms have segmented, flattened, tapelike bodies (**strobila**) with a specialized attachment organ (**scolex**) and suckers at the anterior end. The tip or crown (**rostellum**) of the scolex can have hooks (**armed**) or be smooth (**unarmed**). Tapeworms have no mouth, and absorb nutrients directly through the surface of the worm. Each segment of the worm is hermaphroditic and called a "**proglottid.**" Proglottids near the tail end are mature and filled with eggs. Many eggs have a lidlike structure called an "**operculum.**" After fertilization, eggs (ova) contain embryos ("oncospheres") with six tiny hooks. Embryos develop into larvae called "**cysticerci.**" **Humans are infected by eating food contaminated with encysted cysticerci.** Cysticerci develop into adult worms that attach with their scolex to the small intestines and compete with the host for foodstuffs. Tapeworms can live up to 20 years.

a. *Diphyllobothrium latum* (fish tapeworm, also called "broad tapeworm"): endemic to North and South America, Europe, the Middle East, and Asia.

(1) **Transmission and life cycle.** *D. latum* eggs develop into coracidium (ciliated embryos), which are eaten by water fleas (*Cyclops*), and in turn are eaten by fish. The eggs develop into larvae within the fish flesh. **Humans eat the fish**, and the larvae mature into adults that reside in the small intestines.

(2) **Clinical syndromes**: intestinal symptoms are minimal. *D. latum* competes with the host for vitamin B_{12}; subsequent B_{12} deficiency can cause **megaloblastic anemia**.

(3) **Diagnosis: eggs or proglottids in the feces.**

b. *Taenia saginata* (**beef tapeworm**) and *Taenia solium* (**pork tapeworm**): **worldwide distribution**

(1) **Transmission and life cycle.** Eggs are ingested by cattle or pigs and develop into embryos (oncospheres), which invade the muscles and become larvae ("cysticerci"). **Humans eat the undercooked meat** (beef or "measly" pork) and the larvae mature into adult worms that reside in the small intestine.

(2)   **Clinical syndromes: eating larvae-infested meat causes mild abdominal pain**. However, **ingesting the embryonated eggs of *T. solium*** (or regurgitating gravid proglottids of *T. solium*) causes a potentially fatal disease called **cysticercosis**, in which larvae migrate into the **brain, eye, muscle**, and so on. Up to three-fourths of Mexican patients in some regions who have seizures have cysticercosis of the brain.

(3)   **Diagnosis: proglottids or eggs in the feces; biopsy for cysticercosis; serologic tests** (e.g., ELISA, Western blot) **are diagnostically helpful when there are multiple cysts** (sensitivity is low for single cysts).

  c.   ***Dipylidium caninum*** (dog tapeworm). *D. caninum* has a worldwide distribution, but is uncommon in the United States. Eggs are ingested by dog fleas and develop into larvae. The **dog fleas are ingested by humans** (or dogs) and the larvae become adults that reside in the small intestine. Symptoms include **mild diarrhea** with loss of appetite. Diagnosis is made by identifying **proglottids or egg packets** in the feces.

  d.   ***Hymenolepis diminuta* (rat tapeworm)**. *H. diminuta* has a worldwide distribution, but is uncommon in the United States. Eggs are ingested by **rat fleas or meal worm beetles** and develop into larvae. The insects contaminate flour and are then **ingested by humans** (or rats), and the larvae become adults that reside in the small intestine. Patients are usually asymptomatic, but may have **diarrhea**. Diagnosis is made by identifying **eggs in stool**.

  e.   ***Hymenolepis nana* (dwarf tapeworm)**. *H. nana* has a worldwide distribution, and is the **most common tapeworm seen in the United States**. It commonly infects mice, and is transmitted to humans who consume **food or water that is contaminated** with the fertilized eggs. Clinical syndromes include asymptomatic infections or mild **abdominal pain, diarrhea**, and headache. Diagnosis is made by identifying **eggs in the stool**.

2.   **Pathogenic tissue cestodes (tissue tapeworms)**

  a.   ***Echinococcus* species** (e.g., *granulosus, multilocularis*) causes **"hydatid disease,"** and are endemic to sheep and cattle-raising areas worldwide.

(1)   **Transmission and life cycle**: adult worms reside in carnivores (e.g., wolves) and release eggs with their feces. Herbivores (e.g., sheep) eat vegetation contaminated with the feces. The cycle is completed in nature as infected herbivores are then eaten by carnivores. **Humans become accidental intermediate hosts by ingesting eggs**, which mature into embryos, penetrate the intestines, travel to various organs, and develop into **"hydatid cysts."**

(2)   **Morphology**. Hydatid cysts measure 1–20 cm, have an external fibrous capsule (created by the host) and

an inner **germinal membrane** that produces **"proto-scolices"** (**"hydatid sand"**). The cysts usually form in the liver, but can occur in the **lungs, brain, kidneys**, and so forth. Adult worms cannot develop within humans.

(3) **Clinical syndromes: jaundice** from liver cysts, cough and **hemoptysis** from lung cysts, seizures and **increased intracranial pressure** from brain cysts, for example. If cysts rupture, **anaphylaxis can occur**, and metastatic new cysts can form.

(4) **Diagnosis: serologic tests include ELISA and Western blot. DO NOT BIOPSY.**

C. **Trematodes (flukes)** are **flat, leaflike worms** with an epithelial surface (**no cuticle**), **two suckers** (one for attachment and one for ingesting food), and **a blind gastrointestinal system** (no anus). Flukes are **hermaphroditic except for the *Schistosoma* species**. The flukes usually have a **sexual phase in humans**, and **an asexual phase in snails or other mollusks**. An egg hatches into a **miracidium** (a free-swimming larva) that infects a snail. Within the snail, the second larval stage (cercaria) develops, which then swims to encyst in another mollusk or on vegetation (becoming metacercaria), and finally infects humans when ingested. The cercariae of *Schistosoma* directly penetrate human skin, and the metacercarial stage is omitted.

1. **Pathogenic intestinal and hepatobiliary trematodes**

a. *Fasciolopsis buski* (**giant intestinal fluke**): endemic to India and Southeast Asia; pigs are commonly infected.

(1) **Transmission**: ingestion of fresh-water vegetation (e.g., bamboo shoots, **water chestnut**) with metacercaria. Larvae attach to the small intestinal wall and mature into adults.

(2) **Clinical syndromes: epigastric pain** (particularly in the morning) with diarrhea, intestinal ulceration, and ascites.

(3) **Diagnosis: ova in feces or bile**; serology may be helpful.

b. *Fasciola hepatica* (**sheep liver fluke**): worldwide distribution; sheep and cattle are commonly infected.

(1) **Transmission**: ingestion of fresh-water vegetation (e.g., **watercress**) with metacercaria. The larvae migrate through the peritoneal cavity and penetrate the liver, where they reside as adults in **hepatobiliary ducts**.

(2) **Clinical syndromes**: headache, **substernal pain**, fever and chills, **diarrhea, biliary obstruction**, and jaundice.

(3) **Diagnosis: eggs in feces or bile; serologic tests** (e.g., ELISA, Western blot) may be helpful.

c. *Clonorchis sinensis* (**Chinese liver fluke**): endemic to the Orient.

(1) **Transmission**: ingestion of raw (or smoked) **fresh-water fish** with metacercaria. Larvae migrate up the bile passages, and reside as adults in the **hepatic bile ducts** for up to decades.

(2)   Clinical syndromes: asymptomatic or **abdominal pain**, cirrhosis, **jaundice**, and, rarely, cholangiocarcinoma.

  d.   *Schistosoma* species (from Greek meaning "split body," referring to the groove in the male body): cause **schistosomiasis** (bilharziasis). *Schistosoma* species are the only flukes that have **separate genders**.

    (1)   Transmission: free-swimming cercariae (in snail-infested fresh water) **directly penetrate human skin**, migrate to various organs and reside as adults in veins.

      (a)   *S. mansoni* (endemic to Africa, the Middle East, Caribbean) and ***S. japonicum*** (endemic to the Orient): reside in **large intestinal** and **small intestinal mesenteric veins, respectively**, passing eggs into the feces. *S. japonicum* may disseminate to the brain and other organs.

      (b)   *S. haematobium* (endemic to Africa, the Middle East): resides in the veins of the **urinary bladder**, passing eggs into the urine.

    (2)   Clinical syndromes: inflamed sites of skin penetration (**swimmer's itch**)

      (a)   *S. mansoni* and *S. japonicum*: fever, **abdominal pain, diarrhea**, cirrhosis

      (b)   *S. haematobium*: pelvic pain, **hematuria** (especially at the end of urination), urinary obstruction, urinary bladder **squamous cell carcinoma**

    (3)   Diagnosis: eggs in the stool or urine (early infections). In chronic infections, tissue biopsies are required to visualize the eggs; serologic tests (e.g., ELISA, immunoblot) may be helpful.

  2.   Pathogenic tissue trematode: *Paragonimus westermani* (**lung fluke**) is endemic to Asia, South and North America, North Africa.

    a.   Transmission and life cycle: ingestion of poorly cooked **freshwater crabs** or crayfish containing metacercaria. The metacercariae migrate through the peritoneal cavity and diaphragm into the **lungs** (or rarely the brain), where they reside as adults. Eggs are then coughed up, swallowed, and passed with the feces.

    b.   Clinical syndromes: fever, chills, **cough, hemoptysis**, pleurisy

    c.   Diagnosis: eggs in sputum or feces, worms in surgical biopsies; serologic tests (e.g., enzyme immunoassay, complement fixation) may be helpful.

Arthropods

Jerome Goddard

I. Medical significance of arthropods

A. Introduction. Arthropods can have direct and indirect effects on humans. Direct effects include stings, bites, toxic secretions, and tissue invasion. Indirect effects refer to the transmission of various diseases.

B. Direct effects on health

1. Arthropod stings result **when bees, ants,** and **wasps** defensively attack persons coming near their nests. **Venom** is injected on stinging, which varies from species to species, and contains highly complex mixtures of biologically active agents.

2. Arthropod bites (such as **centipedes, spiders, mosquitoes, bedbugs, lice, fleas, ticks,** and **mites**) cause lesions through immune reactions to arthropod **saliva** or directly through **venoms** in the saliva. Humans may become hypersensitive to salivary secretions (e.g., mosquitoes) after repeated exposure. Spiders inject a venom (ordinarily used for killing and digesting the soft tissues of prey), which can cause neurotoxic effects (e.g., black or brown widow spider venom) or necrotic effects [e.g., fiddle back spider ("brown recluse") venom].

3. Toxic secretions. Blister beetles secrete **"cantharidin"** when they are touched, which can produce large fluid-filled blisters on human skin.

4. Tissue invasion occurs when **scabies** mites, some fleas (e.g., **chigoe**), and fly larvae (maggots) infest the tissues of people or animals. Maggot infestations (**myiasis**) are usually opportunistic, but can be obligate in a few tropical species.

C. Indirect effects on health. Arthropods serve as vectors when they transmit disease organisms to humans (Table 3-28). **Mechanical transmission** occurs when arthropods such as houseflies or cockroaches physically carry pathogens (e.g., cholera, dysentery) unchanged from one place or host to another host. **Biological transmission** occurs when the pathogen develops in the arthropod host (e.g., malaria protozoa).

II. Classification and identification of arthropods. The

Phylum arthropoda includes insects, spiders, mites, ticks, scorpions, centipedes, millipedes, crabs, shrimp, lobsters, sowbugs (rollypollies), and other related organisms. Arthropods have **segmented bodies; paired, jointed appendages** (e.g., legs and antennae); an **exoskeleton**; and **bilateral symmetry** (Table 3-29).

III. Identification tips and where to go for help. The iden-

tification of arthropods should be performed with a stereomicroscope having variable power (7–30×). A good clinical history is essential (Table 3-30). Each clinic or laboratory should have a diagnostic algorithmic key chart for general classification. **Specialists are available** for specific arthropod identification in

Table 3-28.   Common pathogens transmitted by arthropods

Pathogen	Arthropod
Bacteria	
Bartonella	Sandflies, fleas
Ehrlichia	Ticks
Francisella tularensis (tularemia)	Ticks, biting flies
Rickettsia (Rocky Mountain spotted fever, typhus, and so on)	Ticks, mites, lice, fleas
Salmonella, shigella, and so on	Roaches, house flies, and so on
Spirochetes (Lyme disease, relapsing fever)	Ticks, lice
Yersinia (plague)	Fleas
Viruses (including arboviruses, dengue, Colorado tick fever, yellow fever)	Ticks, mosquitoes
Parasites	
Babesia	Ticks
Filarial worms	Mosquitoes
Flukes	Copepods (water fleas)
Leishmania	Sand flies
Plasmodium (malaria)	Mosquitoes
Trypanosoma	Kissing bugs, Tsetse flies
Tapeworms	Fleas, beetles

university entomology departments, extension services, and state health departments.

IV.   Arthropods in the clinical setting. Physicians encounter various arthropod problems—stings or bites, scabies or lice in schools, food products infested with "bugs," myiasis, and imaginary insect infestations. Recently, a tremendous increase in **litigation** has been seen regarding arthropods, especially from specimens found in motels, food products, and so on. **Proper documentation is necessary** because insect samples become integral parts of lawsuits. Clinic personnel should follow the steps listed below.

A.   Make a **careful identification** of the arthropod or submit the specimen to a specialist.

B.   Document all details (who, what, when, where), including food product lot numbers.

C.   Use an **ink pen** and a **bound log book** with consecutively numbered pages.

D.   Retain the specimens **in alcohol** or **in a freezer** for at least 1 year.

E.   Do not stray beyond your area of expertise. Do not comment on the life cycle, ecology, or health effects of a particular insect unless reasonably sure of the facts.

V.   Commonly encountered specimens and clinical situations

A.   Stings. Paper wasps, yellow jackets, honey bees, and **fire ants** (southern United States) are almost ubiquitous, caus-

(*text continues on page 279*)

Table 3-29. Key characteristics of some arthropod groups

Arthropod Group	Class	Characteristics	Remarks
Mites (including chiggers) and ticks	Arachnida	Eight legs One discoid body region	Ticks are essentially "large mites," and transmit several disease agents
Spiders	Arachnida	Eight legs Two body regions	Most bite; black widow and brown recluse are dangerous USA species
Scorpions	Arachnida	Eight legs Flat with tail stinger	One USA dangerous species in Arizona and New Mexico
Insects (includes ants, bedbugs, kissing bugs, bees, beetles, caterpillars, fleas, flies, lice, midges, mosquitoes, wasps)	Insects	Six legs Three body regions Most with wings	Mostly nonharmful, although some species bite or sting
Centipedes	Chilopoda	Two legs per body part Often flattened	Called "hundred leggers" Painful bites, but often harmless
Millipedes	Diplopoda	Four legs per body part Often cylindrical	Called "thousand leggers" Defensive fluids cause skin burns

Table 3-30. Clinical questions for arthropod-related lesions[a]

Question to Ask Patient	Possible Cause
Preliminary general questions	
What is the nature of your work?	Occupational exposure to arthropods (e.g., hunting guide, gardener) or irritating fibers (e.g., fiberglass)
At work, do you sit directly under vents or fans?	Fiberglass or other fibers could be hitting them
Have the curtains/carpets been replaced or cleaned?	Fibers from such items can cause irritation
What time of year did lesions occur?	Spring and summer: arthropods likely
Arthropod-related questions	
Did it look like a worm?	Centipede
Was it firmly attached?	Tick, pubic lice
Did it jump greatly?	Flea
Was it "beetle-like"?	Blister beetle
Was it very tiny (head of a pin or smaller)?	Mite, immature tick
Did it fly off?	Biting fly, mosquito
Environmental-related questions	
Did the lesions occur at night?	If outdoors or in an unscreened house: mosquitoes If indoors: bed bugs
Where were you when these lesions occurred?	Outdoors: biting flies, mosquitoes, fire ants, chiggers Indoors: fleas, mites, bed bugs
Do you have pets (especially ones that go outside)?	Yes: fleas, ticks, mites
Were you hiking, fishing, or hunting?	Yes: ticks, chiggers, biting flies, mosquitoes, etc.
Were you working in the yard, garden, or berry patch?	Yes: ticks, biting flies, mosquitoes, fire ants, chiggers
Were you cleaning out the attic, garage, or shed?	Yes: spiders, mites
Are there bats or bird nests in the attic or eaves?	Yes: mites, soft ticks

[a] Adapted from Goddard; not exhaustive, and intended as a guide only.

ing many stings. Many species of **caterpillars** can produce stings similar to wasp and bee stings. Immediate sting reactions, regardless of species, are usually similar, including **pain, itching, wheal,** flare (generally <5 cm in diameter), and/or pustules, which generally resolve in a few hours. Single stings can also cause **anaphylactic shock** in some patients. Multiple stings (generally several hundred) can produce a **direct toxic reaction. Scorpion stings differ** from wasp and bee stings in that some species (mostly those not found in the United States) have venom potent enough to kill a person outright—without any allergic reaction.

B.   Bites. Arthropod bites cause pathology primarily **through immune responses to arthropod saliva,** and often cause **erythema** or a **wheal** and **flare.** A wide variety of **insects, spiders, and mites** may bite people (Fig. 3-4). **Sucking lice** are an especially common infestation among school-aged children. **Chigger mites** tend to bite in areas of the body where clothing is restrictive (e.g., brassiere straps, waistlines). A series of questions may assist in identifying the general type of arthropod involved (Table 3-30).

Potential **spider-bite lesions** present the physician with difficult choices. Even if it was a spider, it may or may not be a dangerous species. If the spider was a **black widow,** systemic effects such as **pain, nausea, muscle cramps, weakness,** and **tightness in the chest** should soon follow. If exposure was to **brown recluse** (BR) - infected dwellings or property (within the appropriate US geographic region), then a presumptive diagnosis may need to be made and treatment initiated to prevent necrosis, even though current therapies for BR bites (e.g., the leukocyte inhibitor, **dapsone**) can produce severe side effects.

C.   Larval specimens in food products. Immature (and sometimes adult) stages of various arthropods infest food products. Most often, patients complain of "worms" that are usually **beetle, moth,** or **fly larvae.** Even if ingested, these insect larvae are usually harmless.

D.   Specimens from people. Scabies mites ("itch mites") tunnel through the epidermis, particularly **between the fingers** and folds of the wrists. Diagnosis is by skin scrapings (after gently lifting off the tunnel "roofs" with a needle) placed in **20% potassium hydroxide (KOH)** and examined microscopically. **Chigoe fleas (jiggers)** burrow into the skin, particularly **on the feet. Fly larvae (maggots) cause myiasis,** of which there are at least three types. **Obligate myiasis** involves maggots that require a living host for development (e.g., the human bot fly and screwworm flies). **Facultative myiasis** involves maggots that opportunistically feed on human flesh such as a malodorous, neglected wound (e.g., blow and flesh flies, occasionally even house flies). **Accidental myiasis** occurs when a person eats a food product containing fly eggs or larvae: most are killed by stomach acid, but temporary abdominal discomfort can occur.

E.   Delusions of parasitosis (DOP). The condition DOP is characterized by the unshakable belief that tiny bugs are living on the patient, biting them, and making their lives miserable. DOP patients may resort to drastic measures to rid themselves

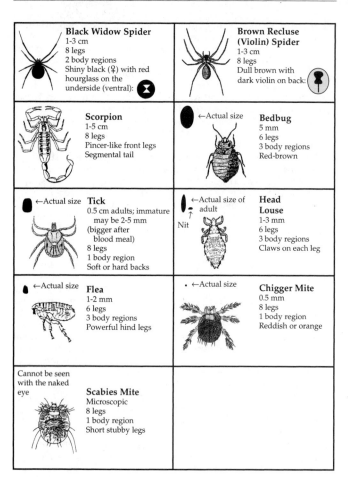

Fig. 3-4. Common arthropods of medical significance (from U.S. Public Health Service).

or their homes of the "bugs." Clinical samples usually consist of tiny bags or jars filled with dust, debris, bits of skin, or even common household insects such as sugar ants or fruit flies.

BIBLIOGRAPHY

Goddard J. *Physician's guide to arthropods of medical importance*, 3rd ed. Boca Raton, FL: CRC Press, 2000.

Pictorial keys to arthropods, reptiles, birds and mammals of public health significance. US Public Health Service; 1969. US Dept of Health, Education, and Welfare PHS publication 1955:1–192.

Infectious Serology

Christine M. Litwin

I. **Practical considerations**
A. **Serology. Use serology when culture is unavailable, impractical, or negative because of antibiotic therapy.**
B. **Key features of an antibody response and its serologic measurement**
1. **Normal antibody response to antigens. In primary infections, the IgM-specific response is usually dominant during the first days or weeks after onset. The IgM response is then replaced by IgG-specific antibodies, which then predominate**. Therefore, a high IgM titer suggests a recent, primary infection; however, IgM titers can occasionally also be elevated in extended infections (see below). **In secondary (anamnestic) responses, the IgG response is faster, more intense, and persists longer than in the primary response** (hence, the purpose for serial vaccinations).
2. **Acute and convalescent samples**. In acute infections, antibodies appear in the first few days and rise sharply over the next 10–21 days. A serum sample collected shortly after the onset of illness (acute) and another collected 2–3 weeks later (convalescent) can be compared quantitatively for changes in antibody titer. **The most reliable evidence of acute infection is seroconversion** (specific antibody is absent from the acute serum but present in the convalescent serum). **A fourfold or higher increase in IgG titer also supports a diagnosis of acute infection. Finally, a high IgM titer is suggestive (but not diagnostic) of an acute infection.**
3. **Problems with measurement of specific antibody responses**
a. **False-positive results can occur** because of cross reactivity (particularly between herpesviruses and between paramyxoviruses), presence of rheumatoid factor, hypergammaglobulinemia, heterophile antibodies against system components [anti-bovine, anti-caprine (goat) or anti-murine antibodies (human anti-murine antibodies: HAMA)], and autoimmune or collagen vascular diseases.
b. **False-negative results can occur** when the antibody response is absent, low, or delayed (especially in immunocompromised hosts such as newborns, patients with the acquired immunodeficiency syndrome, and so on). False negative IgM titers may result from binding of all antigen sites in the test system by a high titer of IgG antibody.
c. **The presence of IgM antibodies is not always an indicator of the acute phase of a primary infection**, because IgM can persist for several months after some acute illnesses, and IgM may be detected in a secondary response to infection as well.

C.   Special considerations in congenital infections (TORCH testing). Prenatal maternal serologic testing can identify infants at risk for infection. However, acute maternal infection does not always result in congenital infection. In suspected congenitally infected infants, **serologic testing should be done on maternal and infant sera collected at the same time. A single neonatal serum sample for IgG titer is not helpful**, because transplacental transmission of maternal IgG antibodies occurs. These maternal antibodies normally decrease and disappear in the infant within 3–6 months. **A fourfold increase in the neonatal IgG titer is suggestive of congenital infection**. Because placental transfer of maternal IgM antibodies does not occur (because of the large size of the IgM), **the presence of IgM antibodies in the infant also supports the diagnosis of congenital infection**.

II.   Assay methods

A.   Agglutination. The cross linking of a particulate antigen and the corresponding antibody are observed as clumping. If red blood cells are used as the particle, this is **hemagglutination**. If latex particles are used, this is **latex agglutination (LA)**. Whole bacteria are often large enough to serve as the particle if the antigen is present on the bacterial surface. Often, the results of agglutination assays are qualitative.

B.   Immunofluorescence. Antibody labeled with a fluorescent dye binds to an antigen. This binding can be detected with a fluorescent microscope. The method is direct if the fluorescent dye is conjugated directly to the antibody. Serology uses **"indirect" immunofluorescence (IFA)** in which the specific antibody is not labeled, but its binding to an antigen is detected in an additional step using a fluorescent-labeled anti-human immunoglobulin antibody.

C.   Immunodiffusion (ID) is the detection of antibody by precipitation of antigen-antibody complexes in a semisolid medium such as agar. The formation of precipitation lines is dependent on relative concentrations of antigen and antibody.

D.   Complement fixation (CF). The fixation of complement occurs during the interaction of antigen and antibodies. All IgM antibodies and many IgG antibodies activate the first component of complement. Antigen and antibody are allowed to react in the presence of a known amount of complement, which is then consumed (fixed). The residual complement activity is then measured with a hemolytic assay. The amount of complement activity remaining after the initial antigen-antibody reaction takes place is inversely related to the number of antibodies in the sample. Results are expressed as the highest serum dilution showing fixation of complement.

E.   Enzyme-linked immunosorbent assay (ELISA). The ELISA method for IgG antibody detection uses antigen immobilized onto a solid surface. Specific antibody in the test serum binds to the antigen. After washing away unbound antibody, the specific antibody bound to antigen is detected with a labeled anti-human indicator antibody followed by a substrate. IgM ELISA methods can use the above-described ELISA method for IgG except that the second antibody is specific for human IgM.

F. Western blot and immunoblot are used to detect and confirm the specificity of antibodies. Antigens are electrophoresed and transferred onto nitrocellulose, or purified antigens are "spotted" onto nitrocellulose. The nitrocellulose is then incubated with patient serum, and patient antibodies to the different antigens are detected by using an anti-human globulin IgG antibody conjugated with an enzyme label.

G. The neutralization test relies on the ability of some serum antibodies to inhibit biologic functions (e.g., growth) of viruses. These neutralizing antibodies are most often indicative of protective immunity. **Hemagglutination inhibition (HI)** relies on the ability of some antibodies to inhibit the ability of some viruses to agglutinate red blood cells from specific animals. Both assays have the potential problem of nonspecific inhibition by serum factors other than antibody.

Table 3-31. Bacterial serologic tests

Organism and/or Disease	Test and Interpretive Clues
Bartonella quintana, *B. henselae* (bacillary angiomatosis, trench fever, cat scratch disease)	**ELISA/IFA:** May cross-react with typhus and scrub typhus sera. Cross-reactions occur between *B. quintana* (trench fever) and *B. henselae* (cat scratch) sera.
Brucella abortus (brucellosis)	**Agglutination:** Titers of ≥1:160 are highly suggestive of active infection. Cross-reactions occur in patients with *Francisella, Yersinia,* or *Vibrio* infections
Chlamydia pneumoniae (pneumonia)	**Micro-IF:** An IgM titer ≥1:20, a four-fold rise in IgG titer, or a single IgG titer ≥1:512, are consistent with acute infection. A panel of chlamydia antigens should be used, and the highest titer is usually seen with the specific infecting species.
Chlamydia trachomatis (lymphogranuloma venereum)	**Micro-IF:** IgM antibody >1:32 and IgG antibody ≥1:2000 (or a fourfold increase in the IgG titer) are consistent with active lymphogranuloma venereum. IgM antibody titers ≥1:128 occur in infants with *C. trachomatis* pneumonitis.
Chlamydia psittaci (pneumonitis, psittacosis)	**Micro-IF:** Presence of IgM antibody or a four-fold rise in IgG titer indicates recent chlamydial infection. *C. psittaci* tests (LGV-1) cross-react with *C. trachomatis* sera.
Coxiella burnetii (Q-fever)	**CF:** <1:8 negative, 1:8–64 suggest infection at undetermined time, ≥1:128 is presumptive evidence of recent or current infection. **IFA or EIA/phase I and II antibodies:** Phase I and II antibodies are useful in serodiagnosis of acute vs. chronic *C. burnetii* infections. Ratio of phase II: phase I >1 in acute disease, ≥1 in subacute disease, <1 in chronic disease.

Francisella tularensis (Tularemia)

Agglutination: Titers ≥1:40–160 indicate past infection; titers ≥1:160 indicate active infection. Minor cross-reactions may occur with Brucella or immunizations.

Helicobacter pylori (gastroenteritis)

ELISA: Antibodies are detectable in almost 100% of duodenal ulcers and 80% of gastric ulcers. Antibodies increase with age (50% of healthy individuals at age 50 have them). Positive results do not confirm *H. pylori*-associated disease, but negative results are evidence against the diagnosis. Antibodies decrease slowly after cure.

IFA: A four-fold rise in IgG titer to 1:128 is indicative of recent infection; however, IgG titers of ≥1:256 may occur in asymptomatic populations.

Legionella pneumophila (Legionaire's disease)

Agglutination: Titers of ≥1:100 (the test measures both IgG and IgM) are indicative of recent or past infection.

Leptospira serovars (aseptic meningitis, renal and hepatic disease)

Mycoplasma pneumoniae

Cold agglutinin test (uses human "O" erythrocytes and measures both IgM and IgG): poor sensitivity (titers rise in only 50% of pneumonia cases), and may rise in cases of hemolytic anemia or liver disease.

CF/ELISA: A positive IgM is consistent with acute infection. High IgG titers may persist for more than 1 year.

Streptococcus (group A)

Streptolysin O (neutralization test), DNAse B (neutralization test): 45% of children with proved group A *streptococcus* (*strep*) pharyngitis have a four-fold rise in antistreptolysin O (ASO) and anti–DNAse B titers (the tests measure both IgM and IgG). ASO is best for pharyngitis or rheumatic fever, and anti-DNAse B is best for strep skin infections or strep-related glomerulonephritis.

Group A extra-cellular proteins [agglutination (streptozyme)] Sensitivity is equivalent to, but the specificity is less than, either ASO or anti-DNAse B. False-positive findings may result from non-group A β-hemolytic streptococci

continued

Table 3-31. *Continued*

Organism and/or Disease	Test and Interpretive Clues
Syphilis	**Nontreponemal (Cardiolipin)** **Rapid Plasma Reagin (RPR) and VDRL:** False positives range from 3–40%. Therefore, positive tests should be confirmed with specific treponemal antigen tests. False positives can occur in the first 3-4 days of life and in patients > 70 years of age, leprosy, acute illnesses, Mycoplasma, pregnancy (0.05%), drug abusers, collagen vascular disease, infectious mononucleosis, etc. Serum RPR is more sensitive (93%) than VDRL. However, for suspected CSF infections, VDRL using CSF should be used rather than RPR. For suspected congenital syphilis, perform serial serologic tests on maternal and neonatal specimens, using both non-treponemal and treponemal tests. **Treponemal (uses Treponema pallidum)** **IF (FTA-ABS IgM and IgG):** IgM is used to diagnose congenital syphilis; it should not be used as a screening tests because of a false positive rate of 10% and a false negative rate ≥ 35%. IgG is used to confirm positive nontreponemal (e.g., reagin) tests. False positives occur in 1%, and are usually due to high immunoglobin levels. **ELISA: IgM & IgG:** comparable to the FTA-ABS test. IgM false negative rate is 20% for congenital syphilis. **HA (MHA-TP):** Used like the FTA-ABS tests to confirm positive nontreponemal tests.
Yersinia enterocolitica, Y. pseudo-tuberculosis	**CF:** Seroconversion or four-fold titer rise indicates recent infection. Primary diagnosis is still by culture. Serology is used as presumptive evidence or for patients with post-infectious manifestations (e.g., Reiter's syndrome, autoimmune disorders, etc.)

Table 3-32. Viral serologic tests

Organism and/or Disease	Test and Interpretive Clues
Adenovirus (pneumonia, gastroenteritis)	**CF:** Titers of ≥1:64 to group-specific antigens are suggestive of active infection. Most cases are diagnosed on clinical grounds alone. Viral culture can be used in selected settings.
Arboviruses (St. Louis, Eastern/Western Equine, California encephalitis)	**IFA:** Significant cross-reactivity exists among the arboviruses, but the titer is usually highest for the specific virus involved. A subsequent infection by another virus within the group will also boost the titer against the initial infecting virus.
Coxsackievirus A 7,9,10,16	**Viral isolation** is the preferred method of diagnosis. Serology (CF) is of limited utility, because of the large number of serotypes, although specific clinical syndromes may narrow the list of suspected serotypes. Single antibody titers ≥1:32 may indicate past or current infection.
Coxsackievirus B 1,2,3,4,5,6	**Viral isolation** is the preferred method of diagnosis. Serology (neutralization) is of limited utility (see above). Single antibody titers ≥1:80 suggest recent infection.
Cytomegalovirus (CMV)	**ELISA, CF, LA:** CMV serologic testing is important in screening blood products for neonates or immunocompromised patients, and in prenatal screening tests. In infants less than 6 months old, IgM is helpful if present, but is not always produced; IgG is meaningless because it may be maternal in origin. For adults with primary CMV infections, tests for IgM are 93%–100% sensitive, or a fourfold increase in IgG titer may be used; however, **culture or antigen detection** is the preferred diagnostic method.
Echovirus (5 serotypes)	**Neutralization:** Titers of ≥1:80 in a single serum specimen strongly suggests current/recent infection, but a fourfold increase in IgG titers is more reliable.

Epstein-Barr (EBV), infectious mononucleosis:

Agglutination tests (uses other species' erythrocytes, and includes the Paul Bunnell test, Davidsohn test, and Monospot). These tests are based on the concept of heterophile antibodies, which are IgM antibodies against EBV that also agglutinate red cells from horses, sheep, and cows. These antibodies are found in up to 90% of EBV infections and may last for 1–2 months. False negatives occur in 10% of cases, especially in children and the elderly.

continued

Table 3-32. *Continued*

Organism and/or Disease	Test and Interpretive Clues

ELISA/IFA tests:

Viral capsid antigen (VCA): Antibodies to EBV VCA arise early in the course of most EBV infections. VCA-IgM antibodies are particularly sensitive and specific. Peak titers of VCA-IgG antibodies occur with the onset of clinical symptoms, and the antibodies are detectable for life.

Early antigen (EA), diffuse and restricted: Antibody titers to EBV EA (EA-diffuse) are seen in the same time frame as VCA-IgM antibodies, and are a sign of active disease. Persistently elevated antibody to EA and EBNA together suggest persistently active, or reactivation of a latent, EBV infection. Antibodies to diffuse EA are also seen in nasopharyngeal carcinoma. Antibodies to restricted EA are also seen in African Burkitt's lymphoma.

Epstein-Barr nuclear antigen (EBNA): A gradual increase in EBNA antibody titer occurs during convalescence, and titers are maintained for life. The appearance of EBNA antibodies in a previously VCA positive and EBNA negative patient is strong evidence of recent infection.

	Monospot	VCA-IgM	VCA-IgG	EA-(Diffuse)	EBNA-IgG
Never exposed	-	-	-	-	-
Incubation	+	+	+	-	-
Acute Infection	+	+	+	+	-
Recovery	-	-	+	-	+
Reactivation of latent infection	+	+	+	+	+

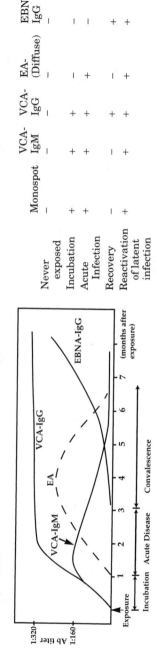

Hepatitis A (HAV)

Hepatitis B (HBV): Surface antigen (sAg), Core antigen (cAg), e antigen (eAg)

Micro-ELISA: Diagnosis of acute HAV infection requires IgM-specific anti-HAV, which appears 4 weeks after infection and persists up to 4 months. Presence of IgG antibody indicates past infection, or immunization and associated immunity.

ELISA: HBsAg (surface antigen) rises within 1–2 months after the onset of infection, and is a sign of active disease (acute or chronic). It disappears with recovery (convalescence). HBeAg (e antigen) rises within 2 months after exposure and lasts for 1 month. It is a sign of active viral replication and the time of greatest infectivity. HBcAb (HB core antibody) rises about the same time as the rise of HBeAg and persists for life. It is used to confirm HBV infection during the "window" between HBsAg and anti-HBs. HBeAb (HBe antibody) rises after HBeAg declines, and is a sign that the infection is resolving. HBsAb (antibody to HB surface antigen) rises after HBsAg decreases, and is a sign of recovery and immunity.

	HBsAg	Anti-HBc-IgM	Anti-HBc-IgG	Anti-HBs	Anti-HBsAg
Never exposed	–	–	–	–	–
Incubation	+	–	–	–	–
Acute or persistent infection	+	+	+	+	+ or –
Asymptomatic carrier	+	–	–	–	–
Early recovery	–	+	+	+	+
Remote exposure (with recovery)	–	–	+	+	+ or –
Immunized	–	–	–	–	+

continued

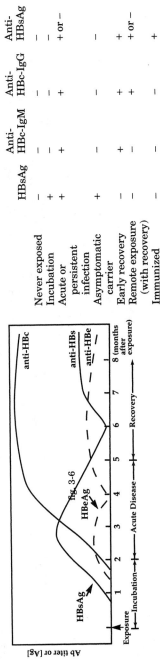

fig. 3-6

Table 3-32. *Continued*

Organism and/or Disease	Test and Interpretive Clues
Hepatitis C (HCV)	**ELISA, recombinant immunoblot:** False positive ELISA results occur when anti-superoxide dismutase is present in the sera. Additionally, 2% of positive results in patients and 40% of positive results in random blood donors are false positives, and are not confirmed by the immunoblot assay.
Hepatitis delta (HDV)	**ELISA:** Serologic diagnosis of hepatitis delta depends upon the finding of HDV antigen and/or the presence of anti-HDV. Patients will almost invariably have hepatitis B surface antigen (HBsAg) and/or antibodies to HBcAg and to HBeAg.
Herpes simplex (HSV) types 1,2	**IFA/ELISA, immunoblot, Western blot:** The major clinical utility for HSV antibody titers is to identify seropositive organ transplant recipients. HSV antibody titer testing is usually too slow for diagnosing acute infections (**viral isolation** is better). Many ELISA tests also show cross reactivity between HSV 1 and 2. Type specific immunoblot and ELISA assays are available.
HTLV 1,2	**ELISA/Western blot:** HTLV-1 may not be distinguished from HTLV-2 with conventional serologic tests, and antibodies may be absent in some cases of adult T-cell leukemia/lymphoma.
HIV	**EIA/ELISA/Western blot:** Polymerase chain reaction (PCR) may detect HIV genetic markers within 20 days of exposure. The presence of HIV antigens symbolizes active infection. HIV-1 antigens (e.g., p24) are detectable by EIA within 28 days. Antibodies to HIV 1 and 2 are first detectable at about 5–8 weeks with full seroconversion at 10–14 weeks. False positive ELISA tests may be due to autoimmune diseases or anti-HLA class II antibodies, heterophile anti-bodies, liver disease, alcoholism, multiparity, hematologic malignancies, influenza immunizations, and Stevens-Johnson syndrome. False negatives may occur in the "window" period (before seroconversion) and late in the disease (when Ab titers are low). All positive ELISA tests should be repeated, and if positive, confirmed with Western blot tests. Two out of three bands (p24, gp41, gp120/160) are required for a positive Western blot test.

Influenza A and B

Virus isolation is the best method. Serology (CF) is too slow. Single antibody titers ≥1:64 suggest past or current infection.

CF, ELISA: CF antibodies appear after several weeks, are generally of low titer, and may not be detected in all cases. ELISA is more sensitive, but cell culture plaque reduction neutralization tests should be used as a supplement.

Lymphocytic choriomeningitis (LCM)

Neutralization/ELISA, IFA/CF/HI: Neutralization is useful to confirm seroconversion after vaccination and in the diagnosis of subacute sclerosing panencephalitis. Measles may be associated with IgM antibodies late during the rash and for 2–3 months later. ELISA and IFA can detect IgM in secondary immune responses. CF is less sensitive.

Measles (rubeola)

ELISA, CF, HI, neutralization: CF has been replaced by sensitive and specific ELISAs. IgM—ELISA has very low cross reactivity with other paramyxoviruses (compared to IgG) and may persist for months.

Mumps

CF, HI, neutralization: Single positive antibody titers ≥1:64 may indicate past or current infection. Infected children less than 6 months old may have lower titers. CF is insensitive. HI and neutralization are not widely available.

Parainfluenza (types 1,2,3), (croup)

ELISA: IgM response occurs 1–2 weeks after disease onset. Absence of IgM with the presence of IgG antibodies indicates past infection. Serology is not recommended for diagnosis in HIV patients, hemoglobinopathy patients during aplastic crises, fetal hydrops, or patients with persistent polyarthropathy.

Parvovirus B19 (fifths disease/erythema infectiosum)

Neutralization: Viral isolation is the preferred method for diagnosis. Serology is used in its absence.

Poliovirus (types 1,2,3)

IFA, ELISA, CF: Diagnosis is often made on clinical and epidemiologic grounds. Serology is more useful for epidemiologic studies than for patient management. Young infants and the elderly may have low titers.

Respiratory synctial virus (RSV)

continued

Table 3-32. *Continued*

Organism and/or Disease	Test and Interpretive Clues
Rubella	**HI, ELISA:** Viral isolation is definitive, but most cases are diagnosed by serology. HAI is the "gold" standard but ELISA is commonly used. IgM antibodies rise within 2–3 days of infection, peak in 1 week, and disappear in 30 days. IgG antibodies also rise within 2–3 days of infection, peak in 1–3 weeks, and remain elevated for life. IgG titers ≥1:8 are evidence of immunity. Vaccinations cause IgG titers ≥1:8, with negative IgM titers. Cross-reactions may occur with infectious mononucleosis, parvovirus infection, and CMV infection.
Varicella-Zoster (VZV)	**FAMA, ELISA, LA:** FAMA is the most sensitive test, but is not widely available. LA is almost as sensitive. ELISA may not detect antibodies caused by the live attenuated varicella vaccine. VZV antibody titers may increase in patients with HSV infection who have previously had varicella.

CF, complement fixation; EIA, enzyme immunoassay; ELISA, enzyme-linked immunosorbent assay; FAMA, fluorescent treponemal antibody absorption; HAI, hemagglutination in-hibition; HI, hemagglutination inhibition; HIV, human immunodeficiency virus; HTLV, human T-cell leukemia virus; LA, latex agglutination.

Table 3-33. Fungal serologic tests

Organism and/or Disease	Test and Interpretive Clues
Aspergillus fumigatus, A. niger, A. flavus	**CF, ID:** Precipitins can be found in 90% of sera in aspergilloma cases and 50%–70% of cases with allergic bronchopulmonary aspergillosis.
Blastomyces dermatitidis	**CF:** Titers of 1:8 to 1:16 are suggestive of active infection. Titers ≥1:32 are indicative of active infection. 40%–80% of blastomycosis cases are negative by CF.
	ID: Precipitins occur in 80% of cases. Cross-reactions occur with histoplasmosis.
Candida albicans	**ID:** Precipitins are found in 20%–30% of the normal population. Therefore, clinical correlation must exist for the test to be meaningful.
Coccidiodes immitis	**CF:** Titer parallels the severity of infection. Titers as low as 1:2 may be seen in active infection. Titers >1:16 indicate active infection. Low titers should be followed by repeat testing at 2–3 week intervals. Cross-reactions occur with histoplasmosis. False-negatives occur in patients with solitary pulmonary lesions.
	ID: Can be used as a screening test. Positives should be confirmed with the complement fixation test. A concentration (8- to 10-fold) of specimen enhances antibody detection.
	LA: Can be used as a screening test in early infections. Diagnostic (but not prognostic) precipitins occur during the first 3 weeks of infection. False-positives are frequent when diluted serum or CSF specimens are used.
Cryptococcus neoformans	**LA or EIA** (uses latex particles coated with anticryptococcal globulin): The presence of cryptococcal polysaccharide in body fluids is indicative of cryptococcosis. Sensitivity in CSF is 95% for meningitis cases (more sensitive than India ink preparations), and 30% for nonmeningitis cases. Disseminated cryptococcus usually has a positive serum test. Decreasing titers indicates regression. Rheumatoid factor (RF) causes false-positive reactions, and an RF-test must be performed as a control.

continued

Table 3-33. *Continued*

Organism and/or Disease	Test and Interpretive Clues
Histoplasma capsulatum	**CF:** Titers of 1:8 to 1:16 are highly suspicious of infection; titers ≥1:32 are indicative of active infection. Cross-reactions occur with aspergillosis, blastomycosis, and coccidiodomycosis, but titers are usually lower. Follow-up serum samples should be tested at 2–3 week intervals. Recent skin tests in persons who have had prior exposure to *H. capsulatum* (20% of tested patients) will cause an elevation in the complement fixation titer. The yeast antigen based test has a sensitivity of 75%–80%; the histoplasmin based test has a sensitivity of only 10%–15%. **ID:** H and M bands appearing simultaneously are indicative of active infection. M band may appear alone and can indicate early or chronic (late) infection, or a recent skin test. The H bands appear, albeit infrequently, in the mid-course of the infection. **LA:** The test is unreliable. Positive test results should be confirmed by the CF test.
Sporothrix schenckii	Agglutination: Titers ≥1:80 indicate active infection. False negatives occur in some skin infections but are rare in extracutaneous infections.

CF, complement fixation; EIA, enzyme immunoassay; ID, immunodiffusion; LA, latex agglutination.

Table 3-34. Parasitologic serologic tests

Organism and/or Disease	Test and Interpretive Clues
Entamoeba histolytica (*amebiasis*)	**IHA:** Titers ≥1:128 suggests active infection. Sensitivity is 100% for amoebic liver abscesses, 98% for amoebic dysentery, and 66% for asymptomatic amoebic cyst carriers.
	IFA: Titers ≥1:256 are diagnostic; available through Centers for Disease Control (CDC).
Babesia microti	
Cryptosporidium	**IFA, ELISA:** Used as an epidemiologic tool. Antibody persistence limits its usefulness in acute infections.
Dirofilaria immitis	**ELISA:** Sensitivity and specificity are inadequate.
Echinococcus granulosis (hydatid cyst)	**ELISA, Western blot:** The test is 80%–100% sensitive and 88%–96% specific for a liver cyst, 50% sensitive for lung cysts, and 25%–50% sensitive for cysts in other organs. Available through CDC.
Filariasis	**Definitive diagnosis is by demonstration of the parasite.** Serology (IHA, ELISA, IFA) does not differentiate between filarial species or between past and current infection
Fasciola hepatica	**Diagnosis is made by finding ova in feces or bile.** Serology (ELISA or Western blot) may play a supportive role.
Giardia lamblia	**ELISA:** The presence or absence of IgM antibodies may distinguish current from past infections, respectively; IgG antibodies remain elevated for a long time. Useful for epidemiology.
Leishmaniasis	**IFA, ELISA:** IFA sensitivity is 89%–96% using amastigotes as the antigen, lower (62%) for promastigote-based tests. ELISA sensitivity is 85% for 2 years after the primary cutaneous lesion. IFA titers fall after successful chemotherapy.
Paragonimus westermani	**Diagnosis is made by finding ova in feces or bile.** CF test may be helpful in ectopic lesions.

continued

Table 3-34. *Continued*

Organism and/or Disease	Test and Interpretive Clues
Schistosomiasis	**ELISA, Immunoblot:** Poor specificity and sensitivity. Useful in follow-up of travelers returning from endemic areas or in individuals with light infections or ectopic schistosomiasis.
Taenia solium (cysticercosis)	**ELISA, Western blot:** Sensitivity is 94% for patients with multiple cysts but only 28% for single or calcified cysts. Other helminthic infections (e.g., cestodes) can cross react. Available through CDC.
Toxocariasis (e.g., *Toxocara canis*: visceral larva migrans)	**ELISA:** Useful in supporting a clinical diagnosis. However, titers vary and cannot establish the diagnosis by themselves.
Toxoplasma gondii	**Sabin-Feldman dye test (SFDT):** The SFDT is a neutralization test and the reference serologic test, but is available in only a few laboratories.
	IFA: The IFA parallels the SFDT titers. False-positives occur in patients with positive ANAs. False-negatives can occur with low titers. Other tests include Agglutination, IHA, CF.
	ELISA, immunosorbent: ELISA is the recommended test of choice. Many commercial kits are available (with variable sensitivity and specificity) for IgG. Double-Sandwich IgM-ELISA is much more sensitive and specific than conventional ELISA or IFA. IgM immunosorbent assays are also sensitive and specific. The presence of IgM in apatient (including newborns) suggests active infection.
Trypanosoma cruzi (Chagas' disease)	**CF, IHA, ELISA:** Widely available in Latin America. IgG titers are used to diagnose chronic disease. False-positives occur with malaria, leishmaniasis, syphilis and other parasites. Use 2 or 3 serological methods to confirm a positive test result.
Trichinella spiralis (trichinosis)	**ELISA, IFA:** 16% of the US population is positive for trichinosis; ELISA is more sensitive. For IFA, titers of ≥1:100 are often observed in patients during the acute phase of illness.

ANA, antinuclear antibody; CF, complement fixation; ELISA, enzyme linked immunosorbent assay; IFA, indirect immunofluorescence (indirect fluorescent antibodies); IHA, indirect hemagglutination.

Table 3-35. Arthropod-borne infectious serology

Organism and/or Disease	Test and Interpretive Clues
Colti virus (Colorado Tick fever)	**HI,IFA,CF, neutralization:** Antibodies often appear late. Test acute and convalescent samples. If initially negative, a late convalescent sample (>30 days) should be tested.
Ehrlichia chaffeensis (Ehrlichiosis: human monocytic ehrlichiosis)	**IFA:** A fourfold increase in *E. chaffeensis* IgG antibody titer (minimum titer 1 : 64), or a single high serum antibody titer (≥1:128) with a consistent history, are diagnostic.
Borrelia burgdorferi (Lyme disease)	**EIA/Western blot:** Many patients (up to 40%) with early disease are seronegative by ELISA at the time they present with erythema migrans. All positive or equivocal ELISA tests should be confirmed by Western blot. In late Lyme disease, IgM Western blot is unreliable; IgG titers should be used.
Rickettsia rickettsii (Rocky Mountain Spotted Fever)	**LA, HI, ELISA:** Diagnostic titers are 1 : 64 for LA and 1 : 128 for IH. Any antibodies to Rickettsia rickettsii also react with the Spotted Fever group (*Rickettsia conorii, Rickettsia sibirica* and *Rickettsia australis*).
Rickettsia tsutsugamushi (scrub typhus)	**Agglutination, micro IFA:** Weil-Felix agglutination is not very sensitive but is used in less developed countries. The indirect microimmunofluorescent test is similar to Weil-Felix in sensitivity and specificity.
Rickettsia typhi (epidemic or louse-borne typhus)	**IFA:** Antibodies to *Rickettsia typhi* also react with the Typhus Fever group (*Rickettsia prowazekii*).

ANA, anti-nuclear antibodies; CA, cold agglutinins; CDC, Centers for Disease Control; CF, complement fixation; cross reactions, false-positive test results due to antibodies against other organisms; CSF, cebrospinal fluid; EIA, enzyme immunoassay; ELISA, enzyme-linked immunosorbent assay; FAMA, fluorescent treponemal antibody-absorption; HA, hemagglutination; HI, hemagglutination inhibition; ID, immunodiffusion; IFA, indirect immunofluorescence (indirect fluorescent antibodies); IHA, indirect hemagglutination; LA, latex agglutination; Micro-ELISA, microparticle ELISA; Micro-IF, micro immunofluorescence; RI, recombinant immunoblot; WB, Western blot

4

Chemistry

Acid-Base Balance

Thomas D. Batiuk

I. Definitions
A. **Acid** is a substance that donates a proton (H^+).
B. **Base** is a substance that accepts a proton (H^+).
C. The **pH** is the negative log of the H^+ concentration ($-\log$ [H^+]). pH = 7.0 = neutral; pH <7.0 = acidic; pH >7.0 = alkaline.
D. **pCO_2**. The partial pressure of CO_2 in the blood (measured in mm Hg) is pCO_2.
E. **[HCO_3^-]**. The concentration of bicarbonate in the blood (measured in mEq/L) is **[HCO_3^-]**.
F. **-emia**. The suffix "-emia" (e.g., acid*emia*, alkal*emia*) refers to **relatively acidity** of blood.
G. **-osis**. The suffix "-osis" (e.g., acid*osis*; alkal*osis*) refers to **processes that cause acid or alkali to accumulate.**
H. **Buffer** is a substance that can accept or donate H^+ ions.

II. pH and the Henderson–Hasselback equation
The acidity of body fluids is expressed by the concentration of hydrogen ions (protons; H^+), most frequently as the negative log of this concentration (pH). The free [H^+] is maintained at a very low level (40×10^{-9} Eq/L; compare with $Na^+ = 140 \times 10^{-3}$ Eq/L or $K^+ = 4 \times 10^{-3}$ Eq/L). H^+ ions are generated from the oxidation of fuels. These are neutralized by HCO_3^- generated by the kidney. The products of $H^+ + HCO_3^-$ is CO_2 and H_2O; CO_2 is eliminated through the lungs. This process can be viewed as:

$$H^+ + HCO_3^- \leftrightarrow H_2CO_3 \leftrightarrow H_2O + CO_2$$

The balance is expressed by the Henderson equation:

$$[H^+] = 24 \times \text{Lungs/Kidneys or } [H^+] = 24 \times pCO_2/[CO_3^-]$$

Normal reference ranges: $H^+ = 40$ mEq/L (range, 36–44); normal p$CO_2 = 40$ mm Hg (range, 35–45); normal $HCO_3^- = 24$ mEq/L (range, 22–26).

The **Hasselbach equation** complicated life by taking logarithms of everything:

$$pH = 6.1 + \log [HCO_3^-]/0.03 \, pCO_2$$

It is easier for most people to visualize too many or too few H^+ than to conceptualize log units. However, because blood acidity is still widely reported as pH, use the following rule of thumb: for every pH change of 0.3, [H^+] changes by twofold (Table 4-1).

III. General features of acid-base disturbances
A. **Classification of acid-base disturbances**. Acid-base disturbances are categorized as ***respiratory* when the initial disturbance involves pCO_2, or as *metabolic* when the initial disturbance affects HCO_3^-.**
B. **Physiologic mechanisms for handling acid-base disturbances**. The body can deal with acid-base disturbances in the following three ways.

Table 4-1.   pH versus [H⁺]

pH	[H⁺]	Condition
6.8	160	Acidemia
7.1	80	Acidemia
7.4	40	Normal (neutral)
7.7	20	Alkalemia
8.0	10	Alkalemia

1.   **Chemical buffering**. Buffers mitigate, but do not completely prevent, changes in [H⁺]. Both cellular and extracellular (EC) buffers help to correct acid-base disorders (Table 4-2); EC buffers (e.g., HCO_3^-) begin working immediately, whereas intracellular buffers may take several hours to work. **EC buffers work well for metabolic acid-base disorders**, because the CO_2 produced can be eliminated through the lungs. In contrast, **intracellular buffers must be used to deal with respiratory acid-base disturbances,** because the lungs are no longer able to release CO_2 appropriately.

2.   **Regulating the P_{CO_2} in blood by varying ventilation**. This process takes minutes to hours. Changes in arterial pCO_2 lead to changes in interstitial [H⁺] within chemosensitive areas of the brainstem and, in turn, directly alter the ventilatory drive. Peripheral O_2 and H⁺ chemoreceptors (e.g., carotid body) also affect the rate of ventilation.

3.   **Controlling plasma HCO_3^- by changing renal H⁺ secretion**. This process takes hours to days. The kidneys excrete acid through active secretion of H⁺ as well as generation of ammonium ions (NH_4^+) from ammonia (NH_3). This latter process also generates new HCO_3^- in the blood, which can further buffer free H⁺. **The generation of NH_4^+ is the chief means of renal compensation for chronic acidosis. In cases of chronic alkalosis, the kidney can compensate by excreting more HCO_3^-.**

C.   **Compensation of acid-base disorders. Compensation, which refers to the physiologic attempts by the body to correct an acid-base disturbance**, uses the three mechanisms discussed above. Chemical buffering is an important immediate process. In addition to buffers, **primary metabolic disorders prompt offsetting compensatory respiratory changes, and primary respiratory disorders lead to offsetting com-**

Table 4-2.   Body buffers

Site	Agent(s)	Characteristics
Extracellular	Bicarbonate, phosphate	Rapid buffering
Intracellular	Proteins, phosphates, hemoglobin	Slower buffering
Bone	Carbonate	Slowest buffering

pensatory metabolic corrections. For example, a metabolic acidosis will stimulate a secondary respiratory alkalosis. With time, these compensatory changes will lead to a normalization of [H⁺]; **the degree of normalization can be a useful clinical indicator of the duration of the primary disturbance**. However, it is important to remember that **compensation will** *never* **overcorrect the [H⁺]**.

D. Ancillary tests to assist in the evaluation of acid-base disorders

    1. Anion gap. An important tool in the evaluation of acid-base disorders is the ***anion gap*** (AG). Positive and negative charges are always balanced in the body; therefore, for every cation there is always an associated anion. The main extracellular cation is Na^+. The main extracellular anions are HCO_3^- + Cl^-. The Na^+ concentration is usually a little higher than the sum of the HCO_3^- + Cl^-; the difference is the anion gap, which **represents other normal anions that are not usually measured**. The AG can be easily calculated:

$$AG = Na^+ - (HCO_3^- + Cl^-)$$

    The "normal" AG is 6–12. **When the underlying disorder is a metabolic acidosis, an increased AG may be caused by increased numbers of organic anions** that are not measured in the typical electrolyte panel (e.g., methanol).

    2. Serum potassium. Serum potassium can be another important clinical measure in the interpretation of acid-base status. K^+ is the chief intracellular cation. Acidemia causes H^+ to be shifted into the intracellular space; K^+ is shifted to the extracellular space to maintain electrical neutrality. Likewise, in cases where K^+ moves out of cells into the extracellular space (e.g., responding to urinary K^+ loss caused by diuretics), H^+ will enter the cell, leading to *intra*cellular acidosis, and extracellular alkalosis.

    3. Blood urea nitrogen (BUN) and creatinine. Levels of these tell if the kidneys are working, and may suggest dehydration if the BUN is elevated out of proportion to the creatinine.

E. Summary of laboratory values needed to interpret acid-base status

- Arterial blood gas to determine arterial [H⁺] and pCO_2
- Plasma electrolytes, BUN, and creatinine
- Urine pH and electrolytes are necessary in some cases

IV. Basic steps to interpret the acid-base status

A. Look at the [H⁺] (or pH) to determine acidemia or alkalemia.

B. Look at the pCO_2 and the HCO_3^- to determine whether the primary disorder is respiratory or metabolic (Table 4-3).

    1. The primary disorder is respiratory if the changes in the Pco_2 are in the same direction as the changes in the [H⁺].

        a. Respiratory acidosis: high pCO_2

        b. Respiratory alkalosis: low pCO_2

Table 4-3. Patterns of acid-base disorders

Condition	[H⁺]	Pco₂	Hco₃⁻
Acidosis			
Acute metabolic	↑	N	↓
Compensated metabolic	N	↓	↓
Acute respiratory	↑	↑	N
Compensated respiratory	N	↑	↑
Alkalosis			
Acute metabolic	↓	N	↑
Chronic metabolic	↓	↑	↑
Acute respiratory	↓	↓	N
Chronic respiratory	N	↓	↓

↑, increased; N, near normal; ↓, decreased.

2. The primary disorder is metabolic if the changes in the pCO_2 are in the opposite direction as the changes in the [H⁺].
   a. Metabolic acidosis: low pCO_2
   b. Metabolic alkalosis: high pCO_2
3. The primary disorder is both respiratory and metabolic (combined) if the changes in the pCO_2 are in the same direction, and the changes in the HCO_3^- are in the opposite direction from the changes in the [H⁺] (e.g., acidemia with a high pCO_2 and a low HCO_3^-).
  C. After determining the primary disorder, check for the presence and degree of compensation.
   a. **Respiratory acidosis**: compensated by an elevated HCO_3^-
   b. **Respiratory alkalosis**: compensated by a decreased HCO_3^-
   c. **Metabolic acidosis**: compensated by a decreased pCO_2 (rule of thumb: the last two digits of the pH will be very close to the value of the pCO_2).
   d. **Metabolic alkalosis**: compensated by an elevated pCO_2 (rule of thumb: the last two digits of the pH will be very close to the value of the pCO_2).
  D. For situations of metabolic acidosis *only*, calculate the AG. If the AG is increased, consider the items in Table 4-4. If the AG is normal, consider the items in Table 4-5, and calculate the urinary anion gap.
  E. Consider changes in K⁺, BUN, creatinine, and so on for further information.
  V. Specific acid-base disturbances
  A. Metabolic acidosis
   1. **Laboratory findings**: ↑[H⁺], ↓pCO_2, urine pH = 4.5–5.0 (if renal function is normal).
   2. **Etiologies**. The AG is very useful in establishing possible causes.
   a. **Increased anion gap** (Table 4-4). Most metabolic acidoses in the emergency room are also associated with an

Table 4-4. **Differential diagnosis of metabolic acidosis with an increased anion gap (AG)**

Etiology	Examples	Usual AG (mEq/L)
Ketoacidosis	Diabetes mellitus	>25
	Alcohol abuse	20–25
	Starvation	5–10
Renal failure		<25
Drug ingestion	Salicylates	5–10
	Methanol	>20
	Ethylene glycol	>20
	Paraldehyde	>20
Lactic acidosis	Tissue hypoxia	>25

increased AG, and the most common causes are listed below in order of incidence.

- **Diabetic ketoacidosis (DKA)**
- **Uremic acidosis**
- **Drug ingestion (salicylates, methyl alcohol, ethylene glycol, ethyl alcohol)**

If these three causes can be ruled out, **lactic acidosis** (LA) must then be considered. LA frequently occurs secondary to **tissue hypoxia**; LA in the absence of apparent tissue hypoxia may be caused by hereditary enzyme defects, **drugs** or **toxins** (including all those causing an increased AG), and common medical problems (e.g., **diabetes mellitus, liver disease, malignancy**). Note that d-lactic acidosis may present as a metabolic acidosis with an increased AG, but with a negative LA blood level, as d-lactic acid is not detected in some clinical assays of LA.

   b.   Normal anion gap (Table 4-5). Sometimes called *hyperchloremic* acidoses, these disturbances usually involve the **gain of an inorganic acid** (e.g., HCL) or the **loss of base**, and are often classified according to the serum potassium

Table 4-5. **Differential diagnosis of metabolic acidosis with normal anion gap**

Potassium Level	Possible Cause of Metabolic Acidosis
Low serum potassium	Diarrhea
	Renal tubular acidosis
	Carbonic anhydrase inhibitors
	Urinary diversion
Normal/high serum potassium	Urinary obstruction
	Hypoaldosteronism
	Renal failure
	Treatment with HCl (or equivalent)

level. The **urine anion gap (UAG) may also be useful**. It is defined as:

$$UAG = [Na^+] + [K^+] - [Cl^-]; \text{ normal } UAG = 0$$

- UAG < 0 in diarrhea, acetazolamide use, proximal renal tubular acidosis
- UAG > 0 in distal renal tubular acidosis, chronic renal failure

B.   Metabolic alkalosis

    1.   Laboratory findings

- $\downarrow[H^+]$; $\uparrow HCO_3^-$ (>30 mEq/L)
- pCO_2 normal or slightly $\uparrow$
- Urine pH >7.0 (unless severe hypokalemia, in which case the pH may be acid)
- Serum K^+ is frequently low because of hypovolemia-induced hyperaldosteronism (causing renal K^+ wasting); urine Na^+ will be <10 mEq/L if volume contracted

    2.   Etiologies. Common causes (Table 4-6) can be characterized clinically as follows.

      a.   Volume contracted: caused by vomiting, diuretic use or abuse, and so forth. Volume depletion causes increased aldosterone production, increased renal Na^+ absorption, and increased renal H^+ secretion. This responds to volume repletion with Cl^- salts.

      b.   Not volume contracted. If hypertension is present, consider hyperaldosterone states. Otherwise, consider magnesium depletion, Bartter's syndrome, or renal failure with HCO_3^- load.

C.   Respiratory acidosis

    1.   Laboratory findings: $\uparrow[H^+]$, $\uparrow pCO_2$, HCO_3^- normal or slightly increased. It takes ~24 hours for renal compensation

Table 4-6.   Differential diagnosis of metabolic alkalosis

Mechanism	Examples
Loss of acid	Vomiting; gastric suction
	Villous adenoma of colon
Excess base administration	Antacids ($NaHCO_3$, milk-alkali syndrome)
	Weak acids (Na lactate; citrate)
Potassium depletion[a]	GI loss (e.g., diarrhea)
	Inadequate intake (e.g., TPN without K^+)
	Diuresis
	Mineralocorticoid excess syndromes (e.g.) aldosteronism, Cushing's syndrome, steroid therapy)

GI, gastrointestinal; TPN, total parenteral nutrition.

[a] Potassium depletion causes a H^+/K^+ shift, as H^+ leaves the extracellular fluids to exchange places with intracellular K^+.

to take effect (increased HCO_3^-). The effect of compensation is as follows:

- In acute respiratory acidosis, $\uparrow[H^+] = 0.75 \times$ each 1 mm Hg $\uparrow Pco_2$
- In chronic respiratory acidosis, $\uparrow[H^+] = 0.3 \times$ each 1 mm Hg $\uparrow Pco_2$

It is important to determine if the degree of compensation is appropriate; if it is not, then a mixed acid-base disorder exists.

2. Etiologies. Respiratory acidosis is caused by **alveolar hypoventilation**. Causes for this can be roughly divided into factors that alter the normal stimulus to breathe, and those that affect the mechanical ability to breathe (i.e., anatomic abnormalities). Examples of these disorders are shown in Table 4-7.

D. Respiratory alkalosis

1. Laboratory findings. $\downarrow[H^+]$; $\downarrow Pco_2$, HCO_3^- is normal or slightly decreased.

It takes ~24 hours for renal compensation to take effect (decreased HCO_3^-). The effect of compensation is as follows:

- In acute respiratory alkalosis, $\downarrow[H^+] = 0.75 \times$ each 1 mm Hg $\downarrow Pco_2$
- In chronic respiratory alkalosis, $\downarrow[H^+] = 0.2 \times$ each 1 mm Hg $\downarrow pco_2$

It is important to determine if the degree of compensation is appropriate; if it is not, then a mixed acid-base disorder exists.

2. Etiologies. Respiratory alkalosis is caused by **alveolar hyperventilation**, and is the most common acid-base

Table 4-7. Differential diagnosis of respiratory acidosis

Mechanism	Examples
Central hypoventilation	Ischemic brain injury
	Cerebral trauma
	Brain tumor
	Drugs (e.g., narcotics, general anesthesia)
	Central sleep apnea
Mechanical hypoventilation	Muscular dystrophy
	Kyphoscoliosis
	Myasthenia gravis
	Guillain–Barré syndrome
	Pneumothorax
	Pneumonia
	Reactive airway disease
	Pulmonary fibrosis (COPD)
	Severe pulmonary edema
	Smoke inhalation
	Airway obstruction

COPD, Chronic obstructive pulmonary disease.

Table 4-8. Differential diagnosis of respiratory alkalosis

Anxiety, hysteria
Pain
Fever
Gram-negative sepsis
Salicylate intoxication
CNS diseases: subarachnoid hemorrhage, cerebrovascular accident,
    trauma, infection, tumor
Intrathoracic processes: CHF, pneumonitis, asthma, pulmonary
    fibrosis, pulmonary embolus
Hypoxemia
Hepatic failure
Pregnancy
Mechanical hyperventilation

CHF, congestive heart failure; CNS, central nervous system.

disorder in patients with serious illnesses. The differential
diagnosis is shown in Table 4-8.

E. Mixed acid-base disturbances. These are defined as
**concurrence of two or three simple acid-base distur-
bances**; a single disturbance with compensation is not considered a mixed disturbance. A **triple acid-base disorder** occurs
when a respiratory disturbance is superimposed on a combined
metabolic acidosis and metabolic alkalosis. These circumstances
must be evaluated in conjunction with clinical evaluation and
other laboratory investigations. Although compensation cannot
overcorrect the [H+], a mixed disturbance can lead to relatively
normal findings in all acid-base laboratory values. Examples of
mixed disorders are shown in Table 4-9.

Table 4-9. Examples of mixed acid-base disorders

Disturbances	Examples
Metabolic acidosis with metabolic alkalosis	Vomiting with diarrhea
Metabolic acidosis with respiratory alkalosis	Salicylate intoxication Gram-negative bacteremia
Respiratory acidosis with metabolic acidosis	Acute pulmonary edema Cardiopulmonary arrest
Respiratory alkalosis with metabolic alkalosis	Hepatic failure with hyper-ventilation, plus diuretics
High anion gap (AG) metabolic acidosis with normal AG metabolic acidosis	Diarrhea complicated by lactic acidosis Ethylene glycol poisoning with lactic acidosis

BIBLIOGRAPHY

Faber MD, Kupin WL, Heilig CW, Narins RG. Common fluid-electrolyte and acid-base problems in the intensive care unit: selected issues. *Semin Nephrol* 1994;14(1):8–22.

Halperin ML, Goldstein MB. *Fluid, electrolyte, and acid-base physiology*, 3rd ed. Toronto: WB Saunders, 1999.

Narins RG. Diagnostic insights from the anion gap-bicarbonate relationship. *Nephrol Dial Transplant* 1999;14(4):1018.

Riley LJ Jr, Ilson BE, Narins RG. Acute metabolic acid-base disorders. *Crit Care Clin* 1987;3(4):699–724.

Rose BD. *Clinical physiology of acid-base and electrolyte disorders*, 4th ed. New York: McGraw-Hill, 1994.

Uribarri J, Oh MS, Carroll HJ. D-lactic acidosis. A review of clinical presentation, biochemical features, and pathophysiologic mechanisms. *Medicine* 1998;77(2):73–82.

Electrolytes and Fluid Balance

Thomas D. Batiuk

I. **Definitions**
A. **Osmolality** is a measure of the ratio between particles and water.
B. **Intracellular space (IC)** refers to the space inside cells.
C. **Extracellular space (EC)** refers to the space outside of cells. This can be further divided into the ***intravascular*** space, which represents the effective circulatory space, and the ***interstitial*** space, which lies between cells, but outside of the vascular space.

II. **Basic science review**
A. **Distribution of water**. Body mass is 50% to 60% water. Of water, 60% is located in the IC space, and 40% is located in the EC space. As the proportion of muscle mass declines (e.g., with age), so does body water. Water crosses membranes rapidly to achieve equal osmolality in all compartments. Therefore, **the distribution of body water is determined by osmotic forces**.
B. **Osmoles** are particles that can be classified as "ineffective" or as "effective." **Ineffective osmoles** are small particles that move freely between compartments (e.g., urea and alcohol) and have equal concentrations in the different compartments. Although they contribute to overall osmolality, they do not cause a movement of water. **Effective osmoles**, which are particles that are not equally distributed among compartments, cause movements of water and, hence, determine the volume of a space or compartment.

The **chief IC cation is potassium (K^+)**. K^+ is held in cells by macromolecular anions and by active transport of K^+ into cells, and it **controls the IC volume**. The chief IC anions are phosphates.

The **chief EC cation is sodium (Na^+)**; Na^+ salts account for 90% of EC osmolality, and they **control the EC volume**. The chief EC anion is Cl^-. EC fluid consists of intravascular (plasma) fluid and interstitial fluid. Accumulation of interstitial fluid can be manifested clinically as edema, ascites, or pleural effusion.
C. **Regulation of water and sodium**. The kidney is the main control center for regulation of both water and sodium. Weight changes in a patient are useful crude overall indicators of salt and water balance.

1. **Water regulation**. Plasma osmolality is very important because it has a large impact on the intracellular volume. The controls for osmolality are very sensitive, responding to changes as small as 1% to 2%. Indeed, the usual osmolality of blood is 280–295 mOsm/kg H_2O, whereas urine osmolality can vary from 40–1,200 mOsm/kg H_2O. **Plasma osmolality is directly affected by the amount of water excreted through the kidneys, and is regulated by antidiuretic hormone (ADH).**

   2. **Sodium regulation**. Because Na^+ salts represent >90% of EC osmoles, control of Na^+ content is an important way to regulate EC fluid volume. **The sodium content in the body is regulated by the kidney, which is primarily influenced by the "effective" EC volume**. Multiple factors control this process. **Aldosterone** is critically important; other factors include various hormones, arterial and venous sensors, and so on. Decreases in the effective EC volume (e.g., dehydration, hemorrhage) cause the kidney to reabsorb more Na^+ (a spot urine $[Na^+]$ will be <10 mEq/L), which in turn will increase the EC volume. Decreases in the *effective* EC volume also occur in common edematous states such as congestive heart failure, advanced liver disease, or nephrotic syndrome; despite the obvious total body Na^+ excess, the vasculature still senses an intravascular volume deficit. In contrast, diuretics prevent renal reabsorption of Na^+, which leads to osmotic losses of water (a spot urine $[Na^+]$ is often >20).

III.   Serum sodium
  A.   Basic review. Serum Na^+ is the primary circulating cation. Because (a) Na^+ is restricted primarily to the extracellular space and (b) water moves to osmotic equilibrium across cell membranes, the *content* of Na^+ determines the EC volume. Because sodium is actively pumped out of cells, the concentration of Na^+ is a reflection of IC volume. **Overall body water content must be established in a careful, targeted physical examination** when assessing both hypo- and hypernatremic states. For example, patients who are hypovolemic may be hypo- or hypernatremic depending on whether free water losses are relatively less or relatively more than sodium losses, respectively.
  B.   Hypernatremia. Causes of hypernatremia are shown in Table 4-10.
  C.   Hyponatremia. In cases of hyponatremia, it is important to **first rule out hyperglycemia, hyperproteinemia, and hyperlipidemia**. Each will reduce the measured plasma $[Na^+]$. In cases of hyperglycemia, $[Na^+]$ decreases by 1.5–2.0 mEq/L for every 100 mg/dL increase in blood glucose. Causes of true hyponatremia are shown in Table 4-11.
  D.   Urinary sodium measurements may be helpful in some circumstances.
     1. **"Spot" $[Na^+]$ can be useful in the evaluation of the effective EC volume**, and also in evaluating causes of acute oliguria. Spot $[Na^+]$ is decreased as a response to a decreased effective EC volume.
     2. **Fractional excretion of sodium (FE_{Na}^+) or urea (FE_{urea})**: these tests can be useful in the evaluation of acute oliguria.
        a.   Decreased renal perfusion (e.g., shock): FE_{Na}^+<1% [except in glycosuria, some preexisting renal diseases, and in some cases of very early acute tubular necrosis (ATN)]; FE_{urea} **<35** (FE_{urea} is more reliable than FE_{Na}^+ if the patient has been on diuretics).
        b.   Acute renal damage (e.g., ATN): FE_{Na}^+ **>2%**
IV.   Serum potassium
  A.   Basic review. Potassium is important for the regulation of intracellular processes such as protein and glyco-

Table 4-10.   Causes of hypernatremia

Clinical Hydration Status	Possible Causes
Hypovolemic patient –Hypotension, tachycardia, poor skin turgor	Renal losses: diuretics, glycosuria, partial urinary obstruction, renal failure Adrenal insufficiency Gastrointestinal losses Skin losses: burns, sweating Pulmonary losses: hyperventilation
Euvolemic patient –Normal blood pressure, pulse, skin turgor, no edema	Diabetes insipidus: central, nephrogenic Skin losses Iatrogenic
Hypervolemic patient –Edema	Iatrogenic Mineralocorticoid excess: aldosteronism, steroid therapy, Cushing's syndrome, adrenal hyperplasia

Table 4-11.   Causes of hyponatremia

Clinical Hydration Status	Possible Causes
Hypovolemic patient –Hypotension, tachycardia, poor skin turgor	Gastrointestinal losses: vomiting, diarrhea Renal losses: diuretics, renal disease, partial urinary tract obstruction, salt-wasting nephropathy, hypoaldosteronism Skin losses: burns, sweating Pulmonary losses: hyperventilation Third space losses: after surgery or trauma
Euvolemic patient –Normal blood pressure, pulse, skin turgor, no edema	Water intoxication Syndrome of inappropriate ADH (SIADH): postoperative pulmonary pathology, malignancy, brain injury, trauma, drugs Renal failure Adrenal insufficiency Hypothyroidism
Hypervolemic patient –Edema	Congestive heart failure Hepatic failure Nephrotic syndrome

ADH, antidiuretic hormone.

gen metabolism. In addition, intracellular K^+ is crucial for the maintenance of the normal resting membrane potential across cell membranes, which is critical to the normal electrical functions of neurons and muscle cells. **Ninety-eight percent of total body K^+ is IC**. This high IC:EC K^+ ratio is maintained by the Na^+/K^+-ATPase pump present in all cells. This pump is influenced by hormones (thyroxine, catecholamines, insulin) and the total K^+ balance. In addition, the IC:EC K^+ ratio can be influenced by exercise, acid-base disorders, and tissue injury. Skeletal muscles release K^+ into the EC in response to exercise. In cases of metabolic acidosis, hydrogen ions (H^+) are buffered by intracellular phosphates and macromolecules. To maintain electroneutrality, K^+ often exits cells in exchange for entering H^+. Finally, any cause of tissue injury or death will result in release of significant K^+ into the EC space. **The kidney is the primary site of overall K^+ regulation**. Renal K^+ excretion is significantly increased by aldosterone.

B. Hyperkalemia. Causes of hyperkalemia are shown in Table 4-12

C. Hypokalemia. Causes of hypokalemia are shown in Table 4-13.

Table 4-12. Causes of hyperkalemia

Mechanism	Examples
"Pseudohyperkalemia"	Blood leukocytosis (>500,000/mm³)
	Blood thrombocytosis (>750,000/mm³)
	Poor venipuncture technique (e.g., use of a small gauge needle, tourniquet ischemia)
	Red blood cell lysis after collection
Redistribution out of cells or excess intake	Acidosis
	Tissue damage: crush injury, hemolysis
	Insulin deficiency
	Drugs: β-blockers, digoxin, succinyl-choline
	Periodic paralysis
	K^+ administration: diet (watch for salt substitutes), recent blood transfusions
Impaired renal excretion	Acute renal failure (especially with oligo- or anuria)
	Advanced chronic renal insufficiency
	Some renal tubular disorders
	Adrenal insufficiency, hypoaldosteronism
	Drugs: spironolactone, triampterene, amiloride, ACE inhibitors, heparin, tacrolimus

ACE, angiotension-converting enzyme.

Table 4-13.   Causes of hypokalemia

Mechanism	Examples
Nonrenal potassium loss	
–Gastrointestinal	Vomiting, diarrhea
	Gastric or biliary suction
	Adenoma or carcinoma of colon
	Zollinger–Ellison syndrome
	Chronic laxative use/abuse
	Uretero-colonic diversion/fistula
–Skin	Excessive sweating
	Burns/wounds
–Cellular shifts	Alkalosis
	Insulin excess
	β-agonists
	Vitamin B_{12}/folate therapy of mega-loblastic anemia
Renal potassium loss	
–Conditions with metabolic acidosis	Renal tubular acidosis
	Diuretic phase following ATN or relief of urinary obstruction
	Chronic pyelonephritis
	Diabetic ketoacidosis
–Conditions with metabolic alkalosis	Diuretics
	Mineralocorticoid excess: (e.g., iatrogenic, tumors, adrenal hyperplasia, exogenous glucocorticoids)
	Licorice excess
	Barter's syndrome
	Drugs: amphotericin B, lithium, gentamicin, carbenicillin

ATN, acute tubular necrosis.

V.   Serum calcium

A.   Basic review. Calcium (Ca^{++}) is of critical importance in normal muscle physiology as well as in bone architecture. Of serum Ca^{++}, 50% is ionized, 40% to 45% is bound to albumin, and 5% to 10% is bound to other anions. **Only the ionized fraction is physiologically active. Vitamin D** enhances gastrointestinal (GI) absorption of dietary Ca^{++}; **parathyroid hormone (PTH), phosphorus**, and vitamin D enhance Ca^{++} reabsorption from bone; PTH enhances renal reabsorption of filtered Ca^{++}.

B.   Hypercalcemia. Causes of hypercalcemia are listed in Table 4-14. Most cases of hypercalcemia are caused by either **hyperparathyroidism** or **malignancy**. Calcium levels >20 mEq/L are almost always associated with **myeloma**.

C.   Hypocalcemia. Causes of hypocalcemia are listed in Table 4-15. When total calcium is low, ionized calcium should be measured. **If total calcium is low, but ionized calcium is normal, diseases causing hypoalbuminemia should be**

Table 4-14.   Causes of hypercalcemia

Mechanism	Examples
Altered bone metabolism	Malignancy Hyperparathyroidism Immobilization Hyperthyroidism Adrenal insufficiency Vitamin A intoxication Aluminum toxicity
Increased intestinal absorption	Hyperparathyroidism Granulomatous diseases: sarcoidosis, histoplasmosis, tuberculosis, coccidiodomycosis Vitamin A or D intoxication Milk-alkali syndrome
Decreased removal from plasma	Thiazide diuretics Adrenal insufficiency Phosphate depletion

Table 4-15.   Causes of hypocalcemia

Serum iPTH	Examples
Low (relative hypoparathyroidism)	Surgical Radiation to neck Infiltrating disorders: amyloid, malignancy Hypomagnesemia Renal wasting (e.g., gentamicin or cis-platin therapy) "Bone hunger" following parathyroidectomy
Elevated	Hyperphosphatemia: rhabdomyolysis, renal failure, cancer chemotherapy Vitamin D deficiency: malabsorption, dietary deficiency, liver disease Pseudohypoparathyroidism Pancreatitis Drugs, gentamicin, colchicine, cis-platin, dilantin, phenobarbital

iPTH, intact parathyroid hormone.

sought. The most common causes of hypoalbuminemia are the nephrotic syndrome and chronic liver failure. Hypocalcemia (ionized calcium) can be associated with **tetany** which, if severe, can be fatal.

VI. Serum phosphorus

A. Basic review. As with potassium, **the bulk of body phosphorus is IC**, with 85% of the total body content in bone and 10% in muscle. Overall phosphorus balance is dependent on GI absorption, which varies widely and is under relatively little control, and renal excretion, which is tightly controlled by many hormones, the most important of which is **PTH**.

B. Hyperphosphatemia. Causes of hyperphosphatemia are shown in Table 4-16.

C. Hypophosphatemia. Causes of hypophosphatemia are shown in Table 4-17. Alkalosis, glucose, and insulin can cause phosphorus to shift from the EC space into the IC space. Thus, it should be noted that therapy of **diabetic ketoacidosis (DKA) almost always causes a precipitous fall in serum phosphorus**. This should be anticipated, and replacement therapy initiated early as severe hypophosphatemia (<1.0 mEq/L) can lead to muscle weakness (with effects on respiration) and rhabdomyolysis.

VII. Serum magnesium

A. Basic review. Unlike the other electrolytes discussed above, magnesium (Mg^{++}) is **not hormonally controlled**. PTH can affect Mg^{++} movement, but concomitant high Ca^{++} levels frequently oppose the effects of PTH. Fluctuations in Mg^{++} are further modulated by movement into and out of bones and soft tissues. Unlike Ca^{++}, only a small amount of Mg^{++} binds to albumin, making changes in serum albumin relatively unimportant in analyzing Mg^{++} concentrations. It is important to **monitor Mg^{++} in patients with renal failure or GI disorders**.

Table 4-16.   Causes of hyperphosphatemia

Mechanism	Examples
Increased renal absorption	Hypoparathyroidism: primary, secondary, "pseudo" Acute or chronic renal failure Sickle cell anemia Acromegaly
Increased gastrointestinal absorption	Enemas, laxatives Vitamin D toxicity Granulomatous diseases (e.g., sarcoid)
Release from intracellular compartment	Bone disease: healing fracture, Paget's disease, multiple myeloma Rhabdomyolysis Hemolysis Chemotherapy Milk-alkali syndrome

Table 4-17.   Causes of hypophosphatemia

Mechanism	Examples
Renal loss	Diuretics
	Hypokalemia, hypomagnesemia
	Acute gout
	Hyperparathyroidism
	Renal tubular disorders: Fanconi's syndrome
Decreased intestinal absorption	Malabsorption
	Vitamin D deficiency
	Malnutrition, vomiting, diarrhea
	Phosphate-binding medications
Intracellular shift	Acidosis (especially DKA)
	Alcoholism
	Nutritional recovery syndrome
	Drugs: insulin, anabolic steroids, androgens, epinephrine, glucagon
	Prolonged hypothermia: open heart surgery

DKA, diabetic ketoacidosis.

B.   Hypermagnesemia. In hypermagnesemic states, renal excretion rises; indeed, hypermagnesemia is **very uncommon in patients with normal renal function**. Causes of high Mg^{++} are shown in Table 4-18.

C.   Hypomagnesemia. In hypomagnesemic states, intestinal absorption increases. Causes of low Mg^{++} are shown in Table 4-19. In addition, note that low Mg^{++} can be a cause of urinary K^+ losses; hypomagnesemia is found in up to 40% of hypokalemic patients. Low Mg^+ can also impair Ca^{++} absorption. Thus, **a low serum K^+ and low serum Ca^{++} strongly suggest a low serum Mg^{++}.**

Table 4-18.   Causes of hypermagnesemia

Mechanism	Examples
Normal renal function	Mg^{++} poisoning
	Laxative and cathartic abuse
	Parenteral nutrition
	Mg^{++} therapy for eclampsia
Reduced renal function	
–Decreased Mg^{++} clearance	Hyperparathyroidism
	Adrenal insufficiency
	Hypothyroidism
–Increased Mg^{++} intake	Antacids
	Enemas

Table 4-19.   Causes of hypomagnesemia

Mechanism	Examples
Gastrointestinal disease	Increased loss: inflammatory bowel disease, carcinoma, laxative abuse Decreased absorption: sprue, enteric fistulas, abdominal radiation
Renal disease	Chronic GN, chronic pyelonephritis, recovery phase of ATN, drugs (diuretics, aminoglycosides, cyclosporine), renal tubular acidosis
Endocrine	Hyperthyroidism, hyperparathyroidism, hypoparathyroidism, diabetes mellitus
Nutritional	Hyperalimentation, starvation, alcoholism
Other	Severe burns, acute pancreatitis, eclampsia, lytic bone tumors

ATN, acute tubular necrosis; GN, glomerulonephritis.

BIBLIOGRAPHY

Faber MD, Kupin WL, Heilig CW, Narins RG. Common fluid-electrolyte and acid-base problems in the intensive care unit: selected issues. *Semin Nephrol* 1994;14(1):8–22.

Halperin ML, Goldstein MB. *Fluid, electrolyte, and acid-base physiology*, 3rd ed. Toronto: WB Saunders, 1999.

Rose BD. *Clinical physiology of acid-base and electrolyte disorders*, 4th ed. New York: McGraw-Hill, 1994.

Renal Function Tests

Martin C. Gregory

I.   Introduction. Reduced to its simplest form, **the kidney functions by a process of copious, nonselective, glomerular filtration, which is followed by tubular reabsorption of an almost equal quantity of salt and water and selective reabsorption of other solutes.** Common tests of renal function can be grouped into tests of glomerular filtration, tests of glomerular permeability (tests for proteinuria), and tests of tubular functions.

II.   Tests of glomerular filtration. The glomerular filtration rate (GFR), which is commonly used as a global measure of renal function, is normally about **125 mL/min**. Glomerular filtration can be assessed by (a) steady-state levels of substances produced in the body and eliminated by glomerular filtration; (b) the rate of disappearance of administered substances that are eliminated by glomerular filtration, and (c) measurement of the clearance of suitable markers.

A.   Steady-state levels of metabolites eliminated by the kidney. Several waste products are produced by the body at nearly a constant rate and are removed mainly by the kidneys. These include **urea, creatinine, and β_2-microglobulin. As renal function declines steadily, the concentration of each of these metabolites rises at an increasingly rapid rate**—in hyperbolic fashion. For example, a fall in GFR from 100 to 75 mL/min can cause serum creatinine to rise from 1.0 to 1.33, whereas a fall to 50 mL/min causes the creatinine to rise to 2.0. The second loss of 25 mL/min in GFR caused twice the rise in serum creatinine as did the first loss. The important clinical conclusion is that **creatinine, urea, and β_2-microglobulin are all relatively insensitive to falls in GFR, and their levels may fail to reveal a 25% to 50% loss of renal function**. A second important point is that these **markers may be misleading if renal function is not in steady-state**. For example, renal function could instantaneously fall to zero and blood urea nitrogen (BUN) and creatinine would initially not budge.

1.   Urea is an end product of protein metabolism, and its production rate depends on dietary protein intake and the balance of protein anabolism and catabolism. For historical reasons, plasma urea is expressed as **blood urea nitrogen (BUN)**. Urea is freely filtered at the glomerulus (i.e., it enters the glomerular filtrate in the same concentration as it is in the plasma), but ~50% is reabsorbed during passage along the nephron. The proportion that is reabsorbed is greater if the urine flow rate is low (i.e., oliguria) or if urea is highly concentrated in the tubular urine.

   a.   Factors that can increase BUN
     (1)   Reduced renal function
     (2)   Renal underperfusion (e.g., **hypovolemia**) will cause an elevation of BUN disproportionate to the eleva-

tion of creatinine. Both BUN and creatinine are increased because of reduced GFR, but BUN is further increased because of enhanced tubular reabsorption of urea during oliguria.

  (3)   Increased dietary protein intake
  (4)   Gastrointestinal bleeding (which can lead to erythrocyte protein breakdown and absorption)
  (5)   Hypercatabolism (e.g., caused by sepsis, steroids, or cytotoxic drugs)
  (6)   Reduced anabolism (e.g., caused by tetracycline)

 b. **Factors that can reduce BUN**
  (1)   Reduced dietary protein intake
  (2)   Anabolism during recovery from illness
  (3)   Severe liver disease that impairs urea production

2. **Creatinine is produced by hydrolysis of creatine.** Creatine phosphate is an important energy substrate stored in muscle, and the rate of creatinine production depends on the quantity of creatine released which, in turn, is **proportional to muscle mass**. The production rate of creatinine is more constant than that of urea. It does not undergo significant tubular reabsorption; thus, in general, it is a better marker of renal function. Still, it has important limitations.

 a. **Factors that can increase serum creatinine**
  (1)   Reduced renal function
  (2)   Urinary tract obstruction
  (3)   Increased total muscle mass (e.g., in athletes)
  (4)   Muscle trauma or rhabdomyolysis. In such cases, colossal quantities of creatine are released, and serum creatinine can increase disproportionately to the degree of renal insufficiency or to the rise in BUN.
  (5)   Drugs. Cimetidine, trimethoprim, triamterene, amiloride, and probenecid can block tubular secretion of creatinine. In a patient with moderately or severely impaired renal function, the serum creatinine will rise within a day or two of starting these drugs. This does not indicate nephrotoxicity.

 b. **Factors that can decrease serum creatinine**
  (1)   Scant muscle mass (e.g., in **frail elderly persons** and **children**). These individuals produce little creatinine. Serum creatinine may be normal or low despite substantial renal dysfunction.
  (2)   Some muscular dystrophies. In latter stages of some muscular dystrophies, creatinine production decreases because of decreased total body muscle mass.

 c. **Additional limitations of creatinine as a marker of glomerular filtration**
  (1)   Creatinine is an imperfect marker of glomerular filtration because there is some tubular secretion, normally amounting to 10% to 20% of total creatinine excreted. In chronic renal disease, the proportion of creatinine excreted by tubular secretion rises and can reach 40%, which can lead to an underestimation of renal dysfunction.

(2)   Some extrarenal elimination of creatinine occurs through the action of creatininases of the intestinal flora. This becomes disproportionately more important as renal function declines.

d.   **Creatinine assays and their problems**. Creatinine can be measured in several ways. Each is subject to errors that can be clinically important. The most common assay uses alkaline picrate (Jaffe reaction).

(1)   **Alkaline picrate method**. Glucose, protein, acetoacetate, pyruvate, uric acid, fructose, and ascorbic acid can all cause color reactions that falsely elevate the result. Several cephalosporins, notably cefazolin and cefoxitin, will do the same.

(2)   The **kinetic or autoanalyzer assay** is less affected by interfering substances, but bilirubin in concentrations above 5 mg/dL will decrease the creatinine by 0.1 to 0.5 mg/dL. This is one of the reasons why serum creatinine can be absurdly low and creatinine clearance ridiculously high in patients with severe liver disease and renal dysfunction.

(3)   **The creatinine imidohydrolase (Ektachem) method** is generally very accurate, but is affected by flucytosine and severe hyperglycemia.

3. β_2**-microglobulin is a constant component of the HLA class I antigen**. In health, it is produced at a constant rate by B lymphocytes, freely filtered at the glomerulus and almost completely reabsorbed and metabolized by proximal tubular cells. **In the absence of neoplastic or immune conditions that elevate production, it is a more precise and reproducible measure of renal function than BUN or creatinine**. It has found some favor in Europe, but has not been widely used in the United States on grounds of cost and the confusing elevations seen in patients whose production is increased by lymphatic malignancies, myeloma, or lupus.

B.   **Plasma disappearance methods. After injection of a substance that is normally removed by glomerular filtration, a period of equilibration occurs, and then the plasma concentration declines in an exponential fashion. The higher the GFR, the more rapidly the plasma concentration declines.** It is most convenient to use a radioactive substance such as ^{51}Cr–EDTA, ^{131}I–iothalamate, or MAG-3, (^{99m}Tc–mercaptoacetyltriglycine). If GFR exceeds about 75 mL/min, it can be estimated by means of a single plasma sample taken at a defined time interval after injection. At lower GFRs, single sample methods have unacceptable errors, and a method using several plasma samples to estimate rate of decay should be used. These isotopic methods offer the advantages of avoiding the analytic problems associated with creatinine measurement as well as the inconvenience and errors in urine collection. Disadvantages include exposure to radiation, cost, and the need to schedule the test. Measurement of GFR can advantageously be combined with imaging procedures.

C.   **Clearance measurements**

1.   **General principles**. For any substance eliminated only by the kidneys, conceive of a volume (C) of plasma containing

the substance in concentration P that is completely emptied or "cleared" of the substance each minute. The quantity of the substance in volume C equals C • P.

If the kidney does not destroy or create the substance being measured, then the quantity removed from the blood (C • P) equals the amount (U • V) that reaches the urine, which contains the substance in concentration U at a flow rate of V mL/min.

$$C • P = U • V, \text{ or}$$
$$C = U • V/P$$

If the substance is freely filtered at the glomerulus and is neither secreted nor reabsorbed by the renal tubule, then the amount leaving the blood via the kidneys equals the amount crossing the glomerular capillary wall which, in turn, equals the amount entering the urine each minute.

$$C • P = GFR • P = U • V, \text{ or}$$
$$\textbf{C = GFR = U • V/P}$$

In this case, the clearance is the same as the GFR. For research purposes, **inulin** can be infused at a constant rate to measure the GFR. For clinical purposes, **endogenous creatinine** is used for this purpose.

   2.   **Limitations of creatinine clearance**
      a.   **Analytic problems in measuring serum creatinine (see above) also apply to creatinine clearance**. When creatinine clearance is nearly normal, errors from overestimation of serum creatinine by the Jaffe method approximately balance the errors from tubular secretion of creatinine. As creatinine clearance falls, the analytic errors in serum creatinine determination become proportionately less and the errors from creatinine secretion proportionately greater. The net result is that **with moderate or severe renal failure, creatinine clearance substantially overestimates GFR.**
      b.   **For patients nearing end-stage renal failure, the arithmetic mean of urea and creatinine clearance gives a value that is fairly close to the true GFR.**
      c.   Measuring creatinine clearance by means of a 24-hour urine sample **requires accurate collection of urine**, which frequently introduces errors.

III.   **Tests for proteinuria**
   A.   **General principles**. In health, a gram or two a day of protein traverses the glomerular capillary wall, and nearly all of this is reabsorbed and catabolized by proximal tubular cells. **Normal proteinuria does not exceed 150 mg/d**. In addition to that crossing the glomerular capillary wall, protein can be added during passage down the nephron, or after urine has left the kidney. Normally, only small quantities of Tamm–Horsfall protein are added in the distal tubule and it is extremely rare for this quantity to be significantly increased. Inflammation or tumors in the lower urinary tract can cause the addition of modest quantities of protein. **For practical purposes, all protein entering the urine has crossed the glomerular capillary wall.**

B. Causes of proteinuria. Proteinuria can be increased by three mechanisms.

   1. Increased glomerular permeability. Glomerular disease of many types can cause proteinuria. The proteinuria can be of any degree, and at times exceeds **3.5 g/d** (nephrotic range proteinuria).

   2. Overflow proteinuria. Patients with **multiple myeloma** can excrete up to several grams a day of **Bence Jones protein**.

   3. Tubular proteinuria. If the tubules fail to reabsorb the protein that normally crosses the glomerular capillary wall, **up to 1.5 g/d** of mostly low molecular weight protein can be excreted.

   4. Microalbuminuria is the excretion of small but nevertheless pathologic quantities of **albumin** even though the total urine protein is not elevated (**dipstick is negative**). These small quantities of albumin are usually measured by an immunochemical method. Although the early stage of any renal disease that can cause proteinuria can result in microalbuminuria, detection of **microalbuminuria is important as the first sign of diabetic nephropathy.**

C. Analytic methods for proteinuria

   1. Dipsticks depend on the protein error of indicators (see chapter 4.4, *Urinalysis*). False-negative results occur in very dilute urine. Tubular proteinuria and overflow proteinuria (low molecular weight proteins) may also escape detection. False-positive results can occur with highly concentrated urine, with very alkaline urine, with phenazopyridine (Pyridium), or if the collection container is contaminated with antiseptic.

   2. Turbidometric methods can be used as semiquantitative tube tests or as common quantitative laboratory tests. Turbidometric methods give false-negative results if the urine is dilute or highly alkaline. They can give false-positive tests with concentrated urine, with large doses of penicillins or cephalosporins, with radiographic contrast media, or with metabolites of sulfisoxazole (Gantrisin).

   3. Electrophoresis is a more specific and accurate method for measuring protein, particularly Bence Jones protein. Electrophoresis is also useful as a measure of selectivity of proteinuria in glomerular disease. **Selective proteinuria**, which means excretion principally of **albumin**, is typically found in **minimal change nephrotic syndrome. Nonselective proteinuria**—excretion of **all serum proteins**—typically indicates a **glomerular lesion more severe than minimal change disease.**

D. Expression of results. Most commonly, protein excretion is expressed as milligrams in a 24-hour specimen. **The normal value is <150 mg/24 hours. Values between 150 and 2,000 mg can represent glomerular, tubular, or overflow proteinuria. Values above 2,000 mg indicate glomerular or overflow proteinuria. Excretion of >3,500 mg/1.73 m^2 occurs in the nephrotic syndrome.**

   To avoid the inconvenience of collecting a 24-hour urine sample, protein and creatinine can be measured on a random urine sample and proteinuria expressed as a protein:creatinine ratio. **Normal excretion is <0.2 mg protein/mg creatinine; light proteinuria is 0.2–2; nephrotic range proteinuria is above 2.**

IV.   Tests of tubular function

A.   General principles. Tests of tubular function can be divided into (a) tests that detect a substance that should normally be absent (or nearly absent) from the urine; (b) and tests that show an inappropriate quantity of a normal constituent. The first type of test is exemplified by tests for **glucose, β_2-microglobulin**, and **amino acids**, which are normally almost completely removed from the urine by the proximal tubule. **Appreciable quantities of these substances indicate proximal tubular dysfunction**. The **second type of test quantitates substances that are normal urine constituents** [e.g., **sodium, hydrogen ion** (H^+)], or total solute concentration (**osmolality**). These tests are most commonly **used to assess distal tubular function**. In most circumstances, it is necessary to load or stress the kidney to interpret the result of a test that quantitates a normal urinary constituent.

When interpreting tests of tubular function, **it is particularly important to consider the physiologic state of the patient, and to compare what the kidney is doing in this circumstance with what would be expected of a normally functioning kidney**. This concept of the appropriateness of renal response is more helpful than trying to compare the result achieved with a "normal" value.

B.   Examples of a few particular tubular function tests

1.   Long ammonium chloride test (used to evaluate distal tubular ability to acidify urine). The patient is given 0.1 g/kg body weight of ammonium chloride daily for 3 days. The urine is then promptly examined for pH using a pH meter. **A normal kidney will reduce urine pH to 5.4 or lower, but this will not be achieved in a patient with distal renal tubular acidosis**. Blood should be obtained for blood gases or venous bicarbonate to prove that a systemic acidosis was achieved.

2.   Urinary concentrating test (used to evaluate distal tubular ability to concentrate urine). The patient is deprived of water for 14 hours and then given an injection of vasopressin. In a patient with a normally functioning kidney, urine volumes will drop progressively and urine osmolality will rise to over 800 mOsm/kg. A patient with **central diabetes insipidus** will not concentrate urine to this degree until the injection of vasopressin is given. A patient with **nephrogenic diabetes insipidus** will concentrate the urine neither after water deprivation nor after vasopressin injection. Care must be taken to supervise the test and to avoid dangerous volume depletion in patients who have a urinary concentrating defect.

3.   Fractional excretion of sodium (FE_{Na^+}). In a patient with acute oliguria, FE_{Na^+} <1% implies renal underperfusion, and FE_{Na^+} >3% implies intrinsic renal damage,

most commonly acute tubular necrosis. FE_{Na^+} is calculated from a simultaneous serum and random urine sample, by dividing the ratio of urine to serum sodium by the ratio of urine to serum creatinine concentration, and then multiplying the result by 100%.

4. Fractional excretion of urea (FE_{Urea}). This is calculated in the same way as FE_{Na^+}. It is generally **<25% in a patient with acute oliguria from renal underperfusion, and >35% in a patient with acute oliguria from acute tubular necrosis**.

Urinalysis

Martin C. Gregory

I. Introduction. Urine is a liquid biopsy, obtained without pain or cost to the patient, that conveys a wealth of diagnostic information (whence the colloquial term "liquid gold"). Indeed, urine is the principal conduit of information from a sick kidney to the physician.

II. Specimen collection. The results of urinalysis are only as good as the specimen collected. The ideal specimen is one that contains the items of interest in greatest concentration with the smallest possible quantity of contaminating material. Generally, this means **a first morning specimen collected as a midstream, clean-catch sample.** The most important aspects of collecting a midstream urine specimen are to expose the urethral meatus and to collect the sample from the midportion of an uninterrupted stream of urine. Urine should be examined as promptly as possible after collection.

III. Macroscopic examination
A. Volume. Wide variation exists in normal 24-hour urine output.
1. Polyuria refers to urine output **>2,500 mL/24 hours**. Among the common causes of polyuria are excessive water intake, diuretics, diabetes insipidus, and chronic renal diseases.
2. Oliguria refers to urine output **<400 mL/24 hours**. **Anuria** refers to **<100 mL/24 hours.** Among the common causes of oliguria are dehydration, urinary tract obstruction, shock, renal tubular necrosis, and acute glomerulonephritis.
B. Color. Normal urine color varies from very pale to dark yellow. Red or brown urine may signify the presence of blood, hemoglobin, myoglobin, or dyes present in food or drugs. Other colors most commonly come from drugs (Table 4-20).
C. Clarity. Turbidity represents undissolved solid material: cells, casts, crystals, bacteria, or amorphous debris. Dissolved substances do not make the urine turbid. Thus protein, even at high concentrations, does not alter the urine clarity.
D. Odor. Infected urine can have a strong odor of ammonia or fish. Some foods can cause a variety of odors (e.g., asparagus). Inherited metabolic disorders (e.g., maple syrup disease) can cause characteristic odors.
E. Measurement of pH. Urine pH is usually between **5.0 and 6.5**; however, the range of normal can extend from 4.5 to 7.8. Among common causes of persistently acidic urine are normal health, respiratory or metabolic acidosis, and some metabolic disorders (e.g., phenylketonuria). Among the common causes of persistently alkaline urine are foods (e.g., excessive ingestion of soda crackers, various fruits and vegetables), urinary tract infection, excessive bicarbonate ingestion, and respiratory or metabolic alkalosis. Alkaline urine can also transiently occur after a large meal.

Table 4-20. Pigments, foodstuffs, and drugs that discolor the urine

Color	Disease or Pigment	Foodstuff	Drug
Red, pink, or orange	Blood Hemoglobin Myoglobin	Red beets Blackberries Food colorings	Phenolphthalein Phenytoin (Dilantin) Deferoxamine (Desferal) Anthracycline Antineoplastics [Doxorubicin (adriamycin, doxil) Daunorubicin (Cerubidine, daunoxomb)] Phenothiazines Rifampin (Rifadin) Phenazopyridine (Pyridium)
Blue or green	Biliverdin (obstructive jaundice) Indigo blue (blue diaper syndrome-intestinal tryptophan malabsorption) Pyocyanin (*Pseudomonas* contamination of diapers)	Food colorings	Anthraquinone laxatives in alkaline urine (cascara, senna) Methylene blue (Urised) Chlorophyll (Clorets) Intravenous cimetidine, promethazine, propofol (phenol preservative) Amitriptyline (Elavil) Flutamide (Eulexin) Methocarbamol[a] (Robaxin)

continued

Table 4-20. *Continued*

Color	Disease or Pigment	Foodstuff	Drug
Black or brown	Melanin[a] (advanced melanoma) Homogentisic acid[a] (alkaptonuria) Porphyrins[a] and PBG[a] (porphyrias) Hemoglobin (acute hemolytic anemia (e.g., malaria)	Rhubarb (in alkaline urine)	Anthraquinone laxatives in alkaline urine (cascara, senna) Iron dextran[a] Levodopa[a] Methocarbamol[a] (Robaxin) Methyldopa (Aldomet) Nitrofurantoin (Macrodantin) Metronidazole (Flagyl)

[a] Color may appear only on standing.

F. Solute concentration. Total urine solute concentration, which is most commonly assessed by **specific gravity (SG)**, is most practicably measured using a refractometer. SD is valuable in a few specific circumstances.

1. In a patient with acute oliguria, relatively high SG (>1.014) implies intact tubular function and suggests renal underperfusion as the cause of the oliguria, whereas isosthenuria (urine SG 1.008–1.012) suggests intrinsic renal damage, most likely caused by acute tubular necrosis.

2. SG can help assess the significance of minor abnormalities in the dipstick or microscopic urinalysis. A borderline increase in protein or cells may be normal if the SG is high. Proteinuria is probably pathologic if the protein concentration (in mg/dL) exceeds the last two figures of the SG (e.g., 30 mg/dL protein by dipstick may be normal if the SG is 1.030, but is likely abnormal at a lower SG).

3. Urine with a SG of <1.010 rapidly lyses red blood cells and dissolves casts, and warns of the possibility of false-negative microscopy findings.

G. Dipstick examination. Semiquantitative chemical analysis by dipstick is readily available, rapid, and informative. Dipsticks consist of an indicator and usually other reagents immobilized on a porous pad attached to a paper or plastic strip. The other reagents are usually enzymes that give specificity to the reaction, and are linked to production of a product that changes the color of the indicator. The color change can be assessed either by visual comparison with a scale, or by automated or semiautomated reflectometry. **Dipsticks degrade with time. Keep them cool, dry, and in a sealed container**. Use or discard them before their expiration date. For most dipstick reactions, **the time of incubation is critical**, and accurate timing is essential to obtain reliable results.

1. Protein

   a. Principle. The principle involved is the protein error of indicators. The color of a pH indicator will vary depending on the solution protein content, because of the net charge on the proteins.

   b. Interpretation. Common causes of proteinuria include **Bence Jones proteins**, Tamm–Horsfall proteins, and **glomerular disorders**. Glomerular disorders can cause **selective proteinuria** (excretion of albumin in minimal change disease) or **nonselective proteinuria** (excretion of protein of all sizes, such as in more serious forms of nephrotic syndrome).

   Strongly buffered alkaline urine can overcome the dipstick buffer and give a spuriously positive test for protein. **Small amounts of Bence Jones proteins may not be detected** by dipsticks (protein electrophoresis with immunofixation is the method of choice). Microalbuminuria (to evaluate early diabetic nephropathy) is best measured with specific immunochemical methods.

2. Glucose

   a. Principle. Double sequential enzyme analysis (uses glucose oxidase and peroxidase).

b. **Interpretation**. The most common causes of glucosuria are **pregnancy** and **diabetes mellitus**. Positive test results should be followed with serum glucose measurements and glucose tolerance tests, if clinically indicated. False-positive test results can occur if the dipsticks are inadvertently stored in an opened jar, or if chlorine or peroxide residues have contaminated the urine container. False-negative results can occur from the ingestion of vitamin C (large amounts), tetracycline, or L-dopa. Sugars such as galactose and fructose are not detected.

3.   Ketones

a. **Principle**. Ketone bodies, products of lipid metabolism, include β-**hydroxybutyric acid, acetoacetic acid, and acetone**. β-hydroxybutyric acid makes up the vast majority of the ketone bodies. **Dipsticks detect acetoacetic acid and acetone**, which react with nitroprusside and create a colored compound.

b. **Interpretation**. Among the common causes of ketonuria are **ketoacidosis** that occurs with **diabetes mellitis** and **alcoholism, fasting states** >18 hours, **high protein diets, high fat/low-carbohydrate diets**, liver damage, heavy exercise, cold exposure, metabolic disorders, febrile infectious disorders during childhood, and normal pregnancy (in some cases). False-positive results can occur from the use of L-dopa or phenolphthalein.

4.   Bilirubin and urobilinogen

a. **Principle. Unconjugated (indirect) bilirubin is the breakdown product of hemoglobin** metabolism by the reticuloendothelial system; it is insoluble in water and is **not excreted in the urine**. Unconjugated bilirubin is conjugated to glucuronic acid in the liver, becoming **conjugated (direct) bilirubin,** which is a water-soluble compound that **can be excreted in the urine and bile**. Conjugated bilirubin is **metabolized by intestinal bacteria to urobilinogen**, some of which is reabsorbed into the circulation and re-excreted in the bile and urine. In dipsticks, bilirubin reacts with diazo compounds to form a colored compound. Urobilinogen reacts with paradiethylaminobenzaldehyde to form a colored compound.

b. **Interpretation**. Increases in serum indirect bilirubin (e.g., from **hemolysis**) **can cause increased urinary urobilinogen, but urinary bilirubin will usually be absent**. Increases in serum direct bilirubin from **complete biliary obstruction can cause increased urinary bilirubin, but urinary urobilinogen will be absent**. Increases in serum direct bilirubin because of **liver injuries can cause increased urinary bilirubin as well as urobilinogen** (because of the liver's decreased ability to excrete it).

5.   Hemoglobin

a. **Principle**. The peroxidaselike activity of hemoglobin acts on a substrate to create a colored compound.

b. **Interpretation**. The most common cause of hemoglobinuria is **intravascular hemolysis**; the hemolysis must surpass the binding capacity of plasma proteins (e.g., haptoglobin) as well as the renal reabsorption threshold. **Hemoglobinuria must be differentiated from hematuria** (whole red blood cells in the urine that are seen in the sediment). Among the common causes of hematuria are calculi, menstrual contamination, urogenital carcinomas, infection, trauma, collagen-vascular diseases, some forms of glomerulonephritis, and high blood pressure. **If red blood cell casts are present, the red cells originated in the glomeruli.**

6. **Leukocyte esterase and nitrite**

   a. **Principle**. Leukocyte esterase reacts with indoxyl esters, which leads to the formation of indigo blue. Nitrate can be reduced to nitrite by many bacteria that are common causes of urinary tract infections, but the urine must be retained for several hours in the bladder for the reaction to have time to occur. Therefore, early morning first voids are the best samples.

   b. **Interpretation**. Leukocyte esterase and nitrite are used as **screens for urinary tract infections, particularly when dilute urine causes lysis of the leukocytes** (which prevents them from being seen in the sediment). **Positive results (particularly with regard to nitrite) strongly suggest a urinary tract infection**. False-positive findings for leukocyte esterase can occur with contamination by vaginal secretions (which contain leukocytes). **Many causes of false-negative results** exist, including infections with low bacterial loads, tetracycline and some cephalosporins, consuming large amounts of tea, urine with a high SG, and so on. False-negative nitrite results can occur with bacteria that do not reduce nitrate to nitrite (e.g., gram-positive cocci), if dipsticks have been inadvertently stored in an open container, with high urinary concentrations of vitamin C, or if the urine was not retained for a sufficient time within the bladder. **Leukocyte esterase and nitrite should never replace urine cultures, microscopy, and Gram's stain.**

IV. **Microscopic examination**

  A. **Specimen preparation**. Examine the specimen as soon after passage as possible. **Gently (1,500 rpm) centrifuge 10–15 mL of urine for 3 minutes**. Always use the same volume, speed, and time. The use of 1,500 rpm for 3 minutes will not precipitate all cells. Higher speed and longer duration will increase the yield, but will pack the pellet and disrupt casts during resuspension.

  B. **Cells**

   1. **Red blood cells**

    a. **Appearance. Erythrocytes originating from glomerular disease will show characteristic distortion (dysmorphism)** when examined by phase-contrast microscopy (Fig. 4-1). Severely dysmorphic red cells can sometimes be distinguished by careful bright-field examination. **Erythrocytes entering the urine below the kidney** (e.g., because of stones, tumor, trauma, infection, or exogenous contamination) **are round or eumorphic (Fig. 4-1).**

    b. **Significance**. If phase contrast microscopy is available, the distinction between dysmorphic and eumorphic

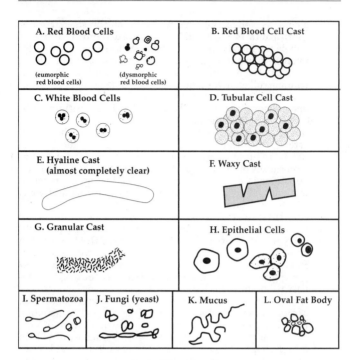

A. Red Blood Cells	B. Red Blood Cell Cast
(eumorphic red blood cells) (dysmorphic red blood cells)	
C. White Blood Cells	D. Tubular Cell Cast
E. Hyaline Cast (almost completely clear)	F. Waxy Cast
G. Granular Cast	H. Epithelial Cells

I. Spermatozoa	J. Fungi (yeast)	K. Mucus	L. Oval Fat Body

Fig. 4-1.

erythrocytes can be **very helpful in deciding between medical and surgical causes of hematuria.**

2. **Leukocytes**

   a. **Appearance**. Urinary leukocytes are typically about one and a half times the diameter of red cells, and contain granular cytoplasm and a lobed nucleus (Fig. 4-1). **Seeing multiple lobes of the nucleus is the key** to identifying a urinary cell as a leukocyte. The most common mistake made in urinalysis is to call renal tubular epithelial cells "white blood cells." In dilute urine, lobes of a polymorphonuclear leukocyte can coalesce and the cell will appear mononuclear.

   b. **Significance**. Urinary tract infection is common, and demonstration of leukocytes in the urine (pyuria) is valuable confirmation of the diagnosis. Nevertheless, **pyuria by itself does not prove infection as pyuria can arise from various noninfectious inflammatory conditions** of the urinary tract, such as interstitial nephritis, calculus, or tumor.

3. **Renal tubular epithelial cells**

   a. **Appearance**. Proximal tubular cells are typically about twice the diameter of a red cell, whereas distal tubular cells are only slightly larger than a red cell. Tubular epithelial cells have a single nucleus and appear similar to lymphocytes.

    b. **Significance**. Renal tubular cells are **shed in most renal parenchymal diseases**. They are not specific for tubulointerstitial disease, but will also appear in glomerulonephritis.

  4. **Oval fat bodies**

    a. **Appearance**. Oval fat bodies are typically two or three times the diameter of a red cell with a very coarsely granular appearance of bright and dark areas (Fig. 4-1). As the fine focus is deftly adjusted, points of light will turn dark and vice versa. Under crossed polarizers, the larger granules will glow as bright "Maltese crosses."

    b. **Significance**. Oval fat bodies are proximal tubular cells that have become stuffed with fat as they incompletely catabolize urinary protein. They signify **prolonged heavy proteinuria** (i.e., nephrotic syndrome).

  5. **Squamous epithelial cells**

    a. **Appearance**. These are large flat polygonal cells with a relatively small nucleus.

    b. **Significance**. Squamous epithelial cells arise from the distal portion of the urethra, vagina, and perineum. **If more than one squame/high power field is seen, the urine has likely been contaminated with vaginal material.**

C. **Casts. A cast is a cylinder of Tamm–Horsfall protein** (synthesized by the loops of Henle and the distal tubules) that has gelled and taken the form of the tubule in which it was born. **It will contain whatever material was in the tubule** at the time it was formed. Because a cast replicates the form of the tubule in which it originated, it will be of constant width, with sides that are parallel or concentrically curved, perhaps replicating the convolutions of the tubule. It is typically about two or three red cell diameters wide, and at least twice as long as it is wide. Usually, the outline of the protein matrix that forms the cast can be clearly seen if the fine focus is adjusted.

  1. **Hyaline casts**

    a. **Appearance**. Hyaline (meaning glassy) casts are very similar in optical characteristics to the urine in which they are suspended, and may be **very hard to see**. Typically, the ends of the casts are **rounded** and a small but variable number of granules, or possibly cells, will be included within the cast.

    b. **Significance**. Normal urine contains a few hyaline casts. More occur in dehydration, physical exertion, fever, and a variety of medical illnesses such as heart failure. They also occur in all types of renal injury. In addition, certain drugs (e.g., gentamicin) can provoke their excretion. Thus, hyaline casts are **very nonspecific and signify significant renal damage only if present in large numbers.**

  2. **Red cell casts**

    a. **Appearance. The cast may be composed entirely of red blood cells (Fig. 4-1), or relatively few red cells are found** within a hyaline cast. Sometimes, a single file of red cells is seen in the cast—a so-called "string cast." The red color of the cells is not usually apparent in bright-field microscopy. As the cast ages, cells break down and cell outlines become less clearly visible. As the cell outlines are lost, the reddish or brownish pigmentation of the cast often becomes more apparent and the red cell cast is then called "a blood cast."

b. Significance. Red cell casts signify glomerular disease. They occur either in proliferative glomerulonephritis or in basement membrane nephropathies, such as Alport's syndrome and familial thin basement membrane disease. Very rarely, red cell casts have been described in tubular necrosis or interstitial nephritis. In any case, **finding a red cell cast establishes that hematuria originates from the kidney and not from lower in the urinary tract.**

3.   White cell casts (leukocyte casts). True leukocyte casts are relatively uncommon. Renal tubular cell casts may be mistaken for leukocyte casts.

a.   Appearance. The cast is typically densely packed with leukocytes, and the **lobed nuclei** of some of these will be apparent with careful adjustment of the fine focus.

b.   Significance. White cell casts signify inflammation. This may represent either renal parenchymal infection (e.g., acute pyelonephritis) or **sterile inflammation** (e.g., allergic interstitial nephritis or interstitial nephritis as a component of lupus).

4.   Tubular cell casts

a.   Appearance. The cast is usually composed almost entirely of renal tubular calls (Fig. 4-1); however, occasionally the tubular cells may be relatively sparse and found in a hyaline cast. Some admixture of red cells or fat bodies may be seen.

b.   Significance. Tubular cell casts indicate significant renal damage, but they are not specific for tubulointerstitial disease; they also occur in glomerulonephritis.

5.   Granular casts

a.   Appearance. A granular cast is similar to a hyaline cast, but is densely packed with fine or coarse granules (Fig. 4-1).

b.   Significance. If more than an occasional granular cast is seen, renal injury is indicated. The injury may be acute or chronic, and can involve the glomeruli or the tubules. Typically, large numbers of pigmented granular casts occur in acute tubular necrosis.

6.   Broad, waxy casts (Fig. 4-1)

a.   Appearance. Waxy casts are superficially similar to hyaline casts, but differ in that they are much **easier to see** because their optical properties differ more sharply from those of the bathing urine. The ends of waxy casts are frequently **fractured** straight across or in a conchoidal fashion similar to that seen at the end of a broken glass rod. Partial fracture lines frequently run across the width of the cast. Broad casts are 8 to 12 red cell diameters wide. Waxy casts are most commonly also broad casts.

b.   Significance. Broad casts arise in dilated tubules. They signify **chronic renal damage** and, thus, are typical of advanced chronic renal disease.

D. Crystals. Many types of crystals can be seen in urine. Because the solubility product for several crystal types is regularly exceeded in normal urine, **crystalluria rarely is of diagnostic importance**. The microscopic appearance of several types of crystal is given in Fig. 4-2. Only two common types, calcium oxalate and uric acid, and one diagnostically important crystal, cystine, will be discussed.

1. Calcium oxalate

a. Appearance. Calcium oxalate dihydrate commonly appears as tetrahedra, which look like **envelopes**

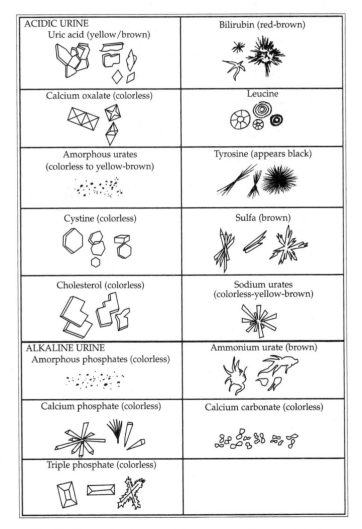

Fig. 4-2. Form of various crystals as seen on microscopy of urine.

when seen straight on. Calcium oxalate monohydrate can assume many forms. **Oval and dumbbell** shapes are typical. The shapes may mimic erythrocytes and aggregates of crystals may look like a cast.

   b.   Significance. In most cases, calcium oxalate crystals are of no significance. They can occur in large numbers, particularly if the urine is not examined when fresh. Large calcium oxalate crystal aggregates are more common in **calcium oxalate stone formers**. In **ethylene glycol poisoning**, many calcium oxalate monohydrate crystals may be excreted.

2.   Uric acid

   a.   Appearance. The most typical form is a **rhomboid** with slightly rounded corners, but barrel shapes and amorphous granular deposits are also common.

   b.   Significance. Small numbers of uric acid crystals are **common and without specificity**. Large aggregates may be found in **uric acid stone formers**. Persistent excretion of uric acid crystals may also be found in uric acid overexcretors—for example those with **hypoxanthine guanine phosphoribosyl transferase deficiency**.

3.   Cystine

   a.   Appearance. Flat hexagonal plates, with very clear straight edges and sharp angles are seen. The plates may overlap one another.

   b.   Significance. Diagnostic of **cystinuria**, an autosomal recessive condition leading to **severe and recurrent stone formation**.

V.   Automated urinalysis. In many large laboratories, an automated process carries out urinalysis. Well-mixed urine is introduced into the analyzer. The analyzer separates aliquots for measurement of specific gravity (by an electrical method), for dipstick analysis (by reflectometry at appropriate time intervals), and for video microscopy. For video microscopy, urine flows through a very narrow flat chamber and images of cells are captured as they pass through this field. A computer sorts the cells into different classes. The images are then presented to a technician for visual verification of the cell type. After the technologist has censored any mislabeled cells, the equipment calculates the precise number of cells in the volume of fluid that was aspirated.

   This equipment provides increased precision in counting cell numbers, but depends on computer algorithms and the expertise of a technician to decide on cell type. Certain **unusual urinary constituents may not be recognized** if they are not part of the embedded algorithms. The same caveats in interpretation of results apply to automated video microscopy and to conventional microscopy.

Serum Enzymes

Joseph A. Knight

I. Basic science review. Enzymes are protein catalysts that increase the rate of a chemical reaction, do not affect the point of equilibrium, and enter into the reaction but are not consumed. These features are indicated in the following equation where E, S, ES, and P represent enzyme, substrate, enzyme-substrate complex, and product, respectively.

$$E + S \leftrightarrow [E\text{-}S] \leftrightarrow P + E$$

Because of the very low concentration of enzymes, they are usually measured by what they do, rather than by the concentration of the enzymes themselves. That is, what is measured is a decrease in substrate concentration, an increase in product concentration, or their cofactors such as oxidized nicotinic acid dehydrogenase (NAD^+)/reduced nicotinic acid dehydrogenase (NADH), expressed in international units (IU). **An IU is defined as the amount of enzyme necessary to convert 1 micro-mole of substrate to product per minute**. International units do **not** define temperature, buffer, pH, concentration of cofactors, and other crucial variables that affect the speed of reactions. Therefore, different analytic methods can produce different reference values. When enzymes exist as different **isoenzymes** (or when isoenzymes exist as different isoforms), they are **numbered based on how fast they travel electrophoretically** from the application point [e.g., lactate dehydrogenase-1 (LD-1) travels faster than LD-2].

II. General considerations. Because of high cell:serum concentration ratios, serum enzyme measurements are highly sensitive (>90%) indicators of disease (Table 4-21). Hence, normal values usually exclude some diseases. For example, serum enzymes may be useful in excluding hepatic disorders (e.g., hepatitis, cholestasis, space-occupying lesions, active cirrhosis), acute myocardial infarction and myocarditis, pancreatitis, hemolytic anemias, rhabdomyolysis, and malignancy, among others.

III. Enzyme testing variables

    A. Specimen and storage variables

        1. Plasma versus serum. Serum is generally used, although no significant differences are found except the following.

            a. Heparin (green top): interferes with acid phosphatase (AcP)

            b. EDTA (purple top): interferes with alkaline phosphatase (ALP)

        2. Capillary versus venous blood. Venous blood is generally used. Capillary blood has increased total LD and an abnormal LD isoenzyme distribution (increased LD-3). This artifact can be overcome by heparinizing the capillary tubes.

Table 4-21.   Clinically useful enzymes

Enzyme	Major Tissue Sources
Acid phosphatase (AcP)	Prostate, erythrocytes, platelets, bone (osteoclasts)
Alanine aminotransferase (ALT)	Liver, heart, muscle, erythrocytes
Aldolase	Muscle, heart
Alkaline phosphatase (ALP)	Liver, bone, intestine, kidneys, placenta, neutrophils
Amylase	Pancreas, salivary glands, ovary
Aspartate aminotransferase (AST)	Heart, liver, erythrocytes, muscle, others
Creatine kinase (CK)	Muscle, heart, brain
Gamma-glutamyltransferase (GGT)	Liver, kidney, endothelium
Lactate dehydrogenase (LD)	Liver, heart, muscle, erythrocytes, leukocytes, etc.
Lipase	Pancreas

   3.   **Hemolysis**
   a.   LD is significantly elevated by "trace" hemolysis (LD activity in erythrocytes is 150 times the serum level).
   b.   Aspartate aminotransferase (AST) is significantly elevated by moderate hemolysis (AST activity in erythrocytes is 15 times the serum level).
   c.   AcP is mildly elevated by hemolysis
   4.   **Storage. Serum or plasma should be separated as soon as possible from red cells.** Enzymes are usually stable 8–12 hours at room temperature, 5–7 days at 4°C, weeks to months at –20°C, and indefinitely at –70°C. **AcP must be kept on ice** and run within 1 hour, or it must be frozen.
B.   **Patient variables**
   1.   **Fasting. ALP can be elevated after eating (the intestines have high levels of ALP).**
   2.   **Age**
   a.   ALP is greatly increased at birth, falls rapidly to two to three times the adult level, **increases during puberty** to three to seven times the adult level, and then decreases to the **adult level by ages 15–17** in females, and ages 18–20 in males.
   b.   AST and ALT are increased at birth to two to three times the adult level, and fall to the **adult level by 2–4 months** of age.
   c.   Gamma-glutamyltransferase (GGT) is greatly increased at birth, and falls to **adult level by about 6 months** of age.
   d.   Aldolase is greatly increased at birth and slowly decreases with age to reach **adult levels by ~16 years** of age.

3. Sex. Creatine kinase (CK) and AcP are higher in males than females.

4. Race and ethnic groups. CK varies with race or ethnic group as follows: black males > Hispanic males > white males $\simeq$ Asian males $\simeq$ black females > Hispanic females > white females $\simeq$ Asian females.

5. Exercise. CK, AST, and LD are increased in untrained individuals following an intense brief workout, and are modestly elevated even in trained athletes following intense prolonged activity (e.g., a marathon).

6. Intramuscular (IM) injections. CK, AST, and LD are increased following IM injections.

IV. Enzymes as diagnostic aids

A. Acid phosphatase, of which there are **five isoenzymes**, catalyzes the hydrolysis of phosphate esters at an **acid pH**, as follows:

$$ROPO_3H_2 + H_2O —AcP \rightarrow ROH + H_3PO_4$$

Increased AcP activity is present in several organs and tissues, primarily **prostate, erythrocytes, platelets, and bone** (osteoclasts) (Table 4-22).

B. Alkaline phosphatase has several isoenzymes, and catalyzes the hydrolysis of various phosphate esters at an **alkaline pH** as follows:

$$ROPO_3H_2 + H_2O —ALP \rightarrow ROH + H_3PO_4$$

1. General. ALP is widely distributed, being present in the **liver** (on membranes between the hepatocytes and bile ducts), **bone, neutrophils, intestine, kidneys, and placenta**. It is particularly helpful as a marker for **obstructive or space-occupying hepatic disorders, and bone disorders (Tables 4-23 and 4-24)**.

2. Weaknesses of ALP as a diagnostic tool

a. Lacks specificity (widely distributed in the body)

b. Marked age variability (greatly increased at birth, falls rapidly to two to three times the adult level, increases during puberty to three to seven times the adult level, and then decreases to the adult level by ages 15–17 in girls

Table 4-22. Diseases/conditions with increased acid phosphatase (AcP) activity

Prostatic carcinoma (increased in 50%–75% of cases with local invasion, >90% of cases with metastases. AcP may be useful when prostatic specific antigen (PSA) is equivocal, but has been almost completely replaced by PSA as a screening test.

Prostatic massage, transurethral resection (TUR), or bladder catheterization

Leukemia (e.g., myelocytic, hairy cell)

Bone disorders [Paget's disease, metastatic carcinoma to the bone (e.g., breast, lung)]

Storage disorders (e.g., Gaucher's disease, Niemann–Pick disease)

Table 4-23. Disorders and conditions associated with increased alkaline phosphatase (ALP)

Nonfasting (ALP increases after a meal)
Liver: lesions that compress, damage, or **block the biliary system:**
–**Obstructive liver disease** (bile stones, hepatic and pancreatic tumors)
–Lesions affecting bile ducts (e.g., sclerosing cholangitis, primary biliary cirrhosis, extrahepatic biliary atresia)
–Drug-induced cholestasis (e.g., phenothiazines)
–**Space-occupying lesions** [primary or metastatic tumors, granulomas (TB, fungal, etc.)]
Bone: metastatic tumors, fractures
Neutrophilia
Pregnancy
Nonhepatic primary tumors (e.g., Regan and Nagao isoenzymes[a])
Benign familial hyperphosphatasemia: autosomal dominant, uncommon cause of persistent ALP elevation (1.5–4.0 times normal), with intestinal ALP being the major component
Hyperphosphatasemia of infancy and early childhood: cause unknown, elevations in ALP may be marked (7–50 times normal), spontaneous return to normal (usually within 4 months), with no known sequelae.

[a] Regan and Nagao isoenzymes are embryonal forms that are structurally related to placental ALP, and seen mainly in undifferentiated tumors (e.g., lung carcinoma).

and 18–20 in boys. Levels slightly increase in women after age 60.

   c.   Normal **reference intervals are skewed** toward higher levels, because 20% to 30% of individuals have a significant (up to 30% of total ALP) intestinal contribution (blood type O or B, and ABH secretors; this is because intestinal ALP strongly binds A red cells and, therefore, more free serum intestinal ALP is present in blood types O or B).

C.   Alanine aminotransferase (ALT) catalyzes the following reversible reaction (equilibrium favors alanine):

L-alanine + alpha-oxoglutarate ←ALT→ pyruvate + L-glutamate

Table 4-24. Disorders associated with decreased alkaline phosphatase (ALP) activity

Hereditary hypophosphatasemia: recessive, failure to calcify bone, causes the chest to collapse during respirations, causing death within first week(s) of life

Vitamin B_{12}, zinc, or magnesium deficiency

Hypothyroidism

1. General. ALT is particularly rich in **hepatocytes**, but is widely distributed (Table 4-21), albeit at lower activity levels than AST. ALT is a very sensitive **indicator of hepatocellular necrosis** (Table 4-25).

2. AST:ALT ratio (DeRitis ratio). The DeRitis ratio derives its utility from the fact that **ALT is a cytoplasmic enzyme primarily found in the liver, whereas AST is both a cytoplasmic and mitochondrial enzyme with a wide distribution in many tissues. Many nonhepatic disorders** (e.g., myocardial infarction, rhabdomyolysis, hemolytic anemia) cause AST to rise further than ALT (**AST:ALT ratio >1.0**), because of AST's wider distribution in the body. **Within the liver, many diseases** cause cytoplasmic damage and have an **AST:ALT ratio <1.0. However, in a few hepatic diseases (primarily involving extensive necrosis or alcohol)**, both cytoplasmic and mitochondrial damage occur, causing AST to rise further than ALT (**AST:ALT ratio >1.0). Liver diseases with AST:ALT ratios >1.0 include** the following.

    a. Severe viral hepatitis with extensive hepatocellular necrosis (poor prognosis)

    b. Alcoholic hepatitis or active cirrhosis

    c. Alcoholic hepatitis in a malnourished patient who has taken small (therapeutic) doses of **acetaminophen**, which can cause extensive liver necrosis with poor prognosis.

D. Aspartate aminotransferase (AST) catalyzes the following reversible reaction (equilibrium favors aspartate):

$$\text{L-aspartate} + \text{alpha-oxoglutarate} \leftarrow\text{AST}\rightarrow \text{oxaloacetate} + \text{L-glutamate}$$

AST is rich in numerous tissues (**heart > liver > muscle > kidney > pancreas**). In addition, AST is rich in **erythrocytes** (15 times the level of serum AST) (Table 4-26).

E. Aldolase catalyzes the following reaction:

$$\text{Fructose 1,6 } (PO_4)_2\text{—aldolase}\rightarrow \text{dihydroxyacetone-} PO_4 + \text{glyceraldehyde-3-}PO_4$$

Aldolase is particularly rich in **skeletal and cardiac muscles**. However, it is also increased in **other tissues**, including liver, erythrocytes, and platelets. **The major clinical use of**

Table 4-25. Major hepatic disorders with increased alanine aminotransferase (ALT)

ALT levels 1.5–8 times the upper reference level are compatible with early, late, and subclinical viral hepatitis, chronic hepatitis, alcoholic hepatitis, chemical hepatitis, passive congestion with centrilobular necrosis, Reye's syndrome, hemochromatosis, cholangitis

ALT levels >8–10 times the upper reference level most often indicate acute viral hepatitis

ALT levels >30 times the upper reference level may be seen in malnourished alcoholics who take small doses of acetaminophen

**Table 4-26.   Major disorders associated with
increased aspartate aminotransferase (AST)**

AST levels 1.5–8 times the upper reference levels are compatible with:

–Liver disorders: Early, late, and subclinical viral hepatitis, chronic hepatitis, alcoholic hepatitis, chemical hepatitis, passive congestion with centrilobular necrosis, Reye's syndrome, hemochromatosis, cholangitis

–Heart disorders: Acute myocardial infarction, pericarditis

–Rhabdomyolysis

–Acute pancreatitis

–Pulmonary infarction

–Hemolytic anemia (or hemolysis for any reason, including traumatic blood draw)

AST levels >8–10 times the upper reference levels usually indicate acute viral hepatitis

AST levels >30 times the upper reference levels may be seen in malnourished patients with alcoholic hepatitis who take small amounts of acetaminophen

---

serum aldolase is for the diagnosis of rhabdomyolysis. However, CK is more sensitive and specific and therefore a better choice for monitoring rhabdomyolysis, muscular dystrophies, and so forth. Serum aldolase can also be significantly elevated in the **eosinophilia–myalgia** syndrome (now rare), which occurs in people taking L-tryptophan that is contaminated with acetaldehyde.

   F.   Amylase catalyzes the hydrolysis of α, 1,4-glucoside bonds in polysaccharides, yielding maltose and maltotriose. **Two amylase isoenzymes** exist: **P-amylase** (40% of total serum amylase), which is essentially limited to the **pancreas**, and **S-amylase** (60% of serum amylase), which is found primarily in salivary glands, ovary, fallopian tubes, small intestine, testes, and bronchial epithelium. **Increases in P-amylase** (measured by electrophoresis or by total amylase with S-amylase inhibition) are **very specific for pancreatic disorders**. Total serum amylase begins to rise within 6–48 hours after the onset of acute pancreatitis (Table 4-27).

   Macroamylasemia is present in ~1% of population, and in **2.5% of patients with hyperamylasemia**. Amylase is **bound to an immunoglobulin**, and the total serum amylase is elevated, whereas **urine amylase levels may be modestly de-**

Table 4-27.   Major disorders with increased serum amylase

P-amylase: Acute and chronic pancreatitis, pancreatic pseudocyst, pancreatic cancer, peptic ulcer

S-amylase: Salivary gland inflammation (e.g., mumps), ovarian carcinoma, pregnancy, acute alcoholism, diabetic ketoacidosis, heroin overdose, bronchogenic carcinoma

creased or normal. A decreased urinary amylase:urinary creatinine ratio may be useful in the diagnosis of macro-amylasemia because the renal clearance of macroamylase is decreased.

G. **Creatine kinase** catalyzes the following reaction:

Creatine + ATP —CK→ creatine phosphate + ADP

CK (Mw: 80,000 d) is a dimer of B (brain) and M (muscle) forms. It is primarily present in **brain, heart, and skeletal muscle. Three major serum isoenzymes** exist, designated **CK-BB (CK1), CK-MB (CK2), CK-MM (CK3). CK-MM is the major serum isoenzyme** in most people, comprising up to 100% of the total serum CK, although very small amounts of CK-MB (<1%–2%) may be present. **CK-MM is particularly rich in skeletal and heart muscle. CK-MB is particularly rich in cardiac muscle (25%–30%** of the CK in the heart), and is found in **low concentrations in skeletal muscle (<3%** of the CK in skeletal muscle). **CK-BB is primarily found in the brain**, with small amounts also present in smooth muscle.

1. **Total CK and acute myocardial infarction (AMI)**

    a. **Sensitivity is ~90%** in AMI cases, but it lacks specificity.

    b. **Total CK begins to rise within 3–8 hours of the attack, peaks in 18–30 hours, and returns to normal within 2.5–3.5 days.**

2. **CK-MB and MI**

    a. **Sensitivity approaches 98%, and is very specific for AMI in the setting "rule out AMI."**

    b. **After AMI, CK-MB begins to rise in 3–6 hours, peaks in 12–24 hours, and returns to normal in 1–3 days.**

    c. Approximately **10% of patients with AMI have a normal total CK but increased CK-MB** ("microinfarc-tion"). Patients are usually older, need more intensive care, have longer hospital stays, and have a higher mortality rate than those with elevated total CK.

    d. CK-MB may be mildly increased in unstable angina or electroshock cardioversion.

    e. **CK-MB mass measurements** are rapid and reliable (normal reference range 0–6 ng/mL). However, these results **must** be interpreted relative to the total CK. Because the units of CK-MB mass (ng/mL) divided by total CK (reported in IU) involve different units, the ratio is called a CK-MB "index" (normal reference range <3.0). In general, myocar-dial injury is associated with a **CK-MB index ≥3.** In some laboratories, a CK-MB mass (≥10 ng/mL **with** an index ≥10 suggests a probable AMI; a CK-MB mass 4–10 ng/mL **with** an index of 4–10 is consistent with an AMI; and a CK-MB mass <4 ng/mL or a CK-MB mass ≥4 ng/mL but **with** an index <4 is negative for AMI.

    f. **In rhabdomyolysis, CK-MB mass is significantly increased as is total CK but the CK-MB index is rel-atively low (<3).**

    g. **Myoglobin** (approximate reference range: 5–90 µg/L; varies with method and can be 25% higher in men than women) and **troponin I** (normal reference range: <0.35 ng/ mL) are usually used to supplement CK-MB as markers for AMI. **Myoglobin is a sensitive (but nonspecific) early marker, whereas troponin I is a specific (but delayed) marker with prolonged elevation.** After AMI, myoglobin begins to increase within 2–4 hours, peaks in 9–12 hours, and returns to normal in 24– 36 hours. After AMI, troponin begins to increase in 4–8 hours, peaks in 12–16 hours, and returns to normal in 5–9 days.

3.   **Creatine kinase isoforms**. Carboxypeptidase hydrolyzes the terminal lysines of CK-MB peptide dimers, resulting in two main isoforms: CK-MB1, and CK-MB2. The normal serum CK-MB2:CK-MB1 ratio is ≤1.5. **After AMI, serum CK-MB2 rapidly increases, and the CK-MB2:CK-MB1 ratio is >1.5**. This isoform ratio is useful as an early marker for AMI, and may be useful in predicting reperfusion after thrombolytic therapy.

4.   **Creatine kinase and rhabdomyolysis**

a.   The diagnosis of rhabdomyolysis is most reliably made when total serum **CK is five or more times normal in the absence of AMI** (CK is more sensitive than aldolase).

b.   The enzyme sensitivity for rhabdomyolysis is **CK > aldolase > AST > LD**.

c.   **CK-MM is more specific than aldolase** for muscular dystrophies.

d.   **CK-MB may be significantly elevated in rhabdomyolysis** but comprises <3% of total CK (**CK index is <3.0**). CK-MB may be significantly elevated in patients with Duchenne muscular dystrophy (and mildly elevated in carriers) (Table 4-28).

5.   **Creatine kinase and malignant diseases**

a.   Total CK can be mildly increased in prostatic carcinoma, in some bronchogenic malignancies, and in a few other malignancies.

b.   Tumor-produced CK-MB or CK-BB may comprise 60% or more of total CK. **If CK-MB exceeds 25% of the total CK, consider a malignancy** as the source.

6.   **Other CK isoenzymes** seen as separate peaks on electrophoresis gels.

a.   **Macro-CK type 1**. Usually **CK-BB is linked to IgG**, and migrates between CK-MM and CK-MB. It occurs in 3%

Table 4-28.   Causes of rhabdomyolysis

Genetic disorders: Muscular dystrophies
Immunologic disorders: Dermatomyositis, polymyositis
Drugs: Ethanol, cocaine, amphetamines, etc.
Toxins: Solvents, venom, CO, $HgCl_2$, etc.
Physical activity: Excessive exercise, seizures
Muscle trauma: Postsurgery, crush syndrome, injections, etc.
Temperature extremes: Hypothermia, hyperthermia
Muscle ischemia: Hypothyroidism, ketoacidosis
Infections: Viral, bacterial

to 4% of hospitalized patients, in females more than males (10:1), and has **no significance** or relationship to any disease.

   b.   Macro-CK type 2. Mitochondrial CK (CK-mt) is part of the mitochondrial membrane. It migrates cathodal to CK-MM, represents **severe cellular injury** [severe AMI, shock, hepatic centrilobular necrosis or metastatic carcinoma (often following radiation or chemotherapy)], and often indicates a poor prognosis.

H.   Gamma-glutamyltransferase is involved in the **transfer of a terminal gamma-glutamyl group from peptides to acceptors**, and is especially involved in the transfer of amino acids across cell membranes. GGT is particularly rich in cell membranes of the **liver, kidney, pancreas, and vascular endothelium (Table 4-29).**

   1.   Advantages of GGT over ALP as a marker of liver disease

   a. GGT correlates with ALP in both obstructive and metastatic liver disease, but **GGT is more sensitive and specific.**

   b. Unlike ALP, **minimal GGT is found in bone, intestines, neutrophils, and placenta.**

   c. Unlike ALP, **GGT is not affected by meals, not increased in ABH secretors, not age-related after ~6–7 months, and shows minimal sex variation.**

   d. GGT is often **elevated in chronic alcoholics** when other tests are normal.

   e. Because of its increased specificity for liver, **GGT helps to evaluate the source of an increased ALP** (i.e., if ALP is increased and GGT is normal, ALP is extrahepatic; if both are increased, ALP is of hepatic origin).

   f. If GGT and ALP are both elevated, but one of the two is disproportionately elevated, suspect drug-induced cholestasis. Also include alcoholism in the differential diagnosis if GGT is the test that is disproportionately high.

   2.   Weaknesses of GGT

   a.   GGT is increased in patients taking **antiepileptic drugs** (e.g., mysoline, phenobarbital, phenytoin).

   b. GGT is **not as specific as desirable** (although it is still more specific than ALP).

I.   Lactate dehydrogenase catalyzes the following reversible reaction:

Lactate + NAD$^+$ ←LD→ Pyruvate + NADH + H$^+$

Table 4-29.   Major causes of gamma-glutamyltransferase elevation

Liver disease: Hepatitis (all etiologies), obstructive jaundice, space-occupying lesions, cirrhosis, etc.

Granulation tissue: Repair processes

Medications: Antiepileptics, warfarin

Alcohol intake

LD is present in the cytoplasm of all body cells where its activity (U/g) is greatly increased over that of serum. The relative tissue activity is **skeletal muscle ≈ liver > heart > kidney > erythrocytes**. LD is a tetramer of peptide chains [chains are H (heart) and/or M (muscle) forms]. As a result, there are **five isoenzymes**:

- LD-1 (H4): rich in heart, red cells, kidney, seminomas
- LD-2 (H3M)
- LD-3 (H2M2): rich in lung, lymphocytes, platelets),
- LD-4 (HM3):
- LD-5 (M4): rich in liver, skeletal muscle, prostate, neutrophils

The normal LD distribution is LD2 > LD1 > LD3 > LD4 ~ LD5. Total LD is a moderately sensitive indicator of numerous disorders. Hence, it is useful in a general chemistry profile (Table 4-30).

1. **Weaknesses of total serum LD**
   a. **Lacks specificity**
   b. **Lacks sensitivity**, especially in hepatocellular disorders.
2. **LD isoenzyme associations with various diseases**
   a. LD-1:LD-2 ratio > 0.80 in myocardial infarction (normal LD-1:LD-2 ratio ≤0.80)
   b. LD-1 ≥LD-2 in hemolytic anemias, including pernicious anemia.
   c. LD-1 increased in renal infarctions and seminomas
   d. LD-3 increased in pulmonary infarction
   e. LD-3 and LD-4 are increased in lymphoproliferative disorders (lymphomas [Hodgkin's and non-Hodgkin's], acute and chronic lymphocytic leukemias); they show a "tenting" pattern (LD-3 is higher than the others). LD-4 may be the major isoenzyme in acute lymphoblastic leukemia.

Table 4-30.   Disorders with increased total lactate dehydrogenase (LD)

Various malignancies: LD is used as a screen for various carcinomas, acute and chronic leukemias, etc. LD is also a good prognostic indicator of lymphoproliferative disorders (e.g., Hodgkin's disease, non-Hodgkin's lymphoma, multiple myeloma), because prognosis varies inversely with LD activity determined at the time of diagnosis.

Acute myocardial or renal infarctions

Hepatocellular necrosis: Hepatitis, centrilobular necrosis

Rhabdomyolysis

Hypothyroidism: Some cases

Hemolysis of any kind: (e.g., trauma during the blood draw, hemolytic anemias), megaloblastic anemias (LD may be extremely high, because of degenerating RBC precursors in the marrow). RBCs have 150 times the LD activity of serum.

LD, lactate dehydrogenase; RBC, red blood cells.

f. LD-5 is increased in various carcinomas (e.g., prostate, colon), hepatitis (including infectious mononucleosis), rhabdomyolysis, and in neutrophilia.

g. Many disorders can cause a nonspecific elevation of all LD isoenzymes.

J. **Lipase** catalyzes the hydrolysis of long chain fatty acids at the carbon 1 and 3 ester bonds, producing free fatty acids and monoglycerides. Lipase is **present primarily in the pancreas**; it is **not present in salivary glands**. As a result, serum lipase is comparable to the measurement of P-amylase (pancreatic amylase) for the diagnosis of pancreatitis and is generally considered to be **superior to total amylase** for this diagnosis. It begins to rise at the same time as amylase (6–48 hours), but remains elevated longer (7–10 days). Prolonged serum lipase elevation suggests either a poor prognosis or the development of a pancreatic pseudocyst. Urine lipase measurements are not useful because lipase is reabsorbed by the proximal tubules.

1. **Disorders with increased serum lipase** include pancreatitis, chronic renal failure, hemodialysis patients, and occasionally in abdominal inflammation (but without pancreatitis).

K. **Miscellaneous serum enzymes**

1. **Enzymes as markers for posthepatic obstruction or hepatic space-occupying lesions** are 5′-nucleotidase (5′-N) and leucine aminopeptidase (LAP).

2. **Enzymes as markers for hepatocellular necrosis** are sorbitol dehydrogenase (SD), guanase (G), isocitric dehydrogenase (ID), and ornithine transcarbamylase (OT).

3. **Enzyme deficiencies in heritable hemolytic anemias**

a. **Glucose-6-phosphate dehydrogenase (G6PD):** sex-linked recessive

   (1) Affects mainly blacks and people of Mediterranean descent (>200,000,000 cases worldwide)

   (2) Hemolysis is usually initiated by acute infectious disorder, oxidant drug medication, or metabolic acidosis.

b. **Pyruvate kinase (PK):** autosomal recessive

   (1) The second most common inherited hemolytic anemia after G6PD

   (2) Can occur in infancy and mimic hemolytic disease of the newborn.

4.6

Body Fluids

Joseph A. Knight

I. Introduction. Appropriate laboratory examination of body fluids is critical in numerous clinical disorders and diseases. In this chapter, appropriate collection and examination of serous, synovial, cerebrospinal, and amniotic fluids will be covered.

II. Serous fluids are those that accumulate in the pleural, peritoneal, and pericardial cavities.

A. Specimen collection and handling. Improper specimen collection, handling, and testing are more common with serous fluids than with other body fluids. Too often, a large vacutainer (that has not been anticoagulated) arrives in the laboratory containing a large fibrin clot that has trapped most of the cells and bacteria. Examination of the clear overlying fluid then results in a false-negative finding on Gram's stain, cytology, or cell count (Table 4-31).

B. The initial classification of a serous fluid as a transudate, exudate, or chylous effusion is clinically useful, cost-effective, and determines whether further testing is recommended (Table 4-32).

   1. Transudates. Among the common causes of transudates are congestive heart failure, hypoalbuminemia (caused by liver failure, nephrotic syndrome, and so on), atelectasis (pleural effusion), peritoneal dialysis (pleural effusion), and myxedema. If a serous fluid is a transudate (as determined by total protein (TP) and lactate dehydrogenase (LD) ratios in Table 4-33), **further testing is rarely needed.**

   2. Exudates. Among the common causes of exudates are trauma, infection (e.g., pneumonia, peritonitis), pancreatitis (10% of cases produce left pleural effusion), infarction (e.g., lung, bowel), collagen-vascular disorders (lupus, rheumatoid arthritis), and malignancy. In contrast with transudates, **all exudates require further testing** to establish their cause.

   3. Chylous effusions. A chylous effusion is one in which **chylomicrons** can be demonstrated by electrophoresis. The presence of chylomicrons is inferred by an **elevated triglyceride level (≥110 mg/dL).** Chylous fluids may or may not have a classic milky appearance. Some serous fluids look milky, however, but have normal triglyceride levels and, hence, are nonchylous by definition). These fluids, called "pseudochylous fluids," are milky because of increased lecithin-globulin complexes. **Among the common causes** of chylous effusions are trauma to lymphatics (usually following surgery), lymphoma, metastatic tumor to lymph nodes, and granulomatous disorders (e.g., tuberculosis, sarcoid).

C. Summary of "routine" serous fluid examination

   1. Collect specimen in appropriate anticoagulant tubes, along with a blood specimen (red or green top tube).

Table 4-31. Desirable collection of serous fluids

Tests	Anticoagulant Tube	Volume (mL)[a]
WBC with differential, RBC, tumor cells	EDTA (purple top)	5–8
Total protein, LD	Heparin (green top)	8–10
Glucose, amylase, Gram's stain, cultures, antigens	Heparin (green top)	8–10
Tumor (Pap stain, cell block)	Heparin (25 U/mL)	25–50

LD, lactate dehydrogenase; RBC, red blood cells; WBC, white blood cells.
[a] 50–100 mL of total fluid is usually adequate. Always draw a simultaneous blood sample in a red top tube.

Table 4-32. Initial classification of serous fluids

Tests	Transudate[a]	Exudate[a]	Chylous[a]
Appearance	Clear	Cloudy	Cloudy to milky
Color	Pale yellow	Variable	Pale yellow to milky
Leukocyte count	<1000/µL	≥1000/µL	≥1000/µL
Differential WBC	Mononuclears	PMNs early, mononuclears late	PMNs early, mononuclears late
Triglycerides	<60 mg/dL	<60 mg/dL	**≥110 mg/dL**
Total protein (TP)	<3.0 g/dL	≥3.0 g/dL	≥3.0 g/dL
Serous fluid TP/serum TP	<0.5	**≥0.5**[b]	≥0.5
Serous fluid LD/serum LD	<0.6	**≥0.6**[b]	≥0.6

LD, lactate dehydrogenase; WBC, white blood cells.
[a] The serous fluid TP/serum TP ratio, serous fluid LD/serum LD ratio, and triglyceride levels are the preferred methods for differentiating transudates, exudates, and chylous effusions.
[b] If either the serous TP/serum TP ratio >0.5 *OR* the serous fluid LD/serum LD >0.6, the fluid is classified as an exudate.

Table 4-33.   Tests to help differentiate benign from malignant peritoneal serous fluids

Tests	Suggests Benign	Suggests Malignant
Serum-ascites albumin concentration gradient[a]	<1.1	≥1.1
Cholesterol	<50 mg/dL	≥50 mg/dL
Fibronectin	<50 µg/dL	≥50 µg/dL

[a] Serum-ascites albumin concentration gradient = serum albumin – serous fluid albumin.

2.   **Determine whether fluid is a transudate, exudate, or chylous effusion.**

3.   **If transudate, no further tests needed unless spontaneous bacterial peritonitis is possible.** Refrigerate in case further testing might be helpful.

4.   **If exudate, establish cause** by systematic examination.

D.   **Follow-up testing of serous fluids**. Exudates and chylous effusions should be further evaluated. Transudates should undergo further evaluation if spontaneous bacterial peritonitis is a possibility. Further testing of serous fluids may provide useful information when the following diagnoses are in the differential.

1.   **Malignancy**

a.   **Cytologic examination** may be definitive, but malignant cells are seen in only 40% to 70% of malignant cases, and a repeat fluid collection for cytologic examination may be needed.

(1)   **The most common malignancies seen in pleural fluid are the breast and lung.**

(2)   **The most common malignancies seen in the peritoneal fluid are the ovary, colon, and pancreas.**

b.   **Tumor markers**. If cytology is negative, but malignancy is still suspected, measurement of tumor markers may be very helpful: **carcinoembryonic antigen** (CEA) (colon), CA-125 (ovary), CA 15-3 (breast), CA 19-9 (pancreas).

c.   **Mucopolysaccharides** (reference range <20 mg/dL): >25 mg/dL suggests mesothelioma.

2.   **Infectious agents**

a.   **Direct examination** (e.g., Gram's stain for bacteria, acid fast stain for tuberculosis)

b.   **Latex fixation** for bacterial antigens

c.   **Cultures** (bacteria, fungi, yeast)

d.   **Spontaneous bacterial peritonitis (SBP)**. The specimen is often a transudate.

(1)   **Total neutrophil count**: 200–500/µL is very suggestive of SBP; ≥500/µL has an excellent correlation with SBP.

(2) **pH ≤7.31** has a very good correlation with SBP; pH ≤7.15 suggests poor prognosis.

e. Organic acids. When the Gram's stain is negative, the presence of **bacterial-produced** organic acids can confirm an infection.

(1) Succinic acid: aerobes and anaerobes

(2) "Volatile" acids (butyric, isobutyric, propionic, isovaleric): anaerobes

f. Adenosine deaminase (produced by T lymphocytes) and **tuberculostearic acid are increased in tuberculous effusions.**

3. Systemic lupus: demonstration of **lupus erythematosus (LE) cell** with Wright-Giemsa stain

4. Acute pancreatitis: 10% to 15% of cases cause **left pleural effusions** and have an **elevated fluid amylase** that correlates with the serum amylase.

5. Ruptured gallbladder: a peritoneal fluid bilirubin: serum bilirubin ratio of ≥1.0 (in the absence of cirrhosis or severe liver disease) suggests gallbladder rupture.

6. Stab-gunshot abdominal wounds. Lavage abdomen with 1,000 mL sterile saline (children, 15 mL/kg body weight), mix well, and submit specimen for **erythrocyte** count.

a. Red blood cell (RBC) count of ≥5,000/μL is very sensitive for bowel perforation in gunshot wounds.

b. RBC ≥10,000–100,000/μL is very sensitive for bowel perforation in stab wounds.

c. RBC ≥100,000/μL is highly specific of bowel perforation in stab wounds.

7. In contrast with cerebrospinal fluid (CSF) and synovial fluid, measuring serous fluid glucose or lactic acid is not useful under any circumstances.

III. Synovial fluid. The laboratory examination of synovial fluid is of **critical importance when infectious or crystal-induced arthritis is suspected** (single joint pain and swelling), because an infected joint can be irreversibly damaged within 24–48 hours (e.g., infection with *Staphylococcus aureus*) (Table 4-34).

A. Specimen collection. Collect three tubes.

1. Tube #1 (for **microbiology**): 3–5 mL in sterile tube; add 25 U heparin/mL fluid

Table 4-34. Normal reference values for synovial fluid

Test	Result
Leukocyte count	0–200 (neutrophils <25%, lymphocytes <30%, monocytes >60%)
Glucose (serum/fluid difference) (mg/dL)	<10
Protein (g/dL)	<3.0
Lactate (mg/dL)	<25
Uric acid (mg/dL)	Males: 2–8 Females: 2–6

2.   **Tube #2** (for **hematology**): 3–5 mL fluid; add 25 U heparin/mL fluid [do NOT use crystalline EDTA (purple top tube), but liquid EDTA is acceptable].

3.   **Tube #3** (for **chemistry**): 3–5 mL in red top tube and observe for clotting (clotting indicates leakage of fibrinogen from the circulation, and is a nonspecific abnormal finding that may also be caused by a traumatic tap).

B.   **Classification of arthritides**

1.   **Noninflammatory (group I)**: osteoarthritis, trauma, neuropathic osteoarthropathy, osteochrondritis dissicans, pigmented villonodular synovitis

2.   **Inflammatory or crystal-induced (group II)**: rheumatoid arthritis, SLE, psoriatic arthritis, ankylosing spondylitis, pseudogout (chondrocalcinosis)

3.   **Septic (group III)**: bacterial, tuberculous, fungal, viral

4.   **Hemorrhagic (group IV)**: trauma, pigmented villonodular synovitis, synovioma

C.   **Routine examination of synovial fluid includes color or appearance, leukocyte count and differential, Gram's stain, culture, examination for crystals, serum, and synovial fluid glucose.**

D.   **Morphologic and chemical clues (Table 4-35)**

1.   **Inflammatory or crystal-induced and septic arthritis (groups II and III)**. Leukocyte counts are significantly increased and **neutrophils predominate**.

2.   **Reiter's syndrome. Reiter's cells** (vacuolated macrophages with blue intracytoplasmic material, representing phagocytosed nuclear material) are often present but not pathognomonic. Usually due to *Chlamydia trachomatis* [polymerase chain reaction analysis is diagnostic].

3.   **Lupus erythematosus. LE cells** (large purple homogeneous cytoplasmic inclusions in phagocytic cells, representing denatured nuclear material damaged by antinuclear antibodies and ingested) are present.

4.   **Rheumatoid arthritis (RA). Ragocytes** (RA cells are neutrophils containing small dark cytoplasmic granules (immune complexes) similar to toxic granules.

5.   **Lyme disease. Eosinophils** (reference range: 3%–4%) may be transiently increased (>35%).

6.   **Gout. Characteristic crystals** are definitive, but increased fluid **uric acid** (monosodium urate) is suggestive of gout, and more sensitive and specific than serum levels.

E.   **Crystal examination**. Proper examination of synovial fluid for crystals requires a microscope fitted with an analyzer, polarizer, and red compensator.

1.   **Uric acid (monosodium urate)** is present in gout. They are **birefringent, needle-shaped** crystals (or may be rod-shaped), 1–20 μ in length, with **characteristic color orientation** (use a **control slide** with known uric acid crystals for comparison).

2.   **Calcium pyrophosphate** is present in chondrocalcinosis (pseudogout). Appears as **birefringent, rod-shaped** crystals (but may be needle-shaped and mimic monosodium urate).

Table 4-35. Usual synovial fluid findings in arthridites

Test	Group I: Noninflammatory	Group II: Inflammatory/ Crystal-Induced	Group III: Septic	Group IV: Hemorrhagic
Color	Yellow	Yellow-white	Yellow-green	Red-brown
Viscosity	High	Low	Low	Low
Leukocytes/μL	<5,000	10,000–100,000	10,000–200,000	50–10,000
Neutrophils (%)	<25	>50	>75	>25
Serum glucose/fluid glucose difference (mg/dL)	<10	>25	>25	<10
Protein (g/dL)	<3.0	>3.0	>3.0	>3.0
Lactate (mg/dL)	Normal	Normal to slightly elevated	110–250: probable >250: positive	Normal

3. **Cholesterol** is common in chronic arthritis. Seen as **birefringent, square platelike crystals with notched corners** (rarely, may be rod-shaped). Steroid crystals may look similar.

4. **Calcium hydroxyapatite** may be present in apatite-associated arthritis, calcific periarthritis, and acute calcific arthritis. **Not birefringent**, but may consist of brownish-yellow aggregates.

F. **Microbiology**

1. **Always do cultures.** *Neisseria gonorrhoeae* is the most common cause of septic arthritis in patients 15–45 years of age. *S. aureus* is the most common cause in patients >45 years of age.

2. **Gram's stain (lacks sensitivity)**: positive in ≤25% of *N. gonorrhoeae* cases, in ≤75% of *S. aureus* cases, and in ≤50% of gram-negative bacilli cases (e.g., *Escherichia coli, Haemophilus influenzae*).

3. **Lactate levels are very helpful** for the early diagnosis of septic arthritis. Gram-positive cocci and gram-negative bacilli significantly increase lactate levels (**caution *N. gonorrhoeae* can cause only mild elevations**). Levels <110 mg/dL are equivocal, 110–250 mg/dL suggest probable infection, levels ≥**250 mg/dL are considered positive**.

4. **Organic acids.** The presence of **valeric acid, hexanoic acid, or succinic acid** is presumptive evidence of infection.

IV. **Cerebrospinal fluid.** The laboratory examination of CSF is critical to establish the diagnosis of various central nervous system (CNS) diseases and disorders that affect both children and adults.

A. **Major CNS diseases and disorders for CSF analysis.** Meningitis [bacterial, viral, and fungal (mainly tuberculosis)], neurosyphilis, multiple sclerosis (MS), CNS hemorrhage (especially small subdural bleeds), and malignancy [primary CNS tumors, leukemia, metastatic carcinoma (lung 65%, breast 30%, melanoma 10%, kidney, colon, pancreas, prostate, stomach, testis)].

B. **Specimen collection**

1. **Collect three tubes** (one for chemistry and immunology, one for microbiology cultures, and one for cell counts and cell morphology).

2. **Never use the first drawn tube for cultures** (contamination is common).

3. **Use the last drawn tube** (the one least likely to be hemorrhagic or contaminated) **for the tests that are most important** and likely to be diagnostic (e.g., chemistry and immunology if MS is suspected) (Table 4-36).

C. **Infectious meningitis.** Despite recent advances in the diagnosis and treatment of infectious meningitis, morbidity and mortality are still relatively high. The major organism in adults is *Streptococcus pneumoniae*, which has high mortality (20%–30%) and neurologic morbidity (50%), including 30% with some hearing loss. The diagnosis of meningitis, particularly bacterial, must not be missed. Although "classic" cases of meningitis have typical clinical and laboratory findings, many do not and may require further evaluation and testing (Table 4-37).

Table 4-36. Normal reference levels for cerebrospinal fluid

Test	Value
Color	Colorless/clear
White blood cells/µL	Term newborn ≤20, premature newborn ≤30, older children and adults ≤5–6
Lymphocytes	≥70%
Monocytes	<30%
Neutrophils	<2%
Protein (mg/dL)	Premature newborn <160, term newborn <100, older children and adults 15–50, elderly (>65 years) <60

1. "Routine" tests for infectious meningitis include total leukocyte count with differential, glucose, total protein, Gram's stain, and bacterial culture.

2. Problems with "routine" tests. They lack sensitivity (except culture) and specificity, and are easily misinterpreted (except culture), and culture takes too long.

D. Diseases with protein abnormalities. An elevated protein level, the most common CSF abnormality, is elevated in most CNS diseases or disorders. Specific analysis of CSF protein is especially useful in the diagnosis of MS, Creutzfeldt–Jakob (C–J) disease, and Alzheimer's disease.

1. Multiple sclerosis is a **demyelinating disease** characterized by a relapsing, remitting course with CNS episodes separated in time and anatomic location. Although the **diagnosis is one of exclusion**, the laboratory plays a highly significant role. Almost all of the following **tests for MS look for increased IgG** production by the CNS (e.g., IgG synthetic rate, IgG:albumin ratio, oligoclonal bands). The presence of **oligoclonal bands** is probably the most important finding. In the absence of oligoclonal bands, elevations in other measures of IgG production have little meaning. CSF IgG can be increased because of a variety of inflammatory or neoplastic disorders with increased antibody production (e.g., viral meningitis, lymphoma, Guillain-Barré, subacute sclerosing panencephalitis). CSF IgG and proteins are also increased when blood contaminates CSF.

    a. Total CSF protein (normal reference range: 15–50 mg/dL)

        (1) Mildly elevated in 25% to 50% of MS cases

        (2) If total protein is >100 mg/dL, MS is probably **not** the diagnosis.

    b. CSF IgG synthetic rate (normal reference range: <3 mg/d); IgG synthetic rate is >3 mg/d in 90% of MS cases.

    c. The following measures of IgG production correct for increased IgG and protein caused by blood contamination (e.g., traumatic tap, defects in blood–brain barrier).

(*text continues on page 358*)

Table 4-37. Causes of infectious meningitis

Test	Bacterial	"Developing"/ "Normocellular" Bacterial	Viral ("Aseptic")	Tuberculous[c]
White blood cells/μL	>500[a]	Normal/minimally elevated[b]	10–200	10–200
White blood cells differential	>75% neutrophils[a]	Normal	>75% lymphocytes	Variably-increased lymphocytes
Protein	Moderate to marked elevation	Normal to mildly elevated	Mildly elevated	Mildly elevated
Glucose (mg/dL)	<40[a]	>40	>40	Decreased or normal
Gram's stain	Positive[a]	±	Negative	Negative
Bacterial culture	Positive	±	Negative	Negative
Fibronectin	Increased	Normal to increased	Normal	Varies
Limulus lysate gelation test[d]	Positive	±	Negative	Negative

Bacterial antigens[e]	Positive	±	Negative	Negative
Lactate[f]	Elevated	Normal to elevated	Normal to slightly elevated	Normal
Adenosine deaminase	Normal	Normal	Normal	Elevated

[a] **A significant number of bacterial meningitis cases have leukocyte counts 100–500/μL, relative lymphocytosis (i.e., >50%), negative Gram's stain (in 20%–30% of the cases), and glucose >40 mg/dL.**

[b] A not uncommon scenario occurs when a patient is sent home after "normal" CSF results, but returns in 12–24 hours with a purulent meningitis.

[c] Often mimics viral meningitis.

[d] **Highly sensitive for gram-negative endotoxin**, but negative for gram-positive organisms.

[e] **Usually positive and highly specific for most bacteria causing meningitis** (i.e., *Neisseria meningitidis, Haemophilus influenza, S. Pneumoniae* (most strains), *Streptococcus agalactica* (group B), but lacks adequate sensitivity/specificity for some organisms (Listeria, tuberculosis, etc.).

[f] Normal range; <25 mg/dL; <45 mg/dL in newborns. **Highly sensitive for bacterial infections** (lactate is elevated), usually normal/equivocal in viral meningitis. Useful when other tests normal/equivocal (the negative predictive value is ≥95%, meaning a 95% probability that, given a normal test result, the patient does not have bacterial meningitis.

(1)   CSF gamma globulin percent of total protein (by protein electrophoresis; normal reference range is <12%–15%); gamma globulin ≥15% in ~65% of MS cases.

(2)   CSF IgG percent of total protein (normal reference range: <10.5%); IgG is ≥10.5% in 70% of MS cases.

(3)   CSF IgG:albumin ratio (normal reference range is <25%–28%); IgG:albumin ratio is ≥28% in ~75% of MS cases.

(4)   CSF IgG-albumin index (normal reference range varies ~0.65–0.81); this index is **the most widely used** of the four tests discussed in this section):

$$\text{IgG-albumin index} = \frac{\text{CSF IgG/plasma IgG}}{\text{CSF albumin/plasma albumin}}$$

(a)   The IgG-albumin index is **elevated in ~85% of MS** cases.

d.   Oligoclonal bands comprise the most important supporting evidence for MS.

(1)   High resolution gel electrophoresis (positive in 90%–95% of MS cases) or **isoelectric focusing** (positive in 95%–98% of MS cases) shows **two or more discrete bands in MS**. Oligoclonal bands are **not pathognomonic** for MS; they may be seen, albeit uncommonly, in some cases of subacute sclerosing panencephalitis, encephalitis, Guillain-Barré syndrome, neurosyphilis, vasculitis, acquired immunodeficiency syndrome (AIDS), and several other disorders.

(2)   A single band should not be interpreted as positive.

e.   Myelin basic protein (MBP). Normal reference range is <4 ng/mL; this is primarily a research tool and is **not of practical usefulness.**

(1)   MBP is elevated in all demyelinating disorders, including MS during relapses.

(2)   MBP is normal to mildly elevated in MS during remission.

2.   Creutzfeldt–Jakob disease (CJD) is a transmissable, subacute spongiform encephalopathy.

a.   Diagnosis of CJD is currently by brain biopsy.

b.   Diagnosis of CJD by combined **polyacrylamide gel or isoelectric focusing**

(1)   The method can identify >300 different CSF proteins.

(2)   Four specific proteins are present in CJD and a few other diseases.

(3)   Increased serum S-100 protein has been reported.

3.   Alzheimer's disease

a.   Amyloid beta-protein precursor levels are decreased.

b.   Tau protein levels are increased.

E.   Diagnosis of CSF leakage (rhinorrhea and otorrhea). Immunofixation electrophoresis is highly sensitive and specific.

1.   All body fluids except CSF show a single transferrin isoform.

   2. CSF fluid (rhinorrhea or otorrhea) shows **two transferrin isoforms**.

F. Diagnosis of Cortical versus Lacunar Stroke

   1. Cortical stroke: elevation of any or all of the following: **lactate dehydrogenase (LD), aspartate aminotransferase (AST), and creatine kinase (CK).**

   2. Lacunar stroke: normal or minimally elevated LD with normal levels of AST and CK.

G. Diagnosis of tumors in CSF

   1. Astroprotein is increased in 40% to 45% of **glial tumors** and in 67% of **glioblastomas.**

   2. Carcinoembryonic antigen is increased in various **carcinomas** (e.g., breast, lung, bowel, stomach), and is a particularly valuable marker in meningeal carcinomatosis where radiologic techniques are not useful.

   3. β_2-microglobulin is increased in **lymphoblastic leukemia, lymphoma**, and some primary brain tumors.

   4. α-fetoprotein (AFP) is increased in **germ cell tumors**.

   5. β-human chorionic gonadotropin is increased in **choriocarcinoma** and gonadotropin-producing **teratomas**.

   6. Lactate dehydrogenase is increased in **leukemia, lymphoma, and metastatic carcinomas.**

   7. Lysozyme is increased in **myeloblastic and monocytic leukemias**, and in some primary and metastatic tumors.

H. Gamma aminobutyric acid (GABA) is decreased in "startle disease" and **Huntington's** disease. May be increased during migraine attacks.

V. Amniotic fluid

A. Reasons to examine amniotic fluid. Amniotic fluid (AF) is examined to diagnosis genetic disorders (including chromosomal anomalies and inherited metabolic disorders), measurement of bilirubin levels in Rh sensitization, diagnosis of chorioamnionitis, assessment of fetal lung maturity, assessment of postdates pregnancies (i.e., >40 weeks), and intrauterine growth retardation (Table 4-38).

Table 4-38. Normal reference values for common amniotic fluid analytes[a]

General Tests	Result
Appearance	Colorless to pale straw, clear
Alpha-fetoprotein	14–16 weeks: <52 mg/L; 22 weeks: <30 mg/L
Bilirubin	28–30 weeks: ΔA450 <0.06 (<0.075 mg/dL)
	40 weeks: ΔA450 <0.02 (<0.025 mg/dL)

Tests for Maturity	Immature	Mature
Lecithin/sphingomyelin (L/S ratio)	<2.0	≥2.0
Phosphatidylglycerol (PG)	Negative	Positive

[a] Screening for neural tube defects, congenital disorders, hemolytic disease of the newborn, and fetal lung maturity—see text for more detailed test values.

B.   Mean Amniotic fluid volume during gestation
- 10 weeks (30 mL)
- 12 weeks (90 mL)
- 14 weeks* (120 mL)
- 16 weeks* (230 mL)
- 18 weeks* (280 mL)
- 20 weeks (320 mL)
- 40 weeks (1,000 mL)

(Asterisks indicate recommended weeks for diagnostic amniocentesis.)

C.   Analyte variation with gestation.
Early in gestation, analyte composition of AF is similar to maternal serum. As gestation progresses, the analytes change as follows.

   1.   Increased: alkaline phosphatase (after ~25 weeks), amylase, creatinine, phospholipids, urea, uric acid.

   2.   Decreased: bilirubin, chloride, glucose, protein, sodium.

D.   Rh sensitization. Amniotic fluid bilirubin
values are used to monitor hemolytic disease of the newborn (HDN). AF is scanned spectrophotometrically over a spectrum of wavelengths, and the bilirubin level is reflected by the absorbance change at 450 nm ($\Delta A450$). The **$\Delta A450$** is then used to predict the severity of the HDN by plotting the $\Delta A450$ on the **Liley graph**. The $\Delta A450$ may be measured once, or may be plotted several times over a period of weeks to detect any trends in the AF bilirubin levels. (Figs. 4-3 and 4-4.)

   1.   Specimen collection. The AF container should be wrapped in **aluminum foil** (bilirubin is light sensitive), refrigerated, and quickly delivered to the laboratory.

   2.   Factors that falsely decrease measured AF bilirubin values: light exposure, polyhydramnios (>1,300 mL dilutes bilirubin), wrong fluid collected (maternal urine, fetal ascitic fluid; placental cyst may be lower or higher than the AF bilirubin).

   3.   Factors that falsely increase measured AF bilirubin values include the following.

   a.   Maternal blood contamination ("bloody tap"): maternal hemoglobin interferes, but laboratory can correct

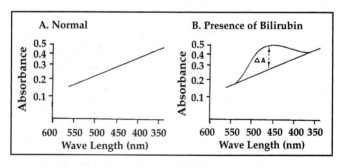

Fig. 4-3. Spectral tracing of amniotic fluid.

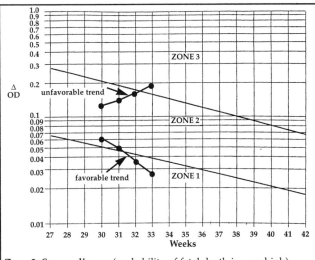

Zone 3: **Severe disease** (probability of fetal death is very high)
Zone 2: **Moderate disease** (fetus should be delivered as soon as lungs mature sufficiently)
Zone 1: **Normal/mild disease** (pregnancy is allowed to go to completion)

Fig. 4-4. Liley graph showing two examples of fetal plots.

by multiplying ΔA410 by 0.05 and subtracting the result from the ΔA450 value.

    b. Fetal blood contamination:

       (1) Fetal hemoglobin interferes with the spectrophotometer measurements at 450 nm, but the laboratory can make appropriate analytic adjustment.

       (2) Fetal bilirubin: 10–100 times higher than AF bilirubin, but cannot be adjusted by the laboratory.

    c. Oligohydramnios (<800 mL concentrates bilirubin)

    d. Jaundice in the mother (caused by hepatitis, S-S/S-C diseases, and so on)

    e. Meconium (no correction factor, but bilirubin can be extracted with organic solvents and the specimen rerun).

E. Genetic disorders (Table 4-39)

F. Congenital anomalies identified by amniotic fluid analysis

    1. Neural tube defects (NTD) occur in 1 of 500 live births.

    a. NTD screening: measures maternal serum AFP in patients with a history of prior pregnancy with NTD (increased risk 10–20 times), or who have a mother, father, or sibling with NTD (or mother, father, or sibling's child with NTD).

Table 4-39. Genetic disorders identified by amniotic fluid analysis

Chromosome anomalies
–Down's syndrome (trisomy 21, 1/500 live births)
–Patau's syndrome (trisomy 13, 1/5,000 live births)
–Edward's syndrome (trisomy 18, 0.3/1,000 live births)
–Turner's syndrome (45 X0, 1/3,000 live births)
–Klinefelter's syndrome (47 XXY, 1/500 male live births)

Metabolic Disorders (Simplified List)	Examples
Amino acid metabolism	Maple syrup urine disease, methyl-malonic aciduria, cystinosis
Mucopolysaccharidoses	Hurler's, Hunter's, and Sanfilippo syndromes
Sphingolipid metabolism	Gaucher's, Niemann–Pick, Tay–Sachs diseases
Carbohydrate metabolism	Glycogen storage diseases, galactosemia
Miscellaneous disorders	Lesch–Nyhan syndrome, adrenogenital syndrome, sickle cell anemia, HgbS-C disease

   b. Algorhythmic steps for NTD diagnosis
     (1) **Maternal serum for AFP** (if AFP elevated, consider repeat verification)
     (2) **Ultrasound examination**
     (3) **Amniotic fluid levels of AFP and acetylcholinesterase (ACHE)**
   c. AFP normal reference ranges are reported in terms of "multiples of the median" (**MoM**); laboratories must establish local reference values.
   d. AFP values must be adjusted for the following.
     (1) **Blacks** (10% higher AFP levels than whites, Hispanics, Asians).
     (2) **Maternal diabetes** (AFP levels 20% higher: multiply results by 0.8 to compare with normal reference ranges).
     (3) **Maternal weight** (the larger the mother, the greater the blood volume and the more AFP is diluted).
   e. Interpretation of AFP values
     (1) **AFP ≥2.5 MoM** identifies 90% of **anencephalics**, 80% of **spina bifidas**.
     (2) **AFP ≥2.0 MoM** identifies essentially 100% anencephalics, 90% spina bifidas.
   f. Acetylcholinesterase is a confirmatory electrophoretic test for NTD when AFP is increased.
     (1) **Normal amniotic fluid has one electrophoretic band**: nonspecific cholinesterase.

(2) **NTD show two electrophoretic bands**: nonspecific cholinesterase and ACHE.

g. **Increased maternal AFP with negative ACHE** is associated with multiple births (twins are the most common cause of increased AFP), intrauterine fetal death, congenital nephrosis, exomphalos or gastroschisis, duodenal or esophageal atresia, and cystic hygroma.

h. **Ultrasound** confirms single fetus, establishes fetal age, establishes fetal viability, and may identify congenital defects.

2. **Down's syndrome and other trisomies**. Women ≥35 years of age should be offered amniotic fluid analysis.

a. **Amniotic fluid chromosome analysis** is the "gold standard" test that should be offered to **all women ≥35 years** of age.

b. **Other screening tests** (the following three tests identify 60% of the trisomies).

(1) **Alpha fetoprotein**. Maternal serum AFP is **decreased in trisomy** gestations.

(a) Median serum AFP for women 32–35 years of age with trisomy gestation is 0.7 MoM.

(b) Median serum AFP for women 25–31 years of age with a trisomy gestation is 0.5 MoM.

(c) **MoM ≥1.0 essentially excludes a trisomic fetus.**

(2) **Unconjugated estriol**. Maternal serum levels are **decreased in trisomy** gestations.

(3) **β-HCG**. Maternal serum levels are **increased in trisomy** gestations.

G. **Fetal lung maturity (FLM)**. The respiratory distress syndrome (hyaline membrane disease) is the second most common cause of death in the newborn period, after birth defects. All of the following tests except the lecithin:sphingomyelin (L:S) ratio are affected by amniotic fluid volume (i.e., polyhydramnios may falsely indicate immaturity, whereas oligohydramnios may falsely indicate maturity). All of the following tests, except phosphatidylglycerol (PG), may indicate false maturity in the presence of amniotic blood or meconium (both are rich in lecithin). **The L:S ratio and the PG are the best two laboratory tests for determination of fetal lung maturity** (Table 4-40).

1. **Lecithin:sphingomyelin ratio**. Lecithin is the major component of the lipid in pulmonary surfactant. Sphingomyelin makes up only 2% of pulmonary surfactant, but the 2% is stable through the third trimester. The L:S ratio is the "gold standard" when it includes a cold acetone precipitation step and is done on thin layer (silica) chromatography. **Of fetuses with L/S ≥2.0, 98% are mature.** L:S ratios are not affected by polyhydramnios or oligohydramnios. **Caution: neonates of diabetic mothers** may still get respiratory distress syndrome when the L:S ratio is ≥2.0

2. **Phosphatidylglycerol** is measured by thin-layer (silica) chromatography, or latex fixation test (AmnioStat FLM). Excellent surfactant, PG is first present at ~35 weeks' gestation, and the percentage increases to 10% of total phospholipids at 40 weeks. Fetuses have **lung maturity when PG is**

Table 4-40. Amniotic fluid tests to determine fetal lung maturity (FLM)

Historical Tests	Value Suggesting Maturity
Creatinine	>2.0 mg/dL
Uric acid	≥8.8 mg/dL
Cytologic examination (Nile blue dye)	≥20% orange-stained epithelial cells
Glucose	<10 mg/dL

Current tests	Value Suggesting Immaturity	Value Suggesting Maturity
Lecithin/ sphingomyelin ratio (L/S ratio)[a]	<2.0	≥2.0 (98% of fetuses are mature)
Phosphatidyl-glycerol (PG)[a]		
–TLC chromatography	Absent	Present
–Latex fixation amniostat (FLM)	No agglutination	Agglutination
Lecithin/albumin ratio (TD × FLM) (mg lecithin/g albumin)	<50 mg/g	≥50 mg/g
Foam shake	Surface foam present <30 sec following 15-sec shake	Surface foam present ≥30 sec following 15-sec shake
Lamellar body count/µL ("amniotic particle counting")	<55,000	≥55,000

TLC, thin-layer chromatography.
[a] The L/S ratio and the PG are the two preferred laboratory tests for assessing lung maturity.

present. **Caution: vaginal amniotic fluid pool** (from ruptured membranes) may give false-positive results because some bacteria reportedly synthesize PG (e.g., *E. coli*, *Listeria monocytogenes*, *Gardnerella vaginalis*).

3. **Lecithin (mg):albumin(g) ratio** ("TD×FLM" by Abbott, using fluorescence polarization). Fetal lung maturity is suggested by a ratio ≥50 mg/g.

4. **Lamellar body count** ("amniotic particle counting"). Lamellar bodies are 2–20 fL in size, and are counted with the platelet channel of a hematology analyzer. Fetal lung maturity is suggested by a count ≥55,000/µL.

5. **Foam/shake test**. Shake a mix of amniotic fluid and 95% ethanol (1:1 ratio) for 15 seconds. Fetal lung maturity is suggested when a surface foam layer is present for ≥30 seconds.

6. Foam stability index. This is a more reliable commercial variant of the foam/shake test.

7. AF absorbance at 650 nm is not recommended; it lacks sensitivity and specificity

H. Miscellaneous disorders and amniotic fluid tests

1. Intrauterine growth retardation (chronic hypoxia) is characterized by fetal hyperlipidemia and hyperketonemia. **Hyperketonemia** is reflected by an increased ($\geq$0.5 mmol/L) AF level of **β-hydroxybutyric acid**.

2. Postdates pregnancy (>40 weeks gestation) are associated with increased AF levels of squalene (product of sebaceous glands). The **squalene:cholesterol** ratio is <0.4 at 40 weeks (term) and **>1.0 at 42 weeks**.

3. Chorioamnionitis

a. Clinical signs and symptoms include maternal fever ($\geq$38°C), foul smelling vaginal discharge, uterine tenderness or irritability, and fetal or maternal tachycardia.

b. Definitive diagnosis is made by histologic examination of placental membranes.

c. Laboratory tests include Gram's stain or bacterial culture. Increased **maternal serum C-reactive protein** precedes clinical signs or symptoms by 12–15 hours.

4.7

Clinical Toxicology

Francis M. Urry, Elizabeth L. Frank,
and Paul I. Brown

I. **Introduction. Clinical laboratory toxicology services
have two principal roles**: monitoring of drugs in patients with
various medical conditions (**therapeutic drug monitoring,
TDM**), and detecting toxic substances in known or suspected poisoning cases (**emergency toxicology, ER tox**). In both TDM and
ER tox, the basics of pharmacokinetics should be understood (see
Bibliography).

II. **Therapeutic drug monitoring**

A. **Objective and rationale for TDM**. Therapeutic drug
monitoring is done **to optimize drug therapy** for the individual patient, by allowing clinicians to achieve effective drug levels while minimizing toxicity. TDM allows time and expense savings through the stabilization of the drug therapy, and allows
detection of patient noncompliance with the dosage regimen. In
addition, TDM facilitates changes in drug dosages to compensate
for patients with poor absorption, altered rates of metabolism,
liver or kidney disease, interactions with other drugs, and so on.

B. **Basic TDM principles**

1. **Steady state** is the condition in repetitive oral drug
administration when the processes of drug accumulation in
the blood (absorption and distribution) are in equilibrium with
the processes of elimination (metabolism and excretion). At
steady state, **the drug concentration remains relatively
constant** during the dosing interval. Steady state occurs after
approximately **five half-lives** of the drug (after the initial
dose). Measuring drug levels for TDM before steady state is
achieved is generally **not** productive.

2. **Drug-receptor action and TDM**. To exert a response,
a drug must penetrate physiologic barriers and bind to receptors in the cells of target tissues and organs. Drug measurement at the receptor is not possible; measurement in the blood
is. At steady state, a correlation exists between drug concentration at the receptor and concentration in the blood, which
is a fundamental principle of TDM.

3. **Total versus free drug concentrations**. Drugs bind
to plasma proteins; the extent varies from zero to nearly 100%.
**The free, nonbound drug is believed to be the active
form**, because it can cross membranes and combine with receptors. In some situations, it is important to measure the
free concentration because the total drug concentration can
remain relatively constant, whereas the percent of free drug
increases significantly (causing toxic effects). Conditions that
reduce protein binding (and therefore increase the percent of
free drug) include the nephrotic syndrome, pregnancy, liver
disease, malnutrition, and interactions between drugs, which
result in the displacement of bound drug from plasma proteins.

Free drug measurements are best suited for drugs that are normally highly bound (>90%) to proteins, because a small decrease in the percent of bound drug results in a significant increase in free drug. Free drug measurements are not useful for drugs that are not highly bound. In general, free drug analysis should be reserved for situations in which the total drug concentration does not explain the patient's condition, or when the patient has a condition that may alter the percentage of free drug.

4. Therapeutic range is the range of concentrations in the blood over which most patients will realize the desired therapeutic effect with little or no toxic effects. Therapeutic ranges can be established from clinical trials, or by the laboratory through evaluation of patient tests. A drug therapeutic range is not equivalent to a reference interval for an endogenous biochemical such as glucose. Clinicians use the therapeutic range as a general guide, in combination with observation of the patient.

5. Critical value is the blood drug concentration above which adverse effects begin to occur more frequently and with increased intensity. These effects range from minor problems to life-threatening crises. Several synonyms are used: toxic level, notification level, alarm level, review level, or panic value (see section II.E below for more details).

C. Major categories of drugs monitored (Table 4-41)

1. Antiepileptic drugs (AED). The major AEDs are **phenytoin, phenobarbital, carbamazepine, and valproic acid.** Epilepsy often requires the addition of a second drug (referred to as "adjunctive therapy"). Several new adjunctive AEDs are now available (e.g., lamotrigine, gabapentin, and topiramate).

2. Cardioregulatory. Digoxin is the major drug monitored in congestive heart failure and atrial fibrillation. Monitoring is essential because of the life-threatening toxicity associated with overmedication. Other cardiac drugs that require monitoring are procainamide and its metabolite N-acetylprocainamide (NAPA), amiodarone, and flecainide (Table 4-41).

3. Psychoactives. This category includes drugs for behavioral abnormalities (e.g., depression, anxiety, mood regulation, obsessive-compulsive disorder, schizophrenia). Many of these drugs have ill-defined therapeutic ranges and critical values; some have serious toxic effects at high levels.

4. Antibiotics. Aminoglycosides (e.g., amikacin, gentamicin, tobramycin) and **chloramphenicol** are monitored for their toxicity, and to see that sufficient drug is being used to treat the infectious disease.

5. Immunosuppressants. TDM is helpful to minimize the prospect of life-threatening and highly costly transplant rejection, and to indicate when toxic concentrations may be present.

D. TDM procedures. The following information is generally applicable, but can vary between individual laboratories (see
(*text continues on page 372*)

Table 4-41. Pharmacokinetics, sample requirements, therapeutic ranges, and critical value information for selected TDM drugs

Drug	Specimen	Half-Life	Time to Steady State	Draw Times	Therapeutic Ranges	Critical Values
Amikacin	S,P	2–3 h	Not applicable	30 min postinfusion 30 min preinfusion	Peak 20–30 μg/mL Trough 4–8 μg/mL	>30 >8
Amiodarone and metabolite	S,P	14–107 d	130–535 d	Trough	1.0–3.0 μg/mL; metabolite parallels drug at steady state	>3
Amitriptyline and nortriptyline	S,P (*no SST*)	9–46 h 15–90 h	7–14 d 4–20 d	Trough	95–250 μg/mL (drug + metabolite)	>500
Caffeine	S,P	41–238 h (neonate)	Not applicable	When toxicity noted or with high doses	6–20 μg/mL	>40
Carbamazepine	S,P	18–65 h	Variable	Trough	4–12 μg/mL	>20
Chloramphenicol	S,P (EDTA or citrate)	2–5 h	10–35 h	Capsule: after 60 min Suspension: 1.5–4 h IV: 30–90 min	10–20 μg/mL	>25

Clomipramine and metabolite	S,P (no SST)	12–36 h	4–6 d	Trough	220–500 ng/mL (drug + metabolite)	>900
Cyclosporine A	WB (no heparin)	10–27 h	2–6 d	Trough	Heart and kidney: (method dependent) 1–3 mo post-transplant 350–525 ng/mL >3 mo post-transplant 145–350 ng/mL Liver: 290–525 ng/mL	>700
Desipramine	S (no SST) P (EDTA)	12–54 h	3–11 d	Trough	100–300 ng/mL	>500
Digoxin	S (no SST) P (EDTA)	30–45 h	7–10 d	Trough or 6 h postdose	0.8–2.0 ng/mL	>2.4
Doxepin and nordoxepin	S (no SST) P	8–25 h	2–5 d	Trough or 10–12 h post single dose	100–300 ng/mL (drug + metabolite)	>400
Flecainide	S,P (no SST)	7–22 h 12–27 h (renal patient)	3–5 d	Trough	0.1–1.0 µg/mL	>1.5
Gabapentin	S,P	5–7 h	1–2 d	Trough	2–10 µg/mL (dose-related range)	Not established

continued

Table 4-41. *Continued*

Drug	Specimen	Half-life	Time to Steady State	Draw Times	Therapeutic Ranges	Critical Values
Gentamycin or tobramycin	S,P(EDTA) *no HEP*	1–3 h	Not applicable	30 min postinfusion 30 min preinfusion	Peak 5–10 µg/mL Trough 0.5–2 µg/mL	>12 >2
Imipramine and desipramine	S (*no SST*) P (EDTA)	6–20 h 12–54 h	2–5 d 3–11 d	Trough	150–300 ng/mL (drug + metabolite)	>500
Lamotrigine	S,P	22–37 h	1.2–14 d	Trough	0.5–4.5 µg/mL (dose-related range for 100–600 mg/d)	Not established
Lithium	S,P (*no Li HEP*)	17–58 h	4–6 d	12 h postdose	0.5–1.5 mEq/L	>1.5
Nortriptyline	S,P (*No SST*)	15–90 h	4–20 d	Trough	50–150 ng/mL	>300
Phenobarbital	S,P	2–6 d	4–20 d	Trough	15–40 µg/mL	>50
Phenytoin	S,P (*no SST; no CIT; no OXA*)	Adt 6–60 h Ch 7–29 h	7–21 d (4–8 d with loading doses)	Trough	>2 mo and adults: 10–20 µg/mL 0–2 mo infant: 6–14 µg/mL	>30 >14

Procainamide and NAPA	S,P	2–5 h 6–11 h	15–25 h	Trough	4–10 µg/mL 10–30 µg/mL	>30 (total)
Tacrolimus	WB (*No HEPARIN*)	6–17 h	72 h	Trough	3–15 ng/mL; target ranges vary with transplant type.	>30
Theophylline	S	3–11 h	14–45 h	Trough	Asthma: 10–20 µg/mL	>25
Valproic acid	S,P (*no CIT; no OXA*)	Adt 8–12 h Ch 7–13 h	48–96 h	Trough	Seizure disorders: 50–100 µg/mL Bipolar disorder: 50–125 µg/mL	>150
Vancomycin	S,P (EDTA)	4–6 h	Not applicable	Trough 30 min preinfusion	5–10 µg/mL	>20

Adt, adult; Ch, child; CIT, citrate; d, day; h, hour; Li HEP, lithium heparin; mo, month; NAPA, *N*-acetylprocainamide; OXA, oxalate; P, plasma; S, serum; SST, serum separator tube; TDM, therapeutic drug monitoring; WB, whole blood.

Table 4-41 in conjunction with the following narrative, and consult your own laboratory for additional specifics).

1.   Collection times. Careful attention must be paid to TDM blood collection times in relation to dosing times. **"Trough" concentrations are the most reproducible values**; they ensure that a therapeutic effect is present throughout the dosing interval. Most TDM specimens should be obtained **within 1 hour of the next dose**. If dosing is once per day, the specimen should be drawn 10–12 hours after the dose. Inconsistency in collection time is a major contributor to failure of effective TDM, and can lead to unnecessary dose adjustment and a worsening of the patient's condition.

2.   Specimen requirements. Some tests are performed on whole blood, because the drug distributes significantly into red blood cells (e.g., cyclosporine A and tacrolimus). **Most tests require serum**, which should be collected in standard clot tubes having no anticoagulant and **no gel** separator. Inaccurate TDM measurements (mostly reduced concentrations) can occur in specimens collected in serum separator or silicon gel tubes, and with some anticoagulants. The minimal required specimen volume varies with the analytic technique and the drug concentration. Some TDM tests may require special handling (consult your laboratory).

3.   Analytic methods. TDM tests are performed by immunoassay on automated chemistry instruments, or by gas chromatography (GC), high performance liquid chromatography (HPLC), or coupled techniques such as GC-MS (mass spectrometry) and HPLC-MS. **Immunoassays are faster, require less specimen volume, and may be offered "stat."** However, some tests are not available by immunoassay, and some immunoassays tend to overestimate the concentration of the drug and active metabolites because some inactive metabolites are included in the measurement. **Chromatographic assays are more specific, can separate active from inactive forms of the drug**, but are more time-consuming and are not as adaptable to stat testing.

4.   Run times. Run times and frequency are based on client service needs, the volume of tests, and instrument and staff availability. A request for stat testing is disruptive to productivity, and should be **restricted to a genuine necessity**. Therapeutically monitored drugs (e.g., **phenytoin, phenobarbital, digoxin, cyclosporine, tacrolimus, lithium, and theophylline) are legitimate candidates for stat testing**; most other TDM drugs are not.

E.   Result interpretation

1.   Result integration. TDM results should be interpreted in conjunction with the patient status. Consult with the laboratory whenever a TDM result appears inconsistent with the patient's condition or the dosing regimen, or for any other reason that may raise doubt about the reliability of the result.

2.   Response to critical values. The laboratory should **notify the attending physician** whenever a result is greater than the critical value, and **the cause should be investigated**. The relationship between the time of the last dose and the specimen collection is vital. A patient who missed a dose may take one just before specimen collection, inadvertently generating a peak concentration instead of a trough. Confirm that the specimen was drawn appropriately (e.g., from a clean or properly flushed intravenous line, in the right collection tube). Is the patient showing toxicity? If not, there may be time to repeat the test with another specimen, making sure that appropriate dosing and collection times are followed.

III. Emergency toxicology (ER tox)

A. Objectives. Poisoned patients may present at any time, day or night. To be useful for diagnosis and management, laboratory ER tox testing must be relevant, consistent, reliable, valid, and available around the clock in a short time frame (within 1 hour of the specimen's arrival in the laboratory).

B. Types of ER tox services. The laboratory should provide three categories of testing: (a) tests when toxicant(s) are known; (b) tests when toxicant(s) are unknown; and (c) additional clinical chemistry tests useful in poisoning cases. Tests should focus on toxicants that are relevant to the diagnosis and management of the patient, which include toxicants that occur with high frequency or that cause serious toxicity. The contents and characteristics of each type of service should be developed with input from the emergency department and a regional poison control center, and should address the needs of the geographical area.

1. Common tests for known toxicant(s) (as determined by history, physical examination, or both). See Table 4-41 for therapeutic drugs that require stat testing (e.g., digoxin, lithium, phenobarbital, and theophylline), and Table 4-42 for other toxicants.

a. Acetaminophen. Serious liver damage can occur from acetaminophen overdose. Laboratory measurement of acetaminophen should be performed **within 4 hours** of ingestion or as soon as possible after that. A **Rumack–Matthew nomogram**, which is a log-linear plot of drug concentration against time, is often used to evaluate the need for treatment with the antidote N-acetylcysteine **(Mucomyst)**. The nomogram is not reliable when the poisoning is caused by extended release products or excessive chronic ingestion. Measurement of a second specimen collected 3–4 hours after the first specimen may be used to estimate the drug half-life. The expected half-life of acetaminophen is 1–3 hours; **a half-life >4 hours may indicate the prospect of hepatic necrosis**.

b. Salicylate. Ingestion of aspirin-containing products or preparations that contain methyl salicylate can cause salicylate toxicity. **Metabolic acidosis and an elevated anion gap** (AG) are seen. **Alkalinization of the urine** with sodium bicarbonate is used to accelerate salicylate excretion.

c. Ethanol. Ethanol increases the severity of intoxication by other central nervous system depressing drugs, and in some situations can be life-threatening by itself. A quantitative plasma, serum, or whole blood ethanol value is of use in the management of many intoxi-

(*text continues on page 376*)

Table 4-42. Frequently encountered toxicants in poisoning cases, associated concentrations, and some specific treatment options

Toxicant	Therapeutic/Expected Ranges	Toxic Levels	Therapy/Antidote
Acetaminophen	10–30 µg/mL	>150 µg/mL within 4 h of ingestion; >37.5 µg/mL within 12 h of ingestion	N-acetylcysteine (Mucomyst)
Barbiturates	Varies with particular agent	Varies	Charcoal hemoperfusion; alkaline diuresis for phenobarbital
Benzodiazepines	Varies with agent	Varies with agent	Flumazenil
Carboxyhemoglobin	0.5%–1.5% sat. of Hb; 4%–9% sat. in smokers	Toxic >20% sat. of Hb Lethal >50% sat. of Hb	100% oxygen gas
Ethanol	None	CNS depression >100 mg/dL Potentially lethal >400 mg/dL	
Ethylene glycol	None	Toxic >20 mg/dL	Ethanol or fomepizole; pyridoxine, thiamine. Hemodialysis

Iron	50–175 µg/dL	Potentially toxic 300–500 µg/dL; toxic >500 µg/dL	Deferoxamine mesylate (Desferal)
Methanol	None	Toxic >20 mg/dL Potentially lethal >40 mg/dL	Ethanol or fomepizole; folinic acid, folic acid; Hemodialysis
Opioids	Varies with agent		Naloxone (Narcan)
Salicylate	<100 µg/mL analgesia, antipyresis; 150–300 µg/mL anti-inflammatory	Toxic >500 µg/mL	Sodium bicarbonate
Tricyclic antidepressants	Varies with particular agent	Toxic >500 ng/mL	Sodium bicarbonate

CNS, central nervous system; Hb, hemoglobin; sat., saturation.
Note: Cocaine also is an important toxicant; however, urine is used to qualitatively identify its presence or absence, and concentrations are not usually provided.

cations. Ethanol concentration also is monitored when it is **used as an antidote** in ethylene glycol or methanol poisoning (ethanol minimizes the formation of toxic metabolites).

d. Ethylene glycol, methanol, and isopropanol. Toxicity is caused by metabolic products (glycolic acid and oxalate; formic acid and formaldehyde; and acetone, respectively), and may be life-threatening. Specific tests by gas chromatography can be used to initiate and monitor therapy, but are not available in every laboratory. However, almost every laboratory can assist in the diagnosis of toxic alcohol poisoning by providing osmolality testing. **Serum osmolality** (measured by the freezing point depression method) **can be used to detect substances such as ethanol, ethylene glycol (EG), and methanol (MeOH)**. Sodium, glucose, and urea nitrogen concentrations can be used to calculate the serum osmolality. The osmolal gap (OG), or difference between the measured and calculated serum osmolality, is used to assess the presence of unmeasured substances. Ethanol is the most common toxic cause of an elevated OG. Both EG and MeOH also produce an elevated OG and metabolic acidosis.

A rapid screening method for serum EG is also available, based on its interference in triglyceride measurements that use glycerol dehydrogenase as a reagent enzyme. If EG toxicity is suspected but the EG screen is unavailable, rule out ethanol by specific testing, and then tentatively diagnose EG based on the findings of metabolic acidosis, an increased AG, and discrepancies between the measured and calculated osmolality. A blood sample can then be sent out for the specific EG test. Ethanol or fomepizole (4-methylpyrazole) are given as antidotes for both EG and MeOH poisoning. Administration of bicarbonate, hemodialysis, or both may be necessary. **Diagnosis of poisoning caused by EG, MeOH, or isopropanol may be aided by the presence of urine calcium oxalate crystals, visual disturbances, or acetonemia/acetonuria, respectively**.

e. Digoxin. Accidental or intentional digoxin overdoses **can be lethal, because of cardiac arrhythmias**. The elderly are particularly susceptible. Immunotherapy with digoxin-specific Fab fragments (**Digibind**) irreversibly removes digoxin from myocardial tissue and other binding sites, and increases its urinary elimination.

f. Theophylline. Theophylline toxicity affects multiple organ systems; it can progress rapidly and **may result in death**. Serial measurements of serum theophylline should be used to establish the extent of the intoxication. Management of the overdose with a **sustained release formulation is particularly important.**

g. Lithium. Lithium has a narrow therapeutic range; the hallmark of intoxication is **neuromuscular irritability. Hemodialysis** may be warranted in symptomatic patients with serum lithium concentrations >**4.0 mm/L at 6 hours** postingestion.

h. Phenobarbital. Overdose may result in extended **respiratory depression, coma, and death**. Phenobarbital levels are useful in making the diagnosis, but may not correlate well with the severity of toxicity. **Hemodialysis or hemoperfusion** may be necessary in the severely toxic patient.

i. Iron. Accidental iron poisoning in children often results from ingesting childrens' chewable multivitamins containing iron, or ingesting adult iron supplements, and is **one of the leading causes of fatal poisoning in children** <6 years of age. Toxicity is caused by direct corrosion of mucosal surfaces, oxidative injury, and free radical damage, and can result in profound shock and metabolic acidosis. Serum iron levels should be drawn every 2 hours for the first 6–8 hours following a toxic ingestion. Chelation therapy with intravenous deferoxamine mesylate (**Desferal**) is used, based in part on the iron concentration.

j. Carbon monoxide (CO). CO binds more tightly to hemoglobin than oxygen does; it displaces the oxygen and causes tissue hypoxia. Symptoms of CO intoxication are highly variable and may not correlate well with the percent of carboxyhemoglobin. Measurement of carboxyhemoglobin requires a **heparinized arterial or venous blood specimen using a spectrophotometric method (Co-oximeter**), and is sometimes performed by a service other than the clinical laboratory. Arterial blood gas assays should **not** be used to evaluate CO exposure. Treatment for CO is administration of 100% oxygen gas.

2. Tests when toxicant(s) are unknown. When an apparent poisoning case has no indication of the specific toxicant(s) involved, a group of tests commonly referred to as a "tox screen" may be helpful. A tox screen may be indicated under the following situations: when the history is unreliable or absent, or the patient is known to have a pattern of intoxications or suicidal gestures; unexplained acidosis or cardiotoxicity; multiple drug ingestion; coma or other altered mental state; seizures of undetermined history; and head trauma with neurologic symptoms. The contents of the tox screen should be **directed toward drugs having specific treatment**, and usually includes quantitative serum testing for acetaminophen, ethanol, and salicylate; the osmolality screen (by freezing point depression) for ethylene glycol, methanol, and isopropanol; qualitative serum testing for tricyclic antidepressants, barbiturates, and benzodiazepines; and qualitative urine testing for cocaine, sympathomimetic amines, and opiates. These tests usually rely on **immunoassay methods** available on automated clinical analyzers, making them available without specialized instrumentation and expertise.

3. Additional clinical chemistry tests. In addition to specific toxicant and freezing point depression osmolality testing, the clinical laboratory performs other important tests that help evaluate conditions such as **metabolic acidosis**. Ethanol, ethylene glycol, iron, methanol, and salicylate are most likely to produce metabolic acidosis and an elevated **anion gap**. Serum electrolyte concentrations can be used to calculate the AG [in general, AG = (sodium) − (bicarbonate + chloride)]. In addition to metabolic acidosis, poisoning can result in excessive vomiting and a serious acid-base and electrolyte imbalance. **Arterial blood gases**, in addition to **electrolytes**, are useful in assessing acid-base balance. Follow-up clinical laboratory tissue and organ function testing is helpful after the emergency has been addressed.

BIBLIOGRAPHY

Therapeutic Drug Monitoring

Evans WE, Schentag JJ, Jusko WJ, eds. *Applied pharmacokinetics: principles of therapeutic drug monitoring*, 3rd ed. Vancouver, WA: Applied Therapeutics, Inc., 1992.

Moyer TP. Therapeutic drug monitoring. In: Ashwood ER, Burtis CA, eds. *Tietz textbook of clinical chemistry*, 3rd ed. Philadelphia: WB Saunders, 1999:862–905.

Emergency Toxicology

Porter WH. Clinical Toxicology. In: Ashwood, Burtis, eds. *Tietz textbook of clinical chemistry*, 3rd ed. Philadelphia: WB Saunders, 1999:906–981.

Viccelho P, ed. *Emergency toxicology*, 2nd ed. Philadelphia: Lippincott-Raven, 1998.

Laboratory Diagnosis of Endocrine Disorders

William D. Odell

I. Introduction. The diagnosis and correct treatment of endocrine disorders require a thorough medical history and a full physical examination. If these suggest a specific diagnosis, then laboratory testing is used to confirm or deny the likelihood of the diagnosis. **The laboratory results should not be used as the sole criterion for a diagnosis.** Be aware that normal and abnormal reference ranges vary according to methodology, instrumentation, and patient populations, and reference ranges should be formulated for each laboratory.

Each physician must be familiar with endocrine physiology and be able to predict expected hormone measurements for a given clinical situation. **"Normal" values are often very abnormal under certain clinical conditions**. For example, a "normal" serum thyrotropin (TSH) in a patient with hyperthyroidism is abnormal. Similarly a "normal" 8 AM serum cortisol level is abnormal if the sample is drawn at 6 PM.

II. The thyroid system

A. Normal physiology

1. Thyronines. The thyroid synthesizes tetraiodothyronine (T_4 or thyroxine) and some triiodothyronine (T_3), which are stored as part of the huge molecule thyroglobulin. T_4 (and to a lesser extent T_3) is then enzymatically cleaved from **thyroglobulin** and secreted into blood. T_4 is a prohormone and may be metabolized to the **more active T_3** in peripheral tissues, or metabolized to **inactive forms** [i.e., **reverse T_3** ($R–T_3$) and T_4 **conjugates** such as T_4 sulphate]. **Almost all of the circulating T_4 and T_3 are bound to proteins,** such as; thyroxine-binding globulin (TBG), thyroxine binding prealbumin (TBPA) and albumin (ALB); and 0.01% of T_4 is unbound or **free** (which is the **biologically active form**). T_4 and T_3 have many body functions, including regulating the basal metabolic rate, bone growth, nervous system maturation, and metabolic processes involving carbohydrates, proteins, and fat. **Thyroid disorders are the second most common endocrine problem** faced by clinicians (diabetes is the first).

2. Regulatory control. Four components comprise the thyroidal system, each connected by neuronal or hormonal signals (Fig. 4-5). The **hypothalamus** secretes thyrotropin-releasing hormone (**TRH**) and somatostatin (**SST**), which stimulate **pituitary** secretion of thyroid-stimulating hormone (**TSH** or thyrotropin). TSH acts on the thyroid gland to (a) stimulate secretion of thyroxine (T_4); (b) stimulate increased iodide trapping and new hormone synthesis; and (c) stimulate thyroid cell hypertrophy (goiter development). T_4 and T_3 provide **negative feedback control** to the pituitary ("gross tuning") and to the hypothalamus ("fine tuning").

thyrotropin = TSH

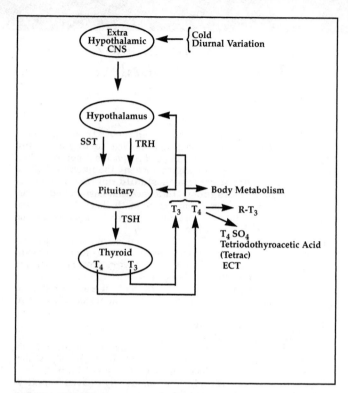

Fig. 4-5. Control of TSH secretion. R-T₃, reverse T₃; TRH, thyrotropin-releasing hormone; TSH, thyroid-stimulating hormone; SST, somatostatin.

Increases or decreases in the amounts of any of the binding proteins described (e.g., increases caused by pregnancy or estrogen therapy, decreases caused by liver disease) will increase or decrease concentrations of *total* T₄, whereas free T₄ and T₃ are maintained at normal concentrations. **Hyperthyroxinemia, which causes no symptoms, should not be mistakenly diagnosed as hyperthyroidism**.

Most TSH is secreted at night (i.e., diurnal variation); however, "normal" TSH reference ranges quoted by laboratories are daytime ranges. In pituitary or hypothalamic causes of hypothyroidism, the nocturnal surges of TSH secretion may be abolished, whereas the daytime TSH secretion is maintained. Hypothyroidism caused by hypothalamic or pituitary disorders, thus, can be associated with a low, free T₄ and a "normal" TSH.

B.   Measurement of thyronines. Relatively inexpensive and accurate **methods of measuring free T₄ are available**, and should be used. This avoids the confusion of using the outdated

T_3 resin uptake and total T_4 measurements to calculate a "free T_4 index," which is only an estimate of free T_4, and is affected by changes in binding proteins.

C. Hyperthyroidism (thyrotoxicosis). Symptoms of hyperthyroidism include nervousness, sweating, tachycardia, increased appetite, weight loss, insomnia, heat intolerance, exophthalmos (in Graves' disease), and pretibial myxedema (in Graves' disease). Causes of hyperthyroidism are listed in Table 4-43. For diagnosing hyperthyroidism, free T_4 and TSH are always recommended. **All of the causes of thyrotoxicosis listed in Table 4-44 should have a suppressed TSH, except a pituitary TSH-producing tumor, which may have a "normal" or elevated TSH.**

  1. Autoimmune thyroid disease. This term includes **Graves' disease, Hashitoxicosis, and autoimmune hypothyroidism**: it includes a spectrum ranging from hypothyroidism to hyperthyroidism, which is determined by the amount and kinds of autoantibodies being produced. **Thyroid-stimulating antibodies** (thyroid receptor antibodies or **TRAB**) cause hyperthyroidism with a diffusely enlarged thyroid gland (goiter) and, in some patients, **exophthalmos**, **pretibial myxedema**, or both. The latter two signs are separate autoimmune manifestations of controversial etiology and, when present, are pathognomonic of Graves' disease. Expected laboratory findings include **elevations in total T_4, total T_3, free T_4, and free T_3, a suppressed and often undetectable TSH, increased thyroid-stimulating immunoglobulin, and normal concentrations of all thyronine-binding proteins**. Radioiodine uptake by the thyroid (^{123}I or ^{131}I) is elevated, and scans generally show **diffuse uptake**. Occasionally, "cold" or irregular areas may be seen because of lymphocyte infiltration. If the history and physical findings are characteristic, laboratory data can be limited to measurement of free T_4, TSH, and radioiodine uptake.

  2. Postpartum hyperthyroidism. Postpartum thyroid disease can cause thyrotoxicosis or, more commonly, hypothyroidism. It occurs in women with a predisposition for autoimmune thyroid disease, but in whom the expression has been

Table 4-43. Causes of hyperthyroidism

Autoimmune thyroid disease
Multinodular goiter
Single toxic nodule
Subacute thyroiditis
Thyrotropin producing pituitary adenoma
Gestational trophoblastic neoplasm
Postpartum thyroid disease
Hyperemesis gravidarum
Exogenous thyroid hormone
Metastatic thyroid cancer
Iodine induced

Table 4-44. Expected laboratory results in hyperthyroidism

Disorder	TSH	Free T4	Other Findings
Autoimmune thyroid disease	Low	High	High TRAB, high iodine uptake
Multinodular goiter	Low	High	Neg TRAB
Single toxic nodule	Low	Normal or high	High T_3, neg TRAB
Subacute thyroiditis	Low	High	Neg TRAB, zero iodine uptake
Thytropin (TSH) pituitary adenoma	Normal or high	High	Neg TRAB, high iodine uptake
Gestational neoplasm	Low	High	Very high hCG
Postpartum hyperthyroidism	Low	High	Thyroid antibodies positive, low iodine uptake
Hyperemesis gravidarum	Low or normal	High	High hCG
Exogenous thyroxine	Low	High	Neg TRAB, low iodine uptake
Exogenous triiodothyronine	Low	Low T_4 and low free T_4	High T_3 and high free T_3, low iodine uptake
Metastatic thyroid cancer	Low	High	
Iodine induced	Variable	High	Low iodine uptake

hCG, human chorionic gonadotropin; TRAB, thyroid receptor antibodies.

suppressed by the normal immune alterations of pregnancy. After delivery, the autoimmune disease emerges, usually transiently.

3. **"Toxic" adenomas and multinodular goiter**. Single "toxic" adenomas produce T_4 or, occasionally, T_3. **In T_3 adenomas, TSH is suppressed; total and free T_4 may be normal, whereas total and free T_3 are increased**. These nodules are usually palpable by the clinician who can distinguish them from the diffuse goiter of Graves' disease or the multinodular goiter. Thyroid scan shows a single "hot" nodule.

4. **Subacute thyroiditis** is a transient viral-related thyrotoxicosis that is often associated with a preceding upper respiratory infection, and spontaneously subsides in several weeks. It causes an uncontrolled release of stored thyroxine, and is not caused by TSH or thyroid-stimulating antibodies. The thyroid is usually tender and may have transient nodules. **Free T_4 is elevated and TSH is suppressed;** in con-

trast to Graves' disease, however, **radioiodine uptake is extremely low**.

    5. Gestational trophoblastic neoplasms (e.g., choriocarcinoma, hydatid mole) can cause hyperthyroidism because of greatly increased production of an altered human chorionic gonadotropin (**CG**), which is biochemically similar to TSH. In any woman of reproductive age who is thyrotoxic, measurement of CG is warranted to diagnose either unexpected normal pregnancy or gestational neoplasm.

    6. Hyperemesis gravidarum can cause transient thyrotoxicosis from unknown mechanisms. The thyrotoxicosis is not usually treated. TSH may be low or normal and free T_4 is increased (note that in normal pregnancy, free T_4 remains normal, whereas *total* T_4 and T_3 increase because of estrogen-induced increases in TBG).

    7. Iodine-induced thyrotoxicosis is a mixture of entities. Some cases involve iodine-induced immune abnormalities that cause thyrotoxicosis. Other cases involve patients with underlying autoimmune thyroid disease who are also iodine deficient (poor diet), and the introduction of dietary iodine allows expression of the disease.

D. Hypothyroidism. Among the symptoms of hypothyroidism are cretinism (if the defect is congenital), lethargy, bradycardia, cold intolerance, hypothermia, and myxedema. Table 4-45 lists the causes of hypothyroidism.

    If hypothyroidism is suspected, measurement of free T_4 and TSH are usually adequate. **In all causes of hypothyroidism (except hypothalamic or pituitary causes), TSH secretion is increased and is a very sensitive indicator for hypothyroidism**. In subclinical hypothyroidism, free T_4 is normal and TSH is minimally elevated (e.g. 5–12 µU/mL). In clinical hypothyroidism, free T_4 is low and TSH more highly elevated. Radioiodine uptake by the thyroid is low in all causes of hypothyroidism except some kinds of goitrogen exposure. For example, compounds that interfere with organification cause increased iodine trapping, but no hormonogenesis, leading to hypothyroidism and an increased TSH.

    In **autoimmune thyroid hypothyroidism**, antibodies such as **antithyroid peroxidase** (antiTPO, a.k.a., **antimicrosomal antibodies**) and **antithyroglobulin** are elevated. This can result in goiter formation from lymphocytic infiltrates and hypertrophy of remaining thyroid cells. Antibodies that prevent

Table 4-45. Causes of hypothyroidism

Autoimmune thyroid disease
Goitrogen exposure
Iodine deficiency
Thyroid ablation (radioiodine or surgery)
Biochemical defects in hormonogenesis
Thyroid agenesis or dysgenesis
Iodine induced
Hypothalamic/pituitary disease

TSH from binding, but do not activate the receptor, can result in hypothyroidism without goiter.

E.   "Goiter" is a term that simply refers to an **enlarged thyroid from any cause** (e.g, inflammatory, neoplastic); function may be normal, increased, or decreased. **Most goiters have normal thyroid function** (e.g., 90% of multinodular goiters and almost all "colloid" goiters).

F.   Euthyroid sick syndrome is also known as "low T_3 syndrome" or "thyroid intensive care unit (ICU) syndrome." Euthyroid sick syndrome is a form of biochemical hypothyroidism produced as T_4 is shifted away from forming T_3 and shifted toward formation of the inert rT_3 and T_4 conjugates. This occurs in simple fasts for 24 hours or more, and shifts fuel utilization from carbohydrates and protein to fatty acids. Oxygen consumption and body temperature also decrease. Total T_4 and TSH usually remain within normal limits.

III.   The adrenal system

A.   Normal physiology

1.   **Adrenal hormones**. The adrenal glands secrete glucocorticoids (e.g., **cortisol**), mineralocorticoids [e.g., **aldosterone (ALDO)**], and **sex steroids** [e.g., dehydroepiandrosterone sulfate (DHEAS) and dehydroepiandrosterone (DHEA)].

    a.   Cortisol. The adrenal does not store cortisol, and requires immediate stimulation by adrenocorticotropic hormone (ACTH or corticotropin) to synthesize it. Cortisol helps the body to adapt to stress; inhibits inflammation; has anti-insulin effects; catabolizes proteins, collagen, bone, and fat; and so forth.

    b.   Aldosterone stimulates Na^+ and water resorption, and K^+ secretion, in the kidneys.

    c.   DHEAS and DHEA are androgen precursors. They are converted in peripheral tissues first to androstenedione and then to testosterone and dihydrotestosterone.

2.   **Regulatory control**. The **hypothalamus secretes corticotropin-releasing hormone** (CRH, Fig. 4-6), which **stimulates pituitary ACTH secretion**; this is greatly augmented by arginine vasopressin (AVP). **ACTH acts on the adrenal cortex to stimulate secretion of cortisol, aldosterone, and sex steroids**. Continued excess ACTH action leads to adrenal hypertrophy. The secretion of aldosterone is also controlled by the renin-angiotensin system, and remains fairly normal in patients with ACTH deficiency. **Cortisol provides negative feedback control** of ACTH by inhibiting pituitary synthesis, and by inhibiting hypothalamic secretion of CRH. Higher central nervous areas also modulate ACTH secretion; **any stress (physical or emotional) increases CRH and ACTH secretion**, overriding cortisol suppression.

Approximately 90% of plasma cortisol is bound to proteins [75% to cortisol-binding globulin (CBG), and 10% to albumin]; **10% of plasma cortisol is free**, which is the biologically active form. Increases in CBG (e.g., caused by estrogen therapy) can increase the total cortisol, but the free cortisol concentration stays the same.

B.   Measurement of ACTH and cortisol. A striking diurnal pattern of ACTH is seen and, hence, cortisol secretion; both reach

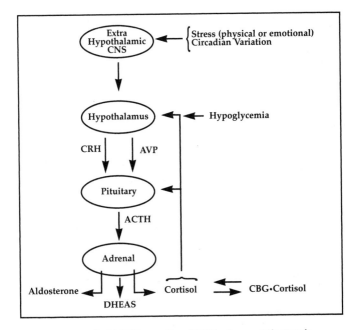

Fig. 4-6. Control of ACTH secretion. ACTH, adrenocorticotropic hormone; AVP, arginine vasopressin; CRH, cortisol-releasing hormone; DHEAS, dehydroepiandrosterone sulfate.

highest blood levels in the early morning (6:00–8:00 AM) and are **lowest in early evening**. Normal cortisol and ACTH reference ranges are available for 6–8 AM, 4–6 PM, and midnight. "Normal" 8 AM cortisol and ACTH concentrations, if present without diurnal change throughout 24 hours, could result in Cushing's syndrome. This scenario is seen in some patients with Cushing's disease, which is the pituitary-dependent form of Cushing's syndrome. Therefore, a single measurement of morning cortisol is not an optimal test for the diagnosis of Cushing's syndrome. Midnight measurements are better screening tests; however, being awakened by an alarm clock can cause transient elevations in cortisol. **The 24-hour urine cortisol test is the best screening procedure for Cushing's syndrome.**

  C. **Cushing's syndrome**

    1. **Definition, symptoms, and causes. Cushing's syndrome refers to the clinical manifestations of excess glucocorticoid action, regardless of the cause.** Symptoms include rounded facies, truncal obesity (with "buffalo hump"), cutaneous striae, osteoporosis, susceptibility to infection, and so on. The causes of Cushing's syndrome are listed in Table 4-46. **Cushing's disease is pituitary (ACTH)-dependent Cushing's syndrome.** Nonpituitary tumor production of ACTH ("ectopic" ACTH syndrome) is another cause of Cushing's syndrome. A small amount of ACTH and ACTH precur-

Table 4-46.   Causes of Cushing's syndrome (CS)

ACTH-dependent causes
–Pituitary dependent: Cushing's disease (65% of patients with CS) and cyclic Cushing's diseases (very rare)
–"Ectopic" ACTH syndrome (20% of CS): Carcinomas of the lung (mostly oat cells; comprises about 50% of ectopic ACTH cases), carcinoma of the thymus (10% of ectopic), medullary carcinoma of the thyroid (5% of ectopic), bronchial adenoma or carcinoid (2% of ectopic), and miscellaneous carcinomas

ACTH-independent (adrenal) causes (10% of CS): Adrenal adenoma, adrenal carcinoma, macronodular hyperplasia, micronodular hyperplasia, ACTH-independent hyperplasia

Miscellaneous causes: Alcoholic pseudo-Cushing's, food-dependent Cushing's, exogenous glucocorticoids

---

ACTH, adrenocorticotropic hormone (corticotropin).
[a] Excluding patients receiving exogenous glucocorticoids (e.g., prednisone).

sors are normally produced by most tissues [e.g., liver, kidney, central nervous system (CNS)] and presumably act as cytokines or neurotransmitters; thus, cancer production of ACTH is not truly ectopic, but increased expression of local tissue production.

   2.   **Laboratory assessment**
     a.   **Midnight cortisol** measurements can be used as a screening test (elevated in Cushing's syndrome). The **"low dose" dexamethasone suppression test** is another screening test. In normal individuals, 1 mg of dexamethasone given at bedtime suppresses the nocturnal rise of ACTH and cortisol, resulting in 8 AM cortisol values <3 µg% (>3 µg% in Cushing's). However, the **24-hour urine cortisol is the preferred diagnostic test.**
     b.   **24-hour urine cortisol. In all causes of Cushing's syndrome** (except administration of exogenous steroids and cyclic Cushing's disease in remission), the 24-hour urine cortisol is elevated (all of which is free cortisol). Both urine creatinine and cortisol should be quantified; the urine creatinine is to assess adequacy of urine collection. In an otherwise healthy outpatient, increased 24-hour urine cortisol indicates Cushing's syndrome, and should be repeated with a second independent collection. Remember that severe stress, including acute psychiatric disease or physical trauma, can increase 24-hour urine cortisol values as well. For children, cortisol:creatinine ratios may be used with short time or spot urine collections.
     c.   **Laboratory investigation of Cushing's syndrome.** Once the presence of Cushing's syndrome has been established, **the next step is to determine whether or not it is ACTH dependent.**
       (1)   **ACTH-independent causes** (Table 4-46). **ACTH is very low** at all times of the day, whereas the **24-hour urine cortisol is increased.**

(a) Adrenal macronodular hyperplasia. The adrenal contains multiple fairly large nodules commonly visible by magnetic resonance imaging (MRI); the cause is unknown.

(b) Micronodular dysplasia is a congenital disorder, involving multiple, small, pigmented nodules; atrophic intervening adrenal tissue; and decreased total adrenal weight. It is often diagnosed in childhood, and can be mistaken for congenital adrenal hyperplasia (CAH).

(c) ACTH-independent, bilateral adrenal hyperplasia, a rare cause of Cushing's syndrome; in some cases, it is caused by ectopically located catecholamine receptors.

(2) ACTH-dependent causes. ACTH is "high normal" or elevated (midnight values are almost always elevated), and the **24-hour urine cortisol is increased**.

(a) Cyclic Cushing's is a very rare entity and probably represents cyclic overproduction of CRH.

(b) Cushing's disease (pituitary-dependent Cushing's syndrome) is caused by **ACTH-secreting pituitary adenomas**. The 8 AM ACTH values are slightly elevated in most patients, but can be in the high "normal" range; midnight ACTH values are almost always increased.

(c) Ectopic ACTH syndrome is characterized by **tumor production (other than pituitary adenomas) of ACTH precursors** that are converted to biologically active ACTH. ACTH precursors are formed by most carcinomas; those causing the "ectopic" ACTH syndrome convert the precursors more efficiently. **ACTH measurements are generally very high— much higher than seen in Cushing's disease**. Other tests that help to distinguish "ectopic" ACTH production from pituitary adenomas (Cushing's disease) include the following:.

- **PROACTH immunoassays**: these help diagnose subtle ectopic ACTH syndromes by identifying the ectopic ACTH precursors.
- **"High"-dose dexamethasone suppression. Normal ACTH-secreting pituitary cells are very "suppressible" by glucocorticoids** (ACTH levels will dramatically decrease). **Pituitary adenomas are mildly suppressible. Ectopic ACTH syndromes are not generally suppressible**. Thus, 4–8 mg of dexamethasone (high dose) given at bedtime will moderately suppress 8 AM ACTH and cortisol from pituitary adenomas, but generally will not do so in "ectopic" ACTH syndrome. However, the "ectopic" ACTH syndrome can be very difficult to distinguish from pituitary adenomas in some cases of bronchial carcinoid or adenoma and CRH-producing tumors, which also show suppression with high-dose dexamethasone.

- **Petrosal vein catheterization with measurement of ACTH** can distinguish pituitary sources of ACTH from ectopic sources. Simultaneous (or as nearly so as possible) blood samples are drawn from both right and left petrosal veins and a peripheral vein. **Pituitary adenomas show a striking ACTH gradient** from the side of the pituitary harboring the adenoma. Ectopic sources of ACTH show no gradient in the pituitary veins.
- **Pituitary and adrenal imaging should be reserved until *after* the laboratory tests** establish the diagnosis of Cushing's syndrome and the probable cause, because incidental pituitary and adrenal adenomas are common in otherwise normal individuals.

(3) **Miscellaneous causes of Cushing's syndrome**

(a) **Food-dependent Cushing's** syndrome appears to be caused by ectopically located gastric inhibitory peptide (GIP) receptors, which cause GIP-stimulated cortisol secretion.

(b) **Alcoholic pseudo-Cushing's** syndrome occurs in some heavy alcoholics. The 24-hour urine cortisol is increased and suppression with high dose dexamethasone is present. Abstinence from alcohol for several weeks reverses these abnormalities. In any alcoholic who is suspected of having Cushing's disease, it is wise to retest cortisol values after alcohol withdrawal.

D. Adrenal insufficiency

  1. Symptoms and causes. Symptoms of acute adrenal insufficiency include shock (e.g., in the Waterhouse–Friderichsen syndrome); among the chronic symptoms are skin pigmentation, fatigue, hypotension, weight loss, hair loss, and menstrual abnormalities. The causes of adrenal insufficiency are relatively few (Table 4-47). Generally, the diagnosis by laboratory testing is easy if performed before treatment.

Table 4-47.   Causes of adrenal insufficiency

ACTH deficiency
Isolated ACTH deficiency
Hypopituitarism
Post-removal of ACTH adenoma
CRH deficiency

Primary adrenal insufficiency
Autoimmune
Agenesis or dysplasia
Adrenoleukodystrophy
Infiltration (e.g., tuberculosis or neoplasm)
Hemorrhage
Surgical removal
Post-treatment of Cushing's syndrome
Enzymatic defects in hormonogenesis

ACTH, adrenocorticotropic hormone (corticotropin); CRH, corticotropin-releasing hormone.

2. ACTH deficiency is relatively common in patients with large pituitary or hypothalamic tumors. In addition, resection of an ACTH-producing adenoma causes transient ACTH insufficiency for weeks or months, because of the prolonged prior suppression of the hypothalamus and the induced insensitivity of the adrenals. When such patients are on hydrocortisone replacement after surgery and the dose has slowly but appropriately been decreased to 10 mg twice daily, simple assessment can be periodically made to ascertain whether endogenous secretion has returned. The patient omits the nighttime dose of hydrocortisone, and ACTH or cortisol is measured the next morning. The metabolism of cortisol is rapid; exogenous cortisol will be undetectable the following day. The presence of any cortisol 24 hours after a 10-mg dose reflects endogenous secretion.

3. Laboratory assessment of adrenal insufficiency. Plasma ACTH and serum cortisol should be measured at 8 AM and, if abnormal, should be followed by ACTH stimulation tests. In an emergency, ACTH and cortisol should be drawn immediately and replacement begun with hydrocortisone before results are known.

  a. ACTH and cortisol tests. If cortisol is very low (<4 μg%) and ACTH is low, ACTH deficiency is likely. If cortisol is low and ACTH is elevated, adrenal insufficiency is likely. Remember, however, that ACTH secretion is pulsatile and single samples can be misleading.

  b. ACTH stimulation tests. Baseline values of cortisol are drawn at 8 AM. Cosyntropin (synthetic ACTH) (1 μg) is then given intravenously (IV), and cortisol is again measured 1 hour following the ACTH. In a healthy individual, the cortisol level should double in 1 hour. **The cortisol level will not significantly increase in cases of adrenal insufficiency**. Diagnosis is difficult in patients with partial ACTH deficiency. They generally have 8 AM cortisol in the low or "low normal" range (e.g., 6–12 μg%). In such patients, either the insulin hypoglycemia provocative test or an overnight metyrapone test can be performed.

  c. The insulin tolerance test is the "gold standard" for assessing possible partial ACTH deficiency. Insulin (0.1 U/kg body weight) is given IV (0.05 U if adrenal insufficiency is highly likely). ACTH and cortisol are measured just before insulin is given and cortisol is measured 30, 60, and 90 minutes following the insulin. In healthy individuals, cortisol is greater than 20 μg% following the test. To be valid, however, glucose must drop significantly, to 40 mg% or lower, and with such decreases all patients have symptoms of hypoglycemia. Once hypoglycemia is achieved, glucose can be given IV without invalidating the test. A physician or highly experienced nurse practitioner should be present during the test.

  d. Metyrapone test. Metyrapone (30 mg/kg body weight; 2 g for a normal adult) is given at 1 PM. Serum cortisol, 11-deoxycortisol (Cmpd S), and plasma ACTH are measured at 8 AM the next day. The assay for cortisol must not cross-react with deoxycortisol. Normal responses include a decrease in cortisol to <5 μg%, with an increase in 11 deoxycortisol to >7–8 µg%. ACTH should increase to high normal or above the normal 8 AM values.

   e.   Any patient with ACTH insufficiency should be evaluated for other anterior pituitary hormone deficiencies, and an MRI scan of the hypothalamus and pituitary are warranted.

IV.   The renin-angiotensin-aldosterone system

   A.   Normal physiology and regulation. Renin is produced by the juxtaglomerular cells (JG cells) on the afferent arterioles of the kidneys (Fig. 4-7). Decreases in perceived pulse pressure in the arteriole leads to increased renin production and secretion. Renin, an enzyme, **acts on angiotensinogen** (produced by the liver) to form **angiotensin I,** a prohormone. Angiotensin I is rapidly cleaved by **angiotensin-converting enzyme** (ACE), which is present on all vascular endothelium, to **angiotensin II, a potent vasoconstrictor**. Angiotensin II also **directly stimulates the secretion of aldosterone** by the adrenal cortex, and independently acts on the kidney to enhance salt and water retention. Although short-term changes in ACTH can modify aldosterone secretion, the main control of aldosterone is mediated by angiotensin.

   B.   Hyperaldosteronism. Hyperaldosteronism can be primary or secondary (Table 4-48). Symptoms of hyperaldosteronism include hypertension and hypokalemic acidosis.

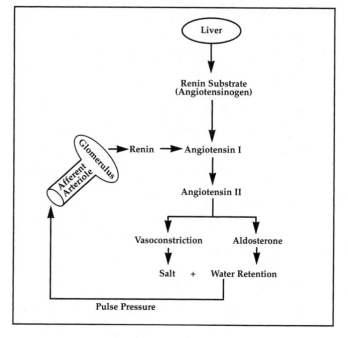

Fig. 4-7.   Renin-angiotensin system.

Table 4-48.   Causes of hyperaldosteronism or excess mineralocorticoid production

Primary hyperaldosteronism (Conn's syndrome)
Adrenal adenoma or carcinoma
Bilateral or unilateral hyperplasia
Glucocorticoid-suppressible or nonsuppressible
11-β hydroxysteroid dehydrogenase deficiency
Licorice ingestion

Secondary hyperaldosteronism
Many causes, including all those of congestive heart failure, hypovolemia, renal artery stenosis, renin-producing tumors, etc.

1.   **Primary hyperaldosteronism**. This rare group of disorders involves primary adrenal disease. Primary hyperaldosteronism is associated with **elevated 24-hour urine aldosterone or mineralocorticoids, with suppressed plasma renin levels**. It is a rare cause of hypertension (<1% of cases). Hypokalemia is present in most patients; therefore, any hypertensive patient with hypokalemia, who is not receiving diuretics, should be evaluated for hyperaldosteronism. Because hypokalemia itself can directly decrease aldosterone secretion, it is wise to restore potassium to normal before measuring aldosterone.

a.   **Adrenal adenomas, carcinoma, or hyperplasia. Solitary adenomas are the most common causes of primary hyperaldosteronism**. Carcinoma and bilateral hyperplasia are rare causes.

b.   **Glucocorticoid-suppressible hyperaldosteronism** is a hereditary disorder associated with abnormal expression of aldosterone synthase. Administration of dexamethasone (0.5 mg every 6 h for 3–4 weeks) will strikingly suppress aldosterone production.

c.   **Hereditary 11-βhydroxysteroid dehydrogenase (11-βOHSD) deficiency**; 11-βOHSD rapidly converts cortisol (which has mineralocorticoid activity) to cortisone (which does not). 11-βOHSD deficiency allows a build-up of the active mineralocorticoid, which then suppresses aldosterone and renin secretion. This disorder is usually detected early in life. Treatment with dexamethasone may reverse the mineralocorticoid effects.

d.   **Licorice ingestion inhibits 11-βOHSD**

2.   **Secondary hyperaldosteronism. Secondary hyperaldosteronism is common and has many causes**, including congestive heart failure, renal hypertension, and hypovolemia. **Renin-producing tumors, which are relatively rare** causes of hyperaldosteronism, are usually renal in origin (e.g., nephroblastomas, juxtaglomerular tumors, rarely hemangiopericytoma), but **extrarenal tumors** have also been described, including adenocarcinomas, hepatomas, paragangliomas, and spindle cell tumors of the ovarian stroma. Some of these tumors respond to postural stimuli of renin or to ACTH stimulation. All causes of secondary hyperaldosteronism are

associated with elevated 24-hour urine aldosterone, with increased plasma renin.

3. **Laboratory evaluation**

a. **24-hour urine aldosterone levels are elevated in primary and secondary hyperaldosteronism.**

b. **Plasma renin and angiotensin levels are suppressed in primary hyperaldosteronism, and elevated in secondary hyperaldosteronism**. Samples are collected after 3 hours in the upright position. Diuretics or any drugs affecting the renin-angiotensin system should be discontinued several weeks before measuring. The **aldosterone:renin ratio (both stated in ng/mL) should be calculated; primary aldosteronism will show a high ratio of more than 20 to 1**.

c. The **saline infusion test** is a confirmatory test for primary hyperaldosteronism. Normal saline is infused at 300–500 mL/h and plasma aldosterone and renin are measured after 4 hours. Normal subjects suppress aldosterone to <10 ng%; those with primary hyperaldosteronism do not.

d. The **Captopril test** is a confirmatory test for primary hyperaldosteronism in patients who cannot tolerate the saline infusion. Captopril (25 mg) is given orally, which inhibits angiotensin formation. In normal subjects, plasma aldosterone falls within 2 hours (<15 ng/dL), but does not decrease in patients with aldosterone-producing adenomas.

e. **CT adrenal scans** should be reserved until **after** primary hyperaldosteronism is confirmed by the aforementioned tests, because incidental adrenal adenomas are found in many normal individuals. The computed tomography (CT) scan often distinguishes an adenoma from bilateral hyperplasia.

f. **18-hydroxy cortisol and 18-oxycortisol** measurements can be useful, as they are usually elevated in aldosterone-producing adenomas but not in bilateral hyperplasia.

g. [131] **I iodomethyl-19-norcholesterol or bilateral catheterization of the adrenal veins** are uncommonly used tests that are useful in some situations.

V. **Hirsutism virilization**

A. **Androgen synthesis and metabolism in women**. Two sources of androgen precursors exist: the **ovarian stroma produces androstenedione, whereas the adrenal cortex produces dehydroepiandrosterone and its sulfate** (Fig. 4-8). These precursors are metabolized within various peripheral tis-

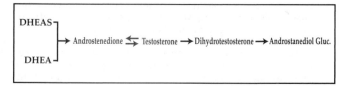

Fig. 4-8. Metabolism of androgen precursors.

sues to testosterone and the potent biologically active androgen—dihydrotestosterone (DHT). DHT is then irreversibly metabolized to androstenediol glucuronide (Adio/Gluc). **Blood and urine Adio/Gluc levels are the tests that best reflect overall DHT production**; they are often highly elevated in disorders of androgen overproduction,and can be used to monitor treatment.

Total and free blood testosterone levels are additional tests that are used to diagnose hirsutism. Blood testosterone is bound to sex hormone–binding globulin (SHBG) which, in turn, is increased by estrogens and decreased by androgens. **Excess testosterone production is best reflected by increases in free or unbound serum testosterone**, which occur in 80% of patients with benign causes of hirsutism [e.g., polycystic ovarian disease (PCO), idiopathic hirsutism or familial hirsutism], and is a more sensitive test than total testosterone.

B. Androgen disorders. Disorders of androgen production or metabolism occur commonly in women. Many causes of hirsutism and virilization are seen (Table 4-49). A good history and physical examination (H&P) can identify some of the causes, such as Cushing's syndrome, acromegaly, galactorrhea-amenorrhea, or a large palpable ovarian tumor. In general, **neoplasms or disorders of ovarian stroma that cause hirsutism or virilization usually have a relatively short history of symptoms** (months to 1–2 years); **cause frank virilization** (deepened voice, android habitus, increased muscle mass, clitoromegaly); and are associated with **high values of total testosterone (>200 ng%)**. Other causes of androgen disorders tend to have a long history (years) of symptoms that often begin shortly after menarche; cause mild hirsutism (without virilization); and are associated with total testosterone levels that are in the upper range of normal or only mildly elevated (i.e. 60–200 ng%). In many cases, increased androgen production directly effects ovarian folliculogenesis and ovulation, and often results in oligomenorrhea, infertility, or amenorrhea.

C. Laboratory evaluation. DHEAS, total and free testosterone, androstanediol glucuronide, luteinizing hormone (LH), and follicle-stimulating hormone (FSH) should be measured.

  1. If total testosterone is >150 ng%, a neoplasm or ovarian stromal disorder is suggested, and a dexamethasone suppression test should be performed.

  2. Dexamethasone suppression test. Dexamethasone (0.5 mg) is given at 10 PM for at least 2 weeks, and DHEAS, total testosterone, and cortisol are then measured at 8 AM. Healthy patients will have suppression of cortisol (<1.0 µg%), DHEAS, and testosterone to very low levels; patients with **neoplasms or ovarian stromal disorders are not expected to show suppression**. The most common causes of hirsutism or virilization (e.g., idiopathic hirsutism, polycystic ovaries, familial hirsutism) will show mild to marked suppression.

  3. **Serum LH and FSH** can be helpful if polycystic ovary disease is suspected, which causes a high normal or elevated LH and a low normal FSH.

Table 4-49.   Causes of hirsutism-virilization

Central nervous system (CNS)–pituitary
Cushing's disease
Acromegaly
Galactorrhea—amenorrhea syndromes
Encephalitis, CNS tumors, etc., causing oligomenorrhea

Adrenal
Adenoma and carcinoma
Enzymatic defects (e.g., 17-ketoreductase deficiency, 21-hydroxylase
  deficiency, 11-hydroxylase deficiency

Ovary
Neoplasms
–Male cell types (arrhenoblastoma, Sertoli–Leydig cell tumors,
  lipoid cell tumors, germ cell tumors, teratomas)
–Female cell types, (granulosa-theca cell tumor, theca cell tumors,
  gynandroblastomas)
Stromal reaction (e.g., adjacent to luteoma of pregnancy or to
  metastatic or primary ovarian neoplasm)
Hyperthecosis
Hilus cell hyperplasia
Polycystic ovaries
Insulin resistance with acanthosis nigricans
Physiologic menopause
Turner's syndrome (rare)

Miscellaneous
Idiopathic hirsutism
Familial
Insulin resistance and hyperandrogenism
Anorexia nervosa
Drugs (e.g., diphenylhydantoin, androgens, contraceptives, minoxidil,
  cyclosporin, diazoxide)
Ectopic corticotropin (ACTH) or CRH production
Male pseudohermaphroditism
Hypertrichosis lanuginosis
Myxedema
Miscellaneous pediatric disorders (Cornelia de Lange syndrome,
  bird-headed dwarfs, trisome E syndrome, Hurler's disease,
  various mucopolysaccharidoses)
Tumors: hypernephroma, adrenal cortical carcinoma of ovary,
  luteoma, adrenal rest tumor, masculinovoblastoma, ovoblastoma,
  androblastoma diffusum

ACTH, adrenocorticotropic hormone; CRH, corticotropin-releasing hormone.

4. Subtle deficiencies in 21-hydroxylase or 11-hydroxylase are easily confused with polycystic ovarian disease or idiopathic hirsutism, and can be detected by measuring **17-hydroxyprogesterone and 11-deoxycortisol before and after ACTH stimulation.**

VI. Disorders of reproduction

A. Normal regulatory control. Figures 4-9 and 4-10 depict schematically the reproductive systems in men and women. In both sexes, **the hypothalamus secretes gonadotropin-releasing hormone (GnRH) in a pulsatile fashion to control pituitary secretion of LH and FSH**. LH concentrations reflect pulsatile GnRH secretion, whereas FSH has a much longer half-life and more stable values. Changes in pulsation frequency, amplitude, or both occur in the different parts of the menstrual cycle in women, and occur in reproductive disorders of both sexes. **In men, LH and FSH control testicular production of testosterone** (T, the predominant steroid). Testosterone is metabolized in peripheral tissues (e.g., fat, muscle, liver) into dihydrotestosterone (DHT) and estradiol (E2). **In women, LH and FSH control follicle development, ovulation, and corpus luteum function which, in turn, produces estradiol (E2) and progesterone (P).**

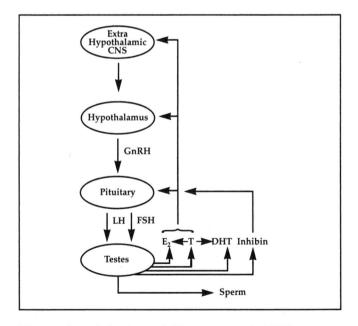

Fig. 4-9. Control of male gonadal hormone secretion. DHT, dihydrotestosterone; E_2, estradiol; FSH, follicle-stimulating hormone; GnRH, gonadotropin-releasing hormone; LH, luteinizing hormone; T, testosterone.

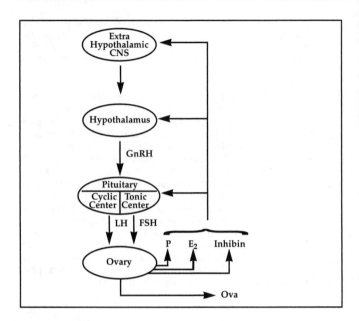

Fig. 4-10. Control of female gonadal hormone secretion. E2, estradiol; FSH, follicle-stimulating hormone; GnRH, gonadotropin-releasing hormone; LH, luteinizing hormone; P, progesterone.

B. Reproduction disorders. Hypogonadism often presents in men as decreased hair growth in the beard, axillary, and pubic regions; and decreased libido. In women, amenorrhea is a common manifestation. Hypogonadism in both sexes can be divided into two broad categories: primary hypogonadism and secondary hypogonadism.

   1. Primary hypogonadism indicates an **abnormality in the ovary or testes** (e.g., menopause, castration) and results in **increased secretion of FSH and LH.**

   2. Secondary hypogonadism includes disorders of hypothalamic or pituitary function that lead indirectly to decreased blood testosterone in men and decreased E2 or progesterone in women. In severe secondary hypogonadism, **LH and FSH may be below normal or even undetectable.** However, in most cases, the LH and FSH are in the "normal" range, which is still inappropriately low given a low T or low E2.

C. Laboratory evaluation. Initial laboratory studies should include serum LH, FSH, and prolactin in both sexes; testosterone and free testosterone in men; and E2 in women. Prolactin is quantified because **hyperprolactinemia is a common cause of gonadal dysfunction**. If LH and FSH are highly elevated (primary hypogonadism), then chromosomal karyotyping should be done to evaluate the gonads. If LH and FSH are "normal" or low, then secondary hypogonadism is suspected and diagnostic attention is directed to the hypothalamus and pituitary gland.

D. Hypogonadism in men. Table 4-50 lists the causes of male hypogonadism. The history and physical examination are as important as the laboratory studies in narrowing the differential diagnosis. In embryologic development of normal male genitalia, DHT is required. Therefore, ambiguous genitalia in males (e.g., hypospadius, bifid scrotum, or other incomplete development) are usually the result of congenital DHT deficiency or resistance. If genitalia are normal, but the individual is eunuchoidal (arm span > height), the abnormality of testosterone production occurred after birth and before puberty. If the individual has normal male genitalia and is not eunuchoid, the abnormality occurred after puberty. Testicular volume or length is also useful; normal length is >4 cm in sexually mature

Table 4-50. Causes of male hypogonadism

Abnormalities in hypothalamic-pituitary function
Panhypopituitarism
GnRH deficiency (Kallman's syndrome)
Hyperprolactinemia
Isolated FSH Deficiency
Isolated LH deficiency
Prader–Willi syndrome
Laurence Moon-Biedl syndrome
Cerebellar ataxia

Primary gonadal abnormalities
Klinefelter's syndrome
XX males (sex reversal syndrome)
True hermaphroditism
Streak gonads XY karyotype
Testicular agenesis (vanishing testes syndrome)
Noonan's syndrome
Sertoli cell only syndrome
Acquired testicular disorders: orchitis, surgical castration, cancer chemotherapy, etc.
Adult seminiferous tubule failure (idiopathic oligospermia or azoospermia)
Testicular mosaichism and infertility
Karazener's syndrome
Myotonia dystrophia
Aromatase deficiency
LH receptor mutations including absent LH receptors
Leydig cell aplasia

Enzymatic defects in androgen synthesis:
20-hydroxylase deficiency (lipoid adrenal hypoplasia)
17, 20-desmolase deficiency
3-β-hydroxysteroid dehydrogenase deficiency
17-hydroxylase deficiency
17-ketosteroid reductase deficiency
5α-reductase deficiency

continued

Table 4-50. *Continued*

Defects in androgen action
Complete androgen insensitivity (testicular feminization)
Incomplete androgen sensitivity

Miscellaneous
Persistent Müllerian duct syndrome
Cystic fibrosis
Hemochromatosis

FSH, follicle-stimulating hormone; GnRH, gonadotropin-releasing hormone; LH, luteinizing hormone.

men. Klinefelter's disease is often associated with very small testes, but in mosaic individuals varying degrees of small testes are found.

If the individual has not gone through normal puberty, or if the laboratory data suggest a primary gonadal cause (low androgens, high LH and FSH), consideration of genetic causes is in order, and karyotyping is required. If the laboratory results suggest hypothalamic or pituitary causes (low androgens, low LH and FSH), then MRI imaging of the hypothalamus and pituitary is required.

If the individual developed normal puberty and had a normal reproductive history and physical examination until adult onset of androgen deficiency, his diagnosis falls into one of only a few categories of acquired hypogonadism. Measurement of LH, FSH, prolactin, and total or free testosterone will localize the likely possibilities. Hyperprolactinemia as a cause of hypogonadism is discussed separately, later in this chapter.

E.   Hypogonadism in women can be divided into primary and secondary causes (Table 4-51). **Primary amenorrhea** indicates a woman who has never had a menstrual cycle. **Secondary amenorrhea** indicates a woman who had menstrual function and then developed amenorrhea. The **most common cause of amenorrhea** in a woman of reproductive age is secondary amenorrhea caused by a normal pregnancy. Thus, the initial test in amenorrheic women should be a **quantitative chorionic gonadotropin (CG)** level in blood or urine. Pregnancy tests are not recommended, because they may not detect mild increases in CG; rare causes of amenorrhea are gestational trophoblastic neoplasms (e.g., hydatid mole, choriocarcinoma), which usually have a high CG but may cause only mild CG elevations. Next, LH, FSH, prolactin, and estradiol tests should be ordered. Another common test is the progesterone withdrawal test, which is used to estimate the amount of circulating estrogen. This test is performed by giving 50–100 µg of progesterone in oil. Withdrawal bleeding is expected shortly after administration, but is not observed in women who are normally pregnant or in individuals with very low estradiol production (e.g. <25 pg/mL).

   1.   Primary amenorrhea is most commonly caused by congenital disorders, of which the most common are Turner's

Table 4-51. Disorders of female reproduction

Abnormalitiees of hypothalamic-pituitary function
Panhypopituitarism (e.g., Sheehan's syndrome, pituitary tumors)
GnRH deficiency (Kallman's syndrome)
Hyperprolactinemia
Cushing's disease
Isolated LH or FSH deficiency
Functional abnormalities in positive feedback stimulation or ovulatory surge
Malnutrition/starvation

Primary gonadal abnormalitiles
Turner's syndrome
Polycystic ovarian syndrome (PCOS)
Gonadal dysgenesis
FSH receptor mutations
Autoimmune oophoritis
Menopause
Inadequate luteal phase
Ovarian neoplasms
Hyperthecosis
Enzymatic mutations (e.g., 17α-hydroxylase, 17-ketoreductase)
Gestational trophoblastic neoplasms

Miscellaneous
Congenital abnormalities in Müllerian development
Obesity
Endometriosis
Disorders of increased androgen production (other than PCOS hyperthecosis)
Androgen resistance
Hypo- or hyperthyroidism
Hemochromatosis

FSH, Follicle-stimulating hormone; GnRH, gonadotropin-releasing hormone; LH, luteinizing hormone.

syndrome (approximately one third) and Kallman's syndrome (approximately one third).

    a. Turner's syndrome. **Gonadal dysgenesis** (streak gonads) causes a lack of estrogen production, resulting in dramatic increases in LH and FSH secretion such as seen in normal menopause. Physical examination usually shows a **short stature**, increased arm-carrying angles, short fourth metacarpals, **webbed neck**, and, at times, cardiovascular abnormalities such as aortic coarctation. Karyotypic abnormalities range from pure **45XO** to various subtle defects and mosaicism.

    b. Kallman's syndrome (GnRH deficiency). LH and FSH concentrations are low or inappropriately "normal" for an amenorrheic woman. Hyposmia or **anosmia** are often present and the patient has **normal stature**, distinguishing Kallman's from Turners.

   c.   **True gonadal dysgenesis** presents as primary amenorrhea caused by ovarian dysgenesis in patients who have a
normal 46XX karyotype; these patients usually develop
eunuchoidism and have a **normal stature.**
   2.   **Secondary amenorrhea. Increased androgens directly interfere with ovarian function**. Most commonly,
this is **polycystic ovary syndrome** (PCOS), but any other
cause (see discussion on hirsutism) may be present. The next
most common causes are **premature ovarian failure** and
hyperprolactinemia. Hyperprolactinemia is associated with
low or "normal" LH and FSH, and low estradiol, and is discussed separately. **Cancer chemotherapy** very commonly
produces direct destruction of ovarian follicles, resulting in
amenorrhea. Premature ovarian failure or early menopause
is an uncommon disorder; various causes exist, including autoimmune oophoritis (usually suspected in women with other
autoimmune endocrine diseases) and mutations in the FSH
receptor.
   F.   **Hyperprolactinemia. Hypersecretion of prolactin
(>50 ng/mL) interferes with reproductive function in both
men and women**. Elevated prolactin levels directly inhibit
LH-stimulated testosterone production by Leydig cells, causing
decreased testosterone levels and decreased libido in men. Increased prolactin levels also interfere with FSH action on the
ovary, inhibiting follicle growth and estradiol production, and
causing amenorrhea in women. In addition, prolactin acts at the
hypothalamic or pituitary area to prevent increases in LH and
FSH secretion. Thus, hyperprolactinemia results in **low testosterone** and decreased libido in men, and **low estradiol** and
amenorrhea in women, in the presence of **low or inappropriately "normal" LH and FSH concentrations**.
   Many causes of hyperprolactinemia are found, including
stress (emotional or physical) and many **medications** (e.g., antidepressants, dopamine agonists such as metoclopramide). Physiologic stimuli such as stress usually increase prolactin only modestly (e.g., to 25–30 ng/mL), whereas **prolactin-producing
tumors cause higher elevations** (e.g., 50–5,000 ng/mL, which
correlate with tumor size). Stimulation and suppression tests are
not generally done. A careful history, particularly of all medications, and physical examination are usually adequate to suggest
the cause. **If no explanation is found for persistent hyperprolactinemia, an MRI scan of the hypothalamus and
pituitary is warranted**. Treatment involves dopamine agonists (e.g., bromocriptine, cabergoline) which usually suppress
prolactin levels to normal and also exert a dramatic antitumor
effect. Transphenoidal surgery is also available and preoperative
staging of the tumor can predict the likelihood of cure (stage I
>90% cure rate). However, the tumors recur within 10 years in
5% to 20% of the patients. Prolactinomas are slow growing and,
in postmenopausal women or women not desiring pregnancy,
some endocrinologists simply follow the patient with repeated
MRIs.
VII.   Disorders of growth hormone (GH) secretion
   A.   **Normal physiology. The hypothalamus secretes
growth hormone-releasing hormone (GHRH), which stim-**

ulates the pituitary to secrete growth hormone (GH) in a pulsatile fashion. The secretion of GHRH is **inhibited by somatostatin (SST), as well as by increased glucose and insulinlike growth factor-I** (IGF-1) concentrations (Fig. 4-11). GH is a **major modulator of metabolism**; it directly stimulates amino acid uptake and protein synthesis in muscle, liver, and other cells, which are anabolic effects augmented by insulin. However, GH has an anti-insulin effect on carbohydrate metabolism, which leads to the development of diabetes mellitus in many acromegalic patients. Thus, a carbohydrate meal stimulates insulin secretion and suppresses GH secretion, and the carbohydrate is used for lipid synthesis. In contrast, amino acids (e.g., a protein meal) stimulate both insulin and GH secretion, which causes new protein synthesis. During a fast, insulin secretion decreases, whereas GH secretion increases, which stimulates the body to use fatty acids rather than glucose as fuel.

B. Acromegaly is generally caused by **hypersecretion of GH by a pituitary adenoma**. Very rarely, a cancer (e.g., pancreatic) secretes GHRH, causing acromegaly.

    1. Common signs and symptoms generally require years to appear. They include general thickening of body skin with acral enlargement, which leads to furrowing of the forehead and posterior neck skin; widening of the nasal margins; increased heel thickness and hand and foot size; arthralgias; and laryngeal enlargement, which causes deepening of the

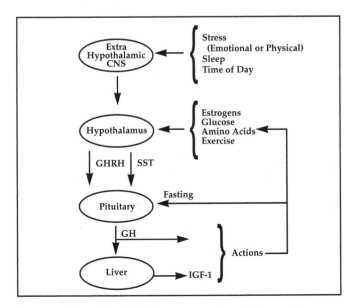

Fig. 4-11. Control of growth hormone secretion. GH, growth hormone; GHRH, growth hormone-releasing hormone; IGF-1, insulinlike growth factor-1; SST, somatostatin.

voice in women. Early symptoms, which are subtle, include fatigue and increased sweating, paresthesias, carpel tunnel syndrome, and hirsutism (in women).

2. Laboratory evaluation. When the disease is suspected, laboratory confirmation is relatively easy. A **glucose tolerance test should be performed with GH and glucose** measured at 0, 30, 60, and 90 minutes following the glucose load. Normal individuals will have suppressed GH values (<1.0 ng/mL), whereas **GH-producing adenomas show no suppression**. Single measurements of GH alone are not recommended, because GH secretion is pulsatile, and peak values in normals overlap with those in acromegaly. Other useful tests include IGF-I concentrations (increased in acromegaly) and IGF-I binding protein-III (useful in patients with equivocal results).

3. Treatment. The optimal treatment of acromegaly is transphenoidal resection of the causative adenoma, but with late diagnosis a successful cure is seen in only about 50% of patients. Other treatments include gamma knife, multiport irradiation (which requires 5–10 years to achieve maximal effects), and SST analogues (SST analogues inhibit GH secretion by adenomas). New long-acting SST analogues require only one dose per month. Currently, the goal of a "cure" is to have GH values of <2 ng/mL, coupled with suppression of GH secretion during a glucose tolerance test.

C. Growth hormone deficiency occurs quite commonly in patients of all ages who have hypothalamic or pituitary masses. In children, a deficiency of GHRH is a common cause of an isolated GH deficiency, which is itself an uncommon cause of short stature or dwarfism.

1. Differential diagnosis. Many illnesses result in decreased growth, including anemia of any cause, gastrointestinal disorders such as regional ileitis or inflammatory bowel disease, Cushing's syndrome, hypothyroidism, cyanotic heart disease, and malnutrition.

2. Laboratory evaluation. In short or dwarfed children whose initial history, physical examination, and laboratory data do not reveal the cause, evaluation of GH secretion is warranted. **Two provocative tests are usually selected** from any of the following: insulin hypoglycemia, arginine stimulation, clonidine stimulation or L-dopa stimulation. GH is measured at 0, 30, 60, and 90 minutes following the stimulus; healthy individuals should show an increase to >8 ng/mL. Because replacement with GH is expensive ($15,000–20,000/y) and must be given and results monitored for years, two abnormal tests are usually required before a diagnosis is made. IGF-I measurements are also useful, but in growth-retarded children or individuals with retarded bone age, assessing age-matched controls can be difficult.

VIII. Disorders of calcium metabolism

A. Normal physiology. Calcium metabolism is closely regulated so that plasma ionized calcium concentrations stay constant. The body requires 1,000 mg of calcium daily to maintain calcium levels; deficits are compensated by slow resorption of bone. Hormonal modulation involves the actions of parathormone (PTH, secreted by the parathyroid glands), vitamins D, and calcitonin. **PTH is the most important regulator of plasma calcium**; it raises plasma (Ca^{++}) by mobilizing bone calcium and stimulating the kidneys to reabsorb more calcium and excrete more phosphorus. **Calcitonin is secreted by the C-cells in the thyroid**, and can decrease plasma (Ca^{++}); however, calcitonin probably has little physiologic role in calcium homostasis in adult humans (total thyroidectomy produces no clinical disorders of calcium homostasis). Vitamin D, particularly in its most potent form, **1,25 dihydroxyvitamin D (1,25 OH D), increases intestinal calcium absorption and works with PTH** to regulate bone calcium metabolism. Vitamin D may be ingested or may be created in the skin by ultraviolet light acting on 7-dehydrocholesterol. Vitamin D is then transformed to 25-hydroxyvitamin D in the liver, and finally to 1,25 OH D in the kidney; this final step is closely regulated and stimulated by PTH itself. Parathormone related protein (PTH-RP) is produced by a wide array of normal tissues (e.g. breast, vascular endothelium, ketatinocytes), and acts as a cytokine in local calcium metabolism.

B. **Hypercalcemia** is a relatively common metabolic abnormality with a number of possible causes (Table 4-52). **The most**

Table 4-52. Differential diagnosis of hypercalcemia

Caused by or related to parathormone (PTH)
Primary hyperparathyroidism
Tertiary hyperparathyroidism
Multiple endocrine neoplasia
Parathyroid carcinoma
Familial hypocalciuric hypercalcemia
Lithium treatment
Cancer production of PTH (very rare)

Hypercalcemia of cancer
Solid tumors (e.g., breast cancer, etc.) that produce parathormone-
    related protein (PTH-RP)
T-cell lymphoma that produces 1,25 OH D
Multiple myeloma
Leukemia: cytokine producing

Miscellaneous causes
Granulomatous diseases (e.g., sarcoidosis, tuberculosis) with 1,25
    OH D production
Vitamin D toxicity
Vitamin A toxicity
Hyperthyroidism
Adrenal insufficiency
Milk alkali syndrome
Aluminum toxicity
Immobilization
Thiazide treatment

1,25 OH D, 1,25 dihydroxyvitamin D.

common cause of hypercalcemia is primary hyperpara-thyroidism, usually caused by a single parathyroid adenoma. Common signs and symptoms involve the heart, musculoskeletal system, gastrointestinal tract, urinary tract, and nervous system.

    1.   **Laboratory evaluation**. The differential diagnosis of hypercalcemia is generally assessed by measuring PTH, 1,25 OH D, and, at times, PTH-RP. It is important to use "intact" PTH third generation assays to quantify PTH; other assays detect circulating degradation products of PTH.

    2.   **Specific causes of hypercalcemia and their laboratory findings.**

        a.   **Vitamin D toxicity**. Blood 1,25 OH D should be measured, and will be elevated.

        b.   **Hyperparathyroidism** results in hypercalcemia, fasting hypophosphatemia, phosphaturia, hypercalciuria, and an increased serum chloride:phosphate ratio. **PTH concentrations are increased or high normal**, when quantified as the "intact" hormone (discussed later). It is always important to **differentiate familial hypocalciuric hypercalcemia from primary hyperparathyroidism** by measuring 24-hour calcium excretion; **calcium excretion is low in the former disorder, and increased in hyperparathyroidism**. PTH concentrations do not distinguish the two disorders. Familial hypocalciuric hypercalcemia is a benign disorder involving changes in calcium channels and requires no treatment. Hyperparathyroidism usually causes slightly increased blood PTH. **Very high PTH concentrations suggest parathyroid carcinoma or tertiary hyperparathyroidism seen in longstanding renal failure.**

        c.   **Hypercalcemia caused by cancer** (other than parathyroid) occurs by three main mechanisms, and is associated with **suppressed blood PTH levels, with or without increases in PTH-RP**.

        (1)   **Most cancers produce PTH-RP**, a protein that is similar to PTH in both structure and function. For example, normal breast tissue secretes PTH-RP into milk, and breast cancers often produce large amounts of PTH-RP.

        (2)   Some neoplasms (e.g., T-cell lymphoma) hydroxylate the 25 hydroxy D (the vitamin D precursor) to **produce increased amounts of 1,25 OH D.**

        (3)   Some neoplasms (e.g., myeloma) produce **cytokines which mobilize bone.**

        d.   The important laboratory findings in all of these cancers are suppressed "intact" PTH, and if the cancer also produces PTH-RP, it too will be elevated. The other miscellaneous causes of hypercalcemia are also associated with suppressed PTH and normal or decreased PTH-RP.

C.   **Hypocalcemia**. Symptoms of hypocalcemia include muscle cramps, tetany, decreased mental acuity (particularly if magnesium deficiency is present), and cardiac arrhythmias. The laboratory evaluation of hypocalcemia is fairly simple, because **only three direct causes exist: (a) deficiency of PTH, (b) defi-**

ciency of vitamin D or vitamin D action, and (c) deficiency of magnesium. Many disorders can lead to one of these three deficiencies, but if hypocalcemia is present it must be mediated by one of these three mechanisms. Which of the three is the likely cause can be suggested by the history and physical findings, and confirmed by measurement of PTH, vitamin D, and magnesium.

    1. **Vitamin D deficiency requires weeks or months to develop** and, thus, is not likely to occur in an acute hospital setting when the patient has been previously healthy. Dietary vitamin D deficiency is manifested by **rickets in children** and is also common in elderly **nursing home patients** (up to 50% in some homes). Other disorders leading to a deficiency of vitamin D (a fat-soluble vitamin) include sprue, short bowel syndromes, and genetic resistance to vitamin D. To determine if dietary vitamin D is adequate, blood levels of **25-hydroxy D should be measured, and will be decreased**. Treatment of dietary deficiency must take place over months by either parenteral or oral vitamin D.

    2. **PTH deficiency** usually occurs as a result of surgical parathyroidectomy, congenital absence of parathyroids, or autoimmune destruction of parathyroids.

    3. **Magnesium deficiency is the most common cause of hypocalcemia in the acute hospital setting**. Hypomagnesemia prevents PTH secretion and inhibits PTH action on bone. Many drugs can cause hypomagnesemia. A low serum magnesium always indicates total body magnesium deficiency. Treatment of hypocalcemia caused by hypomagnesemia must involve intravenous or intramuscular magnesium; simple calcium replacement is ineffectual. Once the magnesium is replenished, PTH will begin to rapidly correct the hypocalcemia. Because magnesium is an intracellular ion, substantial amounts of magnesium may be required.

IX. **Common endocrine disorders of the pancreas**

    A. **Normal physiology**. The pancreatic endocrine cells, which are in the islets of Langerhans, are composed of four main cell types. **Alpha (A) cells produce glucagon; beta (B) cells produce insulin; delta (D) cells produce somatostatin; and pancreatic polypeptide (PP) cells produce a polypeptide that has various effects on the gastrointestinal tract.**

    1. **Glucagon** secretion is stimulated by hypoglycemia, protein meals, and several hormones (e.g., pancreozymin, secretin). Glucagon raises blood glucose levels.

    2. **Insulin** secretion is stimulated by glucose. In turn, insulin facilitates the movement of blood glucose into cells (primarily muscle, connective tissue, and fat), decreasing blood glucose levels. Insulin also has important roles in protein, triglyceride, and nucleic acid synthesis.

    3. **Somatostatin** inhibits both glucagon and insulin.

    B. **Common disorders**

    1. **Diabetes mellitus (DM)** is one of the most common causes of death in the United States. **Type I DM results from the loss of beta cells** because of autoimmunity, viral infection, and so on, whereas **type II DM** ("adult-onset" diabetes) is **the result of abnormal insulin secretion and**

insulin resistance, and is caused by a genetic predisposition coupled with factors such as obesity. Common symptoms include polyuria, polydipsia, polyphagia, and glucose intolerance. Common complications include vascular, neurologic, renal, and optic disease. Laboratory evaluation includes the following tests.

   a. **Glucose tolerance test (GTT)**

     (1) **Nonpregnant individuals**: 75 gm glucose load; the National Diabetes Data Group suggests the following interpretation.

       (a) Fasting glucose >126 mg/dL or 2-hour postprandial >200 mg/dL = DM (no need for GTT); if values are less, perform the GTT.

       (b) A 2-hour post-GTT glucose >200 mg/dL + at least one other glucose value >200 mg/dL = DM.

       (c) A 2-hour post-GTT glucose 126–200 mg/dL + at least one other glucose value >200 mg/dL = glucose intolerance.

     (2) **Pregnant individual** (gestational diabetes: GD): 100 gm glucose load; patient has GD if two or more of the following plasma glucose criteria are met:

       (a) Fasting glucose ≥105 mg/dL

       (b) 1-hour ≥190 mg/dL

       (c) 2-hour ≥165 mg/dL

       (d) 3-hour ≥145 mg/dL

   b. **Long-term laboratory monitoring** of diabetic patients may include blood **glucose, blood urea nitrogen (BUN)**, and **creatinine**; tests for **microalbuminuria**; and glycated hemoglobin (HbA_{1C}). **Increased HbA_{1C} levels reflect elevated blood glucose levels during the previous 2–3 months**, and is a useful test for assessing long-term glucose control.

  2. **Hypoglycemia**

   a. **Normal physiology. Plasma glucose is carefully adjusted in normal individuals**, usually ranging between 60 and 100 mg/dL before meals and up to 150 mg/dL after meals. **Insulin decreases blood glucose** and prevents its elevation to abnormally high values, by decreasing hepatic glucose production and stimulating peripheral glucose utilization. **Several counterregulatory hormones** (e.g., glucagon, growth hormone, ACTH, cortisol, and probably catecholamines) **counteract insulin action** and protect against hypoglycemia. **These same hormones can also act with insulin to modify carbohydrate, lipid, and protein metabolism**, depending on the type of meal ingested and whether a fasting state exists. For example, following a high carbohydrate meal, insulin secretion increases, whereas growth hormone secretion decreases. The insulin causes the glucose from the meal to be used for lipogenesis in adipose tissue and liver. However, a protein-rich meal stimulates the secretion of both insulin and growth hormone, causing the amino acids to be utilized for protein synthesis in liver, muscle, and adipose tissues. During a prolonged fast, insulin secretion decreases, whereas counterregulatory hormone secretion increases; these latter hormones protect against hypoglycemia by attenuating the effects of insulin and by enhancing hepatic gluconeogenesis.

b. Causes of hypoglycemia. The differential diagnosis of fasting hypoglycemia is complex (Table 4-53). **Fasting hypoglycemia can be caused by a deficiency of any of the counterregulatory hormones, such as growth hormone, ACTH cortisol (hypoadrenalism), or catecholamines**. This is a common cause of fasting hypoglycemia, particularly in children. Other causes include any drug that inhibits gluconeogenesis (e.g., **alcohol**) or con-

Table 4-53. Differential diagnosis of hypoglycemia

Postprandial hypoglycemia
Surgical modification of upper gastrointestinal tract
Early type II diabetes mellitus (rare)
Idiopathic or functional hypoglycemia

Fasting hypoglycemia
Counterregulatory hormone deficiency
–Growth hormone (infants and children)
–Catecholamines (infants)
–Glucagon (infants)
–ACTH or cortisol (e.g., adrenal insufficiency, hypopituitarism, isolated ACTH deficiency)
Insulin hypersecretion
–Insulinoma
–Islet cell hyperplasia (nesidioblastosis)
–Factitious insulin injections[a]
–Sulfonylurea ingestion
Cancer-related (excessive production of IGF-II): mesenchymal tumors, hepatic carcinoma, adrenal carcinoma, gastrointestinal carcinoma, hematologic neoplasms
Drugs: ethanol, salicylates, quinine, sulfonylureas (see insulin hypersecretion)
Autoimmune causes
–Insulin receptor antibody hypoglycemia (usually in patients with rheumatoid arthritis treated with penicillanine)
–Autoantibodies to insulin
Miscellaneous causes in infants and children (see also isolated hormone deficiencies)
–Erythroblastosis fetalis
–Small for gestational age
–Enzyme deficiencies involving gluconeogenesis or glycogenolysis
–Defects in amino acid, fatty acid, or ketone metabolism
–Infants of diabetic mothers
Organ failure: severe renal failure, severe congestive heart failure, severe liver failure, and starvation (including anorexia nervosa)

ACTH, adrenocorticotropic hormone (corticotropin); IGF-II, insulin-like growth factor II.
[a] In factitious insulin injections, the patient's C-peptide levels (which are the result of endogenous insulin production, and are not present in exogenous insulin) will be suppressed.

genital defects in any of the hepatic enzymes involved in gluconeogenesis. A rare cause of fasting hypoglycemia is an increase (or a lack of decrease) in insulin secretion during a fast, such as caused by an **insulinoma** or beta cell hyperplasia. **Cancer production of "insulinlike" insulin growth factor II (IGF-II)** also produces fasting hypoglycemia whereas insulin itself is normally suppressed.

c. **Investigation of hypoglycemia**. The clinician must **first separate fasting hypoglycemia from postprandial hypoglycemia**. This can usually be done by history alone. The causes of postprandial hypoglycemia are limited. Postprandial hypoglycemia is found in patients who have undergone **upper gastrointestinal tract surgery**, and (rarely) patients with early type II diabetes (wherein the postprandial glucose is very high, and then falls to low levels after 4–5 hours because of oversecretion of insulin).

The best diagnostic test for hypoglycemia is to measure plasma glucose at times the individual is experiencing possible symptoms of hypoglycemia. A glucose tolerance test may be useful in evaluating postprandial hypoglycemia, but is difficult to interpret because a significant fraction of normal individuals, particularly healthy, young, slender females, may have glucose levels that fall to <50 mg/dL. The GTT is not an appropriate diagnostic test for fasting hypoglycemia.

Fasting hypoglycemia is evaluated by fasting the individual for 72 hours (or less if hypoglycemia occurs). I ask the patient to eat the usual evening meal, and then fast until a clinic visit at 8 AM the next day. The glucose is measured; if it is >50 mg/dL, the fast is continued under clinic observation with glucose measurements every 4 hours, or more frequently if the initial value was 50–60 mg/dL. If (or when) hypoglycemia (glucose, 50 mg/dL) is observed, blood is drawn for measurement of **(a) insulin, (b) proinsulin, (c) "C"-peptide of insulin, (d) growth hormone, and (e) ACTH and cortisol**. If hypoglycemia is not observed by 20–24 hours, the patient is admitted to the hospital, and the fast continued for a maximum of 72 hours under observation. Noncaloric fluids should be consumed all during the fast. Careful interpretation of the results of these hormone measurements will usually lead to the diagnosis. Additional assessments may include measurements of drugs (e.g., oral hypoglycemics), IGF-II (in patients with some tumors), and hormone stimulation tests (if a selective deficiency of a counterregulatory hormone is suspected).

3. **Gastrinoma (Zollinger–Ellison syndrome)**. Gastrin-producing islet cell tumors cause gastric acid hypersecretion with subsequent peptic ulcers, diarrhea, and so forth. Fasting serum **gastrin levels >600 pg/mL suggest a gastrinoma**. Equivocal cases can be evaluated with the **secretin stimulation test**, in which gastrinomas will respond to a secretin provocation by releasing more gastrin.

4. **Multiple endocrine neoplasia (MEN)**. Laboratory evaluation is directed to the suspected organs involved, based

on the history (especially a careful family history) and the physical examination.

X. Disorders of antidiuretic hormone (ADH)

A. Normal physiology. Antidiuretic hormone (ADH or vasopressin) is synthesized by the **hypothalamus** and transported to the posterior lobe of the pituitary for secretion. ADH is secreted in response to hypovolemia and hyperosmolality, and its main effect is to cause **increased reabsorption of water in the renal tubules.**

B. Decreased secretion of ADH causes diabetes insipidus (neurogenic form). Decreased responsiveness of the renal tubules to ADH causes the nephrogenic form of diabetes insipidus. Diabetes insipidus involves the production of **large quantities of dilute urine (polyuria), with subsequent hypernatremia and plasma hyperosmolarity**. Diagnosis is made by demonstrating the production of dilute urine in the face of water restriction, and can be confirmed with decreased serum ADH levels.

C. Increased secretion of ADH causes the syndrome of inappropriate ADH secretion (**SIADH**). Causes include hypothalamic or pituitary tumors, ectopic ADH production by various carcinomas (e.g., bronchial carcinoids), CNS trauma, infections, meningitis, drugs, and so forth. SIADH involves increased reabsorption of water in the renal tubules (causing hyperosmolal urine), expansion of the effective circulating blood volume (overhydration), and subsequent suppression of aldosterone with increased urinary sodium losses (hypernaturia and hyponatremia). Diagnosis is often made by demonstrating **hyperosmolal urine with hyponatremia**, and can be confirmed with increased or inappropriately "normal" serum levels of ADH.

BIBLIOGRAPHY

DeGroot L, Jamison L. *Endocrinology*, 4th ed. Philadelphia: WB Saunders (*in press*).

Felig P, Baxter JD, Frohmen LA. *Endocrinology and metabolism*. New York: McGraw-Hill, 1995.

Kettyle WM, Arky RA. *Endocrine pathophysiology*. Philadelphia: Lippincott-Raven, 1998.

Kyei-Mensah A, Jacobs HS. The investigation of female infertility. *Clin Endocrinol* (Oxf) 1995;43:251–255.

Melmed E. *The pituitary*. London: Blackwell Sciences, 1995.

Wilson J, Foster D, Kronenberg HM, Larsen PR. *Williams textbook of endocrinology*, 9th ed. Philadelphia: WB Saunders, 1998.

Lipids and Lipoproteins

Lily Wu

I. Basic science review. Cholesterol and other lipids are transported through the blood stream by protein carriers, and together are called "lipoproteins." The protein carriers by themselves are called "apolipoproteins" (from Greek, "apo + lipo" = without fat). The detailed mechanism by which the lipids in lipoprotein particles are transported, used, and removed from the body is very complex and involves apolipoproteins, enzymes, receptors, and transfer proteins. Any abnormalities in these components can disturb the balance of the metabolic system and affect the processing of lipids and lipoproteins, which can eventually lead to an increased risk of cardiovascular diseases.

  A. Lipoproteins. Lipoprotein particles are classified on the basis of their density, electrophoretic mobility, and composition of lipid and protein. **Five major classes of lipoproteins** (Table 4-54) exist: **chylomicron**; very low-density lipoprotein (**VLDL**); low-density lipoprotein (**LDL**); high-density lipoprotein (**HDL**); and **lipoprotein(a)**.

   1. Chylomicrons, a major vehicle for transporting fasting blood triglycerides (TG), are formed from dietary (exogenous) triglyceride and released into the lymphatics. Chylomicrons are delivered to skeletal muscle, heart, and adipose tissues, where **lipoprotein lipase** (LPL) on endothelial cells hydrolyzes the particles. This releases free fatty acids and glycerol for energy, or converts them back into triglycerides for storage. The chylomicron remnants, which contain **Apo E**, are cleared by the liver through Apo E receptors. Normally, chylomicrons are absent in 12- to 14-hour fasting blood specimens. Excess chylomicrons form a **creamy layer** on top of serum at 4°C.

   2. VLDL. These particles carry cholesterol and triglycerides synthesized by the liver (endogenous lipids) to peripheral tissues. In peripheral tissues, lipoprotein lipase releases triglyceride from the VLDL particles and **converts them to intermediate-density lipoprotein (IDL)**. Some of the IDL are then converted to LDL, but most of the IDL are cleared from circulation by Apo E receptors in the liver. In Apo E deficiencies, chylomicron remnants and VLDL circulate in excess; they are taken up by macrophages and form foam cells, fat streaks, and eventually **atherosclerosis**. When VLDL is present in excess, the serum is **turbid**.

   3. IDL. This is **not a separate class of lipoprotein**, but the **metabolic intermediate** between VLDL and LDL. Normally, the concentration of IDL in normal plasma is very low.

   4. LDL. The LDL particles, **the major cholesterol carriers in the body, deliver cholesterol to peripheral tissues**. LDL are catabolized mainly by the liver. Excess amounts of circulating LDL particles may be taken up by macrophages (foam cells), leading to **atherosclerosis**.

Table 4-54. Classification and terminology of lipoproteins

Name	Origin	Major Lipids	Electrophoresis Mobility	Apos Major	Apos Minor
Chylomicron	Intestine	Dietary, TG, CE	Origin	B-48; CI,II,III	A-I, II, IV; E
VLDL	Liver	Dietary, CE	Pre-β	B-100	CI, II, III; E
IDL	Catabolism of VLDL	CE, TG	Pre-β/β	B-100	CIII, E
LDL	Liver	CE	β	B-100	C
HDL	Liver, intestine	CE	α	A-I, II	CI, II, II; E, D
Lp(a)	Liver	CE	Sinking Pre-β	B-100, Apo(a)	

Apos, apolipoproteins; CE, cholesterol esters; HDL, high-density lipoprotein; IDL, intermediate-density lipoprotein; LDL, low-density lipoprotein; TG, triglyceride; VLDL, very low-density lipoprotein.

5.   HDL. The HDL particles carry 20% to 35% of total plasma cholesterol. **HDL takes excess cholesterol from the peripheral tissue cells and returns it to the liver for catabolism**, a process that can even **facilitate atheromatous plaque regression**. The major subclasses of HDL are HDL2 and HDL3; **HDL2** is particularly efficient as a cholesterol transporter.

6.   Lipoprotein(a) [Lp(a)] is an LDL-like, cholesterol-rich lipoprotein particle that contains both Apo B and Apo(a). Lp(a) is a risk factor for premature atherosclerosis. The level of plasma Lp(a) is predominately determined **genetically** and seems to be unaffected by gender, age, weight, and most lipid-lowering drugs. Screening for Lp(a) is recommended only for patients with coronary heart disease (CHD) or individuals with a positive family history for CHD, stroke, myocardial infarction (MI), elevated LDL, low HDL, renal dysfunction, or coagulation dysfunction. Patients with elevated Lp(a) should be aggressively treated to eliminate other risk factors.

7.   Apolipoprotein functions include maintaining lipoprotein structure, facilitating lipid transport, serving as receptor-binding ligands, and acting as an activator or inhibitor for the enzymes that participate in the metabolism of lipoproteins. **Elevations in Apo A1, Lp(a), B-100, and E are associated with increased risk for CHD.**

B.   Cholesterol and cardiovascular disease. Elevated cholesterol is a well-established risk factor for cardiovascular disease. Cholesterol and other risk factors (e.g., **homocysteine, fibrinogen, and coagulating factors**) interact synergistically to increase the risk. Common risk factors include **age** (men ≥45 years of age; women ≥55 years of age or postmenopausal without estrogen replacement therapy), **family history of early CHD** (MI or sudden death in first-degree male relatives <55 years of age or in first-degree female relatives <65 years of age), **hypertension** (blood pressure >140/90 mm Hg or on antihypertensive medication), **diabetes mellitus, current cigarette smoking, low HDL** (<35 mg/dL), **elevated LDL, obesity**, and **physical inactivity. High HDL (>60 mg/dL) is protective, and effectively erases one risk factor.**

II.   Diagnosis of lipid abnormalities

A.   Clinical evaluation. Assessments should include personal and family medical histories, physical examinations, prior lipids and medications, current medications, dietary assessments, and appropriate laboratory evaluations. **It is important to determine whether the dyslipidemia is a result of primary (genetic) or secondary (Table 4-55) causes, before beginning antilipidemic therapy.**

B.   Family history and familial lipoprotein disorders. To diagnose familial lipoprotein disorders, having more than two family members' lipid values is very helpful.

1.   Familial hypercholesterolemia (FH, type II hyperlipidemia). **LDL receptor defect** (>300 LDL receptor gene mutations are known); **autosomal dominant**; FH is present in 0.2% to 0.5% of the general population and 3% to 5%

Table 4-55. Secondary causes for hyperlipidemia

HDL-C <35 mg/dL	LDL-C ≥160 mg/dL	Triglyceride >400 mg/dL	
Obesity	Pregnancy	Pregnancy[a]	Pancreatitis
Starvation	Hypothy-	Hypothyroidism	Dysglobu-
Diabetes	roidism	Diabetes	linemia
mellitus	Diabetes	mellitus	Estrogens
β-blocker	Nephrotic	Alcoholism	Steroids
Progestins	syndrome	Obesity	Glycogen stor-
Anabolic	Chronic liver	Chronic liver	age disease
steroids	disease	disease	Lipodystrophy
Lack of	Cushing's	Chronic renal	Acute inter-
exercise	syndrome	failure	mittent
Cigarette	Dysglobu-	Cushing's	porphyria
smoking	linemia	syndrome	β-blocker
Hypertrigly-	Progestins,	Glucocorticoid	
ceridemia	estrogens,	use	
Stress or	β-Blockers	Hypopituitarism	
acute	Steroids	Diuretic drugs	
illness[b]	Hyper-	Gout	
Liver	parathy-		
disease	roidism		
Nephrotic	Acute inter-		
syndrome	mittent		
Uremia	porphyria		
	Dietary fats		

Note: Chem 20 and dipstick urinary analysis are usually sufficient; add other tests based on symptoms.

apo, apoprotein; HDL, high-density lipoprotein; LDL, low-density lipoprotein; TC, total cholesterol.

[a] Total cholesterol, triglycerides, LDL, apo A1 and AII, apo B, and Lp(a) all increase significantly during pregnancy (mainly in the second and third trimester). These tests should be performed at least three months postpartum.

[b] Triglyceride levels rise and TC, LDL, HDL, apo A1 and AII, apo B levels decrease about 24 h after acute myocardial infarction and stay low for 6–8 weeks.

of patients with early CHD; having two or more first-degree relatives with **elevated LDL** is a good indication of FH (Table 4-56).

2. **Familial combined hypercholesterolemia** (FCHL, types IIa, IIb, IV, V hyperlipidemia) is usually **autosomal dominant**; found in 1% to 2% of the general population, and in 20% of patients with early familial CHD. FCHL patients have later onset and less severe CHD than FH. **LDL, VLDL, and chylomicrons are variably elevated. HDL is frequently low**, and children can be affected (but less obvious than with FH).

3. **Polygenic hypercholesterolemia** (type IIa hyperlipidemia) is found in 3% to 5% of the general population and in 5% to 10% of early familial CHD. Usually, all parents and children in the family have **elevated LDL**. Children may not display elevations until adulthood.

Table 4-56. Lipid criteria for diagnosis
of familial hypercholesterolemia (FH)

Criteria	General Population			Within FH Families		
Age group (years)	<18	20	40+	<18	20	40+
TC (mg/dL)	270	290	360	220	240	300
LDL-C (mg/dL)	200	210	260	165	175	215

LDL, low-density lipoprotein; TC, total cholesterol.

4.   **Familial dysbetalipoproteinemia** (type III hyperlipidemia) is an **autosomal recessive** inheritance: >90% of type III patients have **Apo E2-2** genotype. Other environmental or genetic factors are needed for development of type III phenotype. Diagnostic tests include measured-VLDLc/TG >0.3, TG >150, the presence of lipoprotein-remnants (β-VLDL) in serum, Apo E2-2, and a combination of Apo E2-3 or 2-4 (i.e., one copy of E2). LDL receptor defect or other genetic defects and environmental factors also produce type III hyperlipidemia.

5.   **Other familial dyslipidemias**. See Table 4-57.

Table 4-57.   Other familial dyslipidemias

Familial Lipidemia Types and Mode of Inheritance	Risk for CHD	Comments
Hypertri-glyceridemia (type IV); AD	May or may not have increased risk	Population frequency is 2%, and 15% in CHD patients
Hypoalphalipo-proteinemia (low HDL); AD	Some risk	
Hyperalphalipo-proteinemia (high HDL); AD	Usually protected from CHD	
Hypobetalipo-proteinemia; AD	Low risk	Associated with longevity
Abetalipo-proteinemia; AR	Low risk	Low/absent Apo-B-lipoproteins; acanthocytes seen in blood smear
Tangier's disease; AR	Increased risk for cerebrovascular disease	Reticuloendothelial foam cells (e.g. orange tonsils).

AD, autosomal dominant; Apo, apolipoprotein; AR, autosomal recessive; CHD, coronary heart disease; HDL, high-density lipoprotein.

C. **Classification of cholesterol abnormalities**
    1.   **Frederickson phenotypes**. The Frederickson's hyper-
lipidemia phenotypes, are **based on the four major classes
of lipoproteins,** and their determination is **a useful initial
step** to making a diagnosis (Table 4-58). They may also **guide
therapy,** because therapy for a given pattern is essentially
the same, regardless of the underlying causes. Keep in mind
that the Frederickson phenotypes do not (a) take HDL into
consideration, (b) indicate severity, or (c) correspond precisely
with National Cholesterol Education Program (NCEP) guidelines, and (d) they can change after treatment.

III.   **Risk stratification of lipid abnormalities**. In 1993, the
Adult Treatment Panel II (ATPII) suggested that the guidelines
for the classification of lipid abnormalities in adults and children
be followed (Table 4-59).

IV.   **Recommendations for management of lipid abnormalities.** Individuals with potentially atherogenic lipid profiles
should be **managed initially through the introduction of
lifestyle changes and dietary intervention**. However, if these
fail to achieve recommended target values, a **lipid-lowering
drug therapy** should be considered. The decision-making values
and treatment recommendations are listed in Table 4-60.

Additional recommendations for specific lipid abnormalities include the modified NCEP recommendations (Tables 4-61 and 4-62).

V.   **Pearls**
A.   **Lipid and lipoprotein assessment in the future prob-
ably will include total cholesterol (TC), TG, direct LDL-
C, HDL-C, Lp(a)-C, and lipoprotein remnant cholesterol.**
B.   Serum LDL-C is estimated in most laboratories by the
Friedwald equation: LDL-C = TC-HDL-(TG/5). Limitations
to this method include (a) the patient must be fasting, (b) total
TG must be <400 mg/dL for reasonably accurate results, and (c)
the method is inherently imprecise and is not suitable for type
III patient samples. **Direct LDL-C immunoseparation** methods (which can use nonfasting samples) and **homogenous
enzymatic LDL-C** methods (which are not affected by TG up
to 1,000 mg/dL) **are more reliable and accurate methods to
measure LDL-C.**
C.   **Fasting or nonfasting specimens can be used for TC
testing. However, a 12-hour fasting specimen is required
for TG and lipoprotein testing**. Before making a medical decision about further action, **multiple measurements should be
taken within 2 months,** at least 1 week apart. A reduction of
3% to 4% in value is seen in EDTA plasma as compared with
serum.
D.   **A 1% reduction in serum cholesterol is associated
with a 1.5% to 3% reduction in CHD disease.**
E.   **Aggressively lowering LDL-C can reduce the risk for
CHD** morbidity and mortality in both primary and secondary
prevention.
F.   **Serum cholesterol measured at the age of 22 is a
valid predictor of CHD** over the following 40 years. Dietary
and lifestyle modifications instituted while the patient is in the
early 20s can improve the lipid profile and reduce the long-term
risk for CHD in young adults with elevated cholesterol levels.

(*text continues on page 419*)

Table 4-58.   Frederickson classification of the hyperlipidemias

Phenotype	TC	TG	Abnormal Lipoprotein	CAD Risk	Genetic Defects
I	NL to ↑	↑↑↑	Chylomicrons	None seen	LPL; apo C-II
IIa	↑↑	NL	LDL	+++	LDL receptor Familial combined hyperlipidemia Polygenic hypercholesterolemia
IIb	↑↑	↑↑	LDL and VLDL	+++	Familial hypercholesterolemia Familial combined hyperlipidemia
III	↑↑↑	↑↑↑	IDL, remnants	+++	E2, VLDL overproduction Familial dyslipidemia
IV	NL to ↑	↑↑↑↑	VLDL normal to abnormal	+	Familial hypertriglyceridemia Familial combined hypertriglyceridemia
V	NL to ↑	↑↑↑↑	VLDL and chylomicron	+	Familial hypertriglyceridemia Familial multiple hyperlipoproteinemia

CAD, coronary artery disease; IDL, intermediate-density lipoprotein; LDL, low-density lipoprotein; LPL, lipoprotein lipase; NL, normal; TC, total cholesterol; TG, triglyceride; VLDL, very low-density lipoprotein.

Table 4-59. Risk categories for lipid abnormalities in adults, adolescents, and children

Lipid	Desirable	Borderline	High	At risk for pancreatitis
	Risk Category for CHD and Atherosclerosis in Adults (Values for Adolescents and Children Are in Parentheses)			
Cholesterol	<200 (<170)	200–239 (170–199)	≥240 (>200)	No
LDL-C	<130 (<110)	130–159 (110–129)	≥160 >130)	No
HDL-C	≥60	—	<35	No
Triglyceride	<200	200–400	400–1,000	Yes, if TG>1000
TC:HDL[a]	<5.0	5.0–6.0	>6.0	

CDH, coronary heart disease; HDL, high-density lipoprotein; LDL, low-density lipoprotein; TC, total cholesterol; TG, triglyceride.

[a] The ratio of TC:HDL has not been recommended by Adult Treatment Panel II, but it does provide substantial information about CHD risk and is especially useful for individuals with low total cholesterol level. Consider the ratio, TC, TG, HDL, and LDL together for risk assessments.

Table 4-60. NCEP LDL cholesterol decision values (mg/dL) for dietary and drug treatment[a]

CHD Risk Factors	LDL values, Therapy Decisions, and LDL Goals		
No CHD risk and high HDL (≥35)	<160 (try diet)	≥160 (add drug)	Goal = <160
<2 risk factors	≥160 (try diet)	≥190 (add drug)	Goal = <160
≥2 risk factors	≥130 (try diet)	≥160 (add drug)	Goal = <130
CHD or other atherosclerotic disease	≥100 (try diet)	≥130 (add drug)	Goal = <100

CHD, coronary heart disease; HDL, high-density lipoprotein; LDL, low-density lipoprotein; NCEP, National Cholesterol Education Program.

Note: Criteria for adding drug refer to LDL levels after 3–6 months of a lipid-lowering diet.

[a] See common risk factors in section I.B.

Table 4-61.   Primary prevention—in the absence of CHD or other atherosclerotic disease

Laboratory Tests and Decision Values	Recommendation
TC[a] and HDL-C	
TC <200	Repeat testing within 5 yr
HDL-C ≥35	
HDL-C <35	Lipoprotein analysis (see below)
TC 200–239	Repeat testing in 1–2 yr
HDL-C ≥35 and	Increase physical activity, dietary
<2 other risk factors[b]	intervention, risk factor reduction
HDL-C <35 or with	Lipoprotein analysis (see below)
≥2 other risk factors	
TC ≥240	Lipoprotein analysis (see below)
Fasting lipoprotein analysis[c]	
LDL-C <130	Repeat TC and HDL-C testing within 5 yr
TG = 200–1,000, HDL <35	Weight loss, dietary intervention, high-fiber diet
TG>1,000	Prevent pancreatitis, low fat diet (<10% fat), weight loss, increase physical activity
LDL-C = 130–159 with <2 other risk factors	Dietary intervention and physical activity, reevaluate annually, including lipoprotein analysis
With ≥2 other risk factors	Clinical evaluation; initiate dietary therapy
LDL-C ≥160 mg/dL	
TG <200–300	Clinical evaluation; initiate dietary therapy
TG>200–1,000	Rule out type III; clinical evaluation; weight loss, dietary intervention
TG>200–1,000, HDL <35	Clinical evaluation; weight loss, dietary intervention, and drug therapy

CHD, coronary heart disease; HDL, high-density lipoprotein; LDL, low-density lipoprotein; TC, total cholesterol; TG, triglyceride.

[a] Intra-individual total cholesterol variation is from 6%–15% from month to month.

[b] Non-fasting sample can be used here, TC is not affected by food ingestion, but for HDL-C analysis use a method suitable for non-fasting sample.

[c] If fasting sample is used for TC and HDL testing, and if TG <400mg/dL, the calculated LDL-C using Friedwald equation can be used for clinical evaluation (not valid in Type III hyperlipidemia).

Table 4-62. Secondary prevention—in the presence of CHD or other atherosclerotic disease

Test and Decision Values[a] (Fasting Specimens)	Recommendation
LDL-C ≤100	Individualized instruction on diet and physical activity; repeat lipoprotein analysis annually
LDL-C >100	Clinical evaluation; initiate cholesterol-lowering therapy

CHD, coronary heart disease; LDL, low-density lipoprotein.
[a] Average of two determinations 1–8 weeks apart [three if variation is >30 mg/dL (0.8 mmol/L)]

G. Most MIs occur in patients having a 40% to 50% stenosis rather than advanced occlusion; therefore, aggressively lowering cholesterol can stabilize the rupture-prone atherosclerotic plaque to slow down and even reverse the progression of atherosclerosis.
H. Aggressively lowering cholesterol levels can reduce not only coronary mortality but also the all-cause mortality.

BIBLIOGRAPHY

American Heart Association. Consensus Panel Statement. Guide to Primary Prevention of Cardiovascular Diseases. *Circulation* 1997; 95:2330.

Expert Panel on Detection, Evaluation, and Treatment of High Blood Cholesterol in Adults. Summary of the Second Report of the National Cholesterol Education Program (NCEP) Expert Panel on Detection, Evaluation, and Treatment of High Blood Cholesterol in Adults (Adult Treatment Panel II). *JAMA* 1993;269:3015–3023.

Gotto AM Jr. Risk factor modification: rational for management of dyslipidemia. *Am J Med* 1998;104(2A):6S–8S.

Hopkins PN. Hyperlipidemia: detection and treatment. In: Yanowitz FG, ed. *Coronary heart disease prevention. A review towards the 21st century*. New York: Marcel Dekker, 1992:189–249.

Tumor Markers

James T. Wu

I. **Basic science review**
A. **Introduction. The major difference between malignant cells and normal cells is in the control of growth.** Malignant cells have uncontrolled growth that results in dedifferentiation, intensified invasiveness, metastases, and diminished drug sensitivity. Therefore, cancer is a disease of growth regulation. Multiple genetic mutations account for the uncontrolled cellular growth of cancer cells and, thus, cancer is also regarded as a genetic disease.
B. **Terms**
   1. **Hyperplasia**: increased numbers of cells that still respond to normal regulatory mechanisms.
   2. **Hypertrophy**: increased size of a cell.
   3. **Dysplasia** ("premalignant"): cells that do not increase in size or number, but have abnormal morphologic characteristics reflecting genetic damage. Dysplastic cells still respond to some regulatory stimuli, and may or may not progress to cancer.
   4. **Neoplasia**: cells whose growth is no longer under the control of normal biologic mechanisms.
   5. **Malignancy**: neoplastic cells that are monoclonal, grow faster than benign neoplastic cells, can invade and destroy local tissue, and may metastasize.
   6. **Proto-oncogenes**: genes that promote normal cell growth.
   7. **Oncogenes**: altered proto-oncogenes that promote abnormal cell growth.
   8. **Suppressor genes**: genes that suppress abnormal cell growth.
   9. **Differentiation**: how closely the cell resembles (in form and function) mature adult cells.
C. **Cellular growth processes.** Two principal growth processes—namely, **proliferation and differentiation—are involved in the normal growth of cells. Many biological processes control and regulate cell growth**, including growth factors, cell receptors, signal transduction pathways, secondary messengers, nuclear regulatory proteins, and so on. Proliferation and differentiation are well regulated during fetal development and determine the final adult size, shape, and function of various cells, tissues, and organs. After full differentiation of cells occurs, **new growth is either in the form of hyperplasia or neoplasia (tumor)**. All benign tumors are well differentiated, whereas malignant tumors range from being well-differentiated to being undifferentiated.
D. **Genetic aspects of cancer**
   1. **Genetic control of cancer**. Alterations in the genetic components related to cell growth account for all of the differ-

ent behaviors and functions observed in cancer. **Two major groups of genes are responsible for controlling normal cell growth, namely proto-oncogenes and suppressor genes**. Inherited or sporadic mutations in proto-oncogenes, suppressor genes, or both lead to higher risks of the cell transforming into cancer. The **transformation of a normal cell to a malignant cell usually involves multiple steps** and takes years to develop. In general, multiple oncogenes must be activated, at least two suppressor genes must be inactivated, and apoptosis must be suppressed in order for malignancies to develop.

2. **Proto-oncogenes and oncogenes**

   a. **Role of proto-oncogenes.** Proto-oncogenes are **normal genes that regulate cell growth**. Proteins encoded by proto-oncogenes involve growth factors (e.g., platelet-derived growth factor, PDGF; fibroblast growth factor, FGF; and so on), growth factor receptors [e.g., *erb*-B2 (HER-2/*neu*)], signal-transducing proteins [guanosine triphosphate (GTP)-binding protein (e.g., *ras*), tyrosine kinase (e.g., *abl*)], secondary cytoplasmic messengers, and nuclear regulatory factors [e.g., transcription activators (e.g., *myc*)]. **Oncogenes are abnormally activated proto-oncogenes** that produce an abundance of these normal proteins, or proteins that are altered, and the activated or mutated genes **no longer respond to normal physiologic control mechanisms**. Some oncogenes have been named according to the tumors they create when carried by retroviruses (e.g., "**ras**" = **ra**t **s**arcoma).

   b. **Transformation of proto-oncogenes into oncogenes occurs in several ways.**

   (1) **Aging**: cumulative effects of free radicals, and so forth.

   (2) **Heredity**: inherited cancer syndromes (e.g., familial adenomatous polyposis), specific familial cancers (e.g., colon or breast cancer), or defective DNA repair syndromes (e.g., xeroderma pigmentosum, ataxia-telangiectasia).

   (3) **Radiation**

   (4) **Chemical exposures** (e.g., chlorinated hydrocarbons, polyvinyl chloride).

   (5) **Toxins** (e.g., aflatoxin).

   (6) **Viruses** (e.g., human papilloma virus, hepatitis B virus).

   c. **Tumor progression requires additional genetic mutations. In general, once a tumor is formed, it will grow in size and progress through several further stages. Additional genetic mutations must occur** to allow for cell discohesiveness, proteolysis of the basement membrane, attachment of tumor cells to extracellular matrices, locomotion, invasion of vascular structures, and eventually the formation of new tumor cell colonies in distant organs. In general, the more aggressive, the more rapidly growing, and the larger the primary neoplasm, the greater the likelihood that it will metastasize.

3. **Suppressor genes** (anti-oncogenes) code for proteins that regulate normal cell growth by **suppressing excessive growth**, such as **Rb** ("retinoblastoma gene"), **WT-1** (Wilm's tumor gene), and **APC** (adenomatous polyposis coli) gene. Suppressor genes regulate the same processes that oncogenes regulate, but in opposite ways, and their inactivation leads to faster cell growth.

4. **Apoptosis or programmed cell death**. As cells age and gradually accumulate genetic damage, apoptosis occurs, which prevents the cells from passing their genetic damage to progeny cells. For example, **p53** and **bcl-2** are genes that have a major impact on apoptosis. Defects in p53 (which are the most common genetic abnormalities in cancer) allow genetically damaged cells to avoid apoptosis (thereby continuing to live).

II. Tumor markers
A. Basic principles

1. **Diversity of markers and laboratory tests. Almost any molecule can be used as a tumor marker** as long as it reflects tumor cell proliferation, a specific genetic mutation, type of differentiation, tumor aggressiveness, metastatic potential, or responsiveness to therapy. **Many laboratory techniques** are used in tumor marker measurement, including chemical or enzymatic assays, immunoassays based either on competitive binding or sandwich formats, and genetic probes. Some of the most common tumor markers are identified by monoclonal antibodies, without an exact knowledge of the structure of the molecules expressing the target epitope (e.g., CA 125).

2. **Nonspecific proliferation markers**. Many molecules that are **normally found in the blood** circulation can become **elevated in tumors** and, therefore, can be used as tumor markers. Among these are enzymes (e.g., lactate dehydrogenase), serum proteins (e.g., interleukin-2), hormones (e.g., human chorionic gonadotropin), and metabolites (e.g., 5-HIAA). Most markers of this type have **little specificity**, but are still useful to **indicate a rapid new growth** of cells and for tumor monitoring.

3. **Lack of differentiation markers**. In advanced stages of tumors, continued genetic mutations cause dedifferentiation (embryonal-like features), along with the production of **carcinoembryonic proteins** (carcinoembyronic antigen, CEA) or ectopic molecules. These substances occur in normal corresponding fetal tissues, disappear in mature adult tissue, and reappear in tumor tissue.

4. **Genetic markers**. These identify **specific genetic abnormalities that underlie malignancy**, such as oncogenes or damaged suppressor genes, or as a result of overexpression of the gene products. These gene products include growth factors and other molecules involved in specific steps of tumorgenesis, such as membrane receptors, apoptosis, angiogenesis, and cell adhesion.

B. Uses of tumor markers. Tumor markers have multiple applications. **The most successful applications of tumor**

markers are to monitor the course of the cancer during treatment, to access the success of a surgical removal of a tumor, and later for detecting cancer recurrence. A variety of markers have additional uses. Some markers, for example chromogranin A, which is a marker of cells with neuroendocrine differentiation (e.g., carcinoid, small cell carcinoma of the lung), help **identify a malignant cell's line of differentiation**. Some tumor markers help to identify **individuals at high risk** for the development of cancer, such as BRCA 1 and BRCA 2 for inherited breast cancers. High elevations in embryonal tumor markers such as CEA **may support a diagnosis of malignancy** over benignancy. Tumor markers such as alkaline phosphatase isoenzymes can assist in identifying **locations of metastases** (e.g., bone vs. liver). Other tumor markers help to **evaluate a tumor's aggressiveness**, such as HER-2-/*neu*, proliferating cell nuclear antigen (PCNA), or the percent of the cells in S phase. Still other tumor markers can indicate a tumor's **potential responsiveness** to certain therapies, such as a breast cancer's hormone receptor status (estrogen or progesterone status).

C. **General guidelines for interpreting tumor markers**
   1. **No tumor-specific marker has ever been found**. All tumor markers have <100% specificity and sensitivity. Prostate-specific antigen (**PSA**) **is the most organ-specific** (not cancer specific) of current markers, and is the only marker currently approved as a screening tool for cancer in the United States (when used in conjunction with a digital rectal examination).
   2. **Never rely on a single test**. Always order serial instead of single tests to rule out benign diseases (e.g., hyperplasia or inflammation). In general, the phenotypic expression of a cancer cell is fairly similar to that of a normal cell. Therefore, many of the nonspecific tumor marker differences that exist between benign and malignant conditions largely reflect the difference in proliferation rates over time. **Hyperplasia will cause transient elevations in markers, whereas neoplasia will cause long-lasting, progressive elevations in markers.**
   3. **Order the same tumor marker kit from the same laboratory**. Different kits and different laboratories can produce differing values for the same specimen.
   4. **Be sure to select a tumor marker that is elevated before therapeutic surgery.**
   5. **Consider the half-life of the tumor marker when interpreting postoperative levels**. For most tumor markers, **wait at least 2 weeks** (and preferably 1 month) after surgery before repeating the tumor marker test. It takes time for the preoperative level of tumor marker to decline to normal levels, depending on the half-life of the tumor marker in the circulation, and whether transient increases in the serum tumor marker levels occur because of intraoperative manipulation of the tumor.
   6. **Elevated serum or plasma levels of tumor markers can be found in patients with liver or renal disease** even

though they do not have cancer, depending on how the tumor marker is normally metabolized. For example, CEA is normally metabolized by the liver and, therefore, liver disease can cause elevations in CEA. In a similar manner, β_2-microglobulin (β_2-M) is excreted by the kidneys, and renal failure causes increased serum β_2-M levels.

7. Ordering multiple markers may increase the sensitivity and specificity of the tumor markers for diagnosing disease. For example, ordering CA 15-3, CA 19-9, and CA 125 together may show patterns that are helpful in narrowing the list of possible malignancies.

8. Order nonspecific, inexpensive markers [e.g., lipid-associated sialic acid-P (LASA-P)] when the only purpose of the test is to monitor for tumor recurrence.

9. Be aware of the hood effect. Falsely low results from some immunoassay tests can occur in cases of a marked antigen excess. When a tumor marker level is much lower than would be expected based on the patient's extensive tumor load, order the tumor marker assay rerun after doing a **10-to-1 dilution** of the patient's serum.

10. Metastases are generally associated with the highest elevation of tumor markers.

D. Individual commonly used tumor markers

1. α-fetoprotein (α-FP) is the fetal form of albumin and one of the main **carcinoembryonic markers**. It is transiently elevated in pregnancy and liver disease, and increased in many germ cell tumors. Because of increased fucosylation, α-FP has **increased lentil lectin reactivity in hepatocellular carcinoma** (HCC), and the lentil lectin reactivity may help to differentiate between HCC and other benign liver disorders. α-FP is a useful screen for HCC in the Orient, where the incidence of HCC is very high.

2. β_2-Microglobulin (β_2-M) forms the constant (light chain) portion of the human leukocyte antigen **(HLA) class I molecule**, which is concentrated on the surface of lymphocytes. β_2-M is released into the serum when nucleated cells are metabolized. β_2-M, therefore, is a nonspecific, but useful, marker for **monitoring lymphocytic lymphomas and leukemias**, including their response to treatment, recurrences, and involvement of the central nervous system (cerebrospinal fluid β_2-M levels).

3. CA 19-9. "CA" initially stood for "carbohydrate antigen." CA 19-9, a carbohydrate antigen on high molecular weight **mucin**, is defined by monoclonal antibodies. CA 19-9 is elevated in a variety of carcinomas, particularly those of the **pancreas and stomach.** CA 19-9 is **related to Lewis blood group** substances, and only patients with Le (a+ b–) or Le (a– b+) blood are capable of producing the CA 19-9 antigen (even in carcinomas). CA 50 and CA 19-5 may complement the use of CA 19-9, and be present in Le (a– b–) patients. CA 19-9, CA 19-5, and CA 50 **can also be elevated in hepatocellular carcinoma, cholestasis for whatever reason, and colon cancer.**

4.   **CA 125** is a high molecular weight **mucinlike glyco-protein**, elevated in >80% of patients with nonmucinous epithelial **ovarian carcinomas** (e.g., serous, endometrioid, and clear cell carcinomas), and in many **uterine carcinomas**. CA 125 levels can decrease in patients after chemotherapy, even though their ovarian tumors continue to progress.

5.   **CA 15-3**, a **breast cancer**-associated antigen, is also present in a variety of adenocarcinomas such as **lung, colon, ovary, and pancreas**. CA 15-3 is also elevated in benign conditions such as hepatitis, cirrhosis, sarcoidosis, tuberculosis, and systemic lupus.

6.   **CA 72-4** detects an adenocarcinoma-associated antigen, and is associated with TAG-72, a high molecular weight **mucinlike** substance. It is found in fetal serum, is elevated in a variety of carcinomas, and is considered a **carcinoembryonic protein**. Although not very sensitive, it is the most useful marker for monitoring patients with **gastric carcinoma**.

7.   **Calcitonin** is elevated whenever there is increased bone turnover, such as in **bone metastases**. It can also be elevated in bronchogenic carcinomas and medullary carcinoma of the thyroid.

8.   **Carcinoembryonic antigen is a glycoprotein** found in fetal cells and, hence, considered a **carcinoembryonic protein**. It is increased in a variety of adenocarcinomas, particularly in **colorectal cancer**. CEA can be increased in patients with liver disease, and in patients undergoing chemotherapy or radiation therapy.

9.   **C-*erb*B-2 (HER-2/*neu*)** is an oncogene that produces a transmembrane protein similar to the epidermal growth factor receptor. The HER-2/*neu* gene is amplified in 25% to 30% of **breast and ovarian cancers**, and is a poor prognostic sign.

10.   **Chromogranin A (CgA)** is a marker for neuroendocrine cells. CgA can be elevated in a wide variety of **neuroendocrine tumors**, including pheochromocytoma, carcinoids, and small cell carcinoma of the lung.

11.   **Human chorionic gonadotropin (hCG) is a glyco-protein** secreted by placental trophoblasts. It is elevated in **pregnancy, trophoblastic tumors** (e.g., choriocarcinoma), and many **germ cell tumors of the ovary and testes**. In seminomas, βhCG should be ordered. In non-seminomatous tumors, βhCG, free αhCG, and intact hCG should be ordered, as any of the three can be elevated.

12.   **Lipid-associated sialic acid-P (LASA-P)**, a derivative of **neuraminic acid**, is found in a variety of glycoproteins and glycolipids. LASA-P is a **nonspecific** marker that is increased in a variety of inflammatory and malignant processes. It is a nonspecific, but very useful, **inexpensive way to monitor a tumor's response** to therapy or to identify tumor recurrences.

13.   **Neuron-specific enolase** is found in **neurons, neuroendocrine cells**, and a variety of tumors including **neuro-**

endocrine tumors (e.g., small cell carcinoma of the lung, carcinoids).

14.   p53 is a gene on **chromosome 17** that codes for a nuclear suppressor protein. P53 **allows apoptosis** (programmed cell death) when cells accumulate genetic mutations. The **mutated protein** has a much longer half-life than the normal p53 product; it can actually stimulate cell division and is **a poor prognostic indicator.**

15.   Parathyroid hormone-related peptide (PTH-RP) is usually elevated in patients with **hypercalcemia caused by malignancy**. It is also elevated in patients with renal insufficiency.

16.   Prostate-specific antigen (PSA) is produced by prostate glandular tissue, PSA is the **most organ-specific tumor marker** known at this time. It is elevated in a variety of prostate disorders, including infarction, infection, hyperplasia, and malignancy, as well as transiently after prostatic massage. It is currently used as a screen for prostatic cancer (when used in conjunction with, and drawn previous to, a digital rectal examination). PSA is also useful to determine whether or not all of the prostatic tissue has been removed at prostatectomy, and to monitor patients for tumor recurrence. Free PSA (fPSA), as a percentage of total PSA, has been found to be **lower in patients with prostate cancer** than in patients with benign nodular hyperplasia.

17.   Squamous cell carcinoma (SCC). A portion of the tumor antigen TA-4 is identified in squamous cell carcinoma of the uterine cervix. It is elevated in **squamous cell carcinomas** regardless of their location in the body. SCC is also elevated in patients with renal insufficiency.

18.   Tissue polypeptide antigen (TPA) is a **mixture of epithelial cytokeratins**, and elevations reflect increased mitotic activity. It is, therefore, a **nonspecific but useful marker for cancer progression** versus remission. TPA **can also help differentiate between cholangiocarcinomas (TPA elevated) and hepatocellular carcinomas (TPA not elevated)** (Tables 4-63 and 4-64).

E.   Adjunctive tests

1.   S phase (flow cytometry). Analysis of the cell cycle [resting (GO), gap 1 (G1), DNA synthesis (S), gap 2 (G2), and mitosis (M)] offers prognostic information about tumors. **More than 8%** of the cells in the S phase reflects faster tumor growth and is an **adverse prognostic indicator.**

2.   DNA index (image analysis or flow cytometry) equals the DNA content in the tumor cells relative to the DNA in normal human cells. DNA index of one equals diploid (normal); **DNA index <0.9 or >1.19 reflects aneuploidy**, and is a poor prognostic indicator.

3.   C-*erb*B-2 (HER-2/*neu*, immunohistochemical) is similar to the epidermal growth factor receptor. The **greater the amplification**, the more responsive the cell will be to growth factors, and the **worse the prognosis.**

(*text continues on page 431*)

**Table 4-63. Tumor markers associated
with individual malignances**

Malignancy	Tumor Marker*
Bone cancer	*Alkaline phosphatase, serum calcium, free hydroxyproline
Breast cancer	*CA 15-3, CEA, calcitonin, prolactin, LASA-P, CA 549
Carcinoid tumors	*Serotonin, *5-HIAA, *chromogranin A
Cervical cancer	*SCC, CEA, CA 125
Choriocarcinoma	*hCG
Colorectal carcinoma	*CEA, CA 19-9
Cholangiocarcinoma	*CEA, TPA
Chronic myelogenous leukemia	*TdT
Endocrine neoplasia	*Chromogranin A, *specific hormones depending on the tumor
Gastric carcinoma	*CA 72-4, CEA, CA 19-9, CA 50, NSE
Gastrinoma	*Gastrin
Hepatocellular carcinoma	*AFP, CEA, ferritin, γGT, ALP, TPA
Hypercalcemia of malignancy	*PTH-related peptide
Leukemia/lymphoma	
–Monocytic (e.g., FAB M5)	*Lysosyme
–B-cell	*Monoclonal immunoglobulins, β_2M, Ki-67, LASA-P, LDH3
–T-cell/B-cell	*LDH3
–Hairy cell	*IL-2 receptor
Lung cancer	*NSE, ACTH, calcitonin, CA 72-4, CEA, AFP, ferritin, LASA-P
Melanoma	*TA 90, *melanoma-associated antigen, NSE, catecholamines, LASA-P
Multiple myeloma	*Monoclonal immunoglobulins, Bence Jones protein, β_2M
Mesothelioma	*Hyaluronic acid
Neuroblastoma	*Chromogranin A, *VMA, HVA, NSE, cystathionine, metanephrines
Neuroendocrine tumors	*Chromogranin A, NSE
Osteosarcoma	*ALP
Ovarian carcinoma	*CA 125, inhibin, amylase isoenzyme, CEA
Pancreatic carcinoma (exocrine)	*CA 19-9, CA 195, CA 50, CA 72-4, CEA, CK-BB, insulin-like growth factor

continued

Table 4-63. *Continued*

Malignancy	Tumor Marker*
Pancreatic carcinoma (endocrine/islet tumors)	*Insulin, *glucagon, *somatostatin, *pancreatic polypeptide (depending on the type of islet tumor)
Parathyroid tumors	*PTH intact
Pheochromocytoma	*Metanephrine, chromogranin A, catecholamines
Pituitary tumors	*Free α-hCG (in general)
–ACTH secreting	*ACTH
–Gonadotropin secreting	*LH/FSH
–Growth-hormone secreting	*Growth hormone
–Prolactin secreting	*Prolactin
–TSH secreting	*TSH
Placental tumors	*hCG, free α-hCG
Prostate carcinoma	*PSA (and free PSA)
Renal cell carcinoma	*CEA, renin, erythropoietin, interleukin-4, prostaglandin A, CA 15-3
Sarcoma	*β_2M
Splenic tumors	*ferritin
Squamous cell carcinoma	*SCC
Teratoblastoma	*AFP, hCG, ferritin
Testicular cancer	
–Seminoma	*NSE, LDH1
–Non-seminomatous	*AFP, βhCG
Thyroid carcinoma	
Medullary	*Calcitonin, NSE
Papillary and follicular	*Thyroglobulin
Uterine carcinoma	*SCC, CA 125
Waldenström's disease	*Monoclonal IgM, β_2M

*Most important marker.
ACTH, adrenocorticotropic hormone; AFP, alpha-fetoprotein; ALP, alkaline phosphatase; β_2M, beta-2 microglobulin; CA, carcinoma; CEA, carcinoembryonic antigen; CgA, chromogranin A; CK, creatine kinase isoenzymes; γGT, gamma-glutamyl transferase; 5-HIAA, 5-hydroxyindoleacetic acid; FSH, follicle-stimulating hormone; hCG, human chorionic gonadotropin; HVA, homovanillic acid; LASA-P, lipid-associated sialic acid-P; LDH, lactate dehydrogenase; LH, luteinizing hormone; NSE, neuron-specific enolase; PSA, prostate specific antigen; PTH, parathyroid hormone; SCC, squamous cell carcinoma antigen; TdT, terminal deoxynucleotidyl transferase; TPA, tissue polypeptide antigen; TSH, thyroid-stimulating hormone (thyrotropin); VMA, vanillylmandelic acid.

Table 4-64. Summary of commonly used tumor markers

Tumor Marker	Specimen	Assay Method	Reference Range	Interpretation and Artifact
AFP	Serum or plasma	EIA	0–15 ng/mL	Marker for germ cell and hepatic tumors. The normal reference ranges are much higher in infants, then decrease with age. At 8 months, the serum AFP value reaches adult levels.
CEA	Serum	EIA	0–2.5 ng/mL	Marker for colorectal CA. Elevated serum CEA can also be found in other carcinomas and in heavy smokers.
CA 125	Serum	EIA	0–35 U/mL	Marker for ovarian CA. Elevated serum levels are found in serous ovarian CA and in other carcinomas.
CA 19-9	Serum	EIA	0–37 U/mL	Marker for pancreatic CA. Elevated serum levels can be detected in other carcinomas, especially gastric and colon CA.
CA 15-3	Serum	EIA	0–40 U/mL	Marker for breast CA. Elevated serum levels can also be found in other carcinomas.
PSA	Serum	EIA	0–4 ng/mL	Marker for prostate CA. First tumor marker recommended for screening because of its tissue specificity. Slightly higher normal values are found at older ages.
Free PSA (fPSA)	Serum	EIA	<6%	% fPSA = [(fPSA/PSA) × 100]. Less than 6% indicates the presence of prostate CA.
CgA	Serum	EIA	0–99 ng/mL	Marker for neuroblastoma, pheochromocytoma, small cell lung carcinoma and carcinoid tumors. Elevated serum CgA can also occur in nonendocrine tumors
NSE	Serum	EIA	M: 0–14 ng/mL F: 0–11 ng/mL	Marker for neuroendocrine tumors such as neuroblastoma, pheochromocytoma, small cell lung CA, and carcinoid tumors.

continued

Table 4-64. Continued

Tumor Marker	Specimen	Assay Method	Reference Range	Interpretation and Artifact
SCC	Serum	RIA	0–2.5 ng/mL	Marker for squamous cell CA of the lung, cervix, head, and neck.
β_2M	Serum	EIA	1.1–2.4 mg/L	Elevated in CA, malignant lymphoma, and multiple myeloma
β-hCG	Serum		Male: 2–5 IU/L Female: 2–8 IU/L	β-hCG and AFP together have been recommended for staging and management of non-seminomatous testicular tumors. β-hCG could be an indicator of malignant transformation for a wide range of solid tumor.
VMA	Urine	HPLC	0.5–6 mg/g creatinine	Marker for neuroblastoma. Both random and 24-h urine used. Infants have much higher levels (up to 45 mg/g at 3 months) which decline gradually to adult levels at age 1. 5.5% of neuroblastomas have elevated HVA and normal VMA.
5-HIAA	Urine	HPLC	2–15 mg/d	Many medications can cause interference in this measurement (e.g., aspirin thorazine, aldoclor, compazine, mepergan).
Meta-N	24-h urine	HPLC	30–350 µg/d	Diagnosis and follow-up of patients with pheochromocytoma.
CA 72-4	Serum	EIA	0–5.6 ng/mL	Marker for gastric CA. Serum CA 72-4 can also be detected in breast, colon, ovary, and pancreas carcinomas. The test has very poor sensitivity.

AFP, α-fetoprotein; β-hCG, beta unit of human chorionic gonadotropin; β_2M, beta$_2$ microglobulin; CA, carcinoma; CEA, carcinoembryonic antigen; d, day; EIA, enzyme immunoassay; 5-HIAA, 5-hydroxyindoleacetic acid; HPLC, high-performance liquid chromatography; HVA, homovanillic acid; Meta-N, metanephrine; NSE, neural specific enolase; PSA, prostate-specific antigen; RIA, radioimmunoassay; SCC, squamous cell carcinoma antigen; VMA, 3-methoxy-4-hydroxymandelic acid.

   4. **p53** (immunohistochemical, serum). Normally, p53 stimulates apoptosis of defective cells. Amplification of mutant p53 is a **poor prognostic indicator.**

   5. **Ki-67 (proliferating cell nuclear antigen, PCNA), or MIB-1**, immunohistochemical) is a marker for proliferation and aggressiveness. Generally, the **greater the Ki-67, the worse the prognosis (>18% PCNA is a poor prognostic sign).**

   6. **Cathepsin D** (immunohistochemical) is a lysosomal protease capable of digesting basement membranes. High levels of cathepsin D are a **poor prognostic indicator** in breast cancer.

Liver Tests

Brent A. Neuschwander-Tetri

I.   Introduction. Liver enzyme tests are commonly referred to as "liver function tests" or "LFTs"; however, **liver enzyme elevations reflect liver injury or hepatobiliary obstruction, rather than actual liver functions. True tests of liver functions include bilirubin, prothrombin time, and albumin, which measure the ability of the liver to excrete substances and synthesize proteins**. Liver tests are more sensitive and specific when ordered together as a panel, and should always be interpreted in the clinical context.

II.   Enzymes. Serum liver enzymes are the primary means of detecting subclinical liver injury and hepatobiliary obstruction as causes of otherwise nonspecific constitutional symptoms.

A.   Enzymes that indicate hepatocellular injury. Alanine aminotransferase (ALT), aspartate aminotransferase (AST), and lactate dehydrogenase (LDH) are enzymes that identify processes that directly damage hepatocytes. The most common causes of liver cell injury are **viruses** (e.g., hepatitis A, B, and C viruses, Epstein–Barr virus), **drugs, toxins, alcohol, autoimmune hepatitis, metabolic diseases, nonalcoholic steatohepatitis, shock, biliary obstruction, and passive congestion.**

　　1.   ALT (normal range: 10–35 U/L) is found primarily in the liver (with small amounts in heart, muscle, and red blood cells); it is released into the blood when hepatocytes are injured. An elevated ALT is **the best test for identifying the presence of subclinical parenchymal liver disease.**

　　2.   AST (normal range: 20–45 U/L) is found in liver, heart, kidney, brain, pancreas, lung, white and red blood cells, which makes the **AST less specific than the ALT**. The AST and ALT are measured together because of the additional information and confidence gained by having both results.

　　3.   LDH (normal adult range: up to 200 U/L) is **found in most tissues**, and is less useful than ALT and AST because of this nonspecificity. LDH isoenzymes were once obtained to differentiate liver LDH from cardiac LDH, but ALT has largely supplanted this test.

B.   Enzymes that indicate bile duct obstruction or cholestasis. Alkaline phosphatase (ALP), gamma-glutamyltranspeptidase (GGT), and 5′-nucleotidase (5′-NT) are enzymes that detect obstruction of the extrahepatic bile ducts (e.g., tumors, gallstones, sclerosing cholangitis) or obstruction of the intrahepatic bile ducts and hepatocyte bile canaliculi (e.g., granulomas, abscesses, tumors, primary biliary cirrhosis).

　　1.   Alkaline phosphatase (normal adult range: 50–120 U/L)

　　　　a.   Sources. ALP is an enzyme found primarily in **bone, liver, intestine, and placenta** (whence, the acronym

BLIP); it has a circulating half-life of 7 days. The most common sources by far of serum ALP elevations are bone and liver disorders. The highest serum levels are seen in Paget's disease of the bone. Other causes include normal childhood bone growth (ALP can be as high as 1,000 U/L), pregnancy (doubling during the third trimester because of the placenta), chronic renal failure (from build-up of the intestinal isoenzyme), ABH blood group secretors, hypothyroidism, pernicious anemia, zinc deficiency, congestive heart failure, hypophosphatemia, and benign familial elevations.

   b.   Elevations in liver disease. In the liver, ALP is present on bile canaliculi membranes. **Obstruction in the hepatobiliary tree** (partial or complete, focal or global) causes the serum level of ALP to increase. ALP levels can also be increased up to two to three times the upper limit of normal by **parenchymal disease** such as viral hepatitis, alcoholic hepatitis, and established cirrhosis.

   c.   Heat fractionation can help identify the source of an elevated ALP. The serum sample is heated, and the activity is compared with unheated serum. "Bone burns, liver lives" is a common but somewhat misleading adage. Heat stability occurs in 10% of bone ALP, 60% of liver ALP, and 100% of placental ALP. **In practice, GGT (or 5′-NT), liver ultrasound, and bone scans are used to identify the source of elevated ALP.**

   2.   Gamma-glutamyltransferase (GGT) (normal adult range: 2–30 U/L) is an enzyme found in the **kidneys, liver, and pancreas**. The kidney has the highest concentration of GGT, but kidney diseases generally do not increase the serum GGT level. On the other hand, acute pancreatitis can cause GGT elevations. In the liver, GGT is located in the canalicular membrane of hepatocytes and bile ducts. The serum GGT level is **a very sensitive indicator of obstruction**; it is elevated very early in any process that obstructs bile ducts or intrahepatic bile canaliculi. It is also increased by **alcohol use and abuse, drugs** (e.g., dilantin, phenobarbital, tricyclic antidepressants, coumadin, benzodiazepines), **hepatic steatosis, and nonalcoholic steatohepatitis**. Because hepatic steatosis is very common, mild GGT elevations are also very common and **the clinical evaluation of an isolated GGT elevation should be limited.**

   3.   5′-NT (normal range: 5–10 U/L) is an enzyme that is less commonly used for detecting cholestasis. Its use is primarily in establishing the source (e.g., liver) of an elevated alkaline phosphatase.

C.   Pearls for interpreting liver enzyme levels

   1.   The AST:ALT ratio (DeRitis ratio, normally ≈1) can be helpful in certain settings. **Many nonhepatic disorders** (e.g., myocardial infarction, hemolysis) **will cause the AST to rise significantly while the ALT remains normal** or mildly elevated (the AST:ALT ratio is therefore >1). The AST:ALT ratio is also **>1.0 in cases of extensive hepatocellular necrosis** (e.g., drug-induced necrosis, cirrhosis with ongoing liver injury such as in Hepatitis C), and often **>2.0 in alcoholic hepatitis. In nonalcoholic steatohep-**

atitis, the ALT is almost invariably greater than the AST (the AST:ALT ratio is often <0.5). This difference can help identify occult alcohol abuse as a cause of elevated aminotransferases. **Other causes of an AST:ALT ratio <1.0 include chronic viral hepatitis and extrahepatic biliary obstruction.**

2.   **An AST or ALT value that exceeds 2,000 U/L,** which is unusual, is caused primarily by five major insults to the liver worthy of memorizing: **acute viral hepatitis, severe autoimmune hepatitis, shock or ischemic injury, drugs or toxins** (e.g., acetaminophen, mushroom poisoning), and **acute biliary obstruction** (this is the easy one to forget).

3.   **In general, the degree of aminotransferase elevation is of no *prognostic* value.**

4.   **The circulating half-lives of AST (12–18 hours) and ALT (36–48) are important to know.** If a patient has very high enzyme levels (>1,000 U/L) and the cause is uncertain, **serial values that drop according to their respective half-lives indicate that the acute event was either shock** (e.g., acute myocardial infarction) or **toxin** (e.g., acetaminophen) and that there is no ongoing liver injury. The marked elevations seen with viral and autoimmune hepatitis take much longer to resolve (i.e., weeks or months).

5.   **Always interpret the test results within the clinical context.** For example, **elevated aminotransferases that decrease following severe acute injury can indicate recovery, or can indicate that the entire liver has been destroyed** and no more enzymes are available to be released. In this dire situation, the prothrombin time continues to rise and the mental status deteriorates.

6.   **Severe liver dysfunction with mild aminotransferase elevations** (i.e., <400 U/L) **is typical of disorders of mitochondrial dysfunction** (e.g., acute fatty liver of pregnancy, alcoholic hepatitis, Reye's syndrome). In these disorders, indicators of liver function such as the prothrombin time and the degree of encephalopathy provide a much better assessment of the disease than do the aminotransferases.

7.   **Normal AST and ALT values do not completely exclude liver disease or even cirrhosis. Hemochromatosis is the most common example** of a liver disease that can slowly progress to cirrhosis with normal aminotransferases. Other examples include **nonalcoholic steatohepatitis and chronic hepatitis C.** Indeed, **cirrhosis** of any cause is typically associated with normal aminotransferases if the original insult to the liver has resolved. In addition, **dialysis patients** can have a variety of liver diseases with decreased aminotransferase levels. This is because of displacement of the vitamin B_6 cofactor needed for the activity of these enzymes, which cannot be corrected by the laboratory. The aminotransferases, thus, are insensitive tests to identify occult liver disease in this population.

8.   **Elevated liver alkaline phosphatase levels can be associated with normal aminotransferase and bilirubin levels in cases of *partial* biliary obstruction by stones or tumors.**

III. True tests of liver function. The following tests are indicators of the liver's ability to synthesize protein and carry out its normal excretory process.

A. Prothrombin time (PT) is used to assess patients with both acute and chronic liver disease. A persistently rising PT in acute liver disease may suggest the need for liver transplantation. The degree of elevation (in seconds above the upper limit of normal) in chronic liver disease is used in calculating the **Child-Turcotte-Pugh score** (along with ascites, encephalopathy, bilirubin, and albumin); this score can be used to assess general surgical risk and to classify patients for the urgency of liver transplantation. Prothrombin times are also elevated in vitamin K deficiencies, malabsorptive syndromes, and disseminated intravascular coagulation (DIC).

B. Factor V is a short-lived coagulation factor synthesized by the liver (not vitamin K dependent) that gives a more precise "snapshot" of how well the liver is functioning at a specific point in time. Factor V levels are **measured in certain patients with fulminant hepatic failure,** to identify early signs of recovery that could obviate the need for transplantation. If DIC is a potential cause of a low factor V and an elevated PT, measuring factor VIII can be helpful. **Factor VIII, which is not synthesized by the liver and is an acute phase reactant, is usually well above normal in acute liver failure but low in DIC.**

C. Albumin. All things being equal, the albumin level provides **a measure of the liver's synthetic capacity,** especially in chronic liver disease. Unfortunately, things are not always equal and the albumin can be depressed by other factors such as malnutrition, infection, and proteinuria. **Prealbumin (transthyretin)** has a much shorter half-life (2 days) and may be a better indicator of acute loss of hepatic synthetic functions.

D. Ammonia. Derived from protein metabolism, ammonia is converted to urea by the liver. Failure of the liver to metabolize ammonia **causes brain edema, a leading cause of death** in fulminant hepatic failure. Ammonia levels are useful in evaluating patients with altered mental status of unknown cause and monitoring patients with fulminant hepatic failure. Although the brain edema of hyperammonemia causes mental status changes, this is a separate entity from hepatic encephalopathy. **Hepatic encephalopathy in acute or chronic liver disease is caused by many other factors, both known and unknown. Ammonia levels do not correlate** with the degree of mental status alteration caused by hepatic encephalopathy. To evaluate hepatic encephalopathy, **physical examination surpasses all laboratory tests** currently available.

E. Bilirubin is the metabolic byproduct of heme breakdown. Erythrocyte breakdown (either through senescence or hemolysis) accounts for most bilirubin production.

1. Total serum bilirubin (normal adult range: 0.3–1.0 mg/dL; neonatal values are much higher) **reflects both conjugated and unconjugated bilirubin. An elevated bilirubin can be an indication of liver disease, bile duct obstruction, or non-hepatic problems such as hemolysis.**

In the absence of hemolysis, the bilirubin will rise by about 1 mg/dL/d in complete liver failure or when the common bile duct is completely obstructed. Renal excretion compensates for a rising bilirubin, so bilirubin is rarely above 30–35 mg/dL. Scleral icterus occurs when the bilirubin is >3.5 mg/dL.

2.   **Unconjugated bilirubin ("indirect" bilirubin)** is the immediate product of heme breakdown. It has poor solubility, cannot be excreted in the urine, and is transported by plasma proteins such as albumin. More than 70% of the total bilirubin must be unconjugated to ascribe jaundice to unconjugated hyperbilirubinemia. Among the **limited causes of unconjugated hyperbilirubinemia are hemolysis** (e.g., sickle crisis, transfusion reaction), **Gilbert's syndrome, drugs** (e.g., rifampin), and **resorption of large hematomas.**

3.   **Conjugated bilirubin ("direct bilirubin,"** normal adult range: <0.4 mg/dL) has undergone glucuronidation (primarily in the liver) to increase its solubility and facilitate excretion. Conjugated bilirubin levels **rise in obstructive disorders of the hepatobiliary tract (e.g., cholestasis related to drug reactions, Dubin–Johnson syndrome, Rotor syndrome). Surprisingly, massive liver disease, either from severe acute injury or end-stage cirrhosis, does not significantly impair the conjugation of bilirubin**. Thus, despite jaundice because of impaired excretion of bilirubin into bile, most bilirubin remains conjugated in liver disease.

4.   **"Delta" bilirubin**, which is reported by some automated chemistry analyzers, represents albumin-bound, conjugated bilirubin (with the 3-week circulating half-life of albumin). It can remain elevated for weeks after resolution of an acute hepatic disorder, causing persistent jaundice in an otherwise well patient.

5.   **Caveats**

   a.   **Gilbert's syndrome is a common cause of isolated, asymptomatic elevation of bilirubin, which is nearly all unconjugated**. Hemolysis must be excluded as an alternative cause. The syndrome is caused by a polymorphism in the synthesis of the bilirubin-conjugating enzyme and has no pathologic significance.

   b.   **Wilson's disease can be associated with acute liver failure, with markedly elevated total bilirubin values, and low alkaline phosphatase levels.**

   c.   **With passive congestion of the liver, the bilirubin and PT can be elevated out of proportion to the true degree of liver dysfunction**. The reason for this is unknown.

   d.   **Sustained postinjury cholestasis** is common. Following acute liver injury (e.g., acetaminophen toxicity or acute hepatitis A), the bilirubin and alkaline phosphatase may continue to rise before slowly resolving, whereas the aminotransferases and PT begin to improve more quickly.

   e.   **Urine dipstick tests for bilirubin and urobilinogen can be helpful in the workup of a jaundiced patient**, and constitute quick but imprecise substitutes for bilirubin fractionation and imaging of bile ducts, respectively. In a jaundiced patient, **the absence of urinary bilirubin indicates that the jaundice must be caused by indirect bilirubin** (which is not excreted in the urine). The **absence of urinary urobilinogen indicates that the jaundice is caused by complete obstruction of the common bile duct**, because urobilinogen is a reabsorbed bowel-flora metabolite of bilirubin, and will be excreted in the urine if present.

IV. Viral liver disease and laboratory testing. Viral serologies and direct measures of viral RNA and DNA can accurately diagnose acute and chronic viral hepatitis. Numerous tests are available, but a rational approach can be applied (Table 4-65) with the following background.

  A. Hepatitis A (HAV) infection

    1. Anti-HAV total antibody measures neutralizing IgG, IgM, and IgA antibodies. This test is often incorrectly referred to as an IgG test, which ignores the fact that **it will be positive in acute hepatitis because of the presence of IgM. This test is also of value in identifying individuals who might benefit from vaccination** (i.e., whose test is negative). This test remains negative following immune globulin treatment given for postexposure prophylaxis.

    2. Anti-HAV IgM antibody is used to identify acute HAV infection as a cause of markedly elevated aminotransferases. It is positive in 95% of patients with HAV at the time they present with symptoms and elevated liver enzymes, and remains detectable for about 6 months. This test has **no role in evaluating chronic low-level aminotransferase elevations.**

  B. Hepatitis B (HBV) is evaluated by measuring the presence of three viral proteins and the antibody response to these proteins.

    1. HBsAg (surface antigen) is detected early in the course of acute HBV infection, and persists with chronic HBV infection. The diagnosis of acute HBV infection is based on the history (e.g., recent sexual contacts, intravenous drug use) and the presence of anti-HBc IgM. The

Table 4-65. Recommended serologic tests for viral hepatitis

Acute Viral Hepatitis[a]	Chronic Viral Hepatitis[b]
Anti-HAV IgM[c]	HBsAg
HBsAg	Anti-HBs
Anti-HBs	Anti-HBc total
Anti-HBc IgM	Anti-HCV
Anti-HCV	

HAV, hepatitis A virus; HB, hepatitis B virus; HCV, hepatitis C virus.
[a] Acute viral hepatitis is defined as alanine aminotransferase (ALT) usually >400 U/L with jaundice.
[b] Chronic viral hepatitis is defined as mild elevations of ALT (usually normal to 400 U/L) for several months with minimal symptoms.
[c] Unless prior seroconversion is known.

presence of HBsAg ≥6 months after acute onset indicates the development of chronic HBV infection.

2. Anti-HBs (surface antibody) is a neutralizing antibody to HBV. Its presence indicates immunity acquired by prior infection, vaccination, or administration of hepatitis B immune globulin. In some patients (especially dialysis patients), anti-HBs can fall below detectable levels several decades after an episode of acute hepatitis B.

3. HBcAg (core antigen) is a viral protein retained within hepatocytes and, therefore, is not detectable in the blood. However, it can be detected by immunostaining liver biopsies in acute or chronic hepatitis B.

4. Anti-HBc total antibody measures IgG and IgM. This test is often incorrectly referred to as an IgG test, which ignores the fact that **it will be positive in acute hepatitis B** because of the presence of IgM. Anti-HBc IgG is a non-neutralizing antibody that remains measurable many decades after acute hepatitis B has resolved. The **value of this test is to identify people who have had prior hepatitis B**, although it does not distinguish between chronic HBV infection (i.e., HBsAg positive) and full recovery (i.e., anti-HBs positive). **The test is negative in those with immunity because of vaccination.**

5. Anti-HBc IgM antibody is used to identify acute HBV infection as the cause of markedly elevated aminotransferases. It is positive in most patients at the time they present with symptoms and elevated liver enzymes. **The value of this test is in identifying patients with acute hepatitis B at a time when HBsAg has dropped below detectable levels but anti-HBs has not yet risen to detectable levels (the "window" period). This test has no role in evaluating chronic low-level aminotransferase elevations.**

6. HBeAg ("e" antigen) is a viral protein similar to core antigen, but with a signal sequence that destines it for export from the hepatocyte. **In a patient with an established diagnosis of chronic HBV infection (i.e., HBsAg positive for ≥6 months), the presence of HBeAg indicates a state of relatively high viral replication, and is associated with progressive liver disease** and extrahepatic manifestations. Measuring HBeAg has **no value in the initial evaluation of patients** with acute or chronic liver disease.

7. Anti-HBe ("e" antibody) indicates a state of low viral replication in a patient with a known chronic HBV infection. The presence of anti-HBe is usually associated with benign liver histology, although an increased long-term risk exists for hepatocellular carcinoma. Patients with HBsAg and anti-HBe remain infectious to others. Measuring anti-HBe has **no role in the initial evaluation of patients** with acute or chronic liver disease. Patients with chronic HBV infection will have either HBe antigen or anti-HBe, but not both.

C. Hepatitis C (HCV) is evaluated by measuring antibodies and viral RNA.

1. Anti-HCV detects non-neutralizing antibodies of all classes to any of three viral proteins, and is **the mainstay for detecting HCV infection**. This test can take up to 6 months to turn positive after an acute exposure. Approximately 70% of people with anti-HCV have chronic HCV infection (as indicated by the presence of HCV RNA in the blood).

2. **HCV RIBA identifies antibodies to four viral proteins separately. This is a rational confirmatory test for patients with a positive anti-HCV but without identifiable risk factors** for hepatitis C (who may have a false-positive anti-HCV finding).

3. **HCV RNA** can be measured by a very sensitive qualitative polymerase chain reaction (PCR) test **to confirm a positive anti-HCV test in a patient with risk factors**. Quantitative measures can also be obtained and are used primarily in establishing the likelihood of a response to therapy.

Tests for Myocardial Injury

Steven L. Jones

I. Introduction. Cardiac panels to rule out acute myocardial infarction (AMI) usually include total creatine kinase (CK), CK-MB, myoglobin, and cardiac troponin I. Some institutions use CK-MB isoforms (CK-MB 1 and 2) in place of myoglobin as an early indicator of myocardial damage.

II. Individual tests

A. Myoglobin, which is a low molecular weight, heme-containing protein (oxygen-binding) found in cardiac and skeletal muscle, functions as an oxygen carrier. Myoglobin is a sensitive (99%–100%) indicator of early myocardial or skeletal muscle injury. The most important use of myoglobin in cardiac panels is to "rule out" AMI. The negative predictive value is close to 100%: stable, normal myoglobin values 1–3 hours after onset of symptoms makes AMI highly unlikely. False-positive and false-negative findings can occur. The reference range is males: 20–100 ng/mL; females 20–60 ng/mL).

   1. Pattern in acute myocardial infarction: see Table 4-66 and Fig. 4-12.

   2. Causes of increased myoglobin levels include the following.

      a. Myocardial injury (e.g., infarction, contusion, myocarditis, open heart surgery, some cardiomyopathies).

      b. Skeletal muscle injury [e.g., trauma, surgical procedures, hypothyroidism, malignant hyperthermia, exercise, shock, muscular dystrophy (homozygous or carriers), rhabdomyolysis, polymyositis, viral myositis, alcoholic myopathy, intramuscular injections, burns, seizures].

      c. Other (e.g., renal failure, cocaine use, thrombolytic therapy, heterophilic antibodies).

B. Total creatine kinase. Creatine kinase catalyzes the phosphorylation of creatine. It is primarily present in **brain, heart, and skeletal and smooth muscle. Total CK is used as a moderately sensitive (90%) but nonspecific indicator of myocardial or skeletal muscle injury.** The reference range is males: 50–200 U/L; females 40–160 U/L; levels are higher for blacks.

   1. Pattern in acute myocardial infarction (Table 4-66 and Fig. 4-12)

   2. Causes of increased total CK levels are as follows.

      a. Myocardial injury: infarction, contusion, myocarditis, unstable angina (mild increases), electroshock cardioversion (mild increases), and some cardiomyopathies; congestive heart failure can cause mild increases.

      b. Skeletal muscle injury: same as listed under myoglobin.

      c. Smooth muscle injury: bowel infarctions, tumors or ischemia involving organs with smooth muscle (e.g., uterus, prostate), vasculitis, for example.

Table 4-66. Summary of cardiac profile values in acute myocardial infarction

Criteria	Cardiac Profile Changes (Hours After Onset of Acute Myocardial Infarction)				
	Myoglobin	CK-MB Isoforms	CK-MB	Total CK	CTnI
Begins to rise	1–3	2–3	3–6	4–6	4–8
Peaks	9–12	6–12	12–24	18–30	12–18
Returns to normal	12–24	12–24	24–72	48–72	5–10 days[a]

CK, creatine kinase; CK-MB isoforms, CK-MB$_{1,2}$; CTnI, cardiac troponin I.
[a] Second generation CTnT assays may remain elevated for up to 14 days.

    d. Brain injuries (e.g., trauma, strokes, tumors).
    3. Causes of decreased CK levels: decreased muscle mass, alcoholic liver disease, some connective tissue diseases (e.g., rheumatoid arthritis), normal or ectopic pregnancies, steroid use, and inactivity (even temporary bed-rest can decrease levels by 15%–20%).
C. CK-MB. CK is a dimer of B (brain) and M (muscle) forms, and is present as **three major serum isoenzymes**, designated **CK-BB** ("CK-1," high in **brain and smooth muscle**), **CK-MB** ["CK-2," high in **heart and low (<3%) in skeletal muscle**], and **CK-MM** ("CK-3," high in **heart and skeletal**

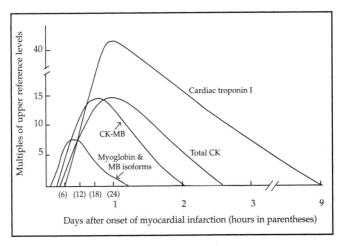

Fig. 4-12. Cardiac profile patterns after acute myocardial infarction.

muscle). In general, **myocardial injury is associated with a CK-MB relative index ≥3.0. In rhabdomyolysis, CK-MB mass is significantly increased as is the total CK, but the CK-MB index remains low (<3).** The reference range is CK-MB (U/L) <0% to 5% of total CK; CK-MB mass (ng/mL) <6 ng/mL; relative index (CK-MB mass divided by total CK) <3.0.

    1.   **Pattern in acute myocardial infarction** (Table 4-66 and Fig. 4-12). Approximately **10% of patients with AMI have a normal total CK but increased CK-MB** ("micro-infarction").

    2.   **Causes of increased CK-MB levels are as follows.**
       (1)   **Myocardial injury**: same causes listed above under total CK.
       (2)   **Skeletal muscle injury**: same causes listed above under total CK, except for intramuscular injections and exercise, which usually do not cause increases in CK-MB. **Remember, whereas the CK-MB mass is increased in skeletal muscle injuries, the relative CK-MB index remains normal.**

    3.   **Mild "smoldering" increases in CK-MB usually represent macro-CK** (see *Enzymes* chapter), which can be confirmed with electrophoresis and does not represent cardiac injury. Persistent mild increases in CK-MB can also be seen in polymyositis (regenerating skeletal muscle produces more CK-MB than mature skeletal muscle tissue).

    4.   **Consistent elevations in CK-MB that are greater than 30% to 40% of the total CK** can represent CK-MB produced by a **malignancy** (the percent of CK-MB in heart muscle generally does not exceed 30% of the total CK in the heart).

    5.   **Note that CK-MB is not increased in cases of pulmonary embolism** (unless the heart is subsequently injured).

D.   **CK-MB isoforms**. The terminal lysines of CK-MB peptide dimers can be hydrolyzed, resulting in two main isoforms, CK-MB_1, and CK-MB_2. The normal serum CK-MB_2:CK-MB_1 ratio is ≤1.5. **After AMI, serum CK-MB_2 rapidly increases, and the CK-MB_2; CK-MB_1 ratio is >1.5.** This isoform ratio is useful as a very early marker for AMI (similar to myoglobin but more specific). Its disadvantage is the need for specialized equipment and its expense.

E.   **Cardiac troponin-I (cTnI).** Troponin is a protein complex that helps regulate contraction in skeletal and cardiac muscle by interacting with tropomyosin and actin. The troponin complex consists of troponin-I (actinomyosin ATPase *i*nhibitory subunit), troponin-C (*c*alcium binding subunit), and troponin-T (*t*ropomyosin binding subunit). Troponin-I has three distinct molecular forms (isotypes), one of which (cardiac troponin-I; cTnI) is found exclusively in the heart. **CTnI is used as a specific marker for myocardial injury. CTnI has a sensitivity that is similar to that of CK-MB, but is more cardiac specific. CTnI values >1.0 ng/mL are consistent with AMI** (range varies with method). Reference range is **<0.06 ng/mL.**

    1.   **Pattern in AMI** (Table 4-66 and Fig. 4-12)
    2.   **Causes of increased cTnI levels**: myocardial infarction (Q wave and non-Q wave), unstable angina, cardiac con-

tusions, myocarditis, cardiomyopathies, and so on. A higher incidence of mortality has been seen in patients with non-Q wave AMI and unstable angina who have increased levels of cTnI. Note: **cTnI values are not increased by skeletal muscle injury and are almost never increased by chronic renal failure**. False-positive results have been reported with some assays because of interference by fibrin or HAMA (human anti-mouse antibodies).

    3. Second generation assays for **cardiac troponin-T (cTnT) may be better than cardiac troponin-I assays**. The new cTnT assays are just as specific for cardiac tissue as cTnI; they are more sensitive and precise at low levels, and remain elevated for a longer period of time (up to 14 days). One disadvantage of the cardiac troponin-T assays is that they are occasionally elevated in patients with renal failure; this phenomenon occurs more often than with the cardiac troponin-I assays.

  F. **Summary of cardiac panel results in acute myocardial infarction**. See Table 4-66 and Fig. 4-12.

III. **Recommendations for serial testing.** Many testing protocols exist. One such protocol is as follows.

  A. **For continued pain with diagnostic electrocardiogram (ECG).** Total CK and troponin at presentation and every 8 hours × 3; then total CK every morning × 3 days.

  B. **For continued or resolved pain with nondiagnostic ECG.** Total CK (with MB) and troponin at presentation, 2 hours, 5 hours, and 9 hours. If the onset of the pain was <6 hours from presentation, also order myoglobin (stat), and repeat at 1 and 2 hours.

IV. **General guidelines**

  A. **Measurement. Never rely on a single measurement**. Acute infarction and contusion show **abrupt increases in cardiac markers followed by appropriate decreases**, whereas other disorders (e.g., myositis, cardiomyopathies, elevations in myoglobin caused by chronic renal failure) show stable, increased levels. If there is any clinical suspicion that the patient's chest pain is cardiac in origin, the patient should be observed for at least 8 hours, and serial cardiac enzymes ordered.

  B. **Trends are just as important as absolute values**. A small, elderly woman with a baseline myoglobin of 10 ng/mL may have a postinfarction value of 70 ng/mL (representing an increase of sevenfold, but which is still "within the normal reference range").

  C. **Blood samples. Collect blood samples as soon as possible to obtain baseline values**. The best reference level for any patient is the patient's own baseline values.

  D. **Cardiac markers. Never diagnose AMI based entirely on cardiac markers.** The World Health Organization requires two of the following to be present to diagnose AMI: chest discomfort of significant duration (>20 minutes), temporal changes in cardiac enzymes, or serial ECG changes consistent with infarction.

  E. **Inconsistent results. Cardiac marker results that are inconsistent with the clinical setting should be**

interpreted with caution. False-positive and false negative findings can occur.

F. Cardiac reperfusion. After thrombolytic therapy, cardiac reperfusion leads to increases in cardiac markers that begin rising much sooner, and peak much higher, than in patients who are not reperfused.

G. Degree of enzyme elevation. Elevations in cardiac panel results tend to correlate with the size of the infarction.

H. Other tests. Older tests that may be helpful include lactate dehydrogenase [an LDH 1:2 ratio >0.8 (isoenzyme "flip") is consistent with myocardial injury], and the aspartate aminotransferase:alanine aminotransferase (**AST:ALT**) ratio (increased ratios in infarction).

5

Immunology

Inflammation and Repair

Darrell D. Davidson

I. **Overview and general principles**
A. **Inflammation. The reaction of vascularized tissue to local injury. Classic signs include rubor (redness), calor (warmth), tumor (swelling), pain (dolor), and loss of function.**
    1. **Acute inflammation** destroys, dilutes, or walls off injurious agents; involves increased blood flow (vasodilation) and vascular permeability; migration of leukocytes (particularly neutrophils) by chemotaxis; and deposition of platelets and fibrin.
    2. **Chronic or systemic inflammation** prepares tissue for healing, and mobilizes systemic resources (e.g., through circulating acute phase reactants that lead to systemic adaptive responses). Involves macrophages, lymphocytes or plasma cells, fibroblasts, and angiogenesis.
B. **Repair is the process of resolving tissue damage by regenerating functional parenchyma or laying down collagen scar tissue.** Repair begins at the time of tissue damage, and persists for months. Repair involves vascular and cellular responses, and the synthesis of a provisional matrix followed by collagen.
II. **Key components of acute inflammation**
A. **Leukocytes** first become **loosely attached** to endothelial surfaces (called "rolling"), and then **tightly attached** to the same surfaces. Attachment, which occurs through the interaction of **adhesion molecules** on both leukocytes and endothelial cells, is mediated by **soluble substances** [e.g., platelet activating factor, IL-1, tumor necrosis factor (TNF)]. Adhesion molecules include **selectins** (similar to lectins), **immunoglobulins**, and **integrins**. Leukocytes then move between endothelial cells (called **diapedesis**), **migrate along chemotactic gradients** toward the site of inflammation, and finally perform **phagocytosis** and other protective functions.
B. **Adhesion molecules**
    1. **LFA-1 (lymphocyte function-associated antigen)** (CD11a/CD18: a β-integrin) **on leukocytes binds ICAM-1** (intercellular adhesion molecule: an immunoglobulin) **on endothelial cells.**
    2. **MAC-1** (CD11b/CD18: one of the β-integrins) **on leukocytes also binds to ICAM-1**
    3. **VLA-4** ($\alpha_4\beta_1$; p150,95: one of the β-integrins) **on leukocytes binds to VCAM-1** (vascular cell adhesion molecule: an immunoglobulin) **on endothelial cells.**
    4. **LAM-1** ($\alpha_4\beta_7$: a selectin) **on leukocytes also binds to VCAM-1.**
    5. **Sialyl-Lewis X glycoproteins on leukocytes bind to E-selectin (ELAM) and P-selectin (GMP-140), which are both on endothelial cells.**

C. Inflammatory mediators are short-lived substances that bind to target cell receptors and cause the target cells to alter their function or produce other mediators (Table 5-1).

D. Chemotactic factors cause locomotion toward an increasing chemical gradient; they include **bacterial N-formyl-methionine peptides, C5a, LTB4, IL-8, and so forth.**

E. Phagocytosis and killing mechanisms involve **opsonization** (e.g., by IgG-Fc, C3b), **attachment to leukocyte receptors** (e.g., FcγR, CR1/2), **engulfment, and killing or degradation** through the oxidative burst and enzymatic proteolysis. The **oxidative burst** involves the production of **superoxides** (O_2^-), **hydroxyl radicals (OH·), hydrogen peroxide,** ($2\ O_2^- + 2\ H+ \rightarrow$ dismutase $\rightarrow$ $\textbf{H}_2\textbf{O}_2 + O_2$), and **hypochlorous acid** (HOCl·; $H_2O_2 + Cl^- \rightarrow$ Myeloperoxidase$\rightarrow$ HOCl·). The strongest killing agent is the HOCl·.

III. Key components of chronic and systemic inflammation

A. Cytokines. At least 56 unique cytokines, and maybe more, are generally grouped into five classes as listed below.

1. Lymphocyte regulators: IL-2 and IL-4 stimulate proliferation; IL-10 and tumor growth factor (TGF)-β are inhibitory.

2. Natural immunity: TNF-α, IL-1, interferon (IFN)-α, IFN-β, IL-6

3. Macrophage activators: IFN-α, TNF-α, TNF-β, IL-5, IL-10, IL-12

4. Hematopoietic growth factors: IL-3, IL-7, c-kit ligand, granulocyte-macrophage colony-stimulating factor (GM-CSF), M-CSF, G-CSF, stem cell factor

5. Chemokines: chemotactic factors, CC or CXC family based on whether two cysteine disulfide bonds are separated by their amino acids.

B. Macrophages accumulate in repair, granulomas, atheromatous plaques, and so on. They are **recruited by C5a, chemokines (MCP-1), platelet-derived growth factors (PDGF)**, transforming growth factor (TGF)-β, fibrinopeptides, and matrix fragments. Macrophages are **immobilized** in an area of chronic inflammation by **macrophage inhibitory factor** (MIF) and oxidized lipids.

C. Acute-phase proteins and systemic inflammatory responses

1. C-reactive protein: described in 1930; name based on reaction with pneumococcal C-polysaccharide; still the **best laboratory monitor** of systemic inflammation (more reliable than ESR)

2. Other acute phase proteins include C3, ceruloplasmin, fibrinogen, factor VIII, plasminogen, haptoglobin, ferritin, α₁-protease inhibitor, lipopolysaccharide (LPS)-binding protein, and serum amyloid A.

3. Plasma proteins that decrease during inflammation include albumin, transferrin, α-fetoprotein, and factor XII.

4. Acute-phase phenomena

a. Neuroendocrine: fever, somnolence, anorexia

b. Hematopoietic: anemia, leukocytosis, thrombocytosis

c. Metabolic: negative nitrogen balance, osteoporosis

Table 5-1. Key soluble inflammatory mediators

Mediator	Function
Nitric oxide	Vasodilation, regulates (limits) leukocyte recruitment, antimicrobial functions (through free radicals)
Histamine	Binds to H_1 receptors, vasodilates arterioles, increases venule permeability
Arachidonic acid metabolites	
$-PGD_2\ PGE_2\ PGF_{2\alpha}$	Vasodilation, mediation of pain (PGE_2) and fever
$-PGI_2$	Vasodilation, inhibits aggregation of platelets
$-TxA_2$	Vasoconstriction, causes aggregation of platelets
$-$Hydroperoxy acids	Chemotaxis
Leukotrienes	
$-LTB_4$	Chemotaxis
$-LTC_4\ LTD_4\ LTE_4$	Slow-reacting substance of anaphylaxis (SRS-A): vasoconstriction, bronchospasm, increased permeability
Complement	
$-C3a$	Increases permeability (anaphylatoxin)
$-C3b$	Opsonizes foreign material
$-C5a$	Increases permeability (anaphylatoxin) and chemotaxis
$-C5b$-9 (MAC)	Lyses target cells
Coagulation	
$-$Thrombin (factor IIa)	Increases leukocyte adhesion, fibroblast proliferation
$-$Fibrinopeptides	Increases permeability, chemotaxis
$-$Factor Xa	Increases permeability, chemotaxis
$-$Fibrin split products	Increases permeability
Kinin system	
$-$Kallikrein	Chemotaxis, activates factor XII and plasmin
$-$Bradykinin	Mediates pain; increases permeability
PAF[a]	Increases permeability, causes endothelial cells to become adhesive
Neuropeptides	
$-$Substance P (SP)	Mediates pain, increases permeability
$-$VIP	Vasodilates, releases histamine from mast cells, chemotaxis
$-$CGRP	Decreases contact hypersensitivity in skin (*i.e.*, anti-inflammatory)

CGRP, calcitonin gene-regulated peptide; PAF, platelet-activating factor; PG, prostaglandin; PGI_2, prostacyclin; TxA_2, thromboxane; VIP, vasoactive intestinal polypeptide.
[a] PAF is formed from phosphatidylcholine, and is 100–10,000 times more potent than histamine.

    d. Hepatic: increased inducible nitric oxide synthetase

    e. Nonprotein plasma components: decreased zinc, iron, copper

IV. Repair

A. "Repair" includes both regeneration and replacement by scar.

  1. Regeneration depends on the regenerating cell type, as well as the extent and type of matrix injury. For parenchymal (epithelial) cells to regenerate, they must be able to migrate, proliferate, and differentiate. Parenchymal cells may have (a) **continual regenerative capacity** (e.g., squamous and mucosal epithelia, bone marrow); (b) **regenerative capacity when stimulated** (e.g., glands, mesenchyme); or (c) **no regenerative capacity** (e.g., neurons, striated muscle). Intact matrix (basement membrane and extracellular matrix) is required for any type of proliferation.

  2. Replacement (by collagen scar) occurs when the matrix is disrupted, the parenchymal cells are unable to proliferate, or there is incomplete resolution of inflammation. Mesenchymal cells (endothelial cells and fibrocytes) migrate, proliferate, and differentiate, producing collagen scar. Early in the process, **granulation tissue** forms [mixed inflammation, edema, collagen type III (reticulin), and angiogenesis], in the zone of resolving inflammation, and then gradually matures to strong type I collagen over a period of 3 months.

B. Growth factors (Table 5-2)

C. Growth inhibitors include the three entities listed below.

  1. Retinoblastoma gene protein Rb: sequesters E2F transcription factors

  2. p53 gene: activated in response to DNA damage; increases CDK inhibitor p21

  3. TGF-β: a stop signal for regenerating tissue; works by increasing CDK inhibitor p27 and decreasing CDK2 activity.

Table 5-2. Growth factors

Name	Subclasses	Activity	Target Cells
EGF/TGF-α		Mitogenic	Fb, Ep
PDGF	AA, AB, BB	Mitogenic, migration	Mp, En, Sm
FGF	Acidic, basic	Angiogenesis, migration, hematopoiesis	En (bFGF), Mp, Fb, En
		Vasculogenesis, angiogenesis	Sk ms, lung, marrow
VEGF	VEGF, VEGF-B, VEGF-C, P1GF	Growth inhibition, migration, collagen synthesis	In utero Repair
TGF-β	TGF-β-1,2		Ep
	TGF-β-3		Fb

EGF, epidermal growth factor; En, endothelial cell; Ep, epithelial cell; Fb, fibroblast; FGF, fibroblast growth factor; PDGF, platelet-derived growth factor; Sk ms, skeletal muscle; Sm, smooth muscle; TGF-α, transforming growth factor-α; VEGF, vascular endothelial growth factor.

Immunity

Timothy R. La Pine and Harry R. Hill

I. Overview of the immune system. Immune responses are generated by **natural and adaptive mechanisms** composed of both **cellular and humoral components**.

A. Natural immunity. Nonspecific, natural immunity is not influenced by prior antigen-antibody interaction; **phagocytic cells, plasma factors, and various barriers** comprise natural immunity.

1. Phagocytic cells, which ingest and destroy pathogenic organisms or foreign material, include **granulocytes** (neutrophils and eosinophils) and **macrophages**.

2. Plasma factors. The **complement system** mediates inflammatory reactions by attracting granulocytes and macrophages, promoting cell-to-cell interactions for antigen processing, and stimulating the lysis of viruses and bacteria. Other plasma proteins also contribute to natural immunity, such as **cytokines, acute-phase reactants**, and the **coagulation cascade.**

3. Barriers include **physical barriers** (e.g., skin, cilia, mucus) and **biochemical barriers** (e.g., gastric acid, lysozyme, lactoferrin, and surfactant protein A).

B. Adaptive immunity is specific; it is characterized by **direct immune responsiveness** as a result of an initial antigen exposure, with memory (**anamnestic**) responses on re-exposure to the antigen; both humoral and cellular responses are recruited.

1. Humoral response involves the production of **immunoglobulins by B-lymphocytes**, which defend against **extracellular bacteria, viruses, and some intracellular pathogens.**

a. Overview. When antigens bind to immunoglobulins (antibodies, Ab) on B-cell surfaces, the B cells develop into mature plasma cells, which secrete antigen-specific antibodies. **IgM is produced first; "class-switching"** can then occur to produce **IgG, IgA, and IgE**. The first reaction to an antigen is the **primary response**, composed of IgM followed by IgG. Re-exposure to the antigen causes a **secondary (anamnestic) response**, with IgM followed by IgG that rises faster, peaks higher, and remains elevated for a longer period of time. The transfer of antibodies to a susceptible host is called **passive humoral immunity** (e.g., antivenom, gammaglobulin therapy, and pregnancy).

b. Immunoglobulin (Ig; a.k.a. antibodies, Ab). An immunoglobulin is composed of **two covalently bonded heavy chains and two light chains**. The immunoglobulin may be one of **five classes** or isotypes, based on the heavy chain.

(1) IgG (75% of serum immunoglobulin): gamma heavy chain; molecular weight = 150,000; normal serum levels = 800–1,500 mg/dL (but vary with age); IgG can freely travel **from vessels into tissues; IgG crosses the placenta** to give passive neonatal immunity; four IgG subclasses exist (with slightly different heavy chains).

  (a)   IgG$_1$: 70% of IgG; **anti-protein antibody**; can **activate complement** (but <IgM)

  (b)   IgG$_2$: 20% of IgG; **anti-polysaccharide antibody** [children <2 years of age do not produce much IgG$_2$ and have more infections with polysaccharide-coated organisms (e.g., *Haemophilus influenzae*, pneumococcus, meningococcus)].

  (c)   IgG$_3$: 5% of IgG; **anti-viral antibody**; can **activate complement** (but <IgM).

  (d)   IgG$_4$: 5% of IgG; involved in skin sensitization.

  (2)   IgA (15%): alpha heavy chain; molecular weight = 350,000; normal serum levels = 80–350 mg/dL; the principal Ab in secretory fluids; **protects mucosal surfaces**; good **anti-viral** activity; exists as a **dimer**, joined to an associated secretory component (that transports and protects the IgA) by a "J" chain; secreted in breast milk and can protect the newborn against gastrointestinal pathogens.

  (3)   IgM (10%): mu heavy chain; molecular weight = 950,000; normal serum levels = 40–160 mg/dL; exists in the serum as a **pentamer** of five monomeric units joined by a J chain, and **remains in the intravascular space** because of its large size; **IgM does not cross the placenta, thus, IgM in the newborn is produced by the newborn, and its presence can suggest congenital infection; one molecule of IgM is enough to activate complement**; IgM is an effective protector against complex polysacharides.

  (4)   IgE (<1%): epsilon heavy chain; molecular weight = 190,000; present in the serum in trace amounts (0.05 mg/dL); found on **mast cell and basophil** surfaces; provides **allergy and parasitic immunity**; antigen-binding and bridging of IgE can initiate **anaphylaxis**.

  (5)   IgD (<1%): delta heavy chain; molecular weight = 180,000; normal serum levels = 3–5 mg/dL; serves as an **early antigen receptor on B cells.**

  c.   Light chains produced by a single cell are either **kappa or lambda, but not both.** The kappa-B-cell: lambda-B-cell ratio is normally **2:1.**

2.   Cellular response: mediated by **T-lymphocytes**, which defend the host against **intracellular pathogens** (e.g., viruses, tuberculosis, *Listeria* spp.) and **fungi**; provide immune surveillance against **malignant and foreign cells** (e.g., allograft rejection, graft-versus-host disease); and are involved in **delayed and contact hypersensitivity** reactions. **T cells also regulate other aspects of immune responsiveness** (including essential roles in regulating B cells and macrophages (Fig. 5-1).

  a.   Subpopulations of T cells have been defined on the basis of function and the presence of characteristic surface antigens.

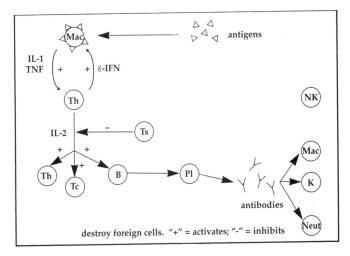

Fig. 5-1. **Cell-mediated immunity. Macrophages (and other antigen-presenting cells) interact with T-helper cells (Th) which, in turn, can "arm" macrophages. Th cells also stimulate other Th cells, cytotoxic T cells (Tc), and B cells. B cells differentiate into plasma cells (Pl), which produce antibodies. Antibodies assist macrophages (Mac), killer cells (K), and neutrophils (Neut) in destroying foreign antigens. T-suppressor (Ts) cells inhibit the immune response. Natural killer cells (NK) work independently of antibodies to destroy foreign cells. +, activates; −, inhibits.**

(1) **Cytotoxic T (Tc) cells** express **CD8**, recognize **HLA class I** antigens, and are responsible for killing cells that express foreign antigens.

(2) **Helper-inducer T (Th) cells** express **CD4**, recognize **HLA class II** antigens (e.g., on macrophages), and enhance the activity of B cells, macrophages, and other T cells.

(3) **Suppressor T (Ts)** cells express **CD8**, and inhibit activities of other immune cells.

b. **T-cell–derived factors**: T cells release **lymphokines**, interleukins (IL), granulocyte-macrophage colony-stimulating factor (GM-CSF), tumor necrosis factor (TNF), and gamma interferon (γ-IFN), which regulate various aspects of the immune response. The cytokines, which are generally classified as either pro-inflammatory or anti-inflammatory, are summarized in Tables 5-3 and 5-4.

II. Leukopoiesis

A. **Leukopoietic stem cells** express CD34 glycoproteins, are regulated by stem cell factors (e.g., GM-CSF, IL-1, and IL-3), and give rise to T cells, B cells, macrophages, and granulocytes. These leukopoietic stem cells are **pluripotent, self-renewing, transplantable**, and show an **asymmetric cell fate** determined by cell trafficking.

Table 5-3. Selected proinflammatory cytokines

Cytokine	Function	Predominant Cell Source
TNF-α	Stimulates IL-6 and CSF. Depresses erythropoiesis, stimulates IL-8 and IL-9. Promotes tumor necrosis and endotoxic shock.	Monocytes and macrophages
IL-1	Stimulates proliferation and differentiation of T and B lymphocytes. Stimulates T lymphocytes to produce IL-2 receptor. Promotes CSF, IL-8, and IL-9 production, and endotoxic shock.	Macrophages, astrocytes, monocytes, fibroblasts, keratinocytes, B cells, corneal epithelium, and other cell types
IL-2	Stimulates growth of T lymphocytes. Stimulates B lymphocyte and monocyte differentiation. Increases cytotoxicity of T lymphocytes and natural killer cells.	Activated T lymphocytes
IL-3	Multipotential hematopoietic cell growth factor, stimulates early B and T lymphocytes. Mast cell growth factor.	Activated T lymphocytes, natural killer cells
IL-8	Stimulates neutrophil, monocyte, and lymphocyte activation chemotaxis.	Monocytes
IL-9	Stimulates neutrophil monocyte and lymphocyte activation chemotaxis. Stimulates erythroid progenitors, helper T lymphocyte growth factor.	T lymphocytes
IL-12	Stimulates helper T lymphocyte differentiation and IFNγ and IL-2 production. Increases cytotoxicity of natural killer cells.	T and B lymphocytes, lymphoblastoid cells
G-CSF	Stimulates neutrophil colony formation	Monocytes and fibroblasts
GM-CSF	Stimulates granulocyte and monocytes formation, induces TNF.	T lymphocytes, natural killer endothelial cells, fibroblasts and keratinocytes
M-CSF	Activates monocytes and granulocytes. Stimulates MC formation. Induces IL-1 and TNF.	Fibroblasts, monocytes, and endothelial cells

G-CSF, granulocyte colony-stimulating factor; IL, interleukin; IFNγ, interferon-gamma; M-CSF, macrophage-colony-stimulating factor; TNF-α, tumor necrosis factor-α.

Table 5-4.   Selected anti-inflammatory cytokines

Cytokines	Function	Predominant Cell Source
IL-4	Stimulates proliferation of T and B lymphocytes, megakaryocytes, and is a growth factor for mast cells and erythroid precursors. Stimulates IgE production.	T lymphocytes
IL-6	Blocks endotoxin induction of IL-1 and tumor necrosis factor B and T lymphocyte-stimulating activity. Stimulates production of acute phase reactants.	Monocytes, and B lymphocytes, fibroblasts, epithelial and endothelial cells
IL-1 Rec antagonist	Binds IL-1 receptors, blocking IL-1 effects.	Monocytes and macrophages
TGF-β	Reduces endotoxin-induced IL-1 and tumor necrosis factor production.	Monocytes and macrophages

IL, interleukin; IL-1 Rec Antagonist, interleukin-1 receptor antagonist; TGF-β, transforming growth factor-beta.
(Adapted from: La Pine T R, Cates K L, Hill H R. Immunodulating agents. In: Feigin R D, Cherry, D (eds.) *Textbook of pediatric infectious diseases,* (4th ed.) Philadelphia: W B Saunders Company, 1998:2719–2729).

B.   Fetal and neonatal leukopoiesis. Leukopoiesis begins in the **yolk sac**. At 6–8 weeks, the **fetal liver** becomes the major site of leukopoiesis, and T- and B-cell precursors are seen. At 8–9 weeks, the **thymus** begins development. By 5 months, the **bone marrow** becomes the major site of leukopoiesis.

C.   T Cells

1.   T-cell development. Bone marrow stem cells that are committed to become T cells migrate to the thymus. Early T-cell progenitors lack CD4 and CD8 before intrathymic maturation. During early thymic maturation, progenitor T cells express both CD4 and CD8. Mature T cells express either **CD4 helper-inducer** or **CD8 cytotoxic-suppressor** glycoproteins, but not both, before migrating to specific lymphoid tissues. T cells have **antigen receptors** that are similar to immunoglobulins, and are composed of alpha and beta chains.

2.   Assessment of T-cell–mediated immunity

a.   Delayed skin hypersensitivity. In normal individuals, intradermal injections of *Candida* spp., mumps, diphtheria, tetanus, and other protein antigens cause **induration** (not just redness) within 24–48 hours, as committed T cells produce cytokines, which **recruit lymphocytes and macrophages to the injection site**.

b.   T cell and T-cell subset quantitation by flow cytometry detects CD2 (pan T cell), CD3 (signal transduction), CD4 (helper), CD8 (suppressor or cytotoxic), CD45RA+ (naive T cell), CD45RO (memory T cell), and so forth.

   c. Mitogenic assays: phytohemagglutinin (PHA, stimulates T cells), **concanavalin A** (stimulates T cells), **pokeweed** (stimulates T cells and B cells), endotoxin, tetanus, and *Candida* spp. antigens stimulate proliferation of T cells, which can be measured by the incorporation of ³H-thymidine into new cellular DNA.

   d. Cytokine production: IL-1, IL-2, TNF, IFN-γ, IL-4, and so on can be assayed by enzyme-linked immunosorbent assay (ELISA).

3. Causes of T-cell immunodeficiency

   a. Defects in the maturation, differentiation, and activation of lymphopoietic **stem cells**

   b. Defects of the **thymus**

   c. Defects in **T cells,** T-cell cytokine receptors, or T-cell intracellular signal transduction

   d. Defective production of **regulatory proteins** needed for T-cell activation

D. B cells

1. B-cell development. B cells develop in the **bone marrow.** Early pre-B cells undergo rearrangements of the mu heavy chain; pre-B cells have cytoplasmic mu heavy chains; **mature B cells have immunoglobulins (IgM or IgD) on their surface membranes**, and then seed the lymphoid tissues. The IgM-bearing B cells undergo **class switching to IgG, IgA, or IgE** bearing B cells, which then **differentiate into antibody-secreting plasma cells with the help of T cells** and T-cell–derived lymphokines. Some B cells further differentiate into small memory B cells for secondary immune responsiveness.

2. Neonatal antibody immunity (passive humoral immunity)

   a. Maternal IgG (all subclasses) crosses the placenta by the eighth gestational week, and the "Brambell receptor" prolongs the IgG half-life. At birth, newborn IgG levels actually exceed maternal IgG levels, but immediately begin to decrease until a **nadir (400 mg/dL) is reached at 3–4 months of age.** At this point, the infant's production of antibodies begins to compensate for maternal Ab loss. Some maternal IgG is still detectable until 10–12 months of age.

   b. Mucosal-associated lymphoid tissue (MALT) and IgA in breastfed infants contributes to postnatal gastrointestinal antibody immunity.

3. B-cell immunodeficiency can result from the following factors.

   a. Defects in the maturation, differentiation, and activation of lymphopoietic **stem cells**.

   b. Defects in B cells (e.g., defects in B-cell signal transduction or antibody isotype switching, or failure of B cells to differentiate into normal, functioning plasma cells).

   c. Any defect in T-cell immunity is also associated with variable degrees of B-cell deficiency, because most of the maturation, differentiation, and activation processes of B cells are mediated by T cells and associated lymphokines.

4. Laboratory testing for B-cell immunity

a. ELISA or nephelometry can quantitate patient antibodies against specific infectious agents (e.g., *S. pneumoniae*, *H. influenza*, measles, human immunodeficiency virus); many false-positive results occur. The ability to produce certain IgG subclasses can be tested by giving the patient the following vaccinations, and measuring the magnitude of the antibody response.

(1) **Diphtheria or tetanus** to evaluate **IgG$_1$** (which responds to protein antigens)

(2) **Pneumococcus** to evaluate **IgG$_2$** (which responds to polysaccharide antigens)

(3) **Influenza** to evaluate **IgG$_3$** (which responds to viruses)

b. Complement fixation is a classic but complicated test based on the principle that antigen-antibody complexes can activate complement. If a patient's serum has an antibody against a specific antigen, complement activation can be induced and measured.

c. Immunofluorescence allows visualization of antibody attachment to bacteria or cell components, by tagging the antibodies with a fluorescent dye.

d. Tests of historical interest include measurement of opsonic activity and viral neutralization.

e. Note: **Do *not* use serum protein electrophoresis to quantitate IgG** and assume that if the total IgG is normal that an IgG deficiency can be ruled out. The total IgG may appear to be normal, but an entire subclass (e.g., IgG$_2$) may be missing, with increased production of the other subclasses.

III. Phagocyte functions. Major phagocytic functions include **adherence to endothelium, aggregation, diapedesis, chemotaxis, phagocytosis, and degranulation, leading to pathogen destruction**. The phagocytic system is one of the first lines of defense against **extracellular bacteria and fungi**, in association with opsonizing antibodies, complement, and some acute-phase reactants.

A. Phagocytic development. Stem cells develop into neutrophils and monocytes within the fetal bone marrow by 5 months of gestation, a process that is regulated by colony-stimulating factors (e.g., GM-CSF, G-CSF), IL-3, and IL-6. Neonatal neutrophils are not fully functional, and show decreased chemotaxis, degranulation, and killing abilities.

B. Normal neutrophil functions

1. Adhesion

a. Sialyl-Lewis X glycoproteins and L-selectin on neutrophils "tether" (loosely bind) the neutrophil to **E-selectin and P-selectin on endothelial cells.**

b. Integrins such as CD11/CD18 [particularly **CD11b/18** (MAC-1)] **on neutrophils** form tight bonds between the neutrophil and receptors on the capillary endothelium [e.g., **intercellular adhesion molecule (ICAM)-1** and **vascular cell adhesion molecule (VCAM)-1**].

2. Migration. Neutrophils are attracted toward sites of infection by chemical factors, including complement **C5a**, bacterial **endotoxin**, and cytokines (e.g., **leukotriene B4**).

3.   **Engulfment** is enhanced by **opsonization**, which is the binding of antibodies and complement (i.e., C3b) onto bacteria and other foreign pathogens.

4.   **Killing-respiratory burst** activity involves the generation of **superoxides** (O_2^-), **hydrogen peroxide** (H_2O_2, through superoxide dismutase), **hydroxyl radicals** ($OH^\cdot$, through H_2O_2 and Fe), and **HOCl$^\cdot$** (through H_2O_2, Cl$^-$), and myeloperoxidase. In addition, IFN-γ stimulates the generation of nitric oxide (from arginine) in macrophages.

5.   **Phagocyte immunodeficiency** can result from stem cell or colony-stimulating factor defects, neutrophil and endothelial cell adhesion defects, migration and chemotactic defects, membrane defects impairing engulfment or degranulation, an absent or incomplete respiratory burst, or deficiencies of the regulatory cytokines.

6.   **Tests of phagocytic function**
  a.   **Absolute neutrophil count**
  b.   Measurement of surface expression of **selectins and integrins** by flow cytometry
  c.   **Chemotactic assays**: Boyden chamber assay, transwell membrane (or agarose) migration assay, Rebuck skin window
  d.   **Respiratory burst assays:** nitroblue tetrazolium (**NBT**), dye reduction, dihydrorhodamine fluorescence, cytochrome C reduction
  e.   **Phagocytosis and killing assays**: colony count reduction

IV. **Complement**
 A. **Function**
  1.   **Lysis of bacteria, tumor cells, and allograft cells**
  2.   **Generates mediators of inflammation and attracts phagocytic cells**
  3.   **Opsonization** and enhancement of phagocytosis
 B. **The complement cascade** is a series of interacting proteins that **promote and greatly amplify the immune response, lyse some bacteria and human cells, opsonize** bacteria, and assist in removing immune complexes. Most components are made by mononuclear phagocytes in the liver and tissues. **Two pathways of complement activation exist: the classical pathway, which is initiated by antibody complexes, and the alternate pathway, which occurs in the absence of antibody complexes and is triggered by complex polysaccharides**. Note that **complement levels in the neonate are only 50% of adult levels**. For more details on the complement system, please see *The Complement System* chapter that follows.

5.3

The Complement System

Steven L. Jones

I. Basic science review

A. Introduction. The complement system is made up of a series of more than **30 heat-labile plasma proteins that play an integral role in the immune system**. The complement system functions as a **cascade** (similar to the coagulation system), in that the individual proteins act in concert, in an orderly fashion, and with amplification. The **amplification** provides one of the most powerful driving forces of inflammation as a whole. Genes for several components (factor B, C2, C4) are found in the major histocompatibility complex (MHC-class III) on chromosome six.

B. The classical and alternative pathways eventually join in a common pathway, and together make up the complement system. The classical pathway proteins are called **components** (and numbered in order of their discovery), whereas those in the alternative pathway are called **factors**. When complement proteins are cleaved and thereby activated, the fragments are given a lowercase letter (e.g., C3a and C3b), and activation is indicated by a line across the top of the component. C1 (composed of q, r, and s subcomponents) is the first component that is activated in the classical pathway, to which are added the components 4, 2, and 3, which then activate 5–9. A small amount of C3b always circulates in the blood, and serves as the initial substrate for the alternative pathway by binding to factor B. Factor D activates factor B, which is then stabilized by properdin, and they in turn activate C3 and C5–C9 (Fig. 5-2).

C. Activation of the complement system

1. **Classical pathway is activated by immune complexes** (Ag-Ab complexes). Only **IgM, IgG₃, and IgG₁ can activate ("fix") the complement**, which occurs as C1 binds to the Fc portion of the immunoglobulins. One IgM molecule can activate the complement cascade, whereas hundreds of IgG may be necessary to activate the cascade.

2. **Alternative pathway (properdin system)** is activated by **gram-negative bacterial cell walls, complex polysaccharides, cobra venom, fungi, viruses, parasites, and IgA aggregates**.

D. Functions of the complement system (Table 5-5) include **chemoattraction** and activation of neutrophils and macrophages, **anaphylaxis** (by causing the release of histamine), **opsonization** of foreign antigens, and **cytolysis** of target cell membranes (e.g., tumors, bacteria). Several functions are **mediated by complement receptors** that exist on many cells of the body. The specific function can vary depending on what cell the complement receptor is on.

E. Serum protein regulators of the complement system

1. **C1 esterase inhibitor: inhibits the classical pathway** by inactivating C1 esterase.

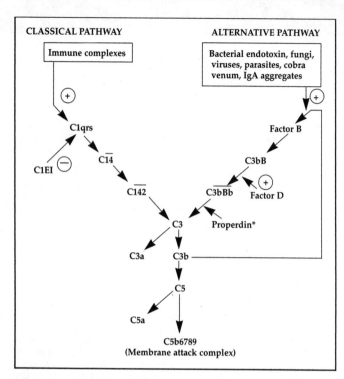

Fig. 5-2. The complement cascade. −, inhibits; +, activates; horizontal lines over a number, activated; *properdin stabilizes C3bBb; C1EI, C1 esterase inhibitor.

    2.   Factors I and H. Factor I inactivates C3b, and factor H dissociates Bb from C3b; both processes **inhibit the alternative pathway.**
F.   Cell membrane regulators of the complement system
    1.   Decay-accelerating factor (DAF or CD 55) inactivates C3 and C4.
    2.   Membrane inhibitor of reactive lysis (MIRL, "protectin," or CD 59) inhibits the formation of the C9 transmembrane pore.
    3.   Homologous restriction factor (HRF) inactivates C8.
II.   Complement system measurement
A.   Total hemolytic complement (CH_{50} and CH_{100}). The functional status of the classical and common pathways is measured by total hemolytic complement. The CH_{50} measures the ability of the patient's serum to lyse 50% of a standard sheep erythrocyte suspension. The amount of complement in the patient's blood is reflected by the number of sheep cells lysed. The CH_{100} is a radial hemolytic assay that records 100%

Table 5-5. Specific complement component functions

Component	Function
C3a	Anaphylatoxin (releases histamine; causes vasodilation, contraction of smooth muscle, and increased vascular permeability)
C3b	Opsonin
C3d	Growth factor for lymphocytes
C4a	Anaphylatoxin, and may neutralize some viruses
C5a	Chemotaxis (attracts neutrophils; causes release of lysozyme, tumor necrosis factor, etc.), anaphylatoxin
C5b6789	"Membrane attack complex" (an amphophilic compound that can lyse cell membranes by forming transmembrane pores, akin to the pores formed by perforin molecules secreted by cytotoxic T lymphocytes).

hemolysis. A normal CH_{50} or CH_{100} indicates that components C1-C9 are present; **they do not quantitate any particular component.**

B.   Other global tests of complement activity. Liposome immunoassay (uses a color change to indicate complement-mediated lysis of liposomes); **enzyme immunoassays** (use monoclonal antibodies to detect the formation of C5b-9 in wells coated with immune complexes).

C.   Alternative pathway hemolytic assay uses rabbit red blood cells to activate and **measure the function of the alternative pathway.**

D.   Individual complement component assays. Often performed by rate **nephelometry**, this assay uses mammal antibody, raised specifically against the human complement factor in question, that is then added to patient serum. The resulting Ab-complement complexes will cause measurable light scattering (nephelometry) that is proportional to the amount of complement in the serum (e.g., **C2, C3, C4, C5, C1 esterase inhibitor, factor B).**

III.   Complement system abnormalities

A.   Increased levels of complement. Several complement proteins (e.g., C3) are **acute phase reactants**, and increases represent nonspecific signs of inflammation (e.g., caused by trauma, subclinical or overt infections, malignancy). They are also elevated in **pregnancy** and in association with **birth control pills.**

B.   Decreased levels of complement or their regulators

1.   Introduction. Most decreases in complement are acquired and caused by excessive consumption (e.g., due to severe inflammation) that causes many of the complement components to be decreased. Occasionally, acquired deficiencies are the result of decreased production, such as in liver disease or severe malnutrition. **Congenital deficiencies are**

rare. Heterozygous congenital deficiencies have ~50% of the normal component level, and usually cause no significant disease. Homozygous deficiencies, which show marked decreases in one component and increased levels of the other components, are often associated with various diseases.

2.   **Neonatal**. Complement components are **normally decreased** in the neonatal period.

3.   **Congenital complement system deficiencies**

   a.   **Deficiencies in C1, C2, or C4** are associated with **connective tissue diseases** [e.g., systemic lupus erythematosus (SLE), rheumatoid arthritis (RA), dermatomyositis]. Almost all patients with homozygous deficiencies in C1 or C4 (and 50% with C2 deficiencies) have SLE.

   b.   **C2 deficiency** is the **most common** congenital deficiency, and in addition to connective tissue diseases, also predisposes the patient to **various infections.**

   c.   **C3 and C4 deficiencies** predispose to **pyogenic infections** with encapsulated organisms such as *Streptococcus pneumoniae*, *Haemophilus influenzae*, and *Neisseria meningitides*.

   d.   **C5-9 (membrane attack complex) deficiencies predispose to infections with** *Neisseria*.

   e.   **Factor I, factor D, properdin, and CR3 (complement receptor 3) deficiencies** predispose to severe **pyogenic infections**.

   f.   **Factor H deficiency** has been associated with hemolytic uremic syndrome.

   g.   **C1 esterase inhibitor deficiency causes hereditary angioedema (HAE). The classical pathway is excessively activated**, consuming various components. This causes massive edema, which can be fatal when the larynx is involved. Of patients with HAE, 85% have a quantitative deficiency of C1 esterase inhibitor, whereas 15% have a functional defect (with normal C1 esterase inhibitor levels).

4.   **Acquired complement system deficiencies**

   a.   **General: most complement deficiencies, which are acquired and the result of excessive consumption, cause multiple components to be decreased. Common causes include autoimmune diseases** (e.g., SLE, RA), **glomerulonephritis** (especially poststreptococcal), **chronic hepatitis, infective endocarditis, disseminated intravascular coagulation (DIC), and immune-complex disease of any cause**. Therefore, autoimmune diseases can be both the cause of acquired complement deficiencies as well as the result of congenital complement deficiencies.

   b.   **C3 nephritic factor (C3nef)** is seen in 70% of patients with **membranoproliferative glomerulonephritis**. C3nef is not a complement component, but is an **IgG antibody** that binds to C3bBb of the alternate pathway, causing prolonged activation and consumption of alternate pathway factors.

   c.   **Decay-accelerating factor (DAF or CD 55), membrane inhibitor of reactive lysis (MIRL), "protectin," or CD 59), or both are decreased in patients with**

paroxysmal nocturnal hematuria (PNH). PNH is an acquired **stem cell disorder** that causes increased red blood cell **sensitivity to complement-mediated lysis**. Complement-mediated lysis can be measured by artificially activating complement with acid or sucrose. PNH increases red cell lysis in the **acidified serum** test (Ham's test) and the **sucrose hemolysis** test. **Flow cytometry** can also identify defects in DAF (CD 55) or MIRL (CD 59).

D. Clues for interpretation

1. **Never rely on a single test**. Perform serial tests to identify trends. For example, in lupus, a "normal" complement level can be part of an upward trend or a precipitous downward trend, depending on at what stage of an acute "flare-up" the patient is.

2. **In the presence of a decreased CH_{50}, normal C3 and C4 values may be a clue that the sample was mishandled, or may indicate a congenital deficiency other than C3 or C4.**

3. **In the presence of a decreased CH_{50}, decreased C3 or C4 values may be seen in any disorder involving immune complexes, or they may be congenital deficiencies**. Decreases in C4 or increases in C3 metabolites (C3a, C3b, C3c, or C3d) are often used to estimate the degree of disease activity. C4 is normally present in smaller concentrations than C3 and, therefore, is a more sensitive indicator of classical pathway consumption than C3. **Extremely low levels of C3 in the setting of an inflammatory or infectious disorder is a dangerous sign that shock may be imminent.**

4. **In the presence of a decreased CH_{50}, decreased C3 with a normal C4 may represent activation of the alternate pathway** (e.g., gram-negative sepsis, fungemia), **hereditary C3 deficiency**, or **immune complex disease.**

5. **In the presence of a decreased CH_{50}, normal C3 with a decreased C4 may be seen in hereditary angioedema, cryoglobulinemia, hereditary C4 deficiency, or immune complex disease**.

Human Leukocyte Antigens (HLA) and Transplantation Immunology

Nancy Higgins and Steven L. Jones

I. Human leukocyte antigens (HLA)

A. Major histocompatibility complex (MHC). The MHC is a group of genes that produce histocompatibility antigens on cell membranes. These antigens help an organism to determine (a) **self from foreign tissue** and (b) compatibility of transplanted tissue. In humans, the antigens are called **human leukocyte antigens** because the antigens are concentrated on white blood cell surfaces. The MHC in humans is located on the short arm of chromosome 6, and is divided into three general groups or classes.

  1. Class 1: A, B, and C genes. Class I antigens are present on **platelets and all nucleated cells** (except trophoblasts, exocrine pancreas, and parotid acinar cells). They are recognized by **CD8+ Tc lymphocytes** (cytotoxic T cells), and are necessary for most **cell-mediated cytotoxic reactions**. Cytotoxic T cells **recognize foreign antigens on cell surfaces** (e.g., viral-infected cells, tumor cells) when the foreign antigens are **placed next to "self" class I antigens** (a process called **MHC restriction**). Approximately 10% of Tc cells can recognize and attack foreign antigens [e.g., foreign HLA antigens in transplants, host HLA antigens in graft-versus-host (GVH) disease] without the need for presentation of the foreign antigen next to self class I antigens (non-MHC restriction). Class I antigens are composed of a **heavy chain** (alpha protein) and a **light chain** (β_2-microglobulin protein).

  2. Class II: D genes (e.g., DP, DQ, DR). Class II antigens are present on **immunocompetent cell surfaces** (macrophages, lymphocytes (B cells and activated T cells), and allow these cells to recognize and communicate with each other. Class II antigens are recognized by **CD4+ Th lymphocytes** (helper T cells), and are necessary for **delayed hypersensitivity** reactions. **Helper T cells recognize foreign antigens** (e.g., tuberculosis, fungal organisms, poison ivy residues) when processed and **placed next to "self" HLA class II antigens on macrophages** (MHC restriction). Approximately 10% of Th cells can recognize and attack a foreign HLA antigen without the need for presentation of the foreign antigen next to self macrophage class II antigens (non-MHC restriction). Class II antigens are composed of two chains **(an alpha protein and a beta protein).**

  3. Class III. These genes code for components of the **complement system** (C2, C4, factor B) and **tumor necrosis factor (TNF).**

B. HLA alleles. Numerous alleles of each HLA gene exist, with at least 30 A alleles, 60 B alleles, 10 C alleles, 24 DR alleles, and 9 DQ alleles, **identified by serologic methods**. Identification of antigens by high resolution, **molecular-level testing shows that many more specific alleles are present**. The total number of possible allelic combinations is astronomic. The different alleles are numbered (e.g., HLA B27). Numbering is generally based on the **serologic identification of the antigen with additional subtypes of the allele as identified by molecular methods**. For example, HLA A1 is a serologically defined antigen. HLA A*0101 and A*0102 are allele subtypes defined by molecular-level testing.

C. Uses of HLA antigen identification. HLA antigen identification is used in **organ transplantation, paternity testing** (although generally replaced by DNA analysis), **selection of platelets for transfusion** into "refractory" patients, **anthropology studies, calculating risk estimates** for certain HLA-associated diseases, and so on.

D. HLA antigen association with disease. Many HLA antigens, particularly the B and D groups, are associated with different diseases (Table 5-6).

II. Transplantation immunology

A. Introduction. Approximately 20,000 organ transplants are performed each year in the United States. On average, 8–10 people who are waiting for transplant organs die in the United States each day. Organs are allocated according to guidelines developed by the transplant community and administered through the United Network for Organ Sharing (**UNOS**). UNOS is the designated Organ Procurement and Transplantation Network for the Department of Health and Human Services. Transplant immunology requirements have been developed by the American Society for Histocompatibility and Immunogenetics (**ASHI**) which, in turn, follows Clinical Laboratory Improvement Amendment (CLIA) and Joint Commission on Accreditation of Healthcare Organizations (JCAHO) requirements. Organs that are currently transplanted in the United States include **kidney, bone marrow, liver, heart, pancreas, combined heart and lung, lung, intestines, stomach, skin, and whole eyes**. Tissues that are currently transplanted include **corneas, powdered bone** (often used in reconstructive surgeries), **long bones, fascia, tendons, arteries and veins, and heart valves**. Grafts can be divided into **autographs** (from self), **syngrafts** (from an identical twin), **allografts** (from a genetically different individual), and **xenografts** (from a different species). Organ placement is administered through UNOS. Allocation algorithms are developed by the transplant community.

B. Organ placement. The allocation algorithms are slightly different for each organ type, but in all the algorithms **a patient is assigned points for each particular donor on the basis of predetermined criteria**, which can include time waiting, disease severity, preformed antibody levels, and HLA matching. Patients are then listed in descending order by number of points. The **organ is offered first to the patient with the highest number of points**. The appropriateness of that particular donor for that particular patient is evaluated by the patient's medical team and either accepted or declined. **If declined,**

Table 5-6. HLA association with disease

HLA Antigen	Related Disease	Relative Increased Risk of Developing the Disease
A3	Hemochromatosis	8 times ($\times$)
B8	Addison's disease (and DR3)	5 $\times$
	Myasthenia gravis (and DR 3)	3 $\times$
	Sjögren's syndrome (and DR3)	3 $\times$
B27	Ankylosing spondylitis	90 $\times$
	Reiter's syndrome	40 $\times$
	Septic arthritis caused by *Salmonella*, *Yersinia*, or *Neisseria* spp.	20 $\times$
	Anterior uveitis	15 $\times$
B35	Subacute thyroiditis	14 $\times$
B38	Psoriatic arthritis	7 $\times$
B47	21-hydroxylase deficiency	15 $\times$
Cw6	Psoriasis vulgaris	13 $\times$
DR2	Goodpasture's syndrome	15 $\times$
	Multiple sclerosis	5 $\times$
DR3	Celiac disease (sprue)	11 $\times$
	Dermatitis herpetiformis	15 $\times$
	Chronic active hepatitis	15 $\times$
	Addison's disease	10 $\times$
	Sjögren's syndrome	10 $\times$
	Systemic lupus erythematosus	6 $\times$
	Grave's disease	4 $\times$
	Myasthenia gravis	3 $\times$
DR3, DR4	Diabetes mellitus (insulin-dependent)	11 $\times$
DR4	Pemphigus	30 $\times$
	Rheumatoid arthritis	5 $\times$
DR5	Pernicious anemia	5 $\times$
	Hashimoto's thyroiditis	3 $\times$

the organ is offered by descending point order until it is accepted. **Organs are first offered within the procuring organ procurement organization's (OPO) area**. If no acceptable recipients are within that area, organs are offered to the region (UNOS regions). After regional offers, organs are offered on a national basis. **One exception to the allocation method is for kidneys, which are compared to patients on the national waiting list.** Donor-recipient kidneys with zero mismatches must first be offered to those patients, no matter where they are located.

C. **Immunogenicity.** Different organs and tissues have different abilities to stimulate an immune response (different immunogenicity): **bone marrow (most immunogenic) > skin > pancreas > heart > kidney > liver > bone > xenographic heart valve > cornea (least immunogenic)**. Therefore, different transplants require different pretransplant workups. **"Privileged tissues" are tissues that are not rejected** when grafted (corneas, bone, tendon, cartilage). **"Privileged sites"** refer to some parts of the body that do not reject grafts (e.g., anterior chamber of the eye, brain).

D.   Overview of transplant compatibility testing. The HLA class I A and B antigens, class II DR antigens, and blood group ABO antigens are viewed as the most important antigens for transplant compatibility. Incompatibility of these antigens may lead to humoral or cellular graft damage or loss. **"Complete" workups may include blood group (ABO), HLA, percent reactive antibody (PRA), and crossmatch.** Different organs, because of their different immunogenicities, may require slightly different workups.

1.   Kidney

   a.   Pretransplant: ABO, HLA type, and PRA are required.

   b.   At transplant: crossmatch required.

2.   Pancreas, heart, lung, liver

   a.   Pretransplant: ABO required, HLA type, and PRA not required but frequently performed

   b.   At transplant: crossmatch if PRA is positive (except in liver)

3.   Bone marrow

   a.   Pretransplant: ABO, HLA Class I (by serology), and class II (by molecular methods) are required, PRA is frequently performed.

   b.   At transplant: crossmatch is recommended.

E.   Blood group compatibility. ABO blood groups must be compatible for graft survival. The same principles of ABO blood transfusion compatibility apply to graft compatibility (e.g., organs from blood group type A donors can be given to blood group type A or AB recipients). Blood group type O donors are universal donors (at least in regard to ABO compatibility) but, in accordance with UNOS guidelines, are not generally transplanted into non-O recipients. Doing so routinely would decrease the supply of type O organs available to type O recipients.

F.   Percent reactive antibodies or panel reactive antibodies. Anti-HLA antibodies can be formed in response to pregnancy, transfusions, or transplanted organs. It is extremely important to screen for preformed antibodies in prospective transplant recipients. Antibodies can be identified by complement-dependent cytotoxicity (CDC), flow cytometry (fluorescence-activated cell sorting, FACS), or ELISA methods. FACS and ELISA are both more sensitive than CDC for identifying IgG antibodies. **PRA is expressed as a percentage of the general population that a specific potential recipient can expect to be reactive against, based on the antibodies present in his or her serum.** When written as two numbers (e.g., 78:32) the left number is the highest percentage that the patient has ever shown. The right number is the current reactivity. For example, a patient may have an antibody to A2 (a common antigen) and be reactive against approximately 35% of the general population, or may have an anti-B51 (a less common antigen) and be reactive against only 5% of the general population. The patient with the anti-A2 will be reactive against a larger percentage of the population and, therefore, it will be more difficult to find a compatible donor. Patients frequently have multispecific antibodies. If a specificity for the preformed antibody can be identified, it will be reported in addition to the PRA percentage. It is very important (and required) to use a PRA screening method that is as sensitive as the final crossmatch method being used.

G.   **Crossmatching. Crossmatches are performed to test for the presence of recipient preformed antibody to specific donor antigens**. Donor lymphocytes and recipient serum are tested together. The most widely used crossmatch techniques are CDC and FACS. **FACS is most sensitive.** Anti-human globulin (AHG) is frequently used to enhance CDC techniques. Autologous crossmatches are generally performed with allo-crossmatches to help in crossmatch interpretation. A number of issues must be clarified before an appropriate interpretation of the crossmatch can be made.

1.   **What organ is being transplanted?** Generally, **HLA alloantibody is a contraindication to transplant for kidney, heart, lung, pancreas, and bone marrow transplant**. Liver transplants can frequently be performed despite the presence of specific anti-donor antibody.

2.   **Is the antibody allo or auto? Autoantibody is not a contraindication to transplant, whereas alloantibodies are generally considered contraindications for transplant (except in livers)**. It is possible for an autoantibody to mask an alloantibody. Care must be taken to differentiate them.

3.   **Is the antibody IgG or IgM? IgG alloantibody is generally considered to be a contraindication** to transplant. Although many (if not most) IgM antibodies are autologous in nature (and therefore not a contraindication to transplant), some IgM antibodies are allogenic and can cause rejection.

4.   **Is the antibody directed against HLA antigens?** When lymphocytes are used as a target cell, it is possible to detect antibodies to antigen systems other than HLA. **Most antibodies to non-HLA antigen systems are not implicated in graft rejection.**

5.   **Is the antibody against class I or class II antigen? Antibody to class I antigen is generally considered to be a contraindication** to transplant. Class II antibody can be difficult to characterize and differentiate from class I or auto-antibody, and can cause graft rejection.

6.   **Current or historic antibody**. Patients who historically have positive serum (generally >12 months old) and are **currently negative** (by very sensitive crossmatch techniques) **can often receive a transplant.**

7.   **Sensitivity of the crossmatch**. In patients having previously received a transplant or those otherwise sensitized, it is very **important to use a sensitive crossmatch technique** such as AHG enhanced CDC or FACS to identify potentially harmful subcytotoxic levels of antibody.

H.   **Frequently used methods for typing and antibody identification**

1.   **Complement-dependent cytotoxicity** is a commonly used technique that uses lymphocytes obtained from periph-

eral blood, lymph node, or spleen. Lymphocytes have a high concentration of HLA antigen on their surface. T and B lymphocytes are easily separated by a variety of methods. **T-lymphocytes have class I antigens and are routinely used for class I typing. B-lymphocytes have class I and class II antigens and are routinely used for class II typing**. The antigens are identified by reacting the cells with panels of different sera having known antibodies against specific HLA antigens. **Sera is obtained commercially from multiparous women**, individuals sensitized by transfusions, or individuals sensitized by a transplant. Monoclonal antibodies against specific HLA antigen epitopes are also available commercially for typing.

After incubating the lymphocytes with the antisera, complement is added. If antibodies in the reagent sera have recognized and become attached to the HLA antigens on the lymphocytes, complement will be activated and the cell wall will be damaged. A stain such as eosin, trypan blue, ethidium bromide, or acridine orange is added as an indicator. Stain will enter damaged cells, which can then be visualized through a microscope. In addition to identifying HLA antigens, the CDC assay can also be used to detect preformed antibody (with known reagent cells and unknown patient sera) or for crossmatching a particular donor and recipient. AHG is frequently added to enhance crossmatch reactivity.

2. **Molecular-level testing**. DNA is isolated from nucleated cells. **DNA copies can then be amplified by using the polymerase chain reaction** in which the DNA chains are denatured and then copied using polymerases and specific primers in the presence of nucleotides. In **sequence specific primer (SSP)** testing, panels of specific sequences are used as primers for unknown DNA. If the primer recognizes a sequence, the product will be amplified. After amplification, the product is visualized by gel electrophoresis or ELISA (spectrophotometric) methods. If no sequence is recognized, there will be no product. In **sequence specific oligo probe (SSOP)** methods, a relatively large portion of DNA is amplified, then applied to a membrane with specific probes attached to it. If the DNA has the same sequence as the probe, it will bind and then can be visualized photographically. **Direct sequencing** can be performed by using DNA as a reagent, and exact nucleotides can be identified and recorded. SSP and SSOP can be used for low or high resolution typing, whereas direct sequencing is performed as a high resolution type.

3. **Mixed lymphocyte culture (or reaction). The patient's in vitro cellular reactivity is measured against potential donor cells**. Reactivity is made one-directional by irradiating one set of cells to remove their ability to respond to stimulus. If cellular recognition occurs, T cells will be activated. Tritiated thymidine in the media is incorporated during activation and subsequent replication, and can then be quantitated. With the development of molecular typing techniques, mixed lymphocyte cultures are rarely used now.

4. **Flow cytometry**. A flow cytometer uses fluids to pass cells in a single line in front of a laser light source. In trans-

plantation, it is **primarily used for antibody identification and crossmatching assays**. Sera and cells are incubated together, then washed. Antibody directed against antigens on the cells is labeled with a goat anti-human IgG or IgM antibody with a fluorescent tag (usually FITC). T and B cells are directly labeled using CD2 or CD3 (T cells) and CD 19 or CD 20 (B cells) each having a different colored fluorescent tag. T and B cells can be differentiated in this three-color system and determined to be positive or negative in comparison with reactivity to normal human serum. This technique has an approximately **10-fold increase in crossmatch sensitivity when compared with CDC methods.**

5. **Enzyme-linked immunosorbent assay** is a solid phase assay using HLA antigens bound to a well in a plate. Patient sera is added and, if it recognizes the antigen, will be bound to the plate. A chromogenically labeled goat anti-human IgG or IgM conjugate is then added, along with a substrate. After development, the color produced can be measured with a spectrophotometer. This assay is currently **used primarily for preformed antibody identification and is about ten-fold more sensitive than CDC methods.**

I. **Post-transplant issues**

1. **Molecular-level tests to monitor hematopoietic cell transplant engraftment**. Amplification of the recipient's DNA, followed by electrophoresis, can be used to identify **single tandem repeats (STR), variable number tandem repeats (VNTR), or restriction fragment length polymorphisms (RFLP)**, all of which may be useful in determining whether the lymphocytes in the peripheral blood of the patient are the patient's native cells, or whether they are from the donor's marrow (and therefore a sign of successful engraftment).

2. **Serologic tests to investigate graft insufficiency**. Testing the recipient for anti-donor antibody formation may help to differentiate between rejection and infection or immunosuppressant drug toxicity. Anti-donor antibody may be bound to the graft, and therefore be undectable in circulating blood.

3. **Graft rejection.** Three main classes of organ rejection are seen.

   a. **Hyperacute: caused by preformed antibodies in the recipient**, particularly antibodies against ABO antigens or HLA class I (A,B,C) antigens. The antibodies **attack the graft as soon as the blood vessels are connected**, damaging endothelial cells and causing inflammation and microthrombi formation. The organ often appears mottled and dusky during the transplant procedure itself. Histologically, microthrombi and neutrophils may be seen within vessels.

   b. **Acute or active**: probably caused by **T-lymphocytes** that develop a sensitization against the organ. This reaction, if it occurs, usually takes at least **1–4 weeks** to develop. Late phases of this type of rejection may involve the development of antibodies to the graft. Histologically, lymphocytes are seen infiltrating the graft's epithelial cells (e.g., renal proximal tubule epithelium).

c. Chronic: probably caused by **a combination of antibodies (against weak antigens) and lymphocytes**, and takes **months to years** to develop. Histologically, fibrosis and vascular arteriosclerosis are often seen, and immunofluorescent techniques can identify deposits of antibodies and complement in subendothelial locations (e.g., in renal glomerular capillaries).

4. **Immunosuppression therapy**. Depending on the organ transplanted, immunosuppression therapy may include corticosteroids, cyclosporin, tacrolimus (FK-506) Prograf, mycophenolate mofetil (RS-61443), antilymphocyte globulin (OKT3), thymoglobulin, interleukin-2 receptor antagonists (Zenapax, Simulect), antimetabolites (e.g., azathioprine) and so on. Blood transfusions before a renal transplant may have an immunosuppressive effect (in part because of the development of blocking antibodies that mask the organ's antigens). The immunosuppressed state **predisposes to infection and certain malignancies** (skin carcinomas, large B cell and immunoblastic lymphomas, Kaposi's sarcoma, and cervical carcinoma are the most common). The malignancies can be the result of dampened tumor immunosurveillance by T cells.

5. **Graft-versus-host disease** is the result of **immunocompetent grafts** (blood transfusions with viable lymphocytes or transplanted organs) **being transplanted into immunosuppressed patients**. It is a particular problem for **bone marrow and liver transplants**. If it occurs, it usually happens within 3–30 days after transfusion or engraftment. The donor's immunocompetent cells attack the recipient's body, particularly the skin, intestines, and liver. This causes skin or mucosal ulceration, diarrhea, and liver failure. The greater the number of mismatched HLA antigens, the greater the risk of GVH disease. **It can be reduced in bone marrow patients by using siblings with identical HLA antigens as donors, or by removing the donor T cells using antithymocyte globulin. GVH disease in blood transfusions can be avoided by irradiating the blood** before transfusion, which damages the lymphocytes and prevents them from dividing. GVH disease in liver transplants is still not well understood, and can occur in patients with relatively well-matched grafts.

Hypersensitivity Reactions

Bruce S. Rabin

I. Introduction. The immune-mediated mechanisms of resistance to foreign antigens ("allergens") are generally protective, but in some cases they can be harmful and cause tissue injury. These mechanisms are frequently referred to as "hypersensitivity reactions" because they reflect heightened immune responsiveness. Hypersensitivity reactions involve various combinations of immune system components, and **Gell and Coombs** divided the reactions into four main types. **Types 1, 2, and 3 are mediated by humoral components (antibodies and complement), whereas type 4 is mediated by cellular components (T-lymphocytes):**

A. Type 1: Immediate Hypersensitivity Reactions
B. Type 2: Cytotoxic Reactions
C. Type 3: Immune Complex-Mediated Reactions
D. Type 4: Cell-Mediated Hypersensitivity Reactions
II. Type 1 (immediate hypersensitivity) reactions
A. Mechanism. Foreign antigens (e.g., pollen, house dust mites, foods, animal hair, insect venoms, drugs) bind to and cause **bridging of IgE** antibodies on the surface of mast cells or basophils. This leads to the release of **histamine**, leukotrienes C4, D4, and E4 (**"slow-reacting substance of anaphylaxis"**), bradykinin, and other soluble mediators that produce clinical reactions commonly referred to as **"allergy"** (or "atopy"). These reactions can range from localized itching, swelling, and redness (wheal and flare) to anaphylactic shock (e.g., hypotension, bronchospasm, laryngeal edema, diarrhea).

B. Common clinical situations involving type 1 reactions. Urticaria (hives), atopic dermatitis (eczema), food allergies, **hay fever**, chronic sinusitis, asthma, bee sting reactions, penicillin reactions, **anaphylactic shock**, are examples of common clinical situation involving type 1 reactions.

C. Laboratory testing. To diagnose the presence of an allergic disease, the presence of an antigen-specific IgE antibody and correlation with a clinical response to the antigen is required. Several methods are used to demonstrate antigen-specific IgE antibodies.

   1. Skin tests. Injection of antigen into the skin, the most common and accurate method of provocative challenge, produces an almost immediate response.

   2. In vitro IgE assay (radioallergosorbent test— RAST). A specific antigen is bound to an insoluble surface (e.g., paper disc) and the patient's serum is added. After washing unbound antibodies away, the amount of the patient's IgE bound to the specific antigen is determined by adding an anti-IgE antibody with an attached marker.

III. Type 2 (cytotoxic) reactions
   A. Mechanism. Type 2 reactions refer to a group of reactions that are initiated by non-IgE antibodies (usually **IgG or IgM**)

that bind to an antigen on cell surfaces. The antigen may be a natural constituent of the cell surface or may be adsorbed onto the cell surface. The interaction of antigen and antibody then causes one of the following complement-mediated or antibody-mediated mechanisms to occur.

1. **The complement system is activated**, leading to the formation and attachment of C3b. **C3b acts as an opsonin, facilitating phagocytosis** of the cell by macrophages, neutrophils, and so on ("opsonin" is Greek, meaning "to obtain victuals" and refers to making an antigen more "palatable" for phagocytosis.)

2. **The complement system is activated**, leading to the formation of C5-9 (membrane attack complex). **C5-9 is capable of causing cell death** by forming "pores" (holes) in the cell membrane.

3. The original **IgM or IgG antibodies** may themselves act as **opsonins, facilitating phagocytosis** of the cell by macrophages and neutrophils, or destruction by natural killer (NK) cells ("antibody-dependent, cell-mediated cytotoxicity").

4. The original **IgM or IgG antibodies** may not cause the cell's death, but may alter its **physiologic function**.

B. **Common clinical situations involving type 2 reactions**. Incompatible **blood group transfusion reactions**, autoimmune hemolytic anemia, drug-induced hemolytic anemia, autoimmune thrombocytopenic purpura, **Goodpasture's disease, systemic lupus erythematosus, autoimmune neutropenia, and Graves' disease**, myasthenia gravis, are among the clinical situations involving type 2 reactions.

C. **Laboratory testing**. Common laboratory tests involve the detection of antibodies against various antigens, or abnormally located complement deposits. **Tests can use patient tissues (e.g., the direct Coombs' test, which uses patient red blood cells) or patient serum (e.g., the test for anti-thyroid peroxidase antibodies that allows patient serum to react with a section of monkey thyroid tissue). Anti-human antibodies (e.g., rabbit antibodies with or without an enzymatic or fluorescent marker) are then added** that bind to human antibodies or human complement. These anti-human antibodies allow the visualization or quantification of the antibody or complement deposit in question.

IV. **Type 3 (immune complex) reactions**

A. **Mechanism. Antigen-antibody (immune) complexes** form when circulating antibodies bind to specific antigens (foreign or self). Macrophages in the spleen, liver, and lung normally remove immune complexes from the circulation. If the macrophages are overwhelmed, the excess immune complexes will become **deposited in tissues**. There, the complement system may be activated, **forming C5a, which attracts neutrophils** to the area. Neutrophils then phagocytose the immune complexes, but in so doing also release **lysosomal enzymes that damage surrounding tissues**.

B. **Factors that influence type 3 reactions**

1. **Size**. Small immune complexes are not deposited in tissue. Large complexes are easily phagocytosed. **Intermediate-sized complexes** in the setting of a moderate antigen excess

can be deposited in tissue, and are most **effective at activating complement** and causing a type 3 reaction.

   2.   Quantity. Immune complexes occur frequently, even after a meal. However, they are only of pathologic significance if **large amounts** accumulate in tissue.

   3.   Location. Immune complexes formed within tissue at the site of an injected antigen lead to a localized type 3 reaction called an **"Arthus reaction."** Immune complexes formed within the blood stream can cause systemic deposition of immune complexes called **"serum sickness."** Immune complexes are deposited in tissues such as skin, renal glomeruli, joints, and blood vessel walls, **causing skin rashes, glomerulonephritis, arthritis, and vasculitis,** respectively.

   4.   Duration. After a single exposure to antigen, tissue injury can reverse and heal. **Persistent exposure** to the antigen with resultant immune complex formation can lead to **tissue injury** and scarring.

C.   **Common clinical situations involving type 3 reactions. Systemic lupus erythematosus (type 2 and 3 reactions are involved), rheumatoid arthritis, and poststreptococcal glomerulonephritis are among the common clinical situations involving type 3 reactions.**

D.   **Laboratory testing.** The clinical history and physical examination are essential in guiding the test selection process. Tests to confirm inflammation (e.g., erythrocyte sedimentation rate, C-reactive protein levels) are often followed by tests, such as anti-nuclear antibody (ANA), anti-streptolysin O (ASO), to rule out certain causes. In some cases, histologic examination of tissue (e.g., skin, renal biopsy) is required to confirm vasculitis or the extent of tissue injury. For example, the classic histologic pattern of poststreptococcal glomerulonephritis is a granular ("lumpy-bumpy") deposition of immune complexes seen with immunofluorescence techniques.

V.   **Type 4 (cell-mediated) reactions**

A.   **Mechanism.** These reactions to antigens are mediated by **T-lymphocytes** and, unlike types 1, 2, and 3 reactions, do not involve antibody or complement. They can be **divided into two groups.**

   1.   Delayed-type hypersensitivity (DH). This reaction to an injected antigen takes **24–48 hours** to reach its maximal intensity. **Primary sensitization** usually occurs in lymph nodes or the spleen, where antigen-presenting cells (e.g., macrophages) express the antigen next to **class II HLA** molecules, and **present the antigen to CD4 Th1 lymphocytes (helper T-lymphocytes).** When the antigen is reintroduced into the host, macrophages present the antigen to previously sensitized CD4 Th1 lymphocytes **which, in turn, attract and activate macrophages to phagocytose** the foreign antigens. During phagocytosis, released lysosomal **enzymes can also damage surrounding tissues.** If the antigen is not easily removed, the macrophages can take on an epithelioid appearance, fuse to form multinucleated giant cells, and aggregate into a granuloma. Multiple cytokines are involved in this process. Macrophages secrete **interleukin-1 (IL-1) and tumor necrosis factor (TNF)**, which stimulate T cells and cause endothelial cells to generate adhesion molecules, respectively. T cells secrete **interferon-gamma and IL-2**, which activate macrophages and other T cells.

  2.   Cytotoxic T-cell responses. Although not technically a true hypersensitivity reaction (it lacks inflammatory cell components that the other reactions involve), it is usually included in type 4 reactions because it is cell-mediated and an important host defense. **Antigen-presenting cells** (macrophages) process and express the foreign antigen adjacent to class I major **histocompatibility complex (MHC)** molecules (unlike delayed hypersensitivity reactions, which involve class II MHC molecules). The macrophages then present the antigen to CD8 Tc lymphocytes (**cytotoxic T lymphocytes**), which become activated. Activated **CD8 lymphocytes** can **then kill the cells** exhibiting the foreign antigen by creating "pores" in the cell membrane (using the protein "perforin"), or by cytolysin.

B.   Common clinical situations involving type 4 delayed hypersensitivity reactions. Localized skin reactions to injected antigens (e.g., tuberculin skin test), chronic intracellular bacterial infections (e.g., *Mycoplasma tuberculosis*, brucellosis), fungal infections (e.g., histoplasmosis granulomas), protozoan infections [e.g., trypanosomes (Chagas' disease)], **contact dermatitis** (e.g., poison ivy), **chronic hypersensitivity pneumonitis**, and so on are among the common clinical situations involving type 4 delayed hypersensitivity reactions.

C.   Common clinical situations involving type 4 cytotoxic T-cell reactions. Viral infections, tumors, transplant rejections, and GVH disease are among the common clinical situations involving type 4 cytotoxic T-cell reactions.

D.   Laboratory tests. Common ways of confirming type 4 hypersensitivity reactions include tissue biopsies (where histologic evidence of granulomas may be seen) and skin testing an injectable antigen. **Skin tests are performed for two main reasons**.

  1.   To find out if the patient's immune system is functional and capable of type 4 reactions, at least **five different common antigens are injected**, each of which the patient is very likely to have been previously exposed to (e.g., *Candida* spp.). A negative response suggests "anergy," the inability to manifest a delayed hypersensitivity skin reaction. This is usually associated with an impairment of CD4 function.

  2.   To find out if the patient has been exposed to a particular antigen through infection or immunization (e.g., tuberculosis, *Leishmania* spp.), **the antigen in question is injected. Skin erythema (redness) during the first few hours** after exposure to the injected antigen is *not* evidence of a delayed hypersensitivity reaction, but may be caused by allergic reactions, for example. For a skin test to be positive, **significant palpable induration** (caused by accumulation of lymphocytes and macrophages) **must be present between 24 and 72 hours** after the skin injection. A positive response indicates that the individual has T-lymphocytes that have been previously sensitized to the antigen.

  Note: Antihistaminic drugs must be discontinued 24 hours before skin testing. Histamine can be administered as a positive control.

Immunodeficiency

Timothy R. La Pine and Harry R. Hill

I. Introduction

A. Initial clinical considerations

1. **It is imperative to remember what is considered normal** for different ages and for different situations. For example, a normal child may have 6–12 infections per year if living at home, and up to 18 infections per year if at a day-care center.

2. **Always perform a careful history and physical examination.** Congenital immunodeficiencies almost always have an associated positive family history. Physical examination may reveal skin scarring from previous infections, eczema, lymphadenopathy, and so forth.

3. **Nonimmunologic defects should always be considered** as potential causes of repeated infections. Structural defects such as eczema, burns, urinary tract obstructions, and asplenia can lead to increased numbers of infections. Recurrent infections in the same location (e.g., right middle-lobe pneumonia) should raise the suspicion of an anatomic defect or a foreign body (e.g., swallowed peanut).

4. **Severe cell-mediated (T cell), phagocytic, and complement deficiencies tend to manifest in the neonatal period. Severe humoral (B cell) deficiencies tend to manifest after 4–5 months of life (after the mother's passively transferred antibodies have decreased).**

5. **Immunoglobulin deficiencies in any patient over the age of 30 should raise the suspicion of multiple myeloma** (see Chapter 2.2, *White Blood Cells*, for workup).

B. Immunodeficiency should be suspected in patients such as those listed below.

1. Those who have an **increased frequency of infections** compared with patients of similar age and exposure risks.

2. Patients who have **unusual or opportunistic infections**, infections with organisms that are usually nonpathogenic or inconsequential, or infections that are unexpectedly severe.

3. Those with infections of **prolonged duration**, and require prolonged antimicrobial therapy or surgical intervention, and are **incompletely cleared** between episodes.

4. Patients with **multiple, complicated infections** involving different organ systems.

C. Functional categories of immunodeficiency

1. **Defects in the T-lymphocyte system** (including T cells and lymphokines).

2. **Defects in the B-lymphocyte system** (including B cells and immunoglobulins).

3. **Defects in the phagocytic system** (including neutrophils and macrophages).

4.   **Defects in the complement system.**

5.   Of congenital immunodeficiencies, ~**50%** are caused by **B-lymphocyte** system defects; other causes include **severe combined immunodeficiencies** (SCIDS, see below) (**25%**); **phagocytic** deficiencies (**15%**), **T-lymphocyte** system defects (**7%**); and **complement defects and miscellaneous defects** (3%).

D.   **Laboratory tests used to confirm and define suspected immunodeficiency.** A general sequential approach to laboratory screening tests is shown in Table 5-7.

1.   **Defects in the T-lymphocyte system (cell-mediated immunity) generally present shortly after birth as severe infections and failure to thrive, or may present as recurrent viral infections, systemic illness, or both after vaccination with live viruses. A complete blood count and differential, quantitation of T cells and T-cell subsets** (CD4 and CD8), **skin testing**, and **mitogen assays** are useful aids in the diagnosis of T-lymphocyte defects.

2.   **Defects in the B-lymphocyte system (humoral immunity) are generally characterized by recurrent sinopulmonary and gastrointestinal (GI) infections presenting** *after the first six months* **of** life. **A complete blood count with differential, quantitation of B cells, quantitation of serum immunoglobulins** (with IgG subclasses), and **IgG challenge testing** (to determine the ability of the patient to mount an IgG response) are useful aids in the diagnosis of B-lymphocyte defects. IgG challenge testing includes vaccination with the following substances, followed by serum titer measurements.

a.   **Diphtheria and tetanus vaccination** and antibody titers: to evaluate IgG_1

b.   **Pneumococcal vaccination** and antibody titers: to evaluate IgG_2

c.   **Influenza vaccination** and antibody titers: to evaluate IgG_3

Note: Do not give *live* **virus vaccines to patients suspected of having immunodeficiencies,** as serious illness may ensue.

3.   **Defects in the phagocytic system are characterized by perianal or periodontal abscesses**, recurrent cutaneous and soft tissue abscesses, with or without **a history of delayed separation of the umbilical cord** (>1 month). **A complete blood count with differential, nitroblue tetrazolium (NBT) test, quantitation of the** β_2 **integrins CD11/ 18**, and **chemotaxis assays** are useful aids in the diagnosis of phagocytic defects.

II.   **Defects in the T-lymphocyte system**

A.   **Clinical findings**

1.   **Severe and recurrent infections, particularly with intracellular pathogens,** include the following.

a.   **Viruses:** herpes, cytomegalovirus (CMV), varicella, respiratory snycytial virus (RSV), rotavirus

b.   **Bacteria:** *Mycobacteria, Listeria*

c.   **Fungi:** *Candida* (especially mucocutaneous), *Cryptococcus, Aspergillus, Pneumocystis carinii*

Table 5-7. Laboratory tests used to confirm and define suspected immunodeficiency

	Laboratory Screening Tests
Tests of cellular (T-cell) immunity	Complete blood count with absolute lymphocyte count Delayed hypersensitivity skin tests to recall antigens (diphtheria, tetanus, candida, PPD, mumps) Quantification of T cells and T-cell subsets by flow cytometry Enzymatic tests: ADA, PNP Cytokine receptor expression: IFNγR, IL-2A, gamma chain, IL-12R Tests of immunoregulation and immunoglobulin synthesis Lymphocyte blast transformation response to mitogens and antigens Mixed lymphocyte culture assays Tests of lymphocyte-mediated cytotoxicity Molecular tests for gene defects Cytokine production assays by ELISA: IL2, IL4, TGF-β, IFNγ, etc. HIV testing as indicated
Tests of humoral (B-cell) immunity	Quantitation of serum immunoglobulins –Isotypes: IgG, IgM, IgA, IgE –IgG subclass levels, IgA subclass levels Tests for functional antibodies –Serum isohemagglutinin levels for IgM antibody response –Patient's IgG antibody response after immunization with diphtheria and tetanus toxoids, or pneumococcal or meningococcal polysaccharide antigens, if older than 2 years Antibody response after infection to respiratory viruses Enumeration and phenotyping of B cells in blood, surface IgG, IgA, IgM, IgE, and IgD Polyclonal B-cell–induced immunoglobulin production in vitro
Tests of phagocytic immunity	Complete blood count with absolute neutrophil count NBT (nitroblue tetrazolium) or dihydrorhodamine fluorescence test for respiratory burst activity Chemotaxis assays Serum IgE levels Phagocytosis and bacterial killing assays. Molecular tests: CGD, LAD, etc. Flow cytometry for leukocyte adhesion molecules CD11/18

continued

Table 5-7. *Continued*

Laboratory Screening Tests

Tests of complement immunity	Total hemolytic complement activity (CH50 for primary complement deficiency)
	Rabbit red blood cell screen for alternative pathway hemolytic activity
	Serum C2, C3, C4, C5, and factor B levels
	Individual component assays
	C1 esterase inhibitor concentrations
	C1 esterase functional activity

ADA, adenosine deaminase; CGD, chronic granulomatous disease; ELISA, enzyme-linked immunosorbent assay; HIV, human immunodeficiency virus; IFN, interferon; IL, interleukin; LAD, leukocyte adhesion defect; PNP, purine nucleoside phosphorylase; PPD, purified protein derivative; TGF, transforming growth factor.

    d.   Protozoa: *Giardia*, toxoplasmosis
  2.   Systemic illness after vaccination with a live virus or bacille Calmette–Guérin (BCG)
  3.   Malignancies and autoimmune disease
  4.   B-cell antibody deficiency (caused by the absence of helper T-cell function)
B.   T-cell deficiency disorders
  1.   Severe combined immunodeficiency syndrome (SCIDS) is a heterogenous group of at least five genetic disorders that result in lymphopenia and multiple defects in both T cells and B cells. SCID diseases lead to **severe and often fatal infections** that usually present **shortly after birth** (e.g., opportunistic infections with a failure to thrive by 3 months of age). SCID variants include the following.
    a.   T-cell receptor defects: autosomal-recessive inheritance
      (1)   Failure to express CD3 glycoproteins (associated with T-cell antigen receptor)
      (2)   Abnormalities in the IL-1 receptor
      (3)   Failure to produce IL-2, or a mutation in the IL-2 receptor γ chain
      (4)   ZAP-70 deficiency, defective T-cell CD8 and CD4 receptor transduction
    b.   Purine metabolic pathway abnormalities.
      (1)   Adenosine deaminase (ADA) deficiency (20% of SCID cases). ADA catalyzes adenosine and deoxyadenosine; absence of ADA leads to the accumulation of **toxic metabolites**, which are capable of killing T-cells, which leads to reduced numbers of T cells and B cells. The genetic defect is chromosome **20 q-13**. Clinical features include recurrent infections, dysostosis, and chondrodysplasia. Treatment involves PEG-ADA, or bone marrow or stem cell transplant. More recently, autologous lympho-

cytes or cord blood stem cells have been corrected in vitro, using **retroviral vectors to insert normal human ADA genes.**

(2)   **Purine nucleoside phosphorylase deficiency** is a disorder that leads to the accumulation of intracellular deoxyguanosine triphosphate, which destroys dividing T cells; the genetic defect is chromosome **14q13.12**. Clinical features include recurrent infections, anemia, and mental retardation.

c.   **Autosomal recessive SCIDS ("bare lymphocyte syndrome")** is caused by **aberrant gene regulation of the major histocompatibility complex** (MHC I and II on B cells, macrophages, and dendritic cells). Lack of MHC antigens interferes with the processes of lymphocyte recognition, regulation, and cytotoxic defense.

d.   **X-linked SCIDS: the most common SCID variant**; due to a mutation in the gene for the **IL-2 receptor. No T-cell growth occurs**, as this receptor is the mediator of T-cell growth by several cytokines.

2.   **DiGeorge's syndrome**
a.   **Pathogenesis: third and fourth pharyngeal pouch developmental abnormalities**, including thymic aplasia or hypoplasia, parathyroid and thyroid abnormalities, cardiovascular abnormalities (interrupted aortic arch, truncus arteriosus), and peculiar facies with micrognathia, cleft palate, and low set ears.

b.   **Clinical presentation. Morphologic abnormalities** (see above); **severe viral, fungal, and bacterial infections from birth; hypocalcemia with tetany** (secondary to parathyroid abnormalities); early onset seizures. Some patients may be asymptomatic.

c.   **Laboratory findings include low absolute lymphocyte counts** (i.e., <1,500/μL) and **borderline-low CD4 cell counts** because of defective T-cell thymic maturation; T cells have depressed antigen and mitogen responses. DiGeorge's syndrome may be associated with monosomy 22q11, diabetes, and isoretinoin exposure.

3.   **Chronic mucocutaneous candidiasis**
a.   **Pathogenesis: antigen-specific immune defect** for *Candida albicans*; may be autosomal recessive or sporadic.

b.   **Clinical presentation. Recurrent skin and mucous membrane *Candida* infections** can occur from birth to the third or fourth decade. Autoantibody production may produce multiple endocrine problems (e.g., hypoparathyroidism, diabetes, and Addison's disease, which is a major cause of death).

4.   **Wiskott-Aldrich syndrome**
a.   **Pathogenesis: an X-linked, combined T-cell (helper), B-cell, and macrophage defect**. Decreased production of anti-polysaccharide antibodies ensues, which can lead to overwhelming **pneumococcal disease** or other encapsulated bacterial infections.

b.   **Clinical presentation. Eczema, thrombocytopenia, infections**; bleeding and bruising occur because of small, poorly functioning platelets.

c. **Laboratory findings**. Patients have **low serum levels of IgM, high serum levels of IgA and IgE, and usually normal IgG.**

5. **Ataxia-telangiectasia**

   a. **Pathogenesis**: an **autosomal recessive** disorder involving **defective DNA repair** processes that causes Purkinje cell degeneration (with progressive cerebellar ataxia), oculocutaneous telangiectasia, and recurrent infections. The genetic defect is located on chromosome **11q22.23**.

   b. **Clinical presentation**. Variable time of onset (usually by 2 years of age); **progressive cerebellar ataxia, occulocutaneous telangiectasia, recurrent sinopulmonary infections**, autoimmune phenomena, and **malignancies** occur (with hypersensitivity to ionizing radiation).

   c. **Laboratory findings. Patients have an antibody deficiency** with decreased IgA (70% of cases), absent IgE (80%), IgG_2 and IgG_4 subclass deficiencies, and **decreased T-cell function and numbers. Serum α-fetoprotein levels are often elevated.**

6. **Acquired immunodeficiencies**. Acquired deficiencies of various immune processes may be seen in several clinical situations, including **drug therapies** (e.g., corticosteroids, cytotoxic drugs, chemotherapies), **alcoholism, diabetes, cachexia, myelophthistic disorders**, various hematologic (e.g., **Hodgkin's** disease) and **nonhematologic malignancies**, and acquired immunodeficiency syndrome (AIDS). **AIDS** is caused by **human immunodeficiency virus** (types I and II, with multiple serotypes). This retrovirus has an envelope containing **gp 120**, which **binds to CD4 antigens on T cells**, macrophages, and central nervous system (CNS) cells. The immune system is damaged as **CD4 T cells diminish**, with subsequent **opportunistic and reactivated infections** (e.g., *Candida*, herpes simplex, *P. carinii*, *Mycobacterium*, *Cryptosporidium*, *Giardia*, *Isospora*, CMV), and various **malignancies** (e.g., Kaposi's sarcoma, large B-cell lymphomas). Diagnosis is by **clinical presentation, ELISA** and **Western blot** identification of viral proteins (e.g., two out of the following three: p24, gp41, gp120/160, etc.), and **PCR** testing for the viral genome.

C. **Treatment of T-lymphocyte defects**

1. **Thymus transplant**. Transplants of fetal thymus <14 weeks of gestational development, or thymic epithelial cells in culture, provide only **temporary benefits.**

2. **Bone marrow transplants**

   a. **HLA-matched sibling donors or matched unrelated donors** can be used.

   b. **Haploidentical marrow from parents** can be used. To prevent graft-versus-host (GVH) disease, the **marrow may have mature T cells removed** by sheep red blood cell rosetting, soybean-lectin absorption, or by treating with monoclonal antibodies against T cells.

   c. **Stem cell transplants** from cord or adult peripheral blood can be used.

3. **Gene transfer** refers to the insertion of a normal gene into the patient's own stem cells. Encouraging results have

been seen with gene transfers in ADA deficiency. **Enzyme replacement** therapies may be helpful in some of the enzyme-deficient disorders.

4. Immunotherapy: recombinant cytokine therapy (e.g., IL-2 in SCIDS variants).

5. Antifungal agents: for chronic mucocutaneous candidiasis.

6. Treatment considerations. Rule out AIDS and zinc deficiency, as indicated, and transfuse with irradiated blood products to avoid GVH disease. Infants with zinc deficiency present with symptoms that are similar to infants who have T-cell deficiencies.

III. Defects in the B-lymphocyte system

A. Clinical findings. The clinical presentation of antibody deficiencies results from a **decreased defense against the extracellular phases of bacterial and viral infections.**

1. Serious recurrent bacterial infections without lymphadenopathy or tonsillar enlargement
   a. Sinopulmonary: 90% to 100%
   b. Gastrointestinal (e.g., chronic diarrhea): 50% to 60%
   c. Systemic: common with encapsulated bacteria

2. Blunted responses to certain vaccinations and viral infections (e.g., enterovirus and rubella encephalitis, paralytic polio, and dermatomyositis)

3. Development of lymphoreticular malignancies (25%)

B. B-cell deficiency disorders

1. Bruton's agammaglobulinemia
   a. Pathogenesis: an X-linked defect in a specific B-cell tyrosine kinase (a.k.a. "Btk"; "Colonel Bruton's tyrosine kinase") that leads to the **arrested development of B-cell precursors**. Pre-B cells are present (with cytoplasmic mu heavy chains); mature B cells are absent or severely decreased, with normal numbers of T cells. The genetic defect is on the long arm of the X chromosome **(Xq2l.3-22)**.
   b. Clinical presentation. Severe infections start at 4–6 months of age, after maternally acquired IgG has significantly decreased. **Sinopulmonary infections with encapsulated bacteria, or GI infections** (e.g., *Giardia* spp.), hallmark the disease; however, patients are also at risk for viral infections, particularly **enterovirus meningoencephalitis** from echo, coxsackie, and polio viruses. **Live polio vaccines should be avoided** in affected patients and their close contacts. Lymphoreticular malignancies and autoimmune diseases also occur in 20% of the patients.
   c. Laboratory findings. Total immunoglobulins are severely decreased (<100 mg%) and **all Ig classes are equally low.**

2. Transient hypogammaglobulinemia of infancy
   a. Pathogenesis. Antibody production (particularly IgG$_2$) is delayed for up to 2 years.
   b. Clinical presentation. Increased numbers of infections are noted from 4 months to 1 year after birth.
   c. Laboratory findings: normal numbers of circulating T cells and B cells, with **decreased levels of IgG$_2$.**

d. Treatment. Vaccinate the patient and check the antibody response—most respond and do not need gamma globulin therapy.

3. Immunoglobulin A deficiency

a. Pathogenesis. This is the most common immuno-deficiency (1 of 700 individuals); **a block exists in the differentiation of IgA plasma cells**. The B cells, other antibody classes, and T cells are usually normal. The susceptibility gene is probably in the **class III MHC** region on chromosome 6.

b. Clinical presentation: atopic diseases, food allergies, autoimmune diseases, arthritis, increased respiratory, and GI infections (30% of patients); two thirds of patients are asymptomatic. Patients with IgA deficiency can develop anti-IgA antibodies, which can cause **severe anaphylactic reactions when they are transfused with blood containing IgA**. Measure anti-IgA antibodies levels before blood transfusions and avoid intravenous immunoglobulin (IVIG) therapy.

c. Laboratory findings. Serum IgA levels are <5 mg/dL and salivary IgA is absent. IgG_2 or IgG_4 subclass deficiencies are found in 20% of IgA-deficient patients with infections.

4. Hypogammaglobulinemia with normal to increased IgM

a. Pathogenesis. X-linked and autosomal recessive forms exist; the defect is **a block in the further differentiation of B-cell IgM isotypes**, and "switching" does not occur to IgG, IgA, and IgE isotypes. A critical **T-cell CD40 ligand (gp 39)** is missing in 80% of the cases, which normally binds to B cells, and class switching does not occur without T-cell help. The genetic defect is at chromosome **Xq26.3-27**. In 20% of the cases, an autosomal recessive CD40 receptor signal transduction defect is present.

b. Clinical presentation: lung, sinus, and middle ear infections; increased frequency of autoimmune disease, lymphoma, cirrhosis.

c. Laboratory findings. Absent or decreased IgG, IgA, and IgE, with normal or increased IgM. Neutropenia is common.

5. Common variable hypogammaglobulinemia ("late-onset hypogammaglobulinemia")

a. Pathogenesis. Several mechanisms cause a late-onset, variable immunodeficiency of B cells (the B cells fail to differentiate into plasma cells), resulting in **a slow decline of all immunoglobulin classes** (IgA levels usually decrease first). Mechanisms include increased T-cell suppressor effects, failure of helper T-cell functions, failure of B cells to terminally glycosylate and secrete immunoglobulins, decreased IL-2 levels, and abnormalities of the CD40 system. A susceptibility gene is located in the **class III MHC** region on chromosome 6 (as in IgA deficiency), and affects both males and females.

b. Clinical presentation. A slow, insidious onset is common during the **second or third decade** of life; however, in some cases, the time of onset can vary from several years after birth until 80–90 years of age. Manifestations include **sinopulmonary infections** (90%–100%), **chronic diarrhea or *Giardia*** (50%–60%), **sepsis**, meningitis, splenomegaly, hepatomegaly, autoimmune diseases (e.g., arthritis, thyroiditis, hemolytic anemia, and so on, particularly in patients with associated T-cell defects), and malignancies (in 20%–25% of the patients).

    c. **Laboratory findings. All immunoglobulin classes are decreased**. Total T-cell and B-cell counts are usually normal.

  6. **IgG subclass deficiencies**

    a. **Pathogenesis. Deficiencies exist in one of the four IgG subclasses: IgG$_1$** (anti-protein antibody), **IgG$_2$** (anti-polysaccharide antibody), **IgG$_3$** (anti-viral and anti-protein antibody), or IgG$_4$ (unclear significance).

    b. **Clinical presentation**. Individuals are **usually asymptomatic**; however, some individuals present with recurrent sinopulmonary infections.

    c. **Laboratory findings**. Diagnosis can be made with **IgG subclass determinations**, plus pre- and postimmunization antibody responses [e.g., tetanus vaccinations (a protein antigen) should stimulate IgG$_1$ and IgG$_3$; pneumococcus vaccinations (a polysaccharide antigen) should stimulate IgG$_2$ production].

    d. **Treatment**. Symptomatic patients may benefit from a trial of prophylactic antibiotics such as trimethoprim-sulfamethoxazole, polysaccharide-protein conjugate vaccines, or IVIG.

C. **Treatment of B-lymphocyte defects**

  1. Treatment is done to prevent life-threatening infections, decrease pulmonary damage, and eradicate localized infections.

  2. **Gamma globulin (IVIG): passive immunotherapy**

    a. 2,000–100,000 donor units are pooled, followed by multistep fractionations and viral inactivation steps (using detergent solvents)

    b. **Disadvantages** of gamma globulin therapy

      (1) **Anaphylaxis** can occur from IgE or IgG$_4$ (against IgA) in IgA-deficient patients.

      (2) **Anaphylaxislike** process can occur from IgG aggregates triggering complement.

      (3) **Pain** (e.g., rate-related headache and backache): "gamma globulin cripple"

      (4) **Viral infection** (e.g., hepatitis C)

      (5) **Aseptic meningitis** (no specific pathogen isolated)

      (6) **Herxheimerlike reactions** can occur from opsonins in the product that cause the release of cytokines

      (7) **Creutzfeldt–Jakob disease**, theoretically, can be transmitted.

      (8) **Cost**

    c. **Indications for gamma globulin therapy: recurrent bacterial infections, significant decreases in IgG, and no antibody formation after immunization**. IgG subclass deficiencies may benefit from gamma globulin therapy. **Avoid gamma globulin therapy in IgA deficiency** except in cases of an associated IgG_2 deficiency.

    3. Immunotherapy with recombinant cytokines: IL-2 as indicated in SCID variants

    4. Antibiotics

IV. Defects in the phagocytic system

  A. Clinical findings

    1. Recurrent cutaneous tissue infections and abscesses

    2. Chronic mucocutaneous *Candida* infections

    3. Recurrent sinopulmonary infections

  B. Neutrophil disorders

    1. Leukocyte adhesion deficiencies (LAD)

      a. Two types of leukocyte deficiency exist: LAD I and LAD II

        (1) LAD I: autosomal recessive; absence of neutrophil **CD11b/CD18**; tight adhesion to endothelial cells does not occur.

        (2) LAD II: autosomal recessive; absence of neutrophil **sialyl Lewis X**; "tethering" (loose adhesion) to E-selectin and P-selectin on endothelial cells does not occur.

      b. Clinical presentation. Delayed separation of the umbilical cord at birth, tissue infections without pus formation, recurrent necrotic soft tissue infections, periodontitis, perioral or rectal abscesses, and severe pulmonary infections.

      c. Laboratory findings

        (1) Histologically, **phagocytes are absent in lesions**, despite high peripheral white blood cell counts.

        (2) Flow cytometry should be used to **assess CD11b/CD18** glycoproteins on the patient's neutrophils. In healthy individuals, CD11b/CD18 expression increases 5–20 times after stimulation with a degranulating agent; the increase does not occur in affected patients.

    2. Chronic granulomatous disease (CGD)

      a. Pathogenesis. CGD is an X-linked or autosomal recessive disorder characterized by an **absent respiratory burst**, which involves a lack of O_2 uptake by granulocytes, absent $O_2^{\bullet-}$, H_2O_2, and $OH^{\bullet}$ generation, and **absent bactericidal activity for catalase-positive bacteria and fungi** (e.g., *Staphylococci*, *Serratia*, *Nocardia*, *Candida*, and *Aspergillus*). Symptom-free carriers of X-linked CGD have a 50% decrease in respiratory burst activity compared with normal controls. Forms of CGD include the following.

        (1) X-linked CGD (66%): caused by a defect in a 91 kd heavy chain of cytochrome B

        (2) Autosomal recessive CGD (33%): caused by an absence of one of two cytosolic factors (47 kd and 67 kd) required for oxidase activation on the light chain of cytochrome B

        (3) G6PD deficiency: mimics CGD because no reduced nicotinamide-adenine dinucleotide phosphate (NADPH) is regenerated by the hexose monophosphate shunt, leading to a shortened respiratory burst.

b. Clinical presentation. Includes **recurrent cutaneous and visceral abscesses, pneumonia** (usually with catalase-positive organisms), osteomyelitis, **granulomas** by 1 year of age, and lymphadenitis at the site of an infection (caused by the poor removal of the infecting agent).

c. Laboratory findings. A negative NBT test after stimulation; impaired dihydrorhodamine fluorescence.

3. Myeloperoxidase deficiency causes delayed microbial killing because of the inability to generate HOCl⁻. Congenital forms (associated with recurrent *Candida* infections in deep tissues) and acquired forms (associated with myelomonocytic leukemia) exist.

4. Chediak–Higashi syndrome

a. Pathogenesis. This syndrome involves **abnormal granules** and **abnormal microtubule** formation. **Giant lysosomal granules** exist in phagocytes, melanocytes, and other cells; they have an **inability to degranulate** and, therefore, have poor bacterial killing abilities. **Defective melanosomes cause partial albinism.** Defective microtubules lead to **decreased chemotaxis, diapedesis, and engulfment** of bacteria.

b. Clinical presentation. Findings include **recurrent bacterial infections and abscess formation**; partial oculocutaneous **albinism**; hepatosplenomegaly, lymphadenopathy, and a bleeding tendency.

c. Laboratory findings. Pancytopenia; large, azurophilic granules in all types of leukocytes; examining hair shafts for giant melanosomes is useful in making the diagnosis.

5. Glutathione synthetase deficiency

a. Pathogenesis. The **absence of glutathione synthetase leads to a deficiency of reduced glutathione** which, in turn, causes H_2O_2 to accumulate. This leads to **hemolytic anemia and poor neutrophil function**, with an increased susceptibility to infection.

b. Clinical presentation. Increased numbers of infections, and tissue injury caused by auto-oxidation from free oxygen radicals (e.g., atherosclerosis, adult respiratory distress syndrome, accelerated aging).

c. Treatment. Vitamin E and other antioxidants may provide some protection.

6. Job's syndrome (hyperimmunoglobulin E)

a. Pathogenesis. An autosomal dominant disorder with incomplete penetrance that causes **hyperimmunoglobulin E with intermittent neutrophil chemotactic defects.**

b. Clinical presentation. Recurrent infections [particularly staphylococcal infections of the soft tissues (**"cold abscesses"**: abscesses without the classic symptoms of inflammation (redness, heat, and pain) and **chronic mucocutaneous candidiasis**], osteopenia and bone fractures, blood and tissue **eosinophilia** with eczematoid dermatitis, and **coarse facies** with a broad nasal bridge and a protruding lower lip.

   c.   Laboratory findings. Blood eosinophilia, high levels of serum IgE (>2,000 IU/mL), and **neutrophil chemotactic defects.**
C.   Treatment of neutrophil defects
   1.   Antibiotics as indicated
   2.   Granulocyte infusions for poorly responding infections
   3.   Gamma-interferon
      a.   Decreases infections in CGD by 70%, perhaps by increasing nitric oxide generation
      b.   May benefit some patients with Job's syndrome with severe eczema or infections
   4.   Bone marrow transplants
   5.   Gene therapy in early stages
   6.   Colony-stimulating factors as indicated for neutropenia
V.   Defects in the complement system
A.   Functions of the complement system
   1.   Amplification of leukocyte-associated inflammatory responses
   2.   Opsonization (e.g., C3b)
   3.   Chemotaxis (e.g., C5a)
   4.   Lysis of pathogens [e.g., C5b-9 (membrane attack complex)]
B.   Symptoms and signs of complement deficiencies
   1.   Recurrent infections with encapsulated bacteria (particularly with deficiencies of C3, C5, and alternate pathway factors)
   2.   Recurrent infections with *Neisseria* species (with deficiencies of C5-8)
   3.   Collagen vascular diseases (associated with hereditary deficiencies of C1, C2, and C4)
C.   Clinical abnormalities of complement
   1.   Decreases in complement levels because of activation and consumption in disease
      a.   Immune complex diseases
      b.   Rheumatoid arthritis: rheumatoid factor (i.e., IgM directed against IgG) can activate the classic pathway; a decrease in the C4 level is the most sensitive indicator.
      c.   Endotoxemia: lipopolysaccharide triggers the alternative pathway, lowering factor B and C3
      d.   Nephritis (C3NEF membranoproliferative type II nephritis): an autoantibody stabilizes C3bBbP and causes continuous activation of alternative pathway
   2.   Hereditary deficiencies of complement
      a.   C1qr, C4, C2: causes "Lupus-like diseases" (e.g., nephritis, arthritis, and facial rashes) **and infections** (usually pneumococcal).
      b.   C1 esterase inhibitor deficiency: causes hereditary angioedema
         (1)   Autosomal recessive: unchecked activation of the complement cascade leads to the production of **anaphylatoxins** (e.g., C3a and C5a), which cause mast cells to release **histamine**, and leads to capillary leakage and **tissue edema.**

(2)   Acquired form: associated with malignancies; absent functional unit of esterase

c.   C3 and C5 deficiency: severe recurrent infections (e.g., pneumonia, sepsis, meningitis, fungal infections)

3.   Terminal component deficiencies (C5, 6, 7, 8): recurrent gonococcal and meningococcal infections because of poor complement-mediated lysis

4.   C9 deficiency: asymptomatic (no clinical significance)

5.   Abnormalities of the alternative pathway

a.   Causes severe, **overwhelming infections with polysaccharide-coated bacteria**

b.   Conditions associated with alternative pathway defects

(1)   **Newborns**: factor B is not fully developed until later

(2)   **Nephrotic syndrome**: factor B is lost in urine

(3)   **Sickle cell disease**: uncertain mechanism, factor D is probably decreased

(4)   **Splenectomy**: uncertain mechanism, factor D is probably decreased

c.   Properdin deficiency (X-linked): causes *Neisseria* infections

d.   Deficiencies of factor H and I: cause continuous activation of the alternative pathway and very low C3 levels, with **recurrent pyogenic infections and nephritis**

D.   Management of complement abnormalities

1.   Vaccination for *Streptococcus pneumoniae, Neisseria meningitidis, H. influenzae*

2.   Antibiotic therapy as clinically indicated.

5.7

Autoimmunity

Bruce S. Rabin

I. Introduction. An autoimmune response occurs when the immune system reacts to self-tissue as if the self-tissue were a foreign antigen. The resultant immune-mediated damage to cells and tissue is considered to be an **autoimmune disease when a causal relationship between the autoimmune response and the tissue damage is established**. Both antibody-mediated (autoantibodies) and cell-mediated (autoreactive T-lymphocytes) immune pathways are involved in the pathogenesis of autoimmune disease.

A variety of mechanisms exists for the activation of autoreactive T and B lymphocytes, which may be responsible for the etiology and pathogenesis of autoimmune diseases. Obviously, because autoimmune diseases can occur, the normal mechanisms for removal (clonal deletion) or inactivation (clonal anergy) of autoreactive lymphocytes must not be absolute. In other words, normal, healthy individuals may have some B-lymphocytes that are capable of producing autoantibodies, and low levels of these autoantibodies may exist in the absence of actual autoimmune disease. Therefore, **the presence of an autoantibody to self-tissue does not always indicate that disease of that tissue is present**. In particular, caution must be exercised when interpreting the clinical implications of antibodies to thyroid antigens, gastric parietal cells, the adrenal gland, smooth muscle cells, pancreatic islet cells, and mitochondria. A stronger disease association is found in patients who have antibodies to the glomerular basement membrane, the acetylcholine receptor, myelin basic protein, skin antigens, the thyroid-stimulating hormone receptor, and gluten. In all cases, **the higher the titer of the antibody, the more likely that tissue disease is present** (a **titer** is the reciprocal of the highest dilution of serum showing a positive reaction: the higher the titer, the higher the number of antibodies). However, the final determination of whether an autoimmune disease is present depends on the evaluation of all clinical, laboratory, and tissue studies.

Many of the established autoimmune diseases are described below. Diagnostic testing primarily involves antibody detection. Although cell-mediated immune mechanisms may be responsible for the pathologic damage to tissue, no reliable assays of cell-mediated immunity to autoantigens are clinically useful.

II. Hashimoto's (lymphocytic autoimmune) thyroiditis
  A. Pathogenesis of disease. Serologic tests show a high concentration of antibodies to antigens specific for the thyroid. High titers of these antibodies indicate a high likelihood of thyroid damage occurring. Histologically, thyroid glands with Hashimoto's thyroiditis are largely replaced with a lymphocytic infiltrate. This indirectly suggests that T cell-mediated immune mechanisms also participate in the destruction of the tissue.

However, tests for T cell-mediated reactivity are not routinely available. The relative contribution of humoral or cell-mediated immunity in the initiation and course of autoimmune thyroiditis is not known.

  B.   Relevant immunologic testing. Assays for antibodies to **thyroglobulin** and the **thyroid peroxidase** enzyme (a.k.a. "antimicrosomal antibodies") are useful to evaluate the likelihood of autoimmune thyroiditis. A negative test for both antibodies virtually excludes thyroiditis because >98% of patients are positive for one of the two antibodies. However, a positive test (usually with low antibody titers), which is relatively nonspecific, may be seen in Hashimoto's thyroiditis, Graves' disease, adenocarcinoma of the thyroid, pernicious anemia, collagen vascular diseases, myasthenia gravis, and at low levels in normal individuals (particularly elderly women). The presence of antibodies to thyroid peroxidase usually rules out hypothyroidism secondary to nonimmune mechanisms.

III.   Graves' disease

  A.   Pathogenesis of disease. Autoantibodies in Graves' disease activate the **thyroid-stimulating hormone (thyrotropin) receptor**, which leads to the release of thyroid hormones from their storage site in the thyroglobulin molecule. The resulting **hyperthyroidism**, which is usually associated with a diffusely enlarged thyroid, provides evidence that some antibodies can upregulate cell functions. Graves' autoantibodies can cross the placenta and cause clinical symptoms of hyperthyroidism in neonates; the symptoms disappear once the antibodies have been catabolized.

  B.   Relevant immunologic testing. Testing for thyrotropin receptor antibodies (TRAb) is currently performed with the thyrotropin binding inhibiting immunoglobulin technique. Approximately 95% of patients with Graves' disease have antibodies to the thyroid-stimulating hormone (TSH) receptor. These antibodies may be present in some patients with other autoimmune thyroid diseases, but are not found in normal individuals. The antibody level often decreases with antithyroid drug therapy.

IV.   Myasthenia gravis (MG)

  A.   Pathogenesis of disease. Myasthenia gravis is caused by an antibody-mediated effect on postsynaptic **acetylcholine receptors**. The disease provides evidence that, in contrast to Graves' disease, antibodies can downregulate cell function. The antibodies cause a reduction of the number of receptors at the **neuromuscular junction**, resulting in easy fatigability of muscles. These antibodies can cross the placenta, causing clinical symptoms in neonates; the symptoms disappear once the antibodies have been catabolized. Approximately 10% of patients with MG have a **thymoma** and, from 15% to 80% of patients with a thymoma have been reported to have myasthenia gravis. Patients with MG also have an increased prevalence of Graves' disease and collagen-vascular diseases.

  B.   Relevant immunologic testing. Of patients with MG, 90% have **antibodies to acetylcholine receptors** solubilized from human muscle (a very specific and sensitive test), which means that 10% of patients with MG do not. Patients with disease onset before 40 years of age have the highest antibody levels. Antibodies to acetylcholine receptors can also be seen in patients with epithelial thymomas, paraneoplastic syndromes, and the **Lambert–Eaton myasthenic syndrome**. An additional **antibody to striated muscles** is also seen in ~90% of patients with MG with a thymoma, and in 50% of patients with MG >60 years of age. A negative antistriated muscle antibody test result is useful in suggesting that the patient with MG does not have a thymoma. A role for this antibody in the pathogenesis of the disease is unclear.

V.   Pernicious anemia (PA)

A.   Pathogenesis of disease. Pernicious anemia results from the destruction of **gastric parietal cells**, with the subsequent loss of intrinsic factor and the ability to absorb vitamin B_{12}. Autoantibodies include antibodies directed against (a) gastric parietal cell antigens; (b) the proton pump that acidifies the stomach lumen (acidity is necessary for B_{12} to be released from its bound salivary protein); and (c) the intrinsic factor binding site for B_{12}. Patients with PA frequently have other autoimmune diseases, including autoimmune thyroiditis, insulin-dependent diabetes, and Addison's disease.

B.   Relevant immunologic testing. Antibodies to gastric parietal cells are usually detected by immunofluorescence using mouse stomach as the substrate. Of patients with PA, ~90% have detectable antibodies to gastric parietal cells; however, these antibodies are relatively nonspecific, and are present in 25% of patients with a variety of other autoimmune disorders. They may occasionally be present in patients with gastric ulcers or gastric cancer, and occur in 15% of healthy elderly individuals. Individuals with antibodies to parietal cells, but who do not have PA, may have early or subclinical parietal cell damage, and should be followed closely. Antibodies to intrinsic factor (IF) are present in almost all children with PA, and in most adults with PA. Anti-IF antibodies, which may be of the "blocking" or the "binding" subtypes, are extremely specific for PA.

VI.   Addison's disease

A.   Pathogenesis of disease. The cause of Addison's disease is immune-mediated damage of the **cortical cells of the adrenal**, possibly occurring from a cell-mediated immune reaction (histologically, the adrenals contain a chronic inflammatory infiltrate). Autoantibodies are also present. However, as with autoimmune thyroiditis, the relative contributions of cell-mediated and humoral immunity to the disease process is not established.

B.   Relevant immunologic testing. Immunofluorescence is commonly used to detect antibodies to cytoplasmic antigens in cells of the adrenal cortex. The target antigen is often the enzyme that converts 17-α-progesterone and progesterone into 11-deoxycortisol and deoxycorticosterone, respectively. The antibody to this enzyme may also react to antigens in the testes (without disease association), ovary (frequently in association with oophoritis), and placenta. In Addison's disease, the antibody is present in 20% of the patients who have no other diseases; in 50% of the patients if they also have autoimmune thyroid disease or hypoparathyroidism with **chronic mucocutaneous candidiasis**; and in 100% of the patients who also have primary amenorrhea.

VII.   Insulin-dependent diabetes mellitus (IDDM)
   A.   Pathogenesis of disease. Probably no other disease has received as much attention of the immunologic research community as has the mechanism of immune-mediated destruction of the insulin-producing cells of the pancreas. A viral infection of the beta islet cells, with subsequent immune-mediated destruction of the cells, likely occurs in many patients (in a manner analogous to hepatitis virus-initiated hepatocyte damage). In other patients, an immune reaction directed to a peptide of insulin may occur. Other patients may develop disease from nonspecific activation of lymphocytes against a pancreatic **super-antigen**, with the resultant cytokine-mediated destruction of the **beta islet cells**. Many patients are found to have an antibody that binds to the cytoplasm of the beta islet cells. High levels of the antibody may be predictive of disease development in a healthy child who has a sibling with IDDM and who shares an HLA-DR3, HLA-DR4, or both MHC antigens with the patient.
   B.   Relevant immunologic testing. Glutamic acid decarboxylase has been identified as an antigen to which islet cell antibodies are directed. However, other antigens, including insulin, may also elicit antibodies in patients with IDDM. The most common method to detect islet cell antibodies is by indirect immunofluorescence using human pancreas as the tissue substrate. In patients who develop IDDM as a result of a viral infection, islet cell antibodies may be present transiently. In patients who develop IDDM in association with **dysregulation of the immune system**, islet cell antibodies may be present for several years before clinical symptoms develop.

VIII.   Goodpasture's disease
   A.   Pathogenesis of disease. Goodpasture's disease is an antibody-mediated disease in which the physiologic function of a cell is not altered, but rather, complement-dependent lesions are produced in the basement membranes of the renal glomerulus and the lung. As a result, erythrocytes and plasma pass into the urine and alveoli. The target antigen is part of type IV collagen.
   B.   Relevant immunologic testing. Biopsies of the kidney or lung can be studied by immunohistochemical procedures to visualize the presence of immunoglobulin or complement on the basement membrane. If present, these reactants form a smooth, linear staining pattern. Serologic tests for basement membrane antibodies are also available [indirect immunofluorescent tests using renal glomeruli, or enzyme-linked immunosorbent (ELISA) assays using purified antigen]. Changes in the titer of the antibody often correlate with changes in disease activity.

IX.   Pemphigus vulgaris (PV)
   A.   Pathogenesis of disease. Pemphigus vulgaris is caused by antibodies against skin keratinocyte desmosomes, which are responsible for intercellular adhesion. These antibodies inhibit the adhesive properties of the desmosome with resultant formation of intraepidermal blisters.
   B.   Relevant immunologic testing. Biopsy of tissue at the edge of a lesion for immunofluorescence analysis reveals IgG and C3 complement in the intercellular spaces of the keratinocytes of all patients with PV. Serologic tests for these antibodies show binding to the **intercellular epithelial area** of normal monkey

esophagus. Antibody is found in all patients with active disease. Changes in the titer of the antibody correspond to changes in clinical activity of the disease. Clinical relapse is associated with an increased antibody titer.

X.   Bullous pemphigoid (BP)

A.   Pathogenesis of disease. Bullous pemphigoid is caused by antibodies against components of the dermoepidermal junction, leading to detachment of the keratinocytes from the basement membrane and subsequent formation of subepidermal blisters. Similar pathologic and immunologic findings are present in patients who have **herpes gestationalis** and **cicatricial pemphigoid**.

B.   Relevant immunologic testing. Immunofluorescence analysis of biopsies, taken from the edge of a lesion, show IgG and C3 complement bound to the basement membrane at the dermoepidermal junction. Serum from affected patients has antibodies that bind to the dermoepidermal junction in normal skin.

XI.   Primary biliary cirrhosis (PBC)

A.   Pathogenesis of disease. The hallmark of PBC is a chronic, progressive obliteration of the **intrahepatic bile ducts** by a granulomatous inflammatory reaction (CD8 lymphocytes and histiocytes are present in a periductular distribution) that leads to cirrhosis. Patients also have serum antibodies against mitochondria, and a marked elevation of IgM. The role of the antibodies in the pathogenesis of disease is not yet established.

B.   Relevant immunologic testing. The presence of antibody to **mitochondria**, which is characteristic of PBC, is found in 90% of patients at diagnosis. At least nine different mitochondrial antigens (e.g., 2-oxo acid dehydrogenase complex) exist to which antibodies can be directed. Of patients with PBC, ~30% also have antibodies to thyroid tissue, cell nuclei (antinuclear antibody—ANA), or reticulin, and rheumatoid factor (IgM directed against IgG) may be present. Mitochondrial antibodies are routinely detected in patient serum by immunofluorescence using rat kidney as the substrate. As the relevant antigens become identified and purified, ELISA procedures to identify specific antibodies in primary biliary cirrhosis will become more common.

XII.   Autoimmune chronic active hepatitis (ACAH)

A.   Pathogenesis of disease. Chronic active hepatitis is a term that encompasses a pathologic process with more than a single cause. Possible mechanisms include persistence of hepatitis B virus or other hepatitis viruses, drug-induced hepatitis, or an autoimmune reaction to liver antigens. The disease may be asymptomatic or progressive.

B.   Relevant immunologic testing. Two patterns of autoantibodies are seen in patients with ACAH. The pattern in ACAH type I (seen in 50% of ACAH patients) consists of antibodies to the **F-actin** molecule in smooth muscle, and an antibody to ANA. The pattern in ACAH type II consists of an antibody called the **liver-kidney-microsomal (LKM)** antibody. This antibody binds to cytochrome P450 in the cytoplasm of hepatocytes and proximal renal tubules. Of patients with chronic hepatitis C, ~7% also develop LKM antibodies. Another antibody, directed to liver-specific membrane lipoproteins, occurs in ~90% of the patients with either type of ACAH.

XIII. Multiple sclerosis (MS)

A. Pathogenesis of disease. Multiple sclerosis is characterized by damage to (a) myelin, (b) myelin-producing **oligodendrocytes**, and (c) axons passing through areas of demyelination. Inflammatory cells (including B- and T-lymphocytes) are present in the evolving lesions.

B. Relevant immunologic testing. Animal models of MS suggest that an immune reaction to **myelin basic protein** (a component of myelin) may participate in the pathogenesis of the disease. Patients with MS often have high levels of these antibodies in the spinal fluid or serum. Increases in the titer of this antibody are often associated with increased disease activity.

XIV. Gluten sensitive enteropathy (celiac sprue)

A. Pathogenesis of disease. Celiac sprue is characterized by a sensitivity to gluten, reflected by small intestine mucosal damage and subsequent malabsorption of nutrients; clinical improvement occurs on gluten withdrawal. Histologically, the villi of the small intestine are infiltrated by T-lymphocytes, although their relative role in the pathogenesis of the disease is uncertain.

B. Relevant immunologic testing. Several antibodies are present in sprue. Both IgG and IgA antibodies to **gliadin** (an extract of gluten), which are present in patients with sprue, can be measured by ELISA. IgA antibodies are more specific (~95% specificity) than IgG antibodies, as IgG antibodies are also present in patients with other diseases. IgA antibody to **endomysium** (an antigen that is associated with smooth muscle bundles) is also present in sprue (>90% of the patients). Although the relationship between this antibody and gluten is not established, the antibody usually disappears within 12 months of the introduction of a gluten-free diet. This antibody is also present in patients with **dermatitis herpetiformis**. In patients with malabsorption, the presence of anti-gliadin and anti-endomysium antibodies make the diagnosis of sprue highly likely.

XV. Circulating blood elements (hemolytic anemia, thrombocytopenia, leukopenia)

A. Pathogenesis of disease. Antibodies can bind to antigens on the membrane of erythrocytes, leukocytes, or platelets. If the antibodies activate the complement system, complement-mediated lysis of the cell may occur. If the antibody does not activate complement, because of a low density of antibodies or the antibody being of a noncomplement-binding class, the cell can be removed from the circulation by adherence of the Fc portion of the antibody to Fc receptors on neutrophils or macrophages. Clinical sequelae are appropriate for the subsequent anemia, agranulocytosis, or thrombocytopenia result. For specific tests regarding the antibodies detected and their interpretation, please see Section 1, *Blood Bank*, and Chapter 2.2, *White Blood Cells*.

Collagen-Vascular Diseases

John F. Bohnsack

I. Introduction. Collagen-vascular diseases (a.k.a., "systemic rheumatic diseases") comprise a group of autoimmune disorders that affect **connective tissue** (particularly joints, but also skin, muscle, and blood vessels), and frequently also affect **the viscera and nervous system.** Autoimmune disorders that affect single organs are discussed separately in chapter 5.7, *Autoimmunity.* The diagnosis of collagen-vascular diseases depends on the recognition of **clinical characteristics, laboratory testing, biopsies** (occasionally), **and exclusion of other diseases** in the differential diagnosis. General guidelines include the following.

A. The anti-nuclear antibody (ANA) test, which uses human tissue culture cell nuclei as a substrate, **is particularly useful as a diagnostic screen, followed by ANA specificities** (Table 5-8 and Fig. 5-3). ANA "specificity" tests use other types of nuclei, cell organelles, or soluble nuclear substances as substrates, and are **used to identify the actual component of the nucleus** that is targeted by the antibody (e.g., anti-dsDNA, anti-histone). ANA tests are reported as a titer (reciprocal of the last dilution of serum that gives a positive result): **the higher the titer, the more antibodies are present. An ANA "pattern" is also reported** (e.g., speckled, centromeric, homogenous, rim), which describes the parts of the nuclei that are highlighted by the fluorescent antibodies.

B. ANA Pattern
The pattern is rarely useful except when it is centromeric[present in the CREST syndrome—calcinosis, **R**aynaud's syndrome, **e**sophageal dysmotility, **s**clerodactyly (symmetric skin fibrosis of the fingers), and the most common finding, **t**elangiectasia**), or is a very high-titered (≥1:1280) speckled pattern, which suggests the presence of a U1-ribonucleoprotein particle (RNP) antibody (mixed connective tissue disease "overlap").**

C. Interpretation. Always interpret a positive ANA in the context of the patient's clinical condition. No single test is 100% sensitive or 100% specific.

D. Specificity. A positive ANA specificity (e.g., anti-dsDNA) **is more suggestive** of a systemic rheumatic disease than a positive ANA screen alone.

E. Titers. In general, **higher titers of an ANA test are more suggestive** of disease than lower titers.

F. Drug history. Always obtain a drug history. Several drugs can cause a lupus-like condition and elevated ANA titers, such as procainamide, para-aminosalicylic acid, chlorpromazine, phenytoin, griseofulvin, hydralazine, isoniazid, penicillin, methyldopa, and others.

G. Rheumatoid factors are relatively nonspecific; they are more significant and suggestive of underlying disease when present in younger patients than in the elderly.

Table 5-8. Summary of commonly used anti-nuclear antibody (ANA) specificities[a]

Specificity	Disease Association
DNA –dsDNA	SLE (50%); titer correlates with disease activity; rare in other disease states except autoimmune hepatitis. Fairly specific for SLE.
–ssDNA	Many rheumatic diseases. Not a useful diagnostic test.
Histones	SLE, RA, and drug-induced LE. May be useful to differentiate drug-induced lupus from idiopathic form of lupus (antihistones are the only positive specificity in drug-induced lupus).
Nuclear proteins –Sm	Specific for SLE, but only present in 30%–40% of the SLE cases.
–U1-RNP	Marker for MCTD (positive in 90%) *if* other ANA specificities are absent; also positive in SLE, but other ANA specificities are usually also present in SLE.
–SS-A/Ro	SLE (30%–40%), Sjögren's syndrome (80%); subacute cutaneous lupus; neonatal lupus with congenital heart block; "ANA-negative lupus"; RA; primary biliary cirrhosis, chronic active hepatitis; lupus of homozygous C2/C4 deficiency
–SS-B/La	SLE (10%–15%); Sjögren's syndrome (70%–80%)
–Scl-70	Diffuse scleroderma (30%)
–Centromere	CREST syndrome (45%); 25% of patients with idiopathic Raynaud's syndrome

MCTD, mixed connective tissue disease; RA, rheumatoid arthritis; SLE, systemic lupus erythematosus.

[a] The ANA specificity refers to the specific antigen with which the ANA reacts. Specificities are ordered when a specific diagnosis is suspected or to further evaluate a markedly positive ANA screen.

II. Specific diseases
A. Systemic lupus erythematosus (SLE)
1. Clinical characteristics. SLE is a systemic autoimmune disease that can affect practically every organ and tissue. The most common initial manifestations are **systemic** (e.g., fatigue, fever, weight loss), **musculoskeletal** (e.g., arthritis), **cutaneous** (e.g., malar rash, photosensitivity, alopecia, vasculitis), **hematologic** (e.g., anemia, leukopenia and thrombocytopenia), and **renal** (e.g., glomerulonephritis). Other organs, notably the **lungs** (e.g., pleuritis, pneumonitis), **heart** (e.g., pericarditis, valvular dysfunction), and **central nervous system** (e.g., stroke, psychosis) can also be involved during the disease course.

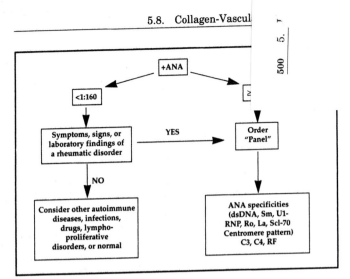

Fig. 5-3. Suggested workup of a positive anti-nuclear antibody (ANA) test. The titers shown are based on the use of a fluorescent ANA test wherein a titer <1:40 is considered negative.

2. **Laboratory results**
   a. **ANA: Almost 100% of the patients with SLE have a positive ANA** (except patients with markedly decreased serum IgG, usually caused by nephrosis); a negative ANA is strong evidence against SLE. ANA specificities include the following.

   (1) **Anti-dsDNA: 50% to 70%** of SLE patients have a positive anti-dsDNA; **very specific** test; rare false-positive findings occur (e.g., autoimmune hepatitis); titers correlate with disease activity.

   (2) **Anti-Sm: 30%** of SLE patients are positive, but this test is **extremely specific** (almost diagnostic) for SLE.

   b. **Direct Coombs' test**: patients may have autoantibodies to red blood cells (RBCs) and hemolytic anemia.

   c. **Anticardiolipin antibodies, lupus anticoagulant**: often present in SLE.

   d. **Serum complement C3, C4**: both are frequently **decreased**, and inversely correlate with disease activity, particularly glomerulonephritis. Hereditary absence of C1, C2, and C4 predispose patients to immune-complex disease that resembles SLE.

   e. **Anti-ribosomal P antibody**: associated with central nervous system lupus (e.g., psychosis).

   f. **Serum immunoglobulins**: frequently are diffusely elevated.

   g. **Complete blood count (CBC)**: anemia, leukopenia (particularly lymphopenia), and thrombocytopenia are common.

    h. **Rapid plasma reagin (RPR)**: a false-positive test result for syphilis is a frequent finding in SLE.

    i. **Renal function tests**: urinalysis and serum albumin, creatinine, and blood urea nitrogen (BUN) are used to determine renal involvement; renal disease is a common cause of SLE-related death.

B. **Primary anti-phospholipid syndrome (PAPLS)**

    1. **Clinical characteristics.** PAPLS is a syndrome of **recurrent vascular thromboses or recurrent fetal loss**, with an **anticardiolipin (ACL) antibody** or **lupus-anticoagulant**. Other clinical characteristics may include transient cerebral ischemia, transverse myelopathy or myelitis, livedo reticularis, cardiac valve disease, chorea, migraine, and a multiple sclerosislike syndrome. By definition, patients with PAPLS do not have SLE or other rheumatologic disorders; by contrast, patients with SLE can have recurrent thromboses and ACL antibodies. PAPLS is diagnosed by the presence of **(a) a primary clinical characteristic and (b) a persistently positive ACL antibody test or lupus anticoagulant.**

    a. **Primary clinical characteristics**

      (1) **Venous, arterial, or small vessel thrombosis in any tissue that is not caused by inflammation**

      (2) **Pregnancy morbidity**: one or more fetal deaths at or beyond 10 weeks of gestation, with normal fetal morphology; or recurrent (3 or more) unexplained, consecutive spontaneous abortions before the 10th week of gestation; or premature birth ($\leq$34 weeks gestation) caused by eclampsia or pre-eclampsia.

    2. **Laboratory results**

    a. **Persistently positive (at least twice, 6 weeks apart) ACL antibody (IgG or IgM**; directed against β_2-**glycoprotein 1; ELISA).** ACL antibodies are also present in 2% to 5% of normal individuals, or following some infections (e.g., hepatitis C), or with some drugs (e.g., phenothiazines, hydralazine, and phenytoin).

    b. **Persistently positive (at least twice, 6 weeks apart) lupus anticoagulant, defined as a prolonged activated partial thromboplastin time (aPTT), kaolin clotting time, or dilute Russell's viper venom test (DRVVT) that does not correct on addition of normal plasma, is corrected with the addition of excess phospholipid, and is not caused by other inhibitors (e.g. heparin, factor VIII inhibitor).**

    c. **Negative ANA** (positive ANA suggests SLE)

    d. Some patients with PAPLS have an **autoimmune hemolytic anemia** (with a positive direct Coombs' test) and **thrombocytopenia**.

C. **Mixed connective tissue disease (MCTD)**

    1. **Clinical characteristics.** MCTD is a controversial multisystem disease with features of **SLE, myositis, and scleroderma.** The major clinical manifestations are **swollen hands or sclerodactyly** (85%), **Raynaud's syndrome** (85%), and synovitis. With time, myositis, acrosclerosis (tightening of the skin on the digits), and systemic sclerosis may develop. Patients develop pulmonary hypertension more frequently than patients with SLE, whereas few develop diffuse proliferative glomerulonephritis, seizures, or psychosis (all common in SLE).

2. Laboratory results

   a. Positive ANA with anti-U1-RNP antibody as the sole ANA specificity. A high titered (≥1:1280) speckled ANA suggests that the ANA is directed against U1-RNP.

   b. Serum immunoglobulins are usually elevated.

   c. Rheumatoid factor is frequently present.

   d. Hematologic abnormalities occur similar to those in SLE [e.g., leukopenia (particularly lymphopenia), thrombocytopenia, Coombs' positive hemolytic anemia].

   e. Serum complement is usually normal.

D. Sjögren's syndrome (SS)

   1. Clinical characteristics. Sjögren's syndrome is **a chronic inflammatory disease of exocrine lacrimal and salivary glands,** causing diminished lacrimal and salivary secretions and resulting in keratoconjunctivitis sicca and xerostomia. Of patients, 90% are women, with a mean age of 50 years. A markedly increased risk for lymphoma is associated with SS. **Primary SS** is not associated with a systemic rheumatic disease, whereas **secondary SS** occurs in association with a systemic rheumatic disease (e.g., rheumatoid arthritis, SLE, MCTD, or scleroderma).

   2. Laboratory results for primary Sjögren's syndrome

      a. ANA is usually positive (≥70%).

      b. Anti-Ro (SS-A) and **anti-La (SS-B)** are frequently positive (80%–90%).

      c. Rheumatoid factor is frequently positive (90%).

      d. Serum immunoglobulins are often (50%) elevated.

   3. Lip biopsy showing lymphocytic infiltration of salivary glands is useful for diagnosis.

E. Systemic sclerosis (scleroderma)

   1. Clinical characteristics. Systemic sclerosis is a **generalized disorder of connective tissue,** characterized by fibrosis and degenerative changes in the blood vessels, skin, synovium, skeletal muscle, and certain internal organs (gastrointestinal tract, lung, heart, and kidney). Systemic sclerosis can be differentiated into three variants.

      a. Diffuse cutaneous: symmetric, widespread skin fibrosis involving distal and proximal extremities, trunk, and face; often with rapid progression and early visceral involvement.

      b. Limited cutaneous (CREST variant): Visceral involvement (e.g., pulmonary hypertension) occurs late.

      c. Overlap: either diffuse or limited cutaneous with typical features of one or more other systemic rheumatic disease (e.g., MCTD).

   2. Laboratory results

      a. ANA: positive in 90% of patients; ANA specificities include the following.

         (1) Diffuse cutaneous: anti-Scl-70, or topoisomerase I (~30% of systemic sclerosis); anti-RNA polymerase I, II, and III (~20%—not usually available in commercial laboratories)

    (2) Limited cutaneous (CREST): centromeric pattern on ANA testing (70%–80%); anti-Th antigen (10%—not usually available in commercial laboratories)

    (3) Overlap: anti-U1-RNP (MCTD); anti-PM-Scl, Ku (myositis-scleroderma overlap—not usually available in commercial laboratories)

F. Inflammatory myopathies (dermatomyositis and polymyositis)

  1. Clinical characteristics. Dermatomyositis (DM) or polymyositis (PM) are inflammatory diseases of striated muscle that cause proximal, symmetric skeletal and oropharyngeal muscle weakness. The peak age of onset is 40–60 years, with a smaller peak in childhood (5–15 years) that is almost entirely DM. DM has a distinctive heliotrope rash on the upper eyelids, a rash over the knuckles or extensor surfaces, and a predilection for various malignancies (in adults). The histology of the muscle biopsy in DM differs from that in PM.

  2. Laboratory results

    a. "Myositis-specific autoantibodies": these are antinuclear and anti-cytoplasmic antibodies that appear to correlate with the clinical syndrome, but the tests are not usually available in commercial laboratories.

      (1) "Anti-synthetase syndrome" (myositis, interstitial lung disease, Raynaud's syndrome, arthritis, fevers): a severe subset of DM or PM, with frequent relapse and persistent disease; PM > DM; Anti-tRNA synthetase antibodies are present (e.g., Anti-Jo-1 in 20% of adult patients).

      (2) Anti-Mi-2 (8%): antigen = helicase; acute onset of disease, V-sign, and shawl rash.

      (3) Anti-signal recognition particle (SRP) (4%): antigen = SRP: severe disease, resistant to therapy (4% of patients with myositis), lacks features of anti-synthetase syndrome.

      (4) Myositis-scleroderma overlap: anti-PM-Scl (8%); anti-Ku (1%); anti-U2-RNP, anti-U3-RNP (<3%).

    b. Muscle-specific substances: the creatine kinase (total and MM fraction), myoglobin, and aldolase are frequently elevated.

  3. Electromyography (EMG) is helpful in the diagnosis.

G. Vasculitides

  1. Clinical characteristics. The vasculitides are a collection of diseases involving **inflammation of blood vessels** (i.e., leukocytes in the blood vessel walls). They are classified according to the size of the blood vessels involved, and whether the vasculitis is primary or secondary to another disorder (e.g., vasculitis is a common secondary characteristic of SLE). The diagnosis is based on the clinical characteristics of the disease, tissue biopsy, and angiography (in some cases). **The laboratory provides general information about the degree of inflammation** (e.g., erythrocyte sedimentation rate) **and organ involvement** (e.g., serum creatinine, urinalysis). In addition, some laboratory tests are helpful in making the specific diagnoses of **Wegener's disease** and **essential cryoglobulinemic vasculitis.**

    a. Wegener's disease is a necrotizing vasculitis affecting the respiratory system (e.g., sinuses, middle ears, lungs) and kidneys, with a mean age of onset of 45 years. Respiratory tissue biopsies reveal necrotizing vasculitis (of small to medium arteries, arterioles, and venules) and granulomas. **Microscopic polyangiitis and idiopathic rapidly progressive (or necrotizing) glomerulonephritis** are related vasculitides involving small blood vessels (venules, capillaries and arterioles) or the glomeruli.

    b. Essential cryoglobulinemic vasculitis results from deposition of immunoglobulins and complement in small blood vessel walls, most frequently caused by a **hepatitis C** infection; it frequently presents as purpuric skin lesions. **Circulating cryoglobulins are present** (immunoglobulins, usually IgM, that precipitate in cold temperatures).

  2. Laboratory evaluation

    a. Anti-neutrophil cytoplasmic antibody—cytoplasmic pattern (C-ANCA; antibodies are directed against neutrophil protease PR-3): C-ANCA is a fairly specific test for Wegener's disease, but the diagnosis cannot be made on the basis of C-ANCA alone. The sensitivity of C-ANCA varies with disease activity.

    b. ANCA—perinuclear pattern (P-ANCA; antibodies are directed against myeloperoxidase and other cytoplasmic proteins): relatively nonspecific, and found in microscopic polyangiitis, rapidly progressive glomerulonephritis, Wegener's disease, ulcerative colitis, primary sclerosing cholangitis, various rheumatic diseases, cystic fibrosis, and Goodpasture's syndrome.

    c. Serum cryoglobulins are present in cryoglobulinemia.

    d. Serum hepatitis C antibody and hepatitis C RNA are sometimes detected in cryoglobulinemic vasculitis.

    e. Serum C3, C4: decreased in cryoglobulinemic vasculitis.

H. Rheumatoid arthritis (RA)

  1. Clinical characteristics. RA is a **symmetric inflammatory peripheral arthritis** that results in erosion of cartilage and bone, with subsequent joint deformity. The diagnosis is based on clinical characteristics and laboratory findings.

  2. Laboratory evaluation. Rheumatoid factor (RF) is usually an IgM (but can be IgG or IgA) directed against the Fc portion of IgG. RF is relatively nonspecific, and found in a variety of conditions, including ~70% of patients with RA, as well as other rheumatic diseases and chronic infections, and in normal individuals (particularly the elderly). No tests are diagnostic of RA, although some tests are useful for monitoring disease activity (e.g., hematocrit, erythrocyte sedimentation rate).

6

Special Topics

Instrumentation

Gabor Komaromy-Hiller

I. **Osmometry and viscometry**
A. **Osmometry**
  1. **Principles.** Osmometry is the measure of the concentration of osmotically active solute molecules. Increased concentration of such molecules results in increased osmotic pressure, lowered vapor pressure, increased boiling point, and decreased freezing point.
  2. **Instrumentation.** Freezing point depression and vapor pressure osmometers are the most commonly used methods in the clinical laboratory.
    a. **Freezing point depression osmometer**: the sample is cooled and the temperature at which it starts to solidify is measured. Osmolality is then calculated.

$$\text{Osmolality (osmol/kg } H_2O) = \frac{\Delta T}{-1.86}$$

  Where ΔT is the observed freezing point in °C, (i.e., depression as compared with the freezing point of water (0°C).
    b. **Vapor pressure osmometer actually measures the decrease in the dew point temperature** of the pure solvent resulting from the decrease of vapor pressure caused by the solutes. This technique is less precise than the freezing point depression osmometer, is nonlinear at osmolalities <200 mOsm/kg H_2O, and does not work well for volatile solutes.
  3. **Applications.** Plasma and urine osmolality measurement is very useful in the assessment of **electrolyte and acid-base disorders.**
B. **Viscometry**
  1. **Principles.** Viscosity is the resistance of matter to flow when subjected to stress or strain. Viscosity is highly temperature dependent and is expressed in poise (P) units.
  2. **Instrumentation**
    a. **Tube viscometer** measures the rate of flow through a tube caused by a known pressure difference. Tube viscometers are very precise, simple, and inexpensive. However, they produce less accurate measurements for the so-called non-Newtonian fluids, such as blood.
    b. **Rotational viscometer**: the fluid is sheared between rotating cylinders, cones, or plates. Blood viscosity can be accurately measured; however, the instruments are more expensive and less precise than tube viscometers.
  3. **Applications.** In clinical practice, **whole blood, synovial fluid**, and serum (rarely) viscosity are measured. Reference ranges are extremely instrument dependent.
II. **Spectrophotometry**
A. **UV-vis.** Ultraviolet (UV) and visible (vis) radiation encompass the portions of the **electromagnetic spectrum between**

180 and 750 nm. UV-vis spectroscopy is **used to analyze compounds that absorb light in this wavelength range**.

1. **Principles. Compounds containing chromophore functional group(s) absorb light in the UV-vis range at one or more specific wavelengths**. Beer's law expresses the relationship between measured absorbance (A) and concentration (c):

$$A = a \times b \times c$$

Where b is the light path, and a is absorptivity (a constant that is compound and wavelength specific).

2. **Instrumentation**. UV-vis instruments have a **light source** or lamp covering the UV-vis wavelength range, a **filter** or monochromator for wavelength selection, a compartment for **sample** and blank solutions, a **detector**, and **electronic circuitry for signal processing and readout** (Fig. 6-1).

   a. **Advantages**: simplicity of methods, inexpensive instrumentation

   b. **Disadvantages:** poor selectivity, analytic sensitivity

3. **Applications**

   a. **UV-vis spectroscopy** is used as a detector for many chromatography or capillary electrophoresis-based separations, and for many enzymatic tests in automated analyzers; and for direct measurement of vitamin C, xylose, urine oxalate, and so forth.

   b. **Urinalysis dip-sticks** are based on a chemical reaction between the analyte and the reagent on the dipstick. The color change in the reaction is compared against a color scale, which provides qualitative or semiquantitative information on the analyte.

B. **Fluorescence**. Fluorescence spectroscopy is similar to UV-vis spectroscopy, and also works in the UV and visible portion of the electromagnetic radiation.

   1. **Principles**

      a. **Fluorescence**. Fluorescence is the selective absorption of a photon (also called excitation), followed by the **return of the compound to its original lower energy**

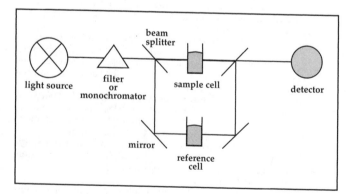

Fig. 6-1. **Block diagram of a double-beam in-time spectrophotometer.**

level, with the **subsequent emission of a fluorescent photon**. Both absorption (excitation) and emission wavelengths are compound specific, and the emission is of a longer wavelength than the excitation wavelength. Intensity of the emitted light (I) depends on many factors, including concentration of the analyte (c):

$$I = k \times c$$

Where k is a constant.

b. Chemiluminescence. In chemiluminescence, **excitation of the fluorescent compound is the result of a chemical reaction**. The emission process is the same as for ordinary fluorescence. Chemiluminescence is also called **cold light** because it does not require the illumination of the chemiluminescent compound.

c. Lifetime measurements. Fluorescent lifetime is the time at which the fluorescence signal decays to 1/e-th of its original value. Fluorescent lifetime is also compound specific.

d. Fluorescence polarization. When the excitation is polarized light, fluorescent emission is partially polarized. **Rotational diffusion results in depolarization of this polarized emission**. The degree of polarization or anisotropy, which depends on the size of the molecule, is the basis of several quantitative immunoassays.

2. Instrumentation is similar to a UV-vis spectrophotometer; however, fluorescence is viewed at 90° with respect to the excitation axis. Instrumentation is more complicated for lifetime or polarization methods.

3. Applications. Fluorescence-based methods are **widely used** in the laboratory. They include measurement of Zn-protoporphyrin, various fluorescent polarization-based drug immunoassays and fetal lung maturity assessment, and chemiluminescent immunoassays. Fluorescence-based detectors are also used in high-performance liquid chromatography (HPLC), capillary electrophoresis (CE), and gel electrophoresis separations.

C. Nephelometry and turbidimetry

1. Principles. Both nephelometry and turbidimetry methods are based on the scattering of radiation by a solution containing particulate matter. The intensity of the scattered radiation depends on several factors, including the wavelength of the incident radiation and the particle size; however, in a given system, **the scattering is directly proportional to the concentration of the particulate matter**.

2. Instrumentation

a. Zero angle scattering. Turbidimetric instruments measure the intensity of the scattered radiation at zero angle relative to the incident radiation. They are more suitable for **high concentration** measurements.

b. Nonzero angle scattering, nephelometric instruments measure the intensity of the scattered radiation at nonzero angle relative to the incident radiation. They are more suitable for measurements at **low concentration**.

3.   Applications. Turbidimetric and nephelometric measurements of molecular complexes (e.g., proteins) **usually follow an immunocomplex formation,** which provides sufficient size for scattering. **Flow cytometers measure scattering from large particles** (see below). **Nephelometers and turbidimeters are used mainly for measurement of various proteins** or protein complexes.

D.   Flow cytometry is the measurement of cells in a flow system.

1.   Principles. Flow cytometry uses scattering and fluorescence from cells to analyze and sort them into various subpopulations. Typically, one to two scattering and three to four different fluorescence signals can be measured simultaneously. **The scattering signals are related to the size and granularity of the cells, whereas the fluorescence signals come from fluorescently labeled antibodies** that are used to selectively label cells based on various antigenic characteristics.

2.   Instrumentation. Figure 6-2 shows the schematic diagram of a flow cytometer. Most modern instruments are multicolor systems (i.e., measure fluorescent signals at multiple wavelengths). The sample cells are **hydrodynamically focused** by the sheath fluid into a very narrow flow, so that **cells can pass through the laser beam one by one.** The scattering and various fluorescent signals are analyzed with very fast electronics. Cell sorting of various subpopulations is also possible. **Gating** refers to the selection of the region of interest in the measured parameters, and simplifies the result display.

3.   Applications. The most common routine application of flow cytometry is the measurement of **cell surface antigens** through immunofluorescence labeling. It is useful in

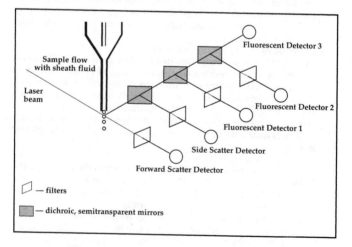

Fig. 6-2.   Block diagram of a flow cytometer.

the lymphocyte subset counting and typing of **leukemias and lymphomas**. Measurement of DNA to evaluate **the cell cycle** and measure cell proliferation and death is the second most common application. Other uses of flow cytometry include measurement of RNA and protein content, membrane permeability and potential, and various intracellular parameters (e.g., calcium ions, pH).

E.   Refractometry is the measurement of refractive index as a light beam passes from one medium to another.

    1.   Principles. Reflectance depends on temperature, wavelength, and pressure. **If solute is added to water, the refractive index of water (1.330 at 20°C) changes.** In a limited range of higher concentration, this change is directly proportional to the amount of dissolved solute.

    2.   Instrumentation. Reflectometers are very simple instruments, usually equipped with temperature control or compensation mechanism. At low concentration, they are likely to be inaccurate.

    3.   Applications. The two most important applications of reflectometers in the clinical laboratory are **quick total protein measurement in serum and estimation of specific gravity of urine.**

F.   Densitometry measures absorbed radiation as a light beam is transmitted through or reflected back from a plate.

    1.   Principle. The basis of densitometry is that the dark and light spots on the plate transmit or reflect light differently to the detector. Therefore, the **measured absorbance is proportional to the darkening of the plate which, in turn, is proportional to the analyte concentration.**

    2.   Instrumentation. In general, densitometers are scanning devices where a plate is moved across a light beam, the transmitted or reflected radiation is measured, and the absorbance is calculated. Some densitometers can determine fluorescing species as well.

    3.   Application. Densitometers are used as detectors for thin-layer chromatography and electrophoresis plates.

G.   Atomic spectroscopy includes the measurement of light absorbed or emitted by atomic species. It is primarily used to determine metals and semimetals in clinical specimens. Because most of these elements are part of molecules, the first step in any kind of atomic spectroscopy method is **atomization.**

    1.   Atomic absorption is analogous to UV-vis spectrophotometry (i.e., it is **based on light absorption by gaseous atomized species**).

        a.   Principle. At characteristic wavelengths, **gaseous atoms absorb light proportionally to the amount of the element of interest in the gas phase** and, subsequently, the concentration of the element in the sample. One notable difference between atomic absorption and UV-vis spectrophotometers is the atomizer, which breaks down the molecules in the sample into elements.

        b.   Instrumentation. Atomic absorption spectrometers are **classified based on the atomization device**. The instruments in general have very low detection limits, which allows trace element determinations in clinical specimens.

(1) Flame atomic absorption. Atomization occurs in a **hot flame** into which the sample or dissolved sample is sprayed.

(2) Electrothermal vaporization. Atomization occurs by an **electrically heated** hot surface, such as graphite platform or cup.

c. **Applications.** Atomic absorption is used for determination of **metals**, including **trace metals**, as well as some nonmetal elements, such as **arsenic**, and **selenium**.

2. **Atomic emission is a thermoluminescence process, where the light emitted by gaseous atoms is measured.**

a. **Principles.** Atomic emission occurs when **atoms that are thermally excited with a high atomizer temperature** (this is different from molecular fluorescence) **emit light**.

b. **Instrumentation.** Atomic emission spectrophotometers are classified based on the atomizer principles.

(1) Flame atomic absorption. The design is similar to flame atomic absorption spectrophotometers.

(2) Inductively coupled plasma is a conducting gaseous mixture maintained by inductive coupling. At the very high temperature of the plasma (6,000–9,000 K), excitation of gaseous atoms occurs more readily than in a hot flame.

c. **Applications. Flame atomic emission is used for sodium, potassium**, and **lithium** analysis, whereas **inductively coupled plasma atomic emission is used for determination of the entire range of trace elements.**

H. **Mass spectrometry (MS) measures ions based on the mass:charge ratio (m:z).** The measured ions can be molecules, molecule fragments, or atoms.

1. **Principles.** The main steps include **ionization and m:z ratio selection**; fragmentation is also important if fragment ions are of interest.

a. **Ionization converts the neutral species into ions.** Ionization can be **"hard,"** when intensive fragmentation accompanies the ion formation, or it can be **"soft,"** when the ionization process preserves the molecular ion.

b. **Fragmentation of each compound is unique**; therefore, this process provides both structural information and compound selectivity.

c. **Mass:charge ratio selection is the most crucial part** of a mass spectrometer, which selectively measures ions with different m:z ratios.

2. **Instrumentation.** Mass spectrometers can be **single stage instruments** (ionization and m:z ratio selection occur only once); or they can be **tandem instruments** (ions selected by the first mass spectrometer are introduced into a second instrument for further fragmentation and analysis).

a. **Single stage instruments** are classified by the type of m:z ratio selection device into quadrupole, ion trap, or time-of-flight mass spectrometers.

b. Tandem instruments. Various combinations of tandem mass spectrometers are available commercially: quadrupole–quadrupole, quadrupole–time-of-flight, and so on.

3. Applications. Mass spectrometers are mainly used as universal, sensitive, and selective **detectors for gas and liquid chromatography, capillary electrophoresis, and inductively coupled plasma** (to measure trace elements). Matrix-assisted laser desorption ionization (**MALDI**) mass spectrometry is used in research laboratories to analyze macromolecules, such as proteins and nucleic acids.

III. Chromatography

A. Basic chromatography principles. Chromatography is composed of a group of separation methods that make use of a so-called stationary phase and a mobile phase. **Separation is based on the difference in migration as the mobile phase** (e.g., helium gas, liquid solvents) **carries the sample components through the stationary phase** (e.g., the polymer coating in a capillary tube, a silica-packed column). Chromatography methods are classified based on either the instrumental platform or the physical principles of the separation mechanism. Our outline follows the much easier classification of instrumental platform.

B. Thin layer chromatography. In thin layer chromatography (TLC), **the stationary phase is thinly spread on a plate** (e.g., silica on aluminum sheet metal). The sample is spotted onto the plate, which is then placed upright in a container with a mobile phase (e.g., methanol) in the bottom.

1. Principles. The mobile phase migrates up through the solid phase by capillary action. The solid phase interacts differently with the various compounds in the sample as they migrate through it. **Separation occurs because of the difference in time a specific compound spends in the mobile versus stationary phase.**

2. Instrumentation. TLC analysis is usually very simple and inexpensive, but is time consuming and requires expertise. **No special instrumentation** is needed. Development of the TLC plates can be done by color reaction with or without subsequent densitometric quantitation of the chromatographic spots. **Two-dimensional TLC** analysis offers improved specificity: a sample is spotted on a TLC plate and developed in one dimension, then the plate is rotated 90° and placed in a different mobile phase for development in the second dimension.

3. Applications. Because of its simplicity, TLC is still widely used for **qualitative amino acid analysis, drug screening, and determination of lecithin:sphingomyelin ratio.**

C. Gas chromatography (GC). The mobile phase of GC is exclusively gas (most often helium). GC is suitable for the analysis of thermally stable volatile or semivolatile compounds.

1. Principles. The stationary phase can be solid or liquid coated on a solid support (e.g., capillary columns). Because most of the analytes in a clinical laboratory are not volatile, a derivatization step precedes the gas chromatographic analysis. GC has excellent resolution for the analysis of highly complex mixtures.

2.   Instrumentation. Temperature and pressure programming are available for optimal separations, and a wide variety of detectors are available to quantitate the separated compounds. Instrumentation requires substantial expertise to run.

3.   Applications. GC is mainly used in **toxicology and therapeutic drug monitoring**, as well as hard-to-analyze compounds such as **organic acids**.

D.   Liquid chromatography. All liquid chromatographic methods have **liquid mobile phases**. By this definition, TLC is also a liquid chromatography technique. Almost anything can be analyzed by a liquid chromatographic system.

1.   Principles. In general, the stationary phase in liquid chromatographic methods is a column packed with tiny particles. High pressures are often required to push the mobile phase through the packed column, hence the name high-performance (high-pressure) liquid chromatography (**HPLC**).

2.   Instrumentation is fairly complex and, because of the high pressure system, not as rugged as gas chromatographs. The selection of stationary phase and mobile phase composition are the most important parameters that affect chromatographic separation. Various detectors are available (Fig. 6-3).

3.   Applications. The major applications of liquid chromatography are in the area of **toxicology and therapeutic drug monitoring**, and in the analysis of small molecular weight compounds such as **metabolites, amino acids, and vitamins**.

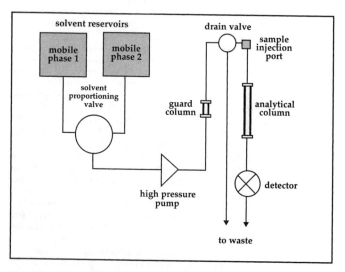

Fig. 6-3.   Schematic diagram of a high-performance liquid chromatography (HPLC) apparatus.

IV. **Electrophoresis is based on the differential migration of charged particles in a liquid media under the influence of an external electric field**. In some forms of electrophoresis, even neutral analytes can be determined. To reduce convection (which would otherwise counteract the separation process), either porous supports or small-bore capillary formats are used.

A. **Gel electrophoresis. Agarose, cellulose acetate, or polyacrylamide gels are used in gel electrophoresis.**

1. **Principles. The rate of migration of ionic particles depends on the electrical field strength, the net ionic charge, and the size of the ion**.

$$v = \frac{X\,Q}{6\pi\,r\,\eta},$$

Where v is the rate of migration, X is the electrical field strength, Q is the net charge of the ion, r is the radius of the particle, and η is the viscosity of the liquid in which separation occurs. Separation occurs because of the difference in migration rate.

To improve resolution, **two-dimensional electrophoresis** and **high-resolution electrophoresis formats** have been developed. **Blotting** refers to the process of transferring the separated analytes from the gel support to a nitrocellulose or nylon membrane for subsequent evaluation and preservation. Three blotting techniques have been developed for **DNA (Southern), RNA (Northern)**, and **protein (Western)** blotting.

2. **Instrumentation**. Essential elements include a stable power supply, a cooling system (to dissipate the generated heat), and a buffer for pH control. The porous support can be **agarose gel** (which has clarity for densitometric measurements), **cellulose acetate gel** (for rapid (<1 hour) separations), and **polyacrylamide gel** (the pore size of which can be regulated by the polymer concentration).

3. **Applications**. Gel electrophoresis is useful for the analysis of macromolecules such as **DNA, RNA, proteins, enzymes**, etc.

B. **Capillary electrophoresis**. The **separation is performed in narrow-bore capillaries**, which reduces convection.

1. **Principles**. The same principles apply as in gel electrophoresis. Support media is not necessary; however, in certain applications, capillary gel electrophoresis can be used.

2. **Instrumentation**. Because capillary cooling is very efficient, **higher electrical fields can be applied** than in gel electrophoresis. This leads to **better resolution** and **reduced analysis time**. The instruments resemble those of liquid chromatography. Generally, anything that can be analyzed in a gel format can also be analyzed in a capillary format.

3. **Applications**. Capillary electrophoresis is not very popular in the clinical laboratory. Its major application is the **automated serum protein electrophoresis**, but it is also used for **DNA fragment analysis** after a polymerase chain reaction (PCR) amplification (mainly in research settings).

V.   Electrochemistry. Electrochemical methods of analysis are based on the **measurement of electric potential, current, or conductance, which is then related to the concentration of the analyte.**

A.   Potentiometry. The potential difference between an indicator electrode and a reference electrode is measured, which is related to the concentration of the analyte.

1.   Principles. A reference electrode with constant potential, a polarizable indicator electrode, and a potentiometer are needed. The measured potential difference is related to the analyte concentration through the Nernst-equation:

$$E = E° - \frac{0.0591}{n} \log \frac{[M_{red}]}{[M_{ox}]}$$

E is the measured potential, $E°$ is the standard potential of the system, n is the number of equivalents of electricity, and $[M_{red}]$ and $[M_{ox}]$ are the concentration of the reduced and oxidized forms of the analyte (one of which is known).

2.   Instrumentation. Instrumentation is very simple. Various electrode designs are available that are selective to one analyte (ion selective electrodes).

3.   Applications. The most well-known application is the pH electrode, which is an H^+-selective electrode with a built-in reference electrode (Fig. 6-4). Other analytes that are measured potentiometrically are Na^+, K^+, Cl^-, free Ca^{++}, and CO_2 (blood gas).

B.   Coulometry, amperometry, and conductometry. Coulometry and amperometry measure the amount of charge or current, respectively, delivered during an electrochemical reaction. This is in contrast to potentiometric measurements that involved no chemical reactions. **Conductometry measures the conductance of a solution, which is related to the analyte concentration.**

1.   Principles

a.   Coulometry. Electrochemical oxidation or reduction occurs at a sufficient potential until all analyte is converted to the new oxidation state. The amount of charge required to accomplish this conversion is measured and related to the mass of the analyte:

$$Q = m \times F \times \frac{FW}{n}$$

Q is the charge measured, m is the mass of the analyte, F is the Faraday constant, FW is the formula weight of the analyte, and n is the number of equivalents of electricity.

b.   Amperometry measures the current delivered during the electrochemical oxidation or reduction of the analyte, which is related to the concentration of the analyte.

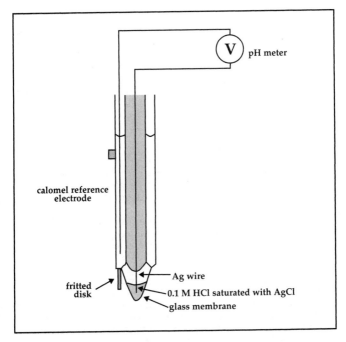

Fig. 6-4. Schematic diagram of a pH electrode.

    c. Conductometry measures the conductance of the analyte solution. This is the least selective of the electrochemical methods.

    2. Instrumentations for coulometric, amperometric, and conductometric measurements, are simple, include electrodes, potentiometers, and amperometers.

    3. Applications. Coulometric and conductometric detectors are widely used in **HPLC** and **CE** separations. A notable example of an amperometric measurement is the P_{O_2} determination with an oxygen-electrode, which is a complete electrochemical cell.

VI. Radiochemistry measures radiation-induced ionization in gases or solids. The amount of ionization is related to the concentration of the analyte.

    A. Principles. Radioactive isotopes spontaneously disintegrate, producing **alpha and beta particles**, as well as **gamma- or x-ray radiation**. When passing through matter, these high-energy particles can **cause excitation and ionization** in the media.

    B. Instrumentation. The radioactive isotopes used in the clinical laboratory emit **beta particles** or **gamma radiation. Beta particles can be counted with gas-filled detectors or scintillation counters; gamma radiation is measured mainly with scintillation counters.**

1.   **Gas-filled detectors (Geiger counter)** are **filled with an inert gas**, and **measure the ionization that is caused by radiation** entering the detector. They are classified as **ionization chambers, proportional counters**, or **Geiger counters**, depending on the amount of voltage used in the detector.

2.   **Scintillation counters. Radiation causes excitation** and ionization within the scintillation detector, and the absorbed energy is dissipated in the form of **measurable UV-vis light**. Scintillation counters can be liquid or crystal scintillation detectors.

C.   **Applications**. Although radioactivity based assays are being rapidly phased out in the clinical laboratory, numerous radioimmunoassay-based procedures are still being used. These include various **steroid hormone** determinations in a competitive or sandwich immunoassay format, or **vitamin B$_6$** determination with radioenzymatic assay.

VII.   **Immunoassays. In immunoassays, the reaction between antigens and antibodies is measured.**

A.   **Principles. Antigen-antibody reactions can lead to lattice formation (precipitin reaction) or can occur at a solid-liquid interface.**

B.   **Qualitative methods: include passive gel diffusion, immunoelectrophoresis, and Western blotting.**

C.   **Quantitative methods. Radial immunodiffusion and electroimmunoassays, turbidimetric or nephelometric** assays (see above), and **labeled immunochemical assays are quantitative methods. Labeled immunochemical assays can be competitive** (limited reagent assays) or noncompetitive (excess-reagent, two-site, or sandwich assays), **simultaneous or sequential, and heterogeneous or homogeneous**. Labeled immunochemical assays include **radioimmunoassays (RIA), enzyme immunoassays (EIA), fluoroimmunoassays (FIA)**, and **chemiluminescence immunoassays.**

D.   **Other methods** include **immunocytochemical** techniques and **agglutination** assays.

E.   **Applications. A wide variety of analytes**, for which antibody is available, can be measured with immunochemical techniques. The technique is not limited to macromolecules or macromolecular complexes (e.g., proteins and lipoproteins), and can also be applied to smaller molecules (e.g., peptides, drugs, and drug metabolites).

VIII.   **Automated analyzers.** Automation refers to a process requiring minimal human intervention. **Each step of the analytic process**, from specimen identification to result reporting, **can be automated.**

A.   **Basic concepts**. The analyzer can be an **open system** (in which user-defined assays can be run), or a **closed system** (in which assay parameters are entered by the manufacturer). Automated analyzers can be **continuous-flow** (samples flow through a common reaction vessel) or **discrete** (each sample has its own reaction vessel). Sample analysis can be **sequential, parallel, batch, or random access.**

B.   **Analyzer Parts**. The major components of automated analyzers can include patient identification, sampling, transport of the sample aliquot, dilution, mixing, incubation, reaction vessels, analytic reaction and measurement, and data analysis and reporting.

C. Measurement approaches. A variety of analytic principles are used, including UV-vis, fluorescence, electrochemiluminescence, spectro- and reflectance photometry, immunochemistry, ion-selective electrodes (potentiometry), and so on.

D. Point-of-care testing (POCT). Point-of-care analyzers are **automated, highly compact devices** designed for use by nonlaboratory personnel at **bedside testing**, screening projects, wellness centers, and physician office laboratories. Most of these devices use disposable cartridges and require <50 µL of blood. These POC analyzers can have an **extensive test menu**, including sodium, potassium, chloride, calcium, glucose, urea, nitrogen, pH, pCO_2, PO_2, hematocrit, and calculated hemoglobin.

IX. Microscopy is the interpretive use of microscopes. **A primary observer is always necessary** to interpret the image.

A. Principles. One important attribute of microscopes is **resolving power** (i.e., the ability to distinguish two points as separate on the image). Other attributes of visibility include correcting for aberrations, focus and focusing depth, illumination, anisotropy, stereoscopy, magnification, and type of radiation used.

B. Light microscopes: use **visible light** for illumination.

    1. Simple and compound light microscopes. Simple microscopes use a one-lens system, whereas compound microscopes use two or more lens systems. The theoretic limit of resolution in light microscopes is **0.2 µm**.

    2. Polarized light microscopy uses polarized light for illumination. If the analyzer is set at 90° relative to the polarizer, only optically active objects can be seen in the microscope.

    3. Dark-field microscopy. The background is dark, and the only light that reaches the observer is visible light that has been scattered from objects in the field.

    4. Near-field scanning light microscopy does not use lenses, but **uses very small holes for focusing**. This prevents aberrations and the resolution is not limited by the wavelength. Resolution of 40 nm has been reported.

C. Electron microscopy. Electron beams have very short wavelengths and can be used as radiation in electron microscopes, which have **better resolution** than light microscopes. **Electromagnetic fields are used as lenses to focus the electron beam.**

    1. Transmission electron microscopy (TEM). Electrons are **transmitted through extremely thin sections** of the specimen to give an image. Additionally, shadows are created on the image by preferentially depositing gaseous metal onto the specimen in high vacuum.

    2. Scanning electron microscopy (SEM). SEM **uses secondary electrons reflected from the surface** of the specimen to form a three-dimensional image; however, resolution is not as good as in TEM.

    3. Electron probe microscopy. Scanning electron probe analyzers are similar to SEM; however, the emitted x-rays (and not the reflected electrons) are monitored. Signal evaluation is focused on chemical elements emitting specific wavelengths.

D.   Other types of microscopy. The techniques discussed below can achieve **resolution down to the atomic scale.**

   1.   Scanning tunneling microscopy uses the tunneling phenomenon of electrons between a very sharp conducting tip and an electrically conducting surface. The tip scans over the surface of the specimen to give a detailed atomic map of the surface. It does not work well for nonconducting surfaces.

   2.   Atomic force microscopy also uses a very sharp tip which is scanned over a surface; however, the tip is in contact with the surface. Laser light is reflected from a tiny mirror on the tip to enhance the displacement of the tip caused by deflections on the surface. With this design, resolutions of 0.01 nm can be achieved.

6.2

Flow Cytometry

John Freedman and Alan H. Lazarus

I. Basic review

A. Introduction. Flow cytometry has major applications across a spectrum of clinical specialties, including hematology and laboratory medicine in particular. The technique uses laser-based cell quantitation and analysis, and has been applied to examine a wide variety of cells in humans and animals, as well as bacteria, viruses, and other particles. A wide range of cellular surface features, functional attributes, and subcellular constituents can be analyzed by flow cytometry (Table 6-1). **The most common use is to examine cell surface proteins (i.e., immunophenotyping), using monoclonal antibodies. Particular advantages of flow cytometry include great sensitivity, specificity, and rapidity (10,000 cells per second measured), multiparameter analyses allowing for correlation of phenotype with functional subsets of cells, and the ability to analyze individual cells and cell populations in a mixture.** On the other hand, the equipment and reagents are expensive, considerable technical expertise is required, and analysis of data should be performed by experienced personnel, taking into account clinical conditions and results of other laboratory tests. Although mostly applied to leukocytes, flow cytometry is increasingly being used to study platelets, red blood cells, and malignant cells. The capacity for rare event analysis is particularly useful in detecting hemolytic transfusion reactions, reticulocyte analysis, fetal-maternal hemorrhage, and residual or recurrent malignancy.

B. Terms

1. FACS. Flow cytometry is often called FACS (*f*luorescence-*a*ctivated *c*ell *s*orting), based on the ability of the technique to sort, isolate, and collect particular cells in a mixture; however, the term is commonly used to include analytic studies such as immunophenotyping without sorting.

2. Forward angle light scatter (FSC) is a measurement indicating dispersal of light in the forward direction, **reflecting relative size of the cell** passing the laser beam (i.e., the larger the value of the FSC, the larger the cell).

3. 90° light scatter is a measurement indicating the relative granularity or number of internal structures within that cell. It is also called **right angle light scatter (RALS) or side scatter (SSC)**.

4. Fluorescence 1, 2 (FL-1, FL-2) indicate **the relative amount of fluorescent light emitted from the cell at specific wavelengths**, as detected by various photodiodes. In immunophenotyping, FL-1 commonly represents staining with an antibody labeled with fluorescein isothiocyanate, whereas FL-2 detects staining with an R-phycoerythrin-labeled antibody. With additional fluorescent detectors in the flow cytome-

Table 6-1.   Some applications of flow cytometry

Parameter Measured	Biologic Property of Interest
Forward light scatter	Cell size, viability, apoptosis
Side scatter	Cell granularity, internal structures
Fluorescence intensity	Surface antigens and receptors: cell populations, functional subsets (e.g., CD4 in HIV, phenotype leukemia/lymphoma, platelet/WBC/RBC phenotyping and antibody-specificity determination, stem cell quantitation).
	Rare event analysis: residual leukemia, minor red cell populations after transfusion
	DNA content: cell cycle analysis, ploidy, apoptosis, chromosome and sperm analysis
	RNA content: reticulocytes, reticulated platelets, proliferation studies
	Cytokines and soluble receptor levels
	WBC function: phagocytosis, respiratory burst
	NK cell function, ADCC, proliferation assays
	Cell activation: B, T, neutrophil, monocyte, platelets
	pH, membrane potential, membrane fluidity, deformability, transport, $[Ca]_i^{2+}$
	Signaling, cell trafficking, cell-cell interaction (e.g., platelet-leukocyte)
	Bacteria, algae and plant quantification
	Intracellular microorganisms and parasites
Image analysis	Correlation of cell image with analytic measurements
Cell sorting	Isolation/purification of population of interest

ADCC, antibody-dependent cell-mediated cytotoxicity; HIV, human immunodeficiency virus; NK, natural killer; RBC, red blood cells; WBC, white blood cells.

ter (e.g., FL-3, FL-4), measurements can be obtained that permit further dissection of multiple parameters on a single cell.

5.   **CD numbers (e.g., CD3, CD4). Cluster of Differentiation (CD) antigens** is the term used to correlate **many monoclonal antibodies produced with different names, but having the same specificity**. The CD antigens are cell surface proteins that are useful in defining a cell population, either alone or in combination with another CD antigen. For example, T-helper cells can be identified by the coexpression of the CD3 and CD4 antigens—anti-CD3 reacts with all T cells, but not monocytes; anti-CD4 reacts with T-helper cells and

with monocytes. Hence, T-helper cells will show co-staining with both antibodies. Table 6-2 shows some of the important CD antigens and their associated cell types.

C. Principles of operation. Flow cytometry is based on the measurement of various parameters as cells flow in a fluid stream past a laser beam. **The cells are hydrodynamically focused to be "interrogated" by the laser as single particles or events.** As the cell passes the laser beam, some of the light will be scattered. **The light scattered in a forward direction is proportional to the size of that cell. The light scattered sideways (90° to the incident light) is proportional to the granularity** within that cell. The flow cytometer contains photodiode detectors that measure light; thus, for each cell passing the laser beam, detectors placed forward and sideways to the incident light will collect data on the size and granularity of the cell. The information is gathered as electronic pulses, which are converted into digital signals and relayed to a computer.

Flow cytometers are also equipped with detectors that measure fluorescent light emitted from the cell at a specific wavelength. A laser light can excite a fluorochrome at a specific wavelength and the fluorochrome will then emit light at a different wavelength. The type of fluorochrome that can be used is dictated by the type of laser available and some flow cytometers now have multiple lasers attached. Fluorochrome bound to the cells (or within a cell) will emit light, as it passes the laser beam, which can be measured by a particular detector. For example, the **commonly employed fluorochromes fluorescein isothiocyanate (FITC) and phycoerythrin (PE)**

Table 6-2. Common CD molecules examined by flow cytometry

Cell Type	Molecules Expressed
Pan-leukocyte	CD45, CD 11a
B cells	CD 19, CD20, CD22, CD23, FMC7, kappa, lambda, cIg, HLA-DR, (B-CLL, CD5+)
T cells	CD 1, CD2, CD3, CD5, CD4 (T helper), CD8 (T cytotoxic), (HLA-DR on activated T cells)
Monocytes	CD 14, CD 11c, CD 13, HLA-DR
Neutrophils	CD15, CD13, CD33, CD11c, (CD14)
Natural Killer cells	CD56, CD57, CD16
Progenitor cells	CD34, (CD33, HLA-DR, TdT)
Platelets	CD41 (gpIIbIIIa), CD42 (gpIb), CD36 (gpIV); activated platelets CD62P, CD63, annexin V
Red cells	Glycophorin
Endothelial cells	CD36, CD54

are both excited by an argon ion laser at 488 nm, but emit light at 520 and 580 nm, respectively, and this, although on the same single cell, can be measured separately by two different detectors. **If the fluorochrome is attached to an antibody that binds to a particular structure on the cell, the amount of fluorescent light measured reflects the amount of antibody bound to the cell**. Thus, if cells are reacted with a saturating amount of anti-CD3 coupled to FITC and also incubated with a saturating quantity of anti-CD4 coupled to PE, then when analyzed on a flow cytometer, information as to size, granularity, and relative number of CD3 and CD4 antigen molecules will be obtained on each cell.

Although cells are sometimes purified before analysis (e.g., mononuclear cell separation by density gradient purification using Ficoll or Percoll), it is now more common to analyze cells in a mixture such as whole blood or bone marrow, distinguishing different cell populations during analysis. The cell population(s) of interest is identified on the basis of light scatter characteristics (e.g., lymphocytes are small and agranular, monocytes larger with some granules, neutrophils have many granules, and blasts are often large agranular cells), or by the use of monoclonal antibodies with specificity for particular cell types. The **population of interest can then be "gated" electronically**, and only these cells analyzed.

Through a series of mirrors and filters, light is directed to specific detectors measuring different properties of individual cells. The data are graded in channels (commonly from 0–1,024 channels) reflecting, for example, gradations from low to high fluorescence. Typically, **the data are displayed as two-dimensional graphs, with each dot representing a single cell or event**. Fig. 6-5 shows how the multiparameter data can be displayed as dot plots or contour plots, or single parameter data displayed as a histogram.

Results are commonly provided as the percent of cells expressing the particular marker. Sometimes, however, it is preferable to examine the mean channel fluorescence (MCF) for the expression of the marker; this reflects the epitope density of the molecule on the cell.

Finally, although flow cytometers are sensitive and perform objective analyses, many factors can adversely affect the final analyses, including (but not limited to) electronic noise, misalignment of the cytometer, probe quenching, cellular autofluoresence, nonspecific antibody binding, improper flow rate, and improper cell or antibody concentration. It is also important to recognize that few of the available monoclonal antibodies uniquely mark a particular cell type, and it is often necessary to use multiple antibodies together, in different combinations, to identify the nature of the cells of interest. Furthermore, when examining malignant cells in particular, it is important to keep in mind aberrant expression of lineage-specific differentiation markers.

D. Submission of samples for flow cytometry. Each laboratory will have different requirements and the physician should prearrange submission of samples for analysis. In general, a flow

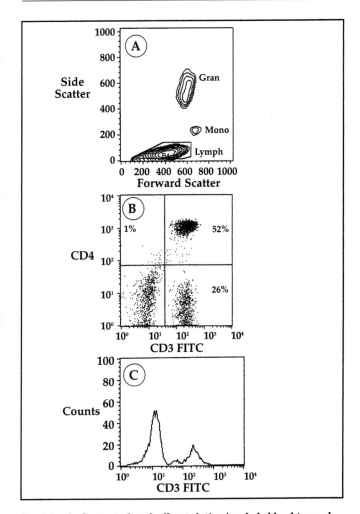

Fig. 6-5. **A.** Contour plot of cell population in whole blood (granulocytes, monocytes, lymphocytes) distinguished on the basis of forward light scatter (size) and side scatter (granularity). **B.** Dot plot of gated lymphocytes showing 52% T-helper cells (CD3+CD4+); the 26% CD3+CD4− cells represent other T cells (e.g., T cytotoxic cells); the CD3− cells represent other cells in the lymphocyte gate (e.g., B cells). **C.** Histogram showing a population of CD3− cells (*left peak*) and CD3+ cells (*right peak*).

cytometry laboratory can analyze most body fluids for cells (e.g., blood, bone marrow, cerebrospinal fluid, pleural fluid).

1. **General principles**

   a.   **The requisition must clearly indicate what analysis or test is being requested** and provide pertinent background information.

   b.   **Some drugs can affect results** (e.g., corticosteroids, antiviral compounds, chemotherapeutics), and should be listed on the requisition.

   c.   **Smoking and exercise cause lymphocytosis.** For CD4 quantitations, ask the patient to refrain from excessive exercise for 12 hours and from smoking for 2 hours before sample withdrawal.

   d.   **B and T cells have a circadian rhythm**, and counts can vary 35% to 70% from the daily mean. For repetitive testing, try to draw blood at the same time of the day.

   e.   **Preferably, samples should be analyzed the same day** as drawn, but some assays can be deferred for analysis for 24–36 hours. Keep samples at room temperature during transport.

   f.   It should be remembered that even preliminary processing is time consuming and **samples should be sent early in the day.**

2. **Guidelines for specific samples**

   a.   **Whole blood**: a 10 mL-draw into EDTA is generally most suitable; add heparin to the sample if mononuclear cell isolation is required.

   b.   **Studies of platelet activation** require particular care and special anticoagulants (Diatube-H, citrate) to avoid in vitro activation. Prompt analysis is required.

   c.   **Bone marrow**: 1 mL is taken into a heparinized tube containing additional anticoagulant (1,000 U heparin in 1 mL bone marrow).

   d.   **Cerebrospinal fluid and pleural fluids** should be added to a heparinized tube.

   e.   **Lymph node biopsies** should be unfixed and added to nutrient media (e.g., 10 mL RPMI-1640).

II.   Clinical uses of flow cytometry

 A.   **Leukocytes** are the cell type most intensely studied by flow cytometry, and many fluorescent reagents are available for use. The relative percentage, or the absolute number of any given leukocyte subpopulation, can be enumerated and compared with the normal range. Specific cell characteristics can also be identified in the following studies.

1. **Lymphocytes**

   a.   **Human immunodeficiency virus (HIV): CD4+ T-helper cell quantitation** (as a percent and as an absolute number) is a prognostic measure of cellular immune function in HIV infections. The absolute level of CD4+ cells is also used as an indicator for starting therapy (e.g., <200/µL for *Pneumocystis carinii* pneumonia, <50–100/µL for *Mycobacterium avium-intracellulare* (MAI) prophylaxis).

   b.   **Lymphomas, leukemias**: flow cytometry is very useful in the diagnosis of leukemias and lymphomas by **establishing the lineage (and clonality)** of the malignant cell, which then is used for prognosis and treatment. The aberrant expression of lineage markers as well as mixed phenotypes is not uncommon. Flow cytometric analyses should always be considered together with morphology, molecular analyses, histochemistry, and chromosomal studies, as appropriate.

  c. **HLA B27**: its presence can be diagnostically helpful in **seronegative arthropathies.**

  d. **Flow cytometric cross match: likely the best cross match method for renal transplantation.**

  e. **Quantification of leukocytes in leukofiltered blood products: $<1 \times 10^6$ per transfusion.**

  2. **Neutrophils**

  a. **Leukemias**: see above.

  b. **Autoimmune neutropenias: direct and indirect antiglobulin assays are available.**

  c. **Transfusion-associated lung injury (TRALI)**: flow cytometry may detect **anti-neutrophil**, (and sometimes anti-lymphocyte) antibodies, usually in **donor plasma**, in this severe adverse transfusion reaction that causes **acute respiratory distress**. When proved, the Blood Bank should be notified to defer the donor.

  3. **Leukocyte function assays. Phagocytosis and respiratory burst functions** can be measured simultaneously in monocytes and in neutrophils. This is useful in congenital and acquired disorders associated with frequent or unusual infections. Commercial kits are available, but are expensive.

B. **Platelets**

  1. **Platelet-associated immunoglobulins (e.g., PAIgG) or complement can be identified in autoimmune thrombocytopenia**, but many factors cause false-positive results (e.g., infection). Interpret with caution.

  2. **Reticulated platelets**, the platelet equivalent of red cell reticulocytes, useful in **differentiating platelet destruction** (which will lead to increased numbers of reticulated platelets) **from lack of production as the cause of thrombocytopenia** (e.g., idiopathic thrombocytopenic purpura, and as an early indicator of bone marrow recovery after chemotherapy).

  3. **Platelet alloantibodies**

  a. **Transfusion issues** include detection of serum anti-HLA or platelet-specific alloantibodies in refractory patients; platelet cross matching; determination of platelet phenotype.

  b. **Neonatal alloimmune thrombocytopenia**: usually caused by mothers who are **HPA-1a (Pl^{A1}) negative**, who have anti-HPA-1a antibodies that attack the baby's platelets. Flow is useful in phenotyping the maternal platelets. Similar studies are used for posttransfusion purpura.

  4. **Heparin-induced thrombocytopenia assay**: flow can evaluate platelets in this condition.

  5. **Platelet activation**: flow cytometry is increasingly used for research or clinical studies of platelet activation, such as in angiography, angina, cerebral ischemia, diabetes,

patients on platelet blockers, monitoring quality of platelet units for transfusion, and so forth.

C.   Red blood cells

1.   Reticulocyte quantitation: thiazole orange staining of RNA; automated, quick, objective.

2.   Hemolytic transfusion reaction: rare event analysis for minor cell populations; survival studies.

3.   Phenotype and zygosity studies: blood group antigens, paternity studies, forensics, paroxysmal nocturnal hemoglobinurin (PNH) diagnosis (e.g., CD55, CD59).

4.   Fetal-maternal hemorrhage: easier, more objective than the Betke–Kleihauer test.

D.   Stem cell identification. Hematopoietic progenitor (stem) cells can be identified and quantified by flow cytometry (**CD34+**) according to standardized protocols that eliminate unwanted committed CD34+ cells. The stem cells are **used to reconstitute patients** recovering from myeloablative protocols.

E.   DNA Ploidy. Propidium iodide (PI) is a fluorescent dye that intercalates with DNA. It can be **used to determine if intact cells are viable** (dead cells are "leaky" and allow the PI to cross cell membranes, bind with DNA, and fluoresce). More commonly, PI is **used in cell cycle analysis** for the diagnosis and evaluation of malignancy. The amount of DNA in the nuclei will be proportional to the amount of PI fluorescence emitted. All normal nondividing cells have the same amount of DNA and, hence, the same level of fluorescence. Dividing cells in the "M" phase of mitosis will have exactly twice the fluorescence as a cell in the resting or "Go" phase of the cell cycle. **Malignant cells can be aneuploid (due to chromosome rearrangements), hypoploid, or hyperploid. The proliferative or "S" (synthesis) phase can also be measured**, providing information useful for making a diagnosis of malignancy and, in some cases, indicating prognosis. Other dyes for such analyses include Hoechst 2322 and BRDU.

III.   Controls for flow cytometry. Appropriate standards and controls are essential. It is critical that the flow cytometer is properly set up, aligned, and calibrated using standardized beads. In addition, antibodies are "sticky" proteins and it is possible that cell staining for a given antibody marker is the result of nonspecific binding. Therefore, it may be important for each analysis to include staining of the same sample with an **isotype control (an irrelevant antibody of the same immunoglobulin class and subclass as the test antibody, but without the same specificity)**. Many laboratories use a commercial two-color isotype control mixture containing an IgG1-FITC and IgG2-PE reagent to determine the level of fluorescence of cells caused by nonspecific binding. The staining of cells with specific antibodies can then be compared with these control cells (often referred to as "isotype controls") and **cells showing more fluorescence than these isotype control cells are designated as positive. Malignant cells, in particular, may show increased nonspecific binding, as well as increased autofluorescence**; they are often also more "sticky" and it is essential to ensure that a single cell suspension is employed. In addition, many assays require samples from normal controls to be run concurrently.

6.3

Cytogenetics

Patricia I. Bader

I. Introduction. Chromosomal abnormalities are arguably the most common causes of death worldwide (if spontaneous abortions are included), and are also implicated in many malignancies. Approximately 50% of all fertilized ova have some form of chromosomal abnormality, and >99% of these abnormal ova will die during gestation. Half of spontaneous abortions, 7% of stillbirths, and 0.5% of all living neonates have a chromosomal abnormality. Cytogenetic analysis can be helpful in prenatal testing, in investigating congenital anomalies, and in the differential diagnosis of neoplasias.

  A. Specific indications for karyotyping
    1. Prenatal testing for patients at risk for familial chromosomal aberrations or advanced maternal age (a risk greater than 1 of 400 for a chromosome abnormality, biochemical abnormality, or for a single gene anomaly detectable by DNA testing).
    2. Infertility or two spontaneous abortions (both partners)
    3. Tissue from a spontaneous abortus, stillbirth, or neonatal death to determine cause of loss
    4. Congenital malformation (especially if more than one organ system is involved)
    5. Features of a specific chromosome abnormality such an trisomy 21, trisomy 13, trisomy 18, Turner's syndrome, Klinefelter's syndrome, poly-X anomalies in females, XYY males, fragile X males or females
    6. Dysmorphic features, especially when combined with developmental delay, mental retardation, or growth retardation
    7. Ambiguous genitalia
    8. Mental retardation or developmental delay of unknown origin
    9. Family history of chromosome translocation. Patients at risk should be tested.
    10. Evidence of mosaicism (some cells are normal, some cells are abnormal) for a particular genetic condition
    11. Bone marrow and peripheral blood studies from patients with leukemia, refractory anemia, myelodysplastic syndromes
    12. Some solid tumors
  B. Cells that may be cultured and examined
    1. Peripheral blood cells
    2. Bone marrow cells
    3. Fibroblasts from skin biopsies
    4. Fibroblasts from amniotic fluid
    5. Fibroblasts from chorionic villus biopsies

6. Blood collected from **PUBS** (percutaneous umbilical blood sampling), also known as periumbilical blood sampling, fetal blood sampling, and cordocentesis

7. Fibroblasts from a **tumor** sample

II. Basic principles of chromosomal analysis

A. Culture and fixation procedure. Cells can be **stimulated to divide** (e.g., lymphocytes are stimulated with phytohemagglutinin), after which **mitotic arrest** is achieved through the addition of colchicine. The chromosomes are then spread out by osmotic swelling in a hypotonic solution. After **fixation** (e.g., Carnoy's solution), the cells are **physically dropped** onto a microscopic slide, which ruptures the cell membranes, and the chromosomes remain in relatively well-defined groups.

B. Staining procedures. Chromosomes are stained with one of various methods that produce a characteristic banding pattern (light and dark) for each chromosome. Different stains will cause different banding patterns, and the stains are often classified according to the total number of bands that are identifiable in a single cell (i.e., "band level" or "band resolution").

1. G (Giemsa) banding is the most common method of banding. The dark bands are rich in the DNA bases adenine and thymidine, whereas the light bands are rich in cytosine and guanine.

2. Q (quinacrine) banding is a fluorescent technique that produces bands analogous to G banding.

3. R (reverse) banding produces a pattern opposite of that seen in G banding.

4. C (constitutive heterochromatin) banding stains the constitutive heterochromatin (noncoding DNA) around the centromeres, polymorphic areas on chromosome 1,9,16, and chromosome Y, which are considered normal human variants.

C. Karyotyping. After the careful microscopic selection of cells with intact chromosomes, each of the chromosomes is counted, identified, and evaluated. A normal cell has **46 chromosomes (22 autosomal pairs and 1 pair of sex chromosomes)**. Each pair of autosomal chromosomes is given a number based on size and shape (the largest is number 1), and each pair of chromosomes is referred to as **homologous** (e.g., two identical chromosomes are seen). The sex chromosomes in a normal female are **XX**, and in a normal male are **XY**. Parts of chromosomes are referred to by the letters "**p**" (for the short arm), "**q**" (for the long arm), and "**c**" (for the centromere). The specific bands on each chromosome are identified by the letter p or q, followed by the **band number** (e.g., 7p2l refers to region 2 and band 1 on the short arm of chromosome 7).

III. Final report. A final report should contain the following information.

A. Number of metaphases examined. Number examined should be 15–20 cells (30–50 cells if mosaicism is suspected).

B. Band level (resolution) and the type of banding. The minimal acceptable number of bands should be at least 400, and most metaphases show 500–550 bands. The number of bands is determined by the length of the chromosome; chromosomes are longest in prometaphase, and will have 850 or more bands. The band number will be approximately equal for G, Q, and R banding, because all three techniques are based on AT and CG areas of the chromosome. C banding shows only centromeres or areas of polymorphic variation, and is helpful in resolving some karyotyping problems.

C.   Number of cells analyzed and karyotyped. The number of cells in each clone should also be listed. By definition, a clone consists of two cells that have the same abnormality(ies), unless the abnormality involves the loss of a chromosome, in which case three cells with the same abnormality(ies) are required.

D.   Karyotypic designation for each clone of cells. The number of chromosomes per cell is listed first in the karyotype (normal = 46), followed by the sex chromosomes. Explanations of any abnormality are listed after the autosomal chromosome number and the sex chromosomes. If two or more cell lines are found in a mosaic patient, the term "mos" will introduce the two karyotypic designations, a slash (/) will separate them, and the number of cells identified with the clonal change will be found in brackets (e.g., mos 45,X[5]/46,XX[25]). **The most common clone is described first**, and so on; however, the normal cell line in always described last. In tumor progression, often several clones of cells are found. The most common clone is called the **mainline** (ml) clone; the original clone is called the **stemline** (sl) clone; and the evolving clones are called the **sideline** (sdl) clones. The stemline clone is listed first with sideline clones of increasing complexity listed next. When it is unclear which clone is the stemline, the mainline clone is listed first.

IV.   Common karyotypic abnormalities (Fig. 6-6)

A.   Hyperploidy ("+"). **Extra chromosomes** exist; examples include hyperdiploidy in some acute lymphoblastic leukemias, and trisomy syndromes (e.g., 47,XX,+21 indicates trisomy 21, Down's syndrome).

B.   Hypoploidy ("−"). **Chromosomes are missing** (e.g., 45,XX,−5 indicates a monosomy 5, such as in some myelodysplastic disorders).

C.   Deletion ("del"). Part of a chromosome is missing (e.g., 46,XY,del(5)(p15) describes a deletion from 5p15 to the 5p terminus).

D.   Mosaic ("mos"). Some cells have the abnormal cytogenetic lesion, whereas other cells do not.

E.   Duplication ("dup"). Part of a chromosome is duplicated.

F.   Insertion ("ins"). Part of a chromosome is repositioned into a different area of the karyotype.

G.   Addition ("add"). A chromosome has additional material attached to it.

H.   Inversion ("inv"). A chromosome abnormality in which **a chromosome segment is reversed in orientation** but not relocated. For example, 46,XY,inv(3)(q21q27), which refers to two breaks that have occurred at 3q21 and 3q27. The segment between the breaks flips over and reattaches in the same chromosome.

I.   Translocation ("t"). A reciprocal balanced exchange of chromosomal segments between two nonhomologous chromosomes, without any gain or loss of material. The

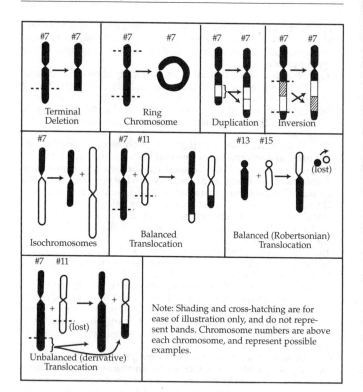

Fig. 6-6.   Common chromosomal abnormalities.

nomenclature is a "t" followed by the two involved chromosomes in parentheses. Following this first parentheses is a second parentheses with the respective break points of the two chromosomes. For example, 46,XX,t(8;l0)(q11;q23) describes a translocation of the end of the long arm of chromosome 8 (breaking at the 11q region) to the long arm of chromosome 10 (which is broken at the q23 region), and vice versa.

J.   Derivative chromosome ("der"). An **unbalanced, structurally rearranged chromosome** that is generated by events involving two or more chromosomes, or by multiple events within a single chromosome. **An unbalanced event means that some genetic material in the cell is either lost or gained**, unlike the balanced translocations (in which chromosomal segments may be exchanged between chromosomes, but the total amount of genetic material in the cell remains the same). Each unbalanced product of a translocation is termed a "derivative chromosome," and is given the number of the chromosome that provided its centromere.

K.   Robertsonian translocation ("rob" or "der"). A special type of balanced chromosomal translocation that only occurs at the centromeres of acrocentric chromo-

somes (i.e., chromosomes 13,14,15,21, and 22). The q arms fuse at the centromere, resulting in one long chromosome composed of two q arms (also called a "derivative chromosome"). The short arms (p arms) are so short that they only contain copies of ribosomal RNA genes. These **short arms are lost** when the translocations occur, and are of **no clinical significance in the affected individual**, although their gametes that are undergoing meiosis may be severely abnormal.

L. Marker chromosome ("+mar"). The uncommon finding of **an extra, abnormal chromosome that is not identifiable** (e.g., 47,XY,+mar).

M. Ring chromosome ("r"). Created by two breaks in a single chromosome, one in the short arm and the other in the long arm. The terminal pieces from the q arm and from the p arm are lost (i.e., both ends of the chromosome are deleted), and the two resulting ends join to each other to **form a circle** or ring chromosome. For example, 46,X,r(X) indicates one normal X and one ring X.

N. Isodicentric chromosome ("idic"). Contains **two copies of the same centromere**. For example, 46,XX,idic13 indicates that one of the thirteenth chromosomes has two 13 centromeres.

O. Isochromosome ("i"). An abnormal chromosome in which **one arm is duplicated and the other arm is lost**. The breakpoint is the centromere (i.e., band p10 or q10), and labeled p or q depending on which arm is duplicated. For example, 46,XX, i (17)(q10) indicates two long arms of 17 and no short arms of 17.

V. Common congenital cytogenetic disorders are discussed below. For common acquired cytogenetic disorders (e.g., neoplasias), please refer to the *Molecular Genetics* chapter. In spontaneous abortions, the most common chromosomal abnormalities are the autosomal trisomies (50%), followed by triploidy (20%), 45,X (15%), tetraploidy (6%), and translocations (3%). In live births, the most common chromosomal abnormality is trisomy 21, followed by an extra sex chromosome (e.g., XXY, XYY, XXX).

A. Autosomal chromosome disorders

  1. Down's syndrome (trisomy 21). Incidence is 1 in 2,000 for mothers <30 years of age, 1 in 50 for mothers >45 years of age, and 1 in 60–100 if the mother has a previous child with Down's syndrome. Features include severe mental retardation, epicanthal folds, oblique palpebral fissures, flat nasal bridge, horizontal palm crease, congenital heart disease [e.g., ventricular septal defect (VSD)], increased risk of leukemia.

  2. Edward's syndrome (trisomy 18). Incidence is 1 in 5,000. Features include severe mental retardation, micrognathia, low set ears, contracted 3rd and 4th fingers with an overlapping 5th, rocker-bottom feet, congenital heart disease (e.g., VSD). Infants usually die within 2–3 months.

  3. Patau's syndrome (trisomy 13). Incidence is 1 in 6,000. Features include severe mental retardation, microcephaly, microphthalmia, hypotelorism, cleft lip or palate, congenital heart disease (e.g., VSD), dextrocardia, polydactaly. Three fourths of the affected individuals die in the first 4 weeks of life.

4. Cri-du-chat syndrome (delection 5p). Incidence is 1 in 50,000. Features include severe mental retardation, a cat-like cry, microcephaly, epicanthal folds, hypertelorism, retrognathia, congenital heart disease (e.g., VSD). Affected individuals may live for decades.

5. Beckwith–Weidemann syndrome (duplication 11p15). Features include macroglossia, ear lobe linear creases, omphalocele, gigantism, capillary hemangioma of the forehead, increased risk for various tumors (e.g., Wilm's tumor, hepatoblastoma, adrenocortical tumors).

6. Trisomy 8 syndrome (trisomy 8 mosaic). Features vary from normal intelligence to severe mental retardation (Warkany's syndrome), and from normal appearing facies to abnormal ears, a prominent bulbous nose, deep palmar and plantar creases, absent patella, various skeletal and joint abnormalities, and so on.

7. Cat-eye syndrome (trisomy 22q11-pter). Features include coloboma (gives the appearance of a cat's eye), anal atresia.

8. Triploidy (e.g., 69,XXY). Features include microphthalmia, coloboma, hypertelorism, and abnormal ear development. Triploidy gestations almost always die *in utero*. Rare live births will usually die within a few hours.

9. Deletion (11p) syndrome. Features include aniridia, ambiguous genitals, and mental retardation (AGR triad), as well as a high incidence of Wilms' tumor, large forehead, and protruding lower lip.

B. **Sex chromosome disorders**

1. Fragile X syndrome. FRAXA (Xq27.3) is the genetic site that is associated with the most common form of familial mental retardation. Affected males have the karyotypic designation of 46,Y,fra(X)(27.3), whereas females who express this trait have the karyotypic designation of 46,X, fra(X)(27.3). The second most common site of fragility in the X chromosome is associated with a mild form of X-linked mental retardation.

2. Klinefelter's syndrome [additional chromosome X (e.g., 47,XXY; other forms include 48,XXXY and mosaic patterns)]. Incidence is 1 in 800 males. Features include testicular atrophy, small penis, infertility, poorly developed secondary sex characteristics, and mild mental retardation.

3. XYY syndrome (47,XYY). Incidence is 1 in 1,000 males. Features include tall stature, acne, and possibly increased aggressiveness.

4. Turner's syndrome [45,X (only one sex chromosome)]. Incidence is 1 in 3,000 females. Features include short stature, webbed neck, broad chest with widely spaced nipples, gonadal dysgenesis and infertility, renal disorders, and cardiovascular abnormalities (e.g., coarctation of the aorta).

5. Triple X syndrome (47,XXX). Incidence is 1 in 1,200 females. Features may include mild mental retardation and infertility.

VI. **Special studies**

A. **Fragile X studies. Fragile sites are specific points on the X chromosome** (usually on both arms of the chromosome)

that do not stain, can only be identified under certain culture conditions (e.g., culture media that is deficient in folic acid), **occur at the same location within members of an affected family, and are inherited in a codominant manner**. Molecular DNA studies are now available that characterize this fragile site more completely.

B. Fluorescent *in situ* hybridization (FISH). The FISH study refers to the binding of labeled, cloned DNA or RNA sequences to cytologic preparations. This technique **allows the localization of specific genes and DNA segments onto specific chromosomes**, determines the position and orientation of adjacent genes along a specific chromosome, and can detect the presence of microdeletions or duplications that lie beyond the resolution of conventional cytogenetics. FISH also facilitates the rapid diagnosis of extra or missing chromosomes (i.e., "aneuploidy").

    1. Terminology. If a karyotype was done before the FISH procedure, a period (.) is used to separate the two parts of the report. After the period, the letters "ish" indicate that a study of *in situ* hybridization has been performed, and the probe is then described in the following manner: the target chromosome number, chromosome band, a series of letters and numbers that indicate whether the probe is DNA or RNA, the actual chromosome involved, the involved segment ("S"), the GDB locus designation of the probe used, and the number of times the probe signal is observed. For example, 46,XX.ish 22q11.2(D22S75x2) indicates a normal result for a patient tested by FISH for the DiGeorge or velocardiofacial syndrome. A patient with the syndrome would have the following report: 46,XX.ish del(22)(q11.2q11.2)(D22S75-), with the "−" reflecting the missing signal.

    2. Relative positions of fluorescent signals. Two different probes (with different genetic sequences and different fluorescent colors) can be used simultaneously in a single cell. If the probes would normally hybridize to sequences on two separate chromosomes, the fluorescent signals in a normal cell would be separated when viewed under the microscope. **Some pathologic disorders cause the signals to appear fused** to each other, and the fusion of the two fluorescent colors is evident both by their proximity and by the blending of their colors into a new and distinct color. For example, in the **Philadelphia chromosome** (written cytogenetically as t(9;22)(q23;q11), a fusion of the BCR/ABL genes is seen, and the fluorescent signals for each gene probe are located next to each other. The cytogenetic designation for such a combination is "con" which stands for "connected." Probe results for the Philadelphia chromosome in a healthy person would read "nuc ish 9q34 (ABLx2),22q11.2 (BCRx2)," which indicates that nuclear *in situ* hybridization was performed using the ABL probe and the BCR probe; two signals from ABL and two signals from BCR did not overlap. A Philadelphia translocation would be described as "nuc ish 9q34(ABLx2),22q11.2 (BCRx2) (ABLcon BCRx1)," which indicates that nuclear *in situ* hybridization was performed, two fluorescent signals for ABL and two fluorescent signals for BCR were seen, and one of the ABL signals and one of the BCR signals were connected.

The opposite situation can occur in some disorders, in which genes that are normally next to each other become separated because of chromosome rearrangement. For example, the STS gene (steroid sulfatase) is normally next to the gene that causes Kallman's syndrome (an infertility and anosmia problem in males) on the X chromosome [i.e., nuc ish Xp22.3(STSx2,KALx2)]. If an abnormal rearrangement of that area is seen (suggesting the possibility of Kallman's syndrome), the two genes can get separated ("sep") and their normally juxtaposed fluorescent signals will be distant from one another [i.e., nuc ish Xp22.3(STSx2, KALx2.) (STS sep KALx1)].

Molecular Genetics

Elizabeth M. Petty

I. Introduction. Discovery of specific disease-causing genetic alterations has accelerated recently, driven by the **Human Genome Project**. Basic recombinant DNA methods were introduced in the 1970s, followed by the polymerase chain reaction (PCR) in the 1980s, and DNA microchip and gene expression microarrays in the 1990s. An increasing array of molecular genetic tests (~1,000) are available for risk assessment, diagnosis, and management of inherited disorders; and for detection of infectious pathogens, tissue typing, and classification of pathologic lesions.

II. Clinical molecular genetic testing: basic considerations

   A. General types of genetic tests. Most often, clinical molecular genetic tests detect **alterations in the DNA** of a particular gene associated with a disease. Other types of genetic tests exist, including **cytogenetic (chromosome) analyses, protein studies, and biochemical assays**. Many metabolic and most chromosome disorders are still best analyzed using these latter assays (e.g., hemoglobinopathies by protein electrophoresis).

   B. Types of familial conditions best evaluated by molecular genetic tests. Cost-effective molecular genetic tests are generally limited to **monogenic conditions** that demonstrate no (or little) locus heterogeneity, and are inherited in classic **Mendelian and mitochondrial maternal or cytoplasmic inheritance patterns**. Genetic tests are not as useful for more complex disorders, which include the **"polygenic"** disorders (i.e., many genes interacting together to cause disease) and the **"multifactorial"** conditions (i.e., disorders caused by multiple interactions between genes and the environment).

   C. Recognition of inherited syndromes or conditions. A detailed family history and review of relevant medical records (Tables 6-3 and 6-4) are helpful in defining the inheritance pattern of a disorder. Sometimes, a clear inheritance pattern is not observed, especially if the family is small, accurate medical histories for relatives are lacking, or incomplete penetrance or variable expression exists.

   D. Types of genetic alterations that cause human disease. A **mutation** simply refers to an alteration of a DNA sequence (Table 6-5). It may be a benign variant (**polymorphism**) or a **disease-causing alteration**. Polymorphisms are defined as DNA variations present in >1% of the population that have no negative impact on biologic well-being. Disease-causing mutations can involve coding regions (**exons**) or noncoding regions (**introns**); lead to a novel aberrant protein or to no protein at all; involve an insertion or a deletion of one or multiple bases; be **"in frame"** (maintains the reading frame) or cause a **"frameshift"** (disrupts the subsequent reading sequences); or be **"missense"** (changes an amino acid) or **"non-**

Table 6-3.   Elements of the family history, medical history, and physical examination to consider before testing

---

FAMILY HISTORY

Evaluate a three-generation pedigree relevant to the "chief complaint/present illness". Obtain detailed information on all first-degree relatives and any additional relatives with similar or related problems. Include current ages, ages of onset for later-onset conditions (e.g., cancers, Alzheimer disease), and age at death and cause(s) of death; racial and ethnic backgrounds; consanguinity; pregnancy losses (i.e., early miscarriages and still-births); mental retardation, birth defects, and other conditions that "run in the family"; and any previous genetic testing of family members if applicable.

Keep the pedigree current by updating it with relevant information

MEDICAL HISTORY

Clarify signs, symptoms, and clinical course of the disorder to confirm the suspected clinical diagnosis. Construct a time-line indicating the onset of specific symptoms and review relevant medical records.

Document any pertinent environmental exposures

Ask about childhood history for disorders with onset before adulthood, including teratogens during pregnancy; any regression of cognitive, motor, or communication skills; physical growth parameters including progression through puberty.

Confirm diagnoses of affected relatives by review of medical records (do *not* rely solely on the patient's recollection)

PHYSICAL EXAMINATION

Evaluate patients and their affected relatives when possible for features suggesting an underlying syndrome (e.g, dysmorphic or atypical features, cutaneous lesions, musculoskeletal or neurocognitive abnormalities)

---

sense" mutations (creates a stop codon and truncates the resulting protein). The significance of the mutation often depends on whether it is located in highly conserved domains with critical functions. **Most inherited disorders are caused by various mutations anywhere within the associated gene.** Huntington's disease and fragile X syndrome are examples of some notable exceptions as one specific mutation accounts for the disorder. In virtually all genetic conditions, **some degree of inter- and intrafamilial variability in phenotypic expression is noted.**

III.   Overview of molecular genetic test methodology. Molecular genetic tests can be considered in three groups: indirect analyses, direct mutation detection methods, and functional assays.

A.   Indirect testing (linkage analysis). When a disease gene is in a well-defined genomic region, linkage analysis can predict whether an individual in an affected family has inherited the disease gene, by **tracking the transmission of polymor-**

**Table 6-4.   Clues suggesting an inherited disorder
for which molecular genetic testing may be available**

A. **The pedigree is consistent with a recognizable inheritance
pattern.** (Note that these patterns may be masked or altered by
incomplete penetrance, variable expressivity, a new mutation in
an individual, gonadal mosaicism in the parent's germline, or
small family size.)

Autosomal dominant. Affected individuals span multiple generations; affected individuals usually have an affected parent;
both sexes transmit the disease equally with 50% probability
of transmitting the disease allele; both sexes are affected
equally—unless the disease is sex-influenced (e.g., breast
cancer) or limited (e.g., ovarian cancer, prostate cancer).

Autosomal recessive. Affected males and females are in sib-
ships or, sometimes, within the same generation (e.g., first
cousins); parents of an affected individual are clinically unaffected but are carriers of the condition with a 25% probability
that each of their offspring will be affected; the condition does
not usually span generations; an increased incidence may be
seen of consanguinity and/or parents of the same ethnic background from the same geographical region.

X-linked recessive. Affected males have unaffected or mildly
affected mothers; in severe disorders, a pattern of early
mortality of males; in mild disorders, affected males may have
unaffected or mildly affected daughters who may have affected
sons; no male to male transmission is seen among first degree
relatives.

X-linked dominant. Similar to X-linked recessive but both
males and females are affected; in some severe X-linked dominant conditions may be found only affected females with a lack
of affected males because of embryonic lethality; all daughters
of affected males will be affected but no sons will be affected.

Mitochondrial/cytoplasmic/maternal. An affected mother
transmits the disorder to all of her male and female offspring,
who will be affected with variable degrees of severity; no children of affected sons are affected, as the mitochondrial genome
are transmitted largely through the cytoplasm of the oocyte,
not the sperm.

B. **The symptoms of disease occur at an earlier age when
compared with the onset of symptoms in the general
population.** For example, the age at which tumors develop
(e.g., breast, colon) in individuals with inherited cancer
syndromes is often much younger than the average age of onset
in the population.

C. **A constellation of multisystem problems or unusual clustering of clinical findings.** For example, multiple primary
tumors in a single individual or bilateral cancers in paired
organs suggest an inherited cancer predisposition.

Table 6-5.   An illustration of different
types of disease-causing DNA mutations

I. First, imagine that the sentence "I like to pat my fat cat" represents the coding sequence (cDNA) of a gene, where each bold phrase in the genomic sequence represents a coding exon, each bold word encodes an amino acid, each letter represents a nucleotide base, and the italicized intron is spliced out during transcription to make the sentence (gene) meaningful:

Genomic DNA
    sequence: **Exon 1**----------*intron*----------**Exon 2**
                         I like to pat   *intron (lay with) intron*   **my fat cat.**
                                              ↓
                                        transcription
                                              ↓
Coding DNA sequence: **I like to pat my fat cat.**
                       Exon1----------**Exon2**

II. Now, the various types of alterations to the sentence (DNA sequence) that may occur are considered:

  A. Nucleotide or base-pair substitutions:
   1. **Missense mutation:** Changes the amino acid, may be a benign polymorphism ("pet vs. pat") or may cause disease ("cat vs. hat")
      - I like to p<u>e</u>t my fat cat.
      - I like to pat my fat <u>h</u>at.
   2. **Nonsense mutation:** Forms a stop codon causing a premature end to the sentence or gene product.
      - I like to pat.
   3. **Examples:** Sickle cell anemia, cystic fibrosis, hemophilia A, thalassemia, familial early onset breast/ovarian cancer genes *BRCA1* and *BRCA2*

  B. Small deletions or insertions involving only a few nucleotides or amino acids:
   1. **In frame:** Maintains reading frame for amino acid translation.
      - I like to ____ my fat cat.
      - I **do not** like to pat my fat cat.
   2. **Frame shift:** Changes reading frame of amino acid translation, and may cause premature stops.
      - I like t<u>p</u> atm yf atc. (the "o" in "to" was deleted)
   3. **Examples:** Cystic fibrosis, familial early onset breast/ovarian cancer genes *BRCA1* and *BRCA2*, hemophilia A, thalassemias

  C. Large deletions of DNA sequence or insertions of DNA sequence from another region:
      - I _____ cat.
      - I like **the cereal box is on the top shelf of the cabinet** to pat my fat cat.

      –**Examples:** Duchenne muscular dystrophy (deletion), Hemophilia A (insertion)

  D. Duplications:
      - I like to pat my fat cat **pat my fat cat.**

      –**Example:** Charcot Marie Tooth Disease type 1A

Table 6-5. *Continued*

E. **Inversions:**
   • I like to **tap** my fat cat.
   –**Example:** Severe hemophilia A

F. **Alternative splice site mutations:**
   • I like to p**lay with** my fat cat.
   –**Example:** Hemoglobinopathies

G. **Trinucleotide repeat expansions:**
   • I like to pat my fat **fat fat fat fat fat fat fat fat fat fat fat fat** cat.
   –**Example:** Huntington disease, myotonic dystrophy, and spinocerebellar ataxias, fragile X syndrome

H. **Noncoding region mutations that modify the gene product:**
   • **I have never seen nor owned a fat cat.** *I like to pat my fat cat.*
   –**Example:** Hemoglobinopathies

---

phic genetic makers located near the specific disease gene. The reliability depends on the recombination rate between markers and the disease locus, which reflects the physical distance between them. Generally, to establish linkage of a disease locus with odds of 1,000 to 1 ("LOD" score of 3.0), analysis of 10 informative individuals is needed. This method will likely have few clinical applications in the future.

B. **Direct mutation detection methods.** The specific method employed often depends on the size of the genetic region being studied, and the type(s) of mutation anticipated. Mutations can be missed as an entire gene is rarely studied, no laboratory technique is 100% sensitive, and technical or human errors can occur. Most mutation detection strategies are rooted in **polymerase chain reaction** methodology. PCR uses synthetic oligonucleotides (primers) that flank a specific DNA sequence of interest, and then synthesizes millions of new copies of the DNA sequence using an enzymatic reaction and cyclic thermal conditions (thermocycling). The DNA product is then most often evaluated with **electrophoresis. The sample can be as small as one cell, and derived from any nucleated tissue.**

C. **Detection of large rearrangements by southern blotting and hybridization.** Restriction digests of genomic DNA are transferred to a nylon membrane (Southern blotting) and hybridized to a **gene-derived specific probe.** A novel or missing band on the blot reveals an alteration of the gene. This is a good, reliable, and relatively inexpensive way to **screen for large genetic alterations** (e.g., rearrangements, large deletions, gene duplications, or inversions).

D. **Screening for "unknown" mutations by sequencing and various PCR-based methods.** High-output, automated, PCR-based sequencing is a sensitive way to detect previously unidentified mutations as well as known alterations. **Several PCR-based screening methods exist**, such as single-stranded conformation polymorphism (SSCP), heteroduplex analysis, conformation-sensitive gradient electrophoresis analysis (CSGE), denaturing gradient gel electrophoresis (DGGE), and restriction endonuclease fingerprinting (REF). These techniques involve the **electrophoresis of single- or double-stranded DNA fragments in various gels**, where the fragments have motilities that differ according to their length, shape (conformation), and denaturing characteristics. These techniques **do not identify the specific genetic mutation**, but simply provide good evidence that such an alteration is present in a specific region of the gene. In contrast, **sequencing the identified region or aberrant band can precisely identify the specific mutation**. Sequencing methods, such as chemical (CMC) or enzymatic mismatch cleavage analysis (EMC), can precisely identify close to 100% of the mutations, with no need for further sequence analysis; however, the techniques are very complex and not widely used.

   E.   Precise Detection of "known" Mutations. Specific, sensitive, and inexpensive **DNA tests are available for disorders where one predominant mutation accounts for virtually all cases of the disease** (e.g., Huntington's disease). Direct DNA tests are often based on **hybridization of complementary DNA strands in a "Dot" or "Slot" blot**, where patient DNA is fixed on a membrane, denatured, and hybridized with a labeled synthetic allele-specific oligonucleotide sequence probe (**ASO**). The ASO is complementary to either the mutant or normal sequence, but not both. DNA from a patient homozygous for two mutant alleles will hybridize with only the mutant ASO probe, an unaffected individual homozygous for normal alleles only with the normal ASO, and a heterozygous individual with both probes. **Reverse Dot or Slot blots** are similar but the synthetic oligonucleotide strands representing the normal and mutant sequences are membrane bound and patient DNA is used as the probe. Other DNA diagnostic methods use specially designed PCR primers to amplify only mutant or normal sequences, use restriction enzymes that will cut only mutant or wild type sequences, or directly compare the sizes of two alleles amplified by PCR.

   F.   Functional detection of mutations. When many different mutations can cause the same disease (e.g., neurofibromatosis), techniques looking beyond the DNA sequence to the **protein product** or its function may be used. Protein truncation–*in vitro* transcription translation assays (**PTT–IVTT**) amplify genes, then transcribe and translate them *in vitro*, and finally electrophorese the protein product for evaluation. **Yeast or cellular expression assays for functional expression of mutations** can also be clinically useful, and are based on the observable alterations in a yeast or cellular phenotype that occur when a mutant human gene is expressed (e.g., *TP53*).

   G.   Future directions in mutation detection methods. Gene microarray and DNA microchip technology can detect literally hundreds of different mutations in several genes in one relatively simple and inexpensive test. This is important because many serious adult diseases (e.g., diabetes, schizophrenia, hypertension, obesity) are complex in origin and involve multiple genetic factors.

IV. Applications of molecular genetic tests in medical practice. The first step is to ensure that the test is really clinically appropriate. The test is probably not indicated when a clinical diagnosis is already well established, when no genotype or phenotype correlations relevant to prognosis or clinical management exist, or when the information will not benefit other family members or have an impact on family planning decisions. The decision to undergo genetic testing must be shaped by the specific concerns and desires of the individual patient.

A. Critical components of the molecular genetic testing process. A comprehensive medical and family history is vital (Tables 6-3 and 6-4). When possible, it is also best to **first define the mutation in an affected family member before testing an asymptomatic individual**. Some diseases are clinically similar and yet can have completely different genetic causes and, unless this is recognized, molecular tests for the "wrong gene" might be obtained. Without establishing the molecular diagnosis in an affected individual, it may be difficult to interpret the significance of negative results in an asymptomatic individual. **Other critical elements** of molecular genetic testing including genetic counseling, patient education, informed consent, interpretation of test results and their implications, conveyance of test results, post-test education and follow-up, management and support, and related ethical issues.

B. Confirmatory molecular genetic diagnostic tests. The most straightforward use of a molecular genetic test is for **diagnostic confirmation or classification** of an already suspected medical disorder (Table 6-5c). Some of the available diagnostic genetic tests more commonly used in medicine are listed in Table 6-6.

C. Molecular genetic testing applications that require special considerations (the 6 Ps). Some uses of molecular genetic tests are relatively unique. It is absolutely essential that the individual freely consents to the test after fully understanding medical risks and benefits, accuracy and limitations, potential result outcomes and their interpretations and implications, potential ramifications for other family members, and other psychosocial concerns.

1. **Preconception testing refers to determining if an individual is at increased risk for having a child with a specific genetic disease**; these test results may be used for family planning.

2. **Population testing**. For serious early onset conditions that are prevalent in certain ethnic or racial groups, **testing can be offered to high-risk populations** to aid in family and or healthcare planning (e.g., Tay-Sachs disease screening in Ashkenazi Jewish communities). Newborn screening programs for severe but manageable inborn errors of metabolism began in the 1960s. Specific molecular genetic tests are now available for common early-onset conditions. Preconception screening programs have begun to focus on additional diseases such as cystic fibrosis in whites of northern European descent, where approximately 1 of 20–25 individuals are carriers.

3. **Preimplantation testing**. Genetic tests for serious childhood conditions can be applied to *in vitro* **embryos**
(*text continues on page 549*)

Table 6-6.   Some of the specific disorders for which direct
molecular genetic tests are clinically available and widely used[a]

Disorders	Inheritance Pattern	Gene(s)	Chromosome Location(s)
Cancer Predisposition Syndromes			
Bloom syndrome	AR	BLM	15q26
Breast/ovarian cancer (familial, early onset)	AD	BRCA1	17q21
		BRCA2	13q12
Familial adenomatosis polyposis colon cancer	AD	APC	5q21–22
Hereditary nonpolyposis colon cancer[b]	AD	MLH1	3p21
		MSH2, Others	2p21–22
Melanoma, familial	AD	CDNK2A	9p21
Medullary thyroid carcinoma (familial)	AD	RET	10q11
Multiple endocrine neoplasia type II	AD	RET	10q11
Multiple endocrine neoplasia type I	AD	MEN1	11q13
Li–Fraumeni syndrome	AD	TP53	17p13
Hereditary retinoblastoma	AD	PB1	13q14
Von Hippel–Lindau syndrome	AD	VHL	3p25–26
Connective tissue disorders and skeletal dysplasias			
Achondroplasia and hypochondroplasia	AD	FGFR3	4p16
Ehlers-Danlos syndrome—arthochalastic type[c]	AD	COL1A1	17q21–22
		COL1A2	7q22
Marfan syndrome	AD	FBN1	15q21
Osteogenesis imperfecta	AD (most cases)	COL1A1	17q21–22
		COL1A2	7q22
Thanatophoric dysplasia	AD	FRFG3	4p16

Craniosynostosis syndromes

Apert syndrome	AD	*FGFR2*	10q26
Craniosynostosis, nonsyndromic	AD	*FGFR3*	4p16
Crouzon syndrome	AD	*FGFR2*	10q26
Jackson–Weiss syndrome	AD	*FGFR2*	10q26
Pfeiffer syndrome	AD	*FGFR1*	8p11
Saethre–Chotzen syndrome	AD	*TWIST*	7p21

Endocrine disorders

Congenital adrenal hyperplasia	AR	*CYP21A2*	6p21
Multiple endocrine neoplasias and medullary thyroid disease (see cancer predisposition syndrome above)			
Prader–Willi syndrome	AD/sporadic	*PWCR*, microdeletions	15q11–12
Sex determination disorders	Y-linked	*SRY* (and cytogenetic analyses)	Yp11
Testicular Feminization syndrome	X-linked	*AR*	Xq11–12

Hematologic disorders

Alpha thalassemia	AR/AD	*HBA1,HBA2*	16p13–pter
Beta thalassemia	AR/AD	*HBB*	11p15
Factor V Leiden mutation	AD	*F5*	1q23
Fanconi anemia	AR	*FANCC*	9q22
Hemoglobin S,C,E	AR	*HBB*	11p15
Hemophilia A	X-linked	*F8C*	Xq28
Prothrombin hypercoagulability	AD	*F2*	11p11–12

continued

Table 6-6. *Continued*

Disorder	Inheritance Pattern	Gene(s)	Chromosome Location(s)
Male infertility			
Azoospermia	Y-linked	*AZF1*	Yq11
		AZF2	Yq
		DAZ	Yq11
		RBMY1A1	Yq11
Congenital absence of the vas deferens	AR	*ABCC7 / CFTR*	7q31
Metabolic diseases and multisystem biochemical disorders			
Alpha-1 antitrypsin deficiency	AR	*PI*	14q32
Canavan disease	AR	*ASPA*	17p13–pter
Cystic fibrosis	AR	*CFTR*	7q31
Familial Mediterranean fever	AR	*MEFV*	16p13
Galactosemia	AR	*GALT*	9p13
Gaucher disease	AR	*GBA*	1q21
Glycogen storage disorder type I/IA	AR	*G6PC*	17q21
Hemochromatosis	AR	*HFE*	6p21
Hereditary fructose intolerance	AR	*ALDOB*	9q22
Krabbe disease	AR	*GALC*	14q31
Long-chain 3-hydroxyacyl-CoA dehydrogenase deficiency	AR	*HADHA*	2p23
MTHFR deficiencies (including homocytinuria)	AR	*MTHFR*	1p36
Phenylketonuria	AR	*PAH*	12q24
Tay-Sachs disease	AR	*HEXA*	15q23–24

Neurologic conditions

Condition	Inheritance	Gene	Locus
Amyotrophic lateral sclerosis	AD	SOD1	21q22
Angelman syndrome	AD	UBE3A or microdeletion	15q11–13
Charcot-Marie-Tooth disease, type I	AD	PMP22	17p11–13
		MPZ	1q22
Charcot-Marie-Tooth, X-linked type	X-linked	GJB1	Xq13
Deafness, AR nonsyndromic	AR	GJB2	13q11–12
Dentatorubral-pallidoluysian atrophy[d]	AD	DRPLA	12p13
Duchenne and Becker muscular dystrophies	X-linked	DMD	Xp21
Dystonia type I	AD	DYT1	9q34
Fragile X syndrome[d]	X-linked	FMR1	Xq28
FRAXE mental retardation syndrome[d]	X-linked	FMR2	Xq28
Facioscapulohumeral muscular dystrophy	AD	FSHMD1A, 1B	4q35
Friedreich ataxia[d]	AR	FRDA	9q13
Hereditary neuropathy with liability to pressure palsies	AD	PMP22	17p11–13
Huntington disease[d]	AD	HD	4p16
Hypokalemic periodic paralysis	AD	CACNA1S	1q32
Leber hereditary optic neuropathy	Cytoplasmic	MTCYB	Mitochondria
		MTND1	
		MTND4	
		MTND6	
Mitochondrial myopathy	Cytoplasmic	MTATP6	Mitochondria
		MTND1	
		MTND4	
		MTND6	
		MTTK	
		MTTL1	
		MTTT	

continued

Table 6-6. *Continued*

Disorder	Inheritance Pattern	Gene(s)	Chromosome Location(s)
Myotonic dystrophy[d]	AD	*DMPK*	9q13
Neurofibromatosis type II	AD	*NF1*	17q12
Neurofibromatosis type II	AD	*NF2*	22q12
Oculopharyngeal muscular dystrophy	AD	*PABP2*	14q11–13
Spinobulbar muscular atrophy	X-linked	*AR*	Xq11–12
Spinocerebellar ataxias[d]			
Type I	AD	*SCA1*	6p23
Type II	AD	*SCA2*	12q24
Type III	AD	*MJD*	14q24–31
Type VI	AD	*CANA1A*	19p13
Type VII	AD	*SCA7*	3p12–21
Type VIII	AD	*SCA8*	13q21

AD, autosomal dominant; AR, autosomal recessive.

[a] This is not an exhaustive chart. Clinicians should consult with geneticists, updated Internet sites (see Table 6–7), and/or diagnostic laboratories to obtain current information about available molecular genetic tests.

[b] Hereditary nonpolyposis colon cancer can also be indirectly assessed through microsatellite instability loci.

[c] Other types of Ehlers-Danlos syndrome such as the vascular type can be detected by biochemical analyses.

[d] Trinucleotide repeat disorders.

when the risk of an affected pregnancy is at least 25%, so that only embryos lacking the genetic alteration are implanted in the uterus.

   4.   Prenatal testing. Molecular genetic tests can be performed on **chorionic villus** placental samples (at 9–12 weeks of gestation), **amniocytes** (after 15 weeks gestation), and **fetal blood or tissue**; the tests are used for disorders that manifest during childhood. Prenatal testing raises sensitive psychosocial and ethical issues related to pregnancy termination, the anticipation of knowingly having and raising a child with serious medical problems, and consideration of experimental *in utero* therapies.

   5.   Presymptomatic testing is used for asymptomatic individuals who are at risk for later-onset conditions (e.g., Huntington's disease).

   6.   Predictive testing (a.k.a. "susceptibility testing"). Whereas presymptomatic testing implies that an individual with a mutation will get the disease (**deterministic**), predictive testing helps more accurately determine *the risk* that an individual will develop the disease (**probabilistic**). Many mutations associated with adult-onset disorders have incomplete penetrance (e.g., hereditary cancer syndromes, such as breast or ovarian cancer caused by *BRCA1, BRCA2* , or both mutations), and testing asymptomatic individuals for these genetic diseases is probabilistic. **For highly penetrant inherited mutations** such as the *RET* or *APC* genes (causing thyroid cancer in multiple endocrine neoplasia type II, and colon cancer associated with classic familial adenomatous polyposis, respectively), **predictive testing for at-risk, first degree relatives is standard practice.**

   Testing minors for adult-onset cancer genes is only encouraged when clear medical benefits are associated with test results, such as in FAP or MEN2, where positive results lead to effective preventative therapies, and negative results spare patients from repeated medical surveillance. It is recommended that predictive genetic tests not be performed before the earliest age at which health benefits can be gained for any particular disorder.

   Risk estimates are influenced by the depth of knowledge about the molecular basis of the disease, the penetrance of the specific mutation, ethnicity, other familial genetic factors, various ill-defined environmental exposures, and so on. Given this complexity, most tests are currently being performed in specialty clinics where coordinated care is provided by medical specialists, specialty nurses, clinical geneticists, genetic counselors, psychologists, and social workers.

   Predictive testing should only be offered (a) with a family history of the condition; (b) with a recognized molecular basis for the condition, and an understanding of what constitutes a disease-causing mutation; (c) the test can be adequately interpreted and is both sensitive and specific; (d) the results of the test will influence someone's medical management, lifestyle or behavioral choices; or (e) the individual is able to make an educated, informed choice.

D.   Evaluating a genetic test. Diagnostic tests should be cost-effective, with a high degree of precision, accuracy, sensitivity, specificity, and predictive value. The **sensitivity** reflects the ability of the test to detect a mutation when a mutation is known to exist. **Specificity** refers to the ability of the test to yield normal results when no mutations exist. A **positive predictive value** estimates the probability that a person with a positive test result (e.g., a mutation was detected) has, or will develop, the disease. Conversely, the **negative predictive value** is the probability that a person with a negative result does not have the disease. **The prevalence of a disorder influences the positive and negative predictive values of a test**. Rare inherited syndromes where the number of affected individuals is small (e.g., 1 of 50,000) yield limited positive predictive values even with highly sensitive and specific tests.

V. Basic mechanics of providing clinical molecular genetic tests

A. Selecting an appropriate laboratory. Molecular genetic tests should be done at specific **laboratories with expertise** in analyzing the gene(s) associated with the disorder being considered. An up-to-date online listing of molecular diagnostic laboratories and the current tests they offer is available through GeneTests on the Internet (http://www. genetests.org/), along with specific contact numbers. It is always preferable to use a **Clinical Laboratory Improvement Amendments (CLIA)-certified** laboratory. Sometimes, testing for rare or newly discovered mutations is only available through a research laboratory; any results from a research laboratory should be interpreted with extreme caution, and should be repeated independently at another laboratory if results will be used for clinical decisions.

B. Specimen and shipping requirements for genetic testing. Each laboratory has specific handling and shipping requirements (e.g., some laboratories only accept samples on certain days). Medical information, family history, and completed informed consent forms must be included. Concurrent tests may be performed that include biochemical tests and cytogenetic studies. **Biochemical tests** use plasma and urine samples (usually kept on ice). **Cytogenetic studies** use any rapidly growing cell or cell that can be cultured, and are often shipped overnight at room temperature. **Molecular genetic DNA-based tests** can be done on any nucleated cell specimens, including blood [often collected in EDTA (purple-topped) or buffered sodium citrate ADC (yellow-topped)], buccal swabs, chorionic villus samples, and so on. Even blood spots dried on filter paper and archival pathologic specimens can be used for many DNA tests. Amniocytes should be placed into sterile tissue culture media. Other tissues can be placed in clean containers for immediate DNA extraction or frozen in liquid nitrogen or dry ice for later use. Samples collected for **forensic analysis** should be handled according to police instructions to avoid invalidating evidential results. Rape collection kits should be available through emergency rooms. For individuals with an inherited syndrome but where DNA tests are not yet available, the option of banking DNA samples for the future is offered by a number of genetic testing laboratories.

C. Documentation. Many laboratories require documentation regarding informed consent, family history, ethnic group, clinical impression, and sometimes genetic counseling (before conducting predictive testing for asymptomatic patients). This also allows the laboratory personnel to suggest appropriate tests. Rather than screening for all mutations at once, it is often more cost-effective to conduct tests in stepwise fashion, starting with a search for the most common mutations for the patient's particular phenotype or those found in the patient's ethnic group.

VI. Genetic counseling, patient education, informed consent, and ethical issues related to clinical molecular genetic testing. Knowledge of one's genes can have great ramifications for oneself, one's children, and for other family members. All efforts must be made to enhance patient benefits, reduce patient risks, and protect patient confidentiality.

A. Pretest genetic counseling and patient education. A respect for autonomy and regard for beneficence are central themes in genetic counseling. Patients must be educated in a style that promotes voluntary, informed decision-making, and that allows patients to incorporate their personal value system into the decision process. Written education materials provided by disease associations can be extremely valuable, as can specific Internet sites. Confirmatory tests for patients with currently suspected disease do not generally require pretest visits and documented informed consent.

B. Posttest counseling. The results of molecular genetic tests should always be disclosed in a face-to-face posttest session to discuss interpretation of results, anticipatory guidance, appropriate medical management, lifestyle modifications, special services or resources that are available, and information about additional medical help, support, and services. Patients should be provided with appropriate referral or consultations for specialty medical, educational, and support care as needed.

C. Ethical, legal, and social issues. Concerns have been raised about predictive genetic tests being used to generate individual genetic profiles which, in turn, may limit their employability, medical insurance, and life insurance. In 1995, the Equal Employment Opportunity Commission stated that a person may not be denied employment because he or she carries a disease susceptibility gene. The Health Insurance Portability and Accountability Act of 1996 expressly recognized genetic information as protected medical information that cannot be used by an employer-based group health plan to deny coverage when a person moves from job to job. Existing laws generally do not prohibit plans from increasing rates, excluding all coverage for a particular condition, or imposing lifetime caps on benefits.

VII. Helpful online molecular genetic testing resources. New molecular tests are continually being developed for diagnostic, predictive, and prognostic purposes. Table 6-7 lists some of the Internet sites that may be particularly useful for current information.

Table 6-7.   Online genetic testing resources

The Alliance of Genetic Support Groups (http://www. geneticalliance.org/): up-to-date listings of support groups

GeneTestsTM (http://www.genetests.org/) and GeneClinics (http://www.geneclinics.org/): user-friendly lists of CLIA-approved laboratories, information about the type of testing done, and synopses of genetic disorders detailing clinical features, molecular genetics, guidelines for diagnostic evaluation, references, and patient support information. It is geared specifically toward healthcare professionals.

Genetics and Your Practice, 3rd ed (http://mchneighborhood. ichp. edu/wagenetics/906317226.html): excellent textbook primer for the practicing physician on genetic principles and conditions (requires Adobe Acrobat).

Genetics Education Center at the University of Kansas Medical Center (http://www.kumc.edu/GEC/prof/geneprof. html): extremely useful for physicians; describes genetics, accessing genetic services, and obtaining genetic tests.

GENOMICS: A Global Resource (http://www.phrma.org/ genomics/ today/index.html): describes current genetic topics in the news; keeps physicians abreast of topics their patients are reading about.

Human Genome Project Information (http://www.ornl.gov/ TechResources/Human_Genome/home.html): excellent educational resources about the Human Genome Project, genetic discoveries, predictions, and related ethical issues.

National Cancer Institute–CancerNet (http://cancernet. nci.nih.gov/): information about various aspects of cancer including genetics.

Spirometry (Pulmonary Function Testing)

Neilsen J. Schulz

I. Introduction. Spirometry, or pulmonary function testing (PFT), measures breathing mechanics such as **volumes, capacities** (which are made up of two or more volumes), and **flows** (which are volumes measured per unit of time). PFTs are very dependent on patient effort. Therefore, patients must be capable of understanding what is required during the tests, and must be willing to give their best efforts. Normal reference ranges for volumes vary according to race, age, sex, and height.

II. Spirograms and flow volume loop diagrams. Spirograms diagram volumes and capacities, whereas flow volume loops diagram flowrates and volumes (Fig. 6-7).

III. Lung volumes and capacities

A. Tidal volume (VT) is the amount of air moved with each resting breath (~5 mL/lb of ideal body weight). The proportion of VT to vital capacity is a good indicator of a patient's ability to do work.

B. Expiratory reserve volume (ERV). The amount of air exhaled from the end-point of normal tidal exhalation to the subjective feeling of total exhalation is the ERV. At this point, only residual volume (RV) remains in the lungs. Chest deformities, lung disease, and a large abdomen (e.g., **obesity**) limit the range potential of the diaphragm, **causing reductions in lung volumes and capacities** [particularly the **ERV**, followed by the forced vital capacity (FVC) and total lung volume (TLC)].

C. Inspiratory reserve volume (IRV) is the volume of air inspired beyond the end-point of normal tidal inspiration to the subjective feeling of maximal breath. The lungs are completely full at IRV.

D. Residual volume (RV). The amount of air that remains in the lung after maximal exhalation is the RV; increases in RV represent air trapping. RV can be measured by washout or dilution techniques. Washout techniques involve breathing 100% oxygen and measuring how long it takes to wash out the nitrogen in the lungs. Dilution techniques involve breathing from a fixed reservoir of helium and oxygen until the percent of helium equilibrates throughout the lungs and the reservoir.

E. Vital capacity (VC). The sum of three lung volumes (tidal, inspiratory reserve and expiratory reserve) represents **the full range of ventilation capability, which is the VC.**

   1. Slow VC: the patient inhales slowly from the point of complete exhalation. This is the most accurate way to measure the VC. Decreases in the SVC provide evidence of restrictive pathologies.

   2. Forced VC measures flows as well as vital capacity (see below under Flows).

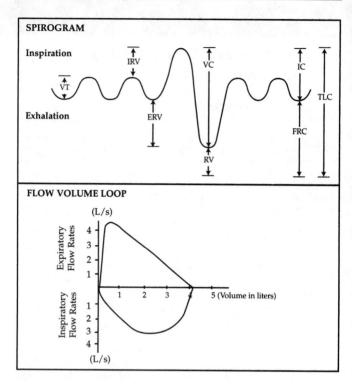

Fig. 6-7.   Spirogram and flow volume loop. ERV, expiratory reserve volume; FRC, functional residual capacity; IC, inspiratory capacity; IRV, inspiratory reserve volume; RV, residual volume; TLC, total lung capacity; VC, vital capacity; VT, tidal volume.

F.   Functional residual capacity (FRC). The sum of expiratory reserve volume (ERV) and residual volume (RV) is the FRC.

   1.   FRC is often increased in obstructive lung diseases. This increase is caused by (a) incomplete lung emptying with subsequent air trapping and (b) collapsing of small airways and asynchronous emptying of lung segments.

   2.   FRC is often reduced in restrictive lung diseases, because of smaller lung volumes (but normal emptying). In pure restrictive pathologies (e.g., interstitial fibrosis), all lung volumes are proportionally decreased. However, mixed obstructive or restrictive pathologies are commonplace and confound easy identification.

G.   Inspiratory capacity (IC). The sum of tidal volume (VT) and inspiratory reserve volume (IRV) denotes IC. IC is equivalent to ~75% of vital capacity, and is a reasonable evaluation of lung volume proportioning. Forced inspired vital capacity is a valuable indicator for upper airway patency, as this maneuver often provokes obstruction of the larynx and large airways in the disease state.

H.   Total lung capacity. The sum of all lung volumes comprises TLC.

    1.   TLC is increased in some obstructive pathologies (e.g., emphysema) and often normal in other obstructive pathologies (e.g., bronchitis or asthma).

    2.   TLC is reduced in restrictive lung diseases. Mixed obstructive or restrictive disorders are more common than pure restrictive disorders, and so some disproportionate decreases in the forced expiratory volume in 1 second (FEV_1) are commonly seen. This evidence of obstruction rules out a wholly restrictive pattern.

    3.   TLC is equivalent to alveolar volume (VA) plus anatomic deadspace (V_{Danat} ~1 mL/lb of ideal body weight).

IV.   Flows

A.   Forced vital capacity. The lungs are forcibly emptied at maximal speed from the point of full inspiration. The FVC measures flows as well as VC, and is expressed graphically as the flow-volume loop. FVC is an **_excellent screening test_** for both obstructive and restrictive pathologies.

    1. FEV_1:FVC is the ratio of the volume expelled in 1 second (FEV_1) divided by the total volume expelled (FVC). Forcibly emptying the lungs provokes diseased small airways to collapse, which decreases the volume expelled in 1 second (FEV_1). Identifying decreases in FEV_1 is the most important reason for performing the FVC. Most healthy lungs have a FEV_1:FVC ratio of ~80%. **FEV_1:FVC ratios <70% are considered obstructive** in most young to middle-aged patients.

    2.   Reductions in the forced expiratory flow (FEF) $FEF_{50\%}$ and $FEF_{75\%}$, with a decreased FEV_1:FVC ratio, represent obstructive defects involving the small airways. Small and medium-sized airway emptying speeds are represented by the 50% and 75% portions of the FVC maneuver. $FEF_{25\%-75\%}$ is the average emptying speed for the middle 50% of the FVC effort.

    3.   Decreases in the FVC, with a normal FEV_1:FVC ratio and decreased RV, represent restrictive defects.

    4.   Peak flow rate (PFR; also called "FEF MAX") is **the fastest airspeed achieved** during the FVC maneuver, and an **inexpensive, convenient screen** for pulmonary function. PFR is a gross indicator of lung-emptying speeds, and is representative of the larger, more stable airways; however, moderate closure of the small airways can also decrease PFR. Decreases in PFR (from an established personal-best PFR) indicate obstructive disorders or poor patient effort (or both).

    5.   FVC testing is often referred to as PFT "screening." It can be performed before and after (usually 10-minute delay) administration of an inhaled bronchodilator to demonstrate drug efficacy in improving air speeds and FEV_1. FVC testing can be done at the bedside in many institutions.

V.   Diffusion tests (DLCO) measure the integrity of the alveolar-capillary interface. They are often performed by inhaling a small known amount of carbon monoxide (CO),

and comparing this with the decreased amount of CO in the exhaled air (the difference representing the CO that diffused through the alveolar-capillary membrane into the bloodstream). A common adult normal reference range for DLCO is 25–30 mL CO/min/mm Hg.

The measurement of diffusion capacity is crucial to the differentiation of lung parenchymal disease from chronic airways obstruction. **In parenchymal diseases (e.g., fibrosis and emphysema), diffusion capacity is markedly reduced**. In obstructive diseases such as asthma and chronic bronchitis, this marked defect is typically not seen. In general, **DLCO is reduced in cases of damage to the alveolar-capillary interface or a decrease in the blood's ability to be oxygenated,** including the following situations.

   A. **Acute pulmonary disorders** (e.g., acute respiratory distress syndrome, pulmonary edema, pneumonia, alveolitis)

   B. **Emphysematous destruction** of the alveolus and its associated capillary system

   C. **Fibrosis** caused by interstitial pneumonitis, radiation therapy, medication-induced changes (e.g., amiodarone)

   D. **Lung parenchymal reduction** from surgery

   E. **Diseases of the heart or vasculature** that cause ventilation–perfusion defects

   F. **Decreased blood volume**, decreased hemoglobin levels (or abnormal forms of hemoglobin with altered affinities), or increased carboxyhemoglobin levels (e.g., in smokers)

   G. **Vascular diseases** (e.g., collagen-vascular disorders, vasculitis)

VI. **Evaluating pulmonary function studies**

   A. **The following general steps may assist in the interpretation of pulmonary function studies.**

     1. **Look at the SVC compared with the FVC**

       a. **If both are equally decreased, and the TLC and RV are also decreased, consider a restrictive defect; confirm with a "normal" FEV_1 : FVC ratio.**

       b. **If the FVC is decreased significantly more than the SVC, consider an obstructive pattern and look at the FEV_1 : FVC ratio** as outlined below.

         (1) If the FEV_1 : FVC ratio is decreased, and if the RV: TLC ratio and the TLC are increased, consider emphysema; confirm with decreased diffusion capacity, history and physical examination, and radiographs.

         (2) If the FEV_1 : FVC ratio is decreased, and the TLC is normal or decreased, consider asthma, chronic bronchitis, or early small airways disease.

           (a) If improvement occurs following bronchodilation, consider asthma or asthmatic bronchitis.

           (b) If no improvement occurs following bronchodilation, consider chronic bronchitis or small airways disease.

              (i) Bronchitis should have a normal diffusion capacity

              (ii) Emphysema should show decreases in the diffusion capacity

         (3) If the FEV_1 : FVC ratio is normal, but the $FEF_{50\%}$ and $FEF_{75\%}$ are decreased significantly (<70% of predicted), consider an obstructive defect involving the small airways (e.g., asthma, bronchiolitis, early small airways disease), and follow steps under A.1.b.2.

2. Evaluate the diffusion studies, and correlate with patient history (e.g., previous spirometry studies, smoking history, recent pneumonia, congestive heart failure) to assess the likelihood of parenchymal damage.

3. Always remember that the most common cause of a falsely abnormal study is **poor patient effort**. Common findings in poor patient efforts include decreased expiratory times (<4 seconds), abrupt irregularities of the flow volume loop (nonsmooth curve), and a subjective appearance of lack of effort (e.g., the patient did not appear to try hard, the patient's face did not turn red). Other common interfering influences are recent (healing) or current pulmonary infections.

B. Common abnormal pulmonary function patterns (Table 6-8 and Fig. 6-8)

1. Obstructive patterns are the most common abnormal patterns; they are caused by **premature closure of the small- and medium-sized airways, with subsequent air trapping**. This leads to hypoxemia, a decreased ability to do work, and an inability to recover from dyspnea. Common obstructive disorders include **emphysema, chronic bronchitis, and asthma**. Classic signs of obstruction include slow

Table 6-8. Common abnormal pulmonary function study findings

Typical obstructive pattern findings
FEV_1 / FVC% of <70%
FEF 25%–75% flow-rates <70% of predicted value
PFR rates less than 80% of predicted value
VT decreased and resting rates increased
VC decreased
RV/TLC ratios >35%
FRC increases >20% of predicted value

Typical restrictive pattern findings
VC <70% of predicted value
All lung volumes <70% of predicted values
Normal or near-normal flowrates
FEV_1 / FVC 80% or greater
Increased resting respiratory rates

Typical mixed obstructive / restrictive pattern findings
VC <70% of predicted value
VT decreased and IRV <70% of predicted values
Decreased air speeds <70% of predicted values
Increase in FRC >30% of predicted value
Increased RV / TLC% >35%

FEF, forced expiratory flow; FEV, forced expiratory volume; FRC, functional residual capacity; FVC, forced vital capacity; IRV, inspiratory reserve volume; PFR, peak flow rate; RV, reserve volume; TLC, total lung capacity; VC, vital capacity; VT, tidal volume.

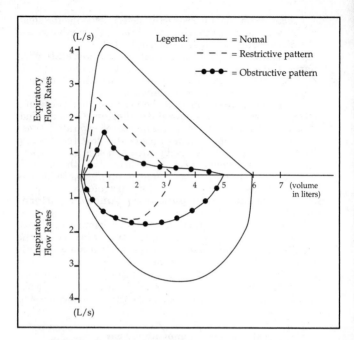

Fig. 6-8. Common abnormal flow volume loop patterns.

air speeds, **low FEV$_1$:FVC%**, decreased VC, **increased RV**, and increased RV:TLC ratio. **The degree of severity may be estimated by looking at the FEV$_1$ as a percentage of its predicted value** (not as a percentage of the FVC): 70% to 80% = mild obstruction, 50% to 70% = moderate obstruction, <50% = severe obstruction.

2.   **Restrictive defects. All volumes are decreased proportionately**. Examples would be chest wall deformity, morbid **obesity, fibrotic lung disease** (e.g., end-stage fibrosis), pneumonia, atelectasis, pleural effusions, **congestive heart failure**, neurologic diseases (e.g., myasthenia gravis, Guillain-Barré). These patients have very high resting respiratory rates, and many have damage to the alveolar-capillary interface with subsequent **decreased diffusion capacity**.

3.   **Mixed obstructive or restrictive patterns** are very common. **Severe emphysema** is the most common example. **Acute severe asthmatic episodes** may also show a combined pattern.

Laboratory Management and Quality Control

Michael S. Brown and Ronald L. Weiss

I. Introduction

A. Role of the laboratory in medical-decision making. Decisions involve **analysis** (based on evidence such as physical examination, laboratory results, and so on) and then **judgment** (based on potential outcomes and individual preferences).

1. The laboratory information and knowledge database. The laboratory provides 70% to 80% of patient care data at 3% to 5% of healthcare costs. The laboratory database is a "gold mine" of clinical information and knowledge creation.

2. Statistical concepts

a. Sensitivity = positivity in disease = "how many of the patients with the disease will the test identify?" = [True Positive]/[True Positive + False Negative] × 100

b. Specificity = absence of disease = "how many of the patients who do not have the disease will the test exclude?" = [True Negative]/[False Positive + True Negative] × 100

c. Predictive value (PV) = value of a laboratory result in assessing disease presence. Positive PV = "given a positive test result, what is the likelihood that the patient actually has the disease?" Negative PV = "given a negative test result, what is the likelihood that the patient does not have the disease?" Unlike sensitivity and specificity, which are not affected by the disease prevalence, the positive and negative predictive values are **strongly influenced by the disease prevalence**. Therefore, physicians may have more confidence in a positive test result when their patient population has a high prevalence of a specific disease (or when using sound clinical judgment in identifying patients with the suspected disease).

(1) Positive PV = [True Positive]/[True Positive + False Positive] × 100, where True Positive = (prevalence of disease) × (sensitivity), and False Positive = (1 − prevalence) × (1 − specificity)

(2) Negative PV = [True Negative]/[True Negative + False Negative] × 100

d. The Bayes theorem refines the probability of disease by adding new information (e.g., likelihood of biopsy-proved breast cancer) **to previous data** (e.g., odds of cancer after a positive mammogram). This is thought of as Odds Ratio After = Odds Ratio Before × Likelihood Ratio.

e. Receiver operating characteristic (ROC) curves graph sensitivity (y-axis) against specificity (x-axis) at different decision cut-off levels (the level at which the test result is considered positive). As the decision cut-off level is moved along the ROC curve to improve sensitivity, the specificity decreases, and vice versa. Decision cut-offs can be moved to favor sensitivity when the disease in question is easily and safely treatable, and the cut-offs can be moved to favor specificity when the disease in question is incurable or the treatment is dangerous. The area under the curve measures test performance (the greater the area, the greater the sensitivity and the specificity).

B. Utilization and outcomes management. Evidence-based methods to optimize utilization and effectiveness, utilization and outcomes management focuses on episodes of acute care (e.g., community-acquired pneumonia) and chronic conditions (e.g. diabetes mellitus). Population-based studies yield implications for individual patient care.

1. Definitions

a. Utilization management: optimal resource utilization to achieve desired results.

(1) Overutilization. Reasons include "desires for diagnostic certainty" (to provide best care), defensive medicine (avoid malpractice), incorrect physician habits and beliefs, patient demands ("consumerism" effect), and teaching practices.

(2) Underutilization and misutilization. Reasons include choosing the wrong test or an obsolete test, and financial incentives not to order diagnostic tests.

(3) Modifying utilization occurs through multidisciplinary consensus, physician education, feedback (e.g., comparison to "best practices"), cost awareness, financial incentives, and administrative change (e.g., requiring prior approval, computerizing order entry rules).

b. Outcomes management: designing practices to achieve desirable outcomes (e.g., longevity, functional status, total cost control, patient satisfaction).

(1) Clinical pathways and "care maps." Institutionally designed, multidisciplinary patient management protocols for specific diseases or episodes of acute care; designed to reduce clinical care variability, optimize outcome, and reduce cost.

(2) Practice guidelines. Recommended approaches based on current knowledge and advice of professional societies (e.g., AMA).

II. Management concepts

A. Human resource management. All decisions and actions affecting the relationship between an organization and its employees comprise human resource management.

1. Management and leadership. Managers guide, handle, control, and direct; leaders provide vision, perspective, inspiration, alignment, and guide the organization through change.

a. Laboratory director: responsible for overall operation and management of the laboratory.

b. Laboratory manager: responsible for the day-to-day operations of the laboratory.

2. Communication and motivation. A manager's expectations are the key to a subordinate's performance and development.

a. Communication: oral, written, and behavioral ("Walk the talk"). It is better to share more than less.

b. Motivation. Assume that people are self-directing, self-controlling, creative, and motivated. Motivators include the following.

    (1) Lower level needs: salary, status, and working conditions.

    (2) Higher level needs: opportunity, achievement, recognition, responsibility, and advancement.

    (3) Set individual goals (expectations), counsel progress, hold accountable for results, and reward accomplishment.

        (a) Maintain equity and fairness.

        (b) Provide regular performance appraisals.

        (c) Counsel substandard performance and dismiss when necessary.

            (i) Comply with applicable union requirements.

            (ii) Document counseling and attempts at remediation.

3. Staffing decisions. Plan staffing to meet workload needs and service expectations with full-time equivalents (FTE): **1 FTE = 40 hours/week for 52 weeks** (2,080 hours).

    a. Cover hours of operation.

    b. Provide necessary level of expertise.

    (1) The laboratory professional staffing mix is based on testing complexity, methods and instrumentation, and any economic constraints.

    (2) Provide necessary training and regularly assess individual competency.

    (3) Meet regulatory (local, state, federal) requirements for supervision.

B. Laboratory service models are used for health systems integration, managed care organizations, and competition-driven restructuring of laboratories.

1. Hospital laboratories: the largest sector; include stand-alone hospitals, integrated hospital systems, and networks of independently owned hospitals.

2. Independent laboratories: include publicly and privately owned regional and national laboratories.

3. Consolidation strategies evolved from pressures to reduce costs, compete for managed care contracts, expand patient access, and improve service.

    a. Networking: networks of laboratories that share testing, and are tied together by service agreements, information technology, and management service organizations.

    b. Core laboratories: consolidation of routine testing and reference testing into one facility to service a group of hospitals; improves economy of scale, centralizes testing, and facilitates standardization of equipment, methods, and reference ranges.

    c. Management contracts: agreements between hospitals and commercial laboratories to manage the laboratory.

III. Financial management

A. Finance and accounting. Sound financial management is necessary for success. Understanding financial statements and accounting principles is vital.

1. **Financial statements** summarize financial information for specific time periods.
   a. **Balance sheet: overall financial structure** (assets, liabilities, and net worth); prepared as of the last day of each month and the end of a fiscal year.
   b. **Income statement: financial performance over a period** (income generated, expenses paid, and net income).
2. **Budgeting and expense management**. A budget is the operating and financial plan, the goal against which actual financial performance is compared, and the tool for fiscal management. It is developed annually, and partitioned into monthly increments of income and expense. Budget variances are used to identify needed improvements; also used to monitor, motivate, or provide incentive to managers.

B. **Cost accounting**. Cost is the expense required to produce a product or service; it is categorized based on behavior and description (e.g., salaries, supplies, utilities). Categories include the following.
   1. **Fixed costs: do not vary with the volume** of tests performed (e.g., rent, utilities, administrative labor, proficiency testing).
   2. **Variable costs: vary proportionately with the volume** of tests performed (e.g., supplies and reagents, quality control materials, testing labor).
   3. **Direct costs: those necessary to produce a test result** (e.g., testing labor, supplies and reagents, quality control materials).
   4. **Indirect costs:** support testing but are not directly attributable to the test results (e.g., rent, utilities, administrative labor).

C. **Pricing decisions**. Laboratory tests are either billable tests or nonbillable tests (e.g., controls and standards, dilutions, repeats). Billable tests are priced by several means: cost-based, competition-based, demand-based.

D. **Capital equipment decisions are expensive (e.g., > \$1,000) items with useful lifetimes of >1 year** (e.g., building, equipment, and instruments).
   1. **Instrumentation**: choosing analytic equipment to automate manual tests, reduce staff, reduce costs, improve analytic quality, improve workflow, or expand test capabilities.
      a. **Financial justification**. Cost-benefit analyses are used to evaluate capital acquisitions and alternatives. The most common methods are as follows.
         (1) **Payback**: time required to recover the initial cost of acquisition.
         (2) **Discounted cash flow** (e.g., net present value): takes into account the costs of acquisition, profits over the useful lifetime, and the discounted (time) value of money.
      b. **Acquisition options**: outright cash purchase, lease, or reagent rental (manufacturer provides "free" use of the instrument and sells test reagents to the laboratory).
   2. **Automation**: instrumentation, informatics, or robotics used to improve the efficiency and effectiveness of part or all of the preanalytic, analytic, and postanalytic processes.

    a. **Total laboratory automation**: integrated modular workstations linked together to transport, process, analyze, store, and so forth.

    b. **Modular automation**: individual workstations to manage one or more components of laboratory workflow.

E. **Reimbursement**

    1. **Medicare**: a governmental insurance program established in 1964 to cover healthcare costs of the elderly.

        a. **Part A: insurance fund to reimburse hospitals for inpatient care. All citizens** >65 years of age are automatically enrolled with no premium cost; a deductible applies and not all services are fully covered. Private ("Medi-Gap") insurance is available to cover the difference.

            (1) Payment to hospitals based on **diagnosis related groups** (DRG).

                (a) Disease or procedure defined.

                (b) Lump sum payment to cover all expenses including laboratory.

        b. **Part B: voluntary participation** to cover physician services, home health and out-patient laboratory services; a monthly premium payment by the beneficiary is required.

            (1) **Physician reimbursement for professional services: governed by a national fee schedule.**

                (a) **Resource-based relative value scale (RBRVS)**: based on service components of work (cognitive or manual), practice expense and malpractice expense relative value units (RVU).

                (b) **Product of the total RVUs and the conversion factor (fixed dollar amount) = fee paid.**

            (2) **Laboratory reimbursement: governed by a national fee schedule** for outpatient laboratory services.

            (3) **Medical necessity requirements: Medicare will only reimburse for services deemed "medically necessary,"** and is based on whether the service provided is appropriate for the medical condition, disease, or symptom, as specified by the attending physician. Required documentation includes the following.

                (a) **International Classification of Disease (ICD)**: coding nomenclature of diseases and symptoms, or

                (b) **A written description.**

        c. **Part C: a managed care option** (see below) established under the Balanced Budget Act of 1997. It is an alternative to traditional fee-for-service, and is sponsored by private health plans.

    2. **Current procedure terminology (CPT)**: nomenclature for medical procedures, including pathology services and laboratory tests. CPT codes are developed, maintained, and annually updated by the American Medical Association, and are used by all insurers (private and governmental) to code services for reimbursement.

    3. **Managed care: healthcare delivery plans** designed to provide quality, cost-effective care to defined populations (members), and which employ a variety of mechanisms to control utilization and reduce cost. Types include the following.

a.   Health Maintenance Organization (HMO): delivers comprehensive health services on a prepaid basis to members.

b.   Preferred Provider Organization (PPO): a group of independent providers who contract with health plans or employers to provide health services.

c.   Exclusive Provider Organization (EPO): similar to a PPO, but if plan members seek care outside of the EPO they are personally responsible for costs.

d.   Individual Practice Association (IPA): an association of individual physicians who contract to provide care to plan members.

4.   **Capitation**: a prepayment method that gives a provider **a fixed amount per health plan member** (i.e., PMPM = per member per month) to provide services.

IV.   Regulatory compliance

A.   CLIA 1988. Clinical Laboratory Improvement Amendments of 1988 were enacted to specify the performance requirements of all laboratories that examine human specimens; effective September 1, 1992.

1.   **Scope. Any laboratory involved in the diagnosis, prevention, or treatment of any disease or human impairment**; includes Registration and Certification requirements, Proficiency Testing, Patient Test Management, Quality Control, Personnel requirements, Quality Assurance and Inspection provisions.

2.   **Test categories: four categories of test systems, based on levels of complexity.**

a.   Waived: so simple and accurate as to have negligible likelihood of error, or pose no harm if incorrect [e.g., urine dipstick, urine pregnancy test, erythrocyte sedimentation rate (ESR), fecal occult blood].

b.   Moderate complexity: includes most common laboratory tests (e.g., complete blood count, differential, chemistry tests, some routine microbiology).

c.   High complexity: highly specialized tests requiring extensive knowledge, training and experience (e.g., cytogenetics, histopathology, cytology, microbiology).

d.   PPMP: category for **Provider** (e.g., physician) **Performed Microscopy Procedures** (e.g., wet mounts, KOH preparations, pin worm examinations, urine sediment).

3.   **Inspections and deemed status**: CLIA 1988 requires that **all patient-testing laboratories be regularly (e.g., annually) inspected** to assure laboratory-wide quality. CLIA 1988 grants "deemed status" to existing inspection and accreditation programs (e.g., CAP, JCAHO, COLA, AABB, New York State) to act in lieu of a CLIA inspection.

a.   CAP: The College of American Pathologists Laboratory Accreditation Program is the most widely used. CAP processes employee checklists based on standards for the following.

(1)   Laboratory director

(2)   Physical facilities and safety measures

(3)   Quality control and performance improvement program

(4)   Analytic methods

b. JCAHO: The Joint Commission on Accreditation of Healthcare Organizations administers a voluntary inspection and accreditation program; includes laboratory inspection similar to the CAP process.

c. COLA: Commission on Laboratory Accreditation, a nonprofit, physician-directed, national accrediting organization for physician office and hospital laboratories; **COLA is the preferred route for physician office laboratories**, and accredits the following specialties.

  (1) Chemistry, endocrinology, and toxicology

  (2) Hematology and coagulation

  (3) Microbiology (including bacteriology, mycology, parasitology, and virology)

  (4) Immunology and syphilis serology

  (5) Immunohernatology and transfusion services

d. Miscellaneous

  (1) For histocompatability and cytogenetics laboratories: American Society of Histocompatibility and Immunogenetics (ASHI), American College of Medical Genetics

  (2) States with deemed status exemptions from CLIA 1988: New York, Oregon, Washington

B. Medicare compliance. Medicare and Medicaid programs protect against fraudulent and abusive practices. Laboratories are strongly encouraged to have **a compliance plan in place.**

  1. Fraud and abuse. Fraud is defined by Medicare as an "intentional deception or misrepresentation" knowingly made. Abuse is "practice inconsistent with sound medical, business, or fiscal practice." Important examples include the following.

  a. Kickbacks: unlawful payments (monetary or in kind) made in return for referral of patients or medical services (e.g., laboratory tests).

  b. Fraudulent billing practices: filing false claims for services (e.g., services not performed, upcoding or unbundling claims for higher reimbursement, double billing, medically unnecessary services).

  2. Self-referral prohibitions ("Stark" laws). Physicians are prohibited from making Medicare or Medicaid referrals to entities (including laboratories) in which they have a "financial relationship."

  3. Compliance plan. A comprehensive strategy to ensure compliance with all applicable regulatory and reimbursement requirements. Model plans are written for hospitals, clinical laboratories, nonhospital providers (e.g., pathologists), and for billing services.

C. State reporting. State Health Departments and the Association of Public Health Laboratories require laboratories to report a variety of test results for disease surveillance purposes (e.g., infectious diseases, lead poisoning). States differ regarding specific reporting requirements.

D. Transfusion services

  1. FDA. The US Food and Drug Administration inspects and licenses all blood banks and donor centers that produce human blood products.

    2. AABA. The **American Association of Blood Banks** is a voluntary inspection and accreditation agency for blood banks.

V. Laboratory operations

  A. Quality is usually defined as a degree of excellence, conforming to specifications or standards, and meeting the needs and requirements of users of laboratory services in a systematic fashion. Components include the following.

    1. Quality control (QC). Monitoring analytic procedures with materials of known analyte concentration (e.g., manufactured controls and calibrators, previously analyzed patient samples) to set method tolerance levels. "Out of control" QC failures should lead to rejection of contemporaneously tested patient samples.

      a. Levey-Jennings (control) charts. Plotting single analyte control values over time on a graph with the expected mean and ±1, 2, or 3 standard deviations from the mean.

      b. Westgard rules (Table 6-9) are a series of control rules developed to minimize the probability of falsely rejecting patient samples because of apparent QC failures. The rules reduce the number of situations where the inherent imprecision or statistical random error of a method would invalidate otherwise acceptable patient results. Control values that exceed rules 1:3s and R:4s are consistent with **random types of error** (increased variability); control values that exceed rules 2:2s, 4:1s, and 10:mean are con-

Table 6-9. Westgard's rules

1:2s	Warning sign: control value is greater than ±2 SD from the mean[a]
1:3s	Reject the run when one control value is greater than ±3 SD from the mean
2:2s	Reject the run when two consecutive control values are >2 SD above the mean, or both controls <2 SD below the mean
R:4s	Reject the run when one control value is >2 SD above the mean and another control value <2 SD below the mean (a 4 SD difference between controls)
4:1s	Reject the run when four consecutive control values are >1 SD above the mean, or all four control values are <1 SD below the mean
10:mean	Reject the run when ten consecutive control values are above the mean, or all ten control values are below the mean

SD, standard deviation.

[a] The 1:2s rule is used as an initial "gatekeeper rule" if a manual approach to quality control is used: if the control value is within the 1:2s rule, then the run is accepted; if the control value exceeds the 1:2s rule, then the other Westgard rules are applied to determine whether or not the run should be accepted. If a computerized approach is used, the 1:2s rule may be discarded, and the other Westgard rules are automatically applied to every run.

sistent with **systemic types of error** [e.g., **a trend** (progressive movement of values) **or a shift** (abrupt movement of values)].

    c. **Patient control data analysis** is the use of individual patient or multiple patient results to monitor test quality and identify possible problems.

        (1) **Individual patients: clinical correlations by attending physicians** (discordance between laboratory result and patient's condition), **correlation with other laboratory results, and "delta checks"** (significant changes in test result values in the same patient over a specified length of time, usually ≤3 days).

        (2) **Multiple patients: statistical analysis** of test result distribution over a significantly large number of patients.

  2. **Quality assurance. A systematic approach to designing quality into processes** through the establishment of minimal performance standards (e.g., indicators), identification of outliers, and problem solving.

  3. **Quality improvement. An organization-wide approach to managing quality**, meeting user requirements, and finding opportunities to improve processes. Focuses on interdepartmental dependencies and cross-functional improvements (i.e., the team approach).

  4. **Proficiency testing (PT)**. An **external, unbiased audit system** to assure analytic accuracy through interlaboratory comparisons. PT must encompass all tests regardless of complexity. Available programs are developed by states (e.g., New York State Department of Health) and private agencies (e.g., College of American Pathologists Surveys). Results must be monitored and corrective actions documented.

B. **Safety**

  1. **Goals of a laboratory safety program**

    a. Reduce losses from occupational illnesses and injuries.

    b. Maintain regulatory and safety-related compliance.

    c. Promote a healthy and positive work environment.

  2. **Regulatory organizations involved in regulation of workplace safety**

    a. Occupational Health and Safety Administration (OSHA)

    b. Environmental Protection Agency (EPA)

    c. Department of Transportation (DOT)

  3. **Safety plan**

    a. **Engineering controls**: built-in design or construction features (e.g., protective equipment) and general facility or environmental controls, as well as process-specific controls for the individual workstations, employees, and functions.

    b. **Procedural controls.** Policies and procedures to reduce the likelihood of undesired incidents.

        (1) General safety policies for the entire organization

        (2) Policies and procedures specific to individual work areas

        (3) Procedures specific to individual processes

4. Carrying out the safety plan
   a. **Risk assessment and monitoring**
      (1) **Proactive**: workplace hazard assessment
      (2) **Reactive**: incident reporting, recording, and tracking
   b. **Routine data evaluation** identifies areas of high risk, helps set priorities, and increases effectiveness.
5. Examples of common safety plans in the laboratory environment: chemical hygiene plan and Material Safety Data Sheets (MSDS), exposure control plan (biological hazards), radiation safety plan, disaster plan

C. Test performance characteristics. Analytic features should be evaluated for each laboratory test and instrument.
   1. **Precision**: repeatability of an assay
   2. **Sensitivity**: lowest detectable level of an analyte
   3. **Accuracy**: ability to measure closest to a true analyte concentration; measured by the following.
      a. Use of reference standards
      b. Assessing assay linearity
   4. **Validation**: comparing an assay method to a reference method ("gold standard")

D. Procedure manual. The procedure manual is a compendium of a laboratory's method descriptions. Standard operating procedures should include the principle of use, supplies, equipment, calibrators, control standards, step-by-step performance, result reporting, reference intervals, interpretation, safety precautions, and references.

E. Risk management involves an organization-wide program to assess sources of risk and likelihood of occurrences, minimize or prevent risk, respond to events and claims, and fund (insure) for loss.
   1. **Risk assessment** should be applied to staff (especially professional staff), physical facility, policies and procedures, hazardous materials, and business practices. Areas of risk include reporting and documenting critical values, erroneous results and diagnostic errors, blood component transfusions, mislabeled specimens, and lost or compromised specimens.
   2. **Monitoring and incident reporting**
      a. **Monitoring**: quality assurance indicators, adverse events, and so forth
      b. **Reporting occurrences**: appropriate use of factual and timely incident reports, timely and appropriate communication, confidential documentation, and consultation with legal counsel
   3. **Risk (damage) control**: DO's and DON'Ts of when a claim is filed
      a. **DO**: notify your insurer as soon as possible, cooperate with your insurer and defense counsel, gather all relevant records, address a summary of the incident to your legal counsel (invoke "attorney-client privilege protection"), and respond to all inquiries only through your counsel.
      b. **DON'T** change records, discuss the case with anyone except legal counsel, or over-react.

F. Productivity Assessment. Methods for monitoring the effective and efficient use of resources comprise productivity assessment. Source of measures include internally or externally developed programs and products (e.g., CAP, LMIP); monitor for trends and compare to peer organizations or "best practices."

1. Productivity = output/input.

2. Identify critical performance attributes (e.g., financial, service, quality).

3. CAP, LMIP. Laboratory Management Index Program categorizes participants by peer group based on test volume and complexity. Quarterly data are collected for comparison with previous quarters and to use in benchmarking to peers. This is used to evaluate and improve operational financial performance.

G. Reference laboratories are used to meet esoteric testing needs, to provide higher quality (experience, proficiency, turnaround time), to be more cost-effective, and to provide consultative assistance.

1. "Make versus buy." Is it cheaper to send testing to an outside laboratory or perform it in house? Is there the required expertise in house to be proficient? Does any necessary instrumentation already exist in house? What are the service needs for turnaround time? Is specimen transport and integrity an issue?

2. Requests for proposal (RFP) is a formal request for a bid to perform reference laboratory services. Should contain contractual terms as well as service terms.

3. Selection and assessment. The laboratory should establish the selection criteria, selection process, and mechanism for assessing acceptable performance of the reference laboratory.

a. Selection criteria include analytic quality, methodologies, instrumentation, and facilities capabilities; test menu and frequency schedule; personnel qualifications; specimen collection criteria; logistics and specimen transport criteria; licensure and accreditation documentation; fee schedule and pricing policies; reputation and references; reporting processes; billing processes; client services support and responsiveness, and so on.

b. Selection process. Design and distribute the RFP; review subsequent bid proposal(s); contact references; perform a site visit and inspection; make final decision; and conduct initial performance evaluation.

c. Performance assessment. Define required attributes of successful performance and penalties for unacceptable performance. Areas to assess include turnaround time compliance, frequency of lost and compromised specimens, frequency of missed orders, frequency and nature (e.g., clerical, analytic) of corrected reports, responsiveness, and satisfaction.

VI. Information systems (IS)

A. Laboratory information systems (LIS). The success of the healthcare enterprise depends on good information systems and management.

1. Stand-alone systems are individual hospital departmental systems that often do not communicate with each other.

2. **Integrated systems. Network technology provides a communication infrastructure** for exchange of information. Integration now includes physician offices, other laboratories, clinics, managed care organizations, and home health organizations.

   a. **Levels of information integration** include the following.

      (1) **Information integration** brings together data, information, knowledge, and expertise from multiple sources for simultaneous use by clinicians.

      (2) **Process integration** couples laboratory information with hospital processes to improve efficiency.

      (3) **Enterprise integration** integrates multiple locations across physical distances.

   b. **Standards for integration of information systems.** Health Level 7 (1-11-7), Logical Observation Identifier Names and Codes (LOINC), and Systemized Nomenclature for Human and Veterinary Medicine (SNOMED).

B. **LIS models.** LIS systems are often multitiered. The complexity requires that LIS hardware capacity be doubled every few years.

   1. **Single-tier system,** a single location for programs and data [e.g., a personal computer (PC)]; has low complexity, easy implementation, low data capacity, limited user access to data, cumbersome system backup.

   2. **Single-tier plus systems** are composed of individual locations for programs and shared location for data. **Local area network (LAN),** with model microcomputers (PCs) that are interfaced with the mainframe. This provides multiple-user access to data, easier system backup, and moderate data capacity, but requires dealing with more than one vendor.

   3. **Two—or more—tiered systems** involve individual locations for programs and intelligent shared location for data (LAN plus client and server model). This provides intelligently administered data, multiple-user access to data, easier system backup, and a high data capacity; however, it also requires multiple vendor involvement and two or more programming languages.

C. **Basic issues involving LIS**

   1. **Security goals**

      a. **Confidentiality** of medical information

      b. **Data integrity**: ensures that data cannot be accidentally or maliciously altered; involves data backup and system files, physical protection (e.g., fire, water) and power protection.

      c. **Data security**: prevents unauthorized accidental or intentional access.

   2. **Result reporting** (in order of increasing cost and efficiency)

      a. Print reports in laboratory and distribute manually.

      b. Fax and printer located at patient-care site.

      c. Upload information into PC-based system.

      d. Direct interface to other computer systems.

3. Intranet, Internet

    a. Intranet: links heterogeneous computing resources within an organization. Protected from Internet access by a software-hardware "firewall."

    b. Internet: publicly links heterogeneous computing resources between organizations, individuals [e.g., the world-wide web (www)].

    c. Networking standards that allow different computers to communicate: Transmission Protocol/Internet Protocol (TCP/IP), HyperText Transfer Protocol (HTTP), HyperText Markup Language (HTML), Extensible Markup Language (XML).

4. Electronic medical record and web-based reporting issues

    a. Data integrity involves issues regarding the use of electronic signatures and the integrity of information between systems.

    b. Security involves issues regarding authentication of users, access control, audit trails, secure messaging or encryption, and physical security.

D. LIS future. Integrated LIS of the future will do the following.

    1. Provide integrated, longitudinal presentation of data on patients at the patient care site

    2. Allow on-site correlation of results with all clinical data

    3. Provide clinicians with practice parameters, flow charts, and diagnostic and management algorithms

    4. Perform all QC/QA functions for the laboratory

    5. Keep track of supplies and orders for the laboratory

    6. Perform all of the financial functions for the laboratory

    7. Carry out billing and ensure proper coding

    8. Provide laboratory utilization analysis tools for the managed care environment

VII. Strategic planning

A. Strategic planning focuses organizational resources in the competitive marketplace, and creates opportunities for continued success and future growth. It is integrally involved with marketing. Planning horizons are from **1–5 years**.

    1. Mission and vision statements

        a. The **mission statement** describes the business' motives and objectives, reasons for an organization's existence, scope of activities, sense of overall direction and priorities, foundation for development of objectives, and product strategies.

        b. Vision statement: describes the organization's desired strategic advantage.

    2. SWOT analysis is an in-depth assessment of **strengths** (internal), **weaknesses** (internal), **opportunities** (external), and **threats** (external).

    3. The **business plan** projects the marketing, operational, financial, and personnel needs of a company; and coordinates the plans of the individual units in the competitive environment; it should be communicated to all employees.

4.   Tracking progress and performance. Tracking is critical to prioritize goals, identify areas in need of more resources, and reassess the plan. Measures should be regularly distributed for all to see. Among the examples of measures are:

- Revenue sources
- Total revenues
- Salaries, wages, and benefits as a percent of revenue
- Supply costs as a percent of revenue
- Income percentage before taxes (profit margin)
- Monthly volume growth
- Test cost
- Monthly billed units per FTE
- Test turnaround times
- Customer/client service measures
- Quality measures

VIII.   Marketing

A.   Definition. Marketing is the managerial process of designing programs to serve the customers' needs and to communicate the substance of the company. Marketing goals include the following.

1.   Seek voluntary exchange of something of value

2.   Carefully select target markets

3.   Ensure survival and growth through more effective service

4.   Design offerings in terms of target market's needs

5.   Produce results to influence buying behavior

6.   Align technologic capabilities of the organization with market needs

B.   Marketing plan. The marketing plan outlines everything to know about the business, how and why the company is in business, what markets are targets, and how customers should be pursued. The plan also **defines the strategy** relating to customers and markets, product and service offerings, pricing and revenue, and distribution of services. The plan includes the following.

1.   Marketing strategies include product development (expanding current capabilities and services), market development (selling services to a new market), product penetration (expanding sales in an existing market), and selling new products in new markets.

2.   Background assessment involves current market composition, including competitors, sales costs, current technology, trends in market, life cycles of products, and services.

3.   Tactical components include sales strategies, advertising and publicity tactics, and sales promotion plan.

4.   Financial statements define financial objectives, investment necessity, and how money is to be used and controlled.

5.   Growth and contingencies comprise a plan for the company to handle growth, hiring, and expansion.

C.   Market analysis. The following items are involved in market analysis.

1.   Current environment: managed care, cost reduction, utilization reduction, improved outcomes and patient satisfaction, capitation and decreased reimbursement, and clinical pathways or algorithms.

2. Potential customers: physician offices, hospital laboratories, multispecialty groups, regional laboratories, managed care organizations, and patients and their families.

3. Competition: commercial reference laboratories, regional laboratories, physician office laboratories, and at-home testing options.

D. Implementation of the marketing plan

1. Product development and management: competitive and strategic pricing, profitability, proposals, technical information, and laboratory user guide.

2. Promotion and advertising: brochures, pamphlets, flyers.

3. Sales support and management: sales representatives.

4. Client support: client staff, problem resolution services, responsiveness, professional interactions.

Appendix–Representative Laboratory Test Values

Representative chemistry blood test values

Component	Conventional Units	SI Units
Albumin, serum	3.5–5.0 g/dL	35–50 g/L
Alkaline phosphatase	20–130 IU/L at 37° C	20–130 U/L at 37° C
Ammonia, plasma	15–48 µg/dL (method dependent)	9–28 µmol/L
Amylase, serum	20–100 units/dL	37–185 U/L
Base excess, whole blood	–3 to +3 mEq/L	–3 to +3 mmol/L
Bicarbonate, plasma	20–30 mmol/L	20–30 mmol/L
Bilirubin, serum		
–Total	0.1–1.3 mg/dL	2–22 µmol/L
–Direct (conjugated)	<0.4 mg/dL	<7 µmol/L
–Indirect (unconjugated)	0.1–1.1 mg/dL	2–19 µmol/L
Blood gases, whole blood		
–Arterial		
—pH	7.35–7.45	7.35–7.45
—Pco_2	35–40 mm Hg	4.7–5.3 kPa
—Po_2	80–95 mm Hg	11–12.7 kPa
–Venous		
—pH	7.36–7.41	7.36–7.41
—Pco_2	40–45 mm Hg	5.3–6.0 kPa
Calcium, serum		
–Total	9.0–11.0 mg/dL	2.25–2.74 mmol/L
–Ionized	3.8–4.8 mg/dL	0.95–1.20 mmol/L
Carbon dioxide (CO_2)		
–Arterial, whole blood	20–25 mmol/L	20–25 mmol/L
–Venous, serum	24–30 mmol/L	24–30 mmol/L
Carboxyhemoglobin, whole blood (carbon monoxide hemoglobin)		
–Nonsmokers	<2%	<0.02
–Smokers (<2 packs/d)	<5%	<0.05
–Smokers (>2 packs/d)	<9%	<0.09
Ceruloplasmin, serum	20–50 mg/dL	200–500 mg/L
Chloride, serum	95–105 mEq/L	95–105 mmol/L
Cholesterol, serum	150–200 mg/dL	3.88–5.17 mmol/L
Chorionic gonadotropin, serum (nonpregnant)	<3 mIU/mL	<3 IU/L
Copper, serum		
–Male	70–150 µg/dL	11–23 µmol/L
–Female	80–160 µg/dL	13–25 µmol/L
Cortisol, plasma		
–8 AM–10 AM	5–25 µg/dL	138–690 nmol/L
–4 PM–6 PM	3–13 µg/dL	83–359 nmol/L
Creatine kinase (CK), serum		
–Male	50–170 U/L	50–170 U/L
–Female	30–135 U/L	30–135 U/L

Continued

Component	Conventional Units	SI Units
Creatinine, serum		
–Adults	<1.2 mg/dL	<106 µmol/L
–Children (<2 years)	<0.5 mg/dL	<44 µmol/L
Creatinine clearance, serum		
–Male	90–130 mL/min/ 1.73 mm^2	1.50–2.17 mL/s/ 1.73 mm^2
–Female	80–120 mL/min/ 1.73 mm^2	1.33–2.00 mL/s/ 1.73 mm^2
Electrophoresis, serum protein		
–Total protein	5.9–7.8 g/dL	59–78 g/L
–Albumin	3.5–5.6 g/dL	35–56 g/L
–Alpha-1	0.1–0.3 g/dL	1–3 g/L
–Alpha-2	0.4–1.0 g/dL	4–10 g/L
–Beta	0.5–1.0 g/dL	5–10 g/L
–Gamma	0.5–1.5 g/dL	5–15 g/L
Ferritin, serum		
–Male	15–225 ng/mL	15–225 µg/L
–Female (<40 years)	12–150 ng/mL	12–150 µg/L
Fibrinogen, plasma	200–400 mg/dL	2.00–4.00 g/L
Folate, serum	5–20 ng/mL	11–45 nmol/L
Folate, red cell	160–640 ng/mL	375–1,450 nmol/L
Globulins, total serum	2.3–4.2 g/dL	23–42 g/L
Glucose, fasting serum	70–115 mg/dL	3.9–6.38 mmol/L
Glucose tolerance test, serum		
–Fasting	70–110 mg/dL	3.9–6.1 mmol/L
–30 min	30–60 mg/dL above fasting	1.7–3.3 mmol/L above fasting
–60 min	20–50 mg/dL above fasting	1.1–2.8 mmol/L above fasting
–90 min	10–25 mg/dL above fasting	0.55–1.39 mmol/L above fasting
–2 h	5–15 mg/dL above fasting	0.3–0.8 mmol/L above fasting
–3 h	≤fasting level	≤fasting level
Glucose: 6-phosphate dehydrogenase (G6PD), erythrocytes	250–5,000 units/ 10^6 cells	250–5,000 µunits/cell
Gamma-glutamyltransferase (GGT), serum		
–Male	5–55 IU/L	5–55 U/L
–Female	5–45 IU/L	5–45 U/L
Growth hormone, serum		
–Male	<10 ng/mL	<10 µg/L
–Female	<13 ng/mL	<13 µg/L

continued

Continued

Component	Conventional Units	SI Units
Haptoglobin, serum	60–250 mg/dL	0.6–2.5 g/L
Hemoglobin (Hb)		
–Plasma	0.5–7.0 mg/dL	5–70 mg/L
–Whole blood		
–Male adult	13.5–18.0 g/dL	135–180 g/L
–Female adult	12.0–16.0 g/dL	120–160 g/L
17-Hydroxycortico-steroids, plasma, (8 AM)		
–Male	7–25 µg/dL	193–640 nmol/L
–Female	9–27 µg/dL	248–691 nmol/L
Immunoglobulins, serum		
–IgG	600–1800 mg/dL	6.0–18.0 g/L
–IgA	100–600 mg/dL	1.0–6.0 g/L
–IgM	50–300 mg/dL	0.5–3.0 g/L
–IgD	0–10 mg/dL	0–100 mg/L
–IgE	<0.04 mg/dL	<0.4 mg/L
Insulin, plasma	20–35 µIU/mL	144–243 pmol/L
Iron, total serum	60–170 µg/dL	10.7–30.4 µmol/L
Iron-binding capacity, serum	250–450 µg/dL	44.8–80.6 µmol/L
Iron saturation	20%–55%	0.20–0.55 of total iron-binding capacity
Ketone bodies, serum	Negative	Negative
17-Ketosteroids, plasma	25–125 µg/dL	866–4334 nmol/L
Lactic acid, whole blood		
–Venous	5–20 mg/dL	0.6–2.2 mmol/L
–Arterial	5–10 mg/dL	0.56–1.11 mmol/L
Lactate dehydrogenase (LDH), serum	100–200 U/L (lactate to pyruvate at 37°C)	100–200 U/L (lactate to pyruvate at 37°C)
	185–640 U (pyruvate to lactate at 30°C)	90–310 U/L (pyruvate to lactate at 30°C)
Lead, whole blood	<20 µg/dL	<0.96 µmol/L
Lipase, serum	15–250 mIU/mL	15–250 U/L
Lipids, serum		
–Cholesterol	100–200 mg/dL	2.58–5.17 mmol/L
–Triglycerides	<200 mg/dL	<2.26 mmol/L
–HDL	≥35 mg/dL	<0.9 mmol/L
–LDL	0–130 mg/dL	0–3.36 mmol/L
Luteinizing hormone		
–Male	8–30 mIU/mL	8–30 IU/L

Continued

Component	Conventional Units	SI Units
–Female		
—Premenopausal	<30 mIU/mL	<30 IU/L
—Postmenopausal	>35 mIU/mL	>35 IU/L
Magnesium, serum	1.8–2.6 mg/dL	0.74–1.06 mmol/L
Methemoglobin, whole blood	<1.5% of total hemoglobin	Fraction of total hemoglobin is <0.015
Myoglobin, serum		
–Male	<100 µg/L	<100 µg/L
–Female	<70 µg/L	<70 µg/L
5′-Nucleotidase, serum	0–1.5 U (at 37°C)	0–1.5 units (at 37°C)
Osmolality, serum	275–295 mOsm/kg	275–295 mmol/kg
Oxygen, whole blood		
–PO_2 arterial	80–95 mm Hg	11–12.7 kPa fraction saturated: 0.94–1.00
–Saturation, arterial	94%–100%	
Parathyroid hormone, serum (intact)	10–50 pg/mL	1.1–5.3 pmol/L
pH, whole blood		
–Arterial	7.35–7.45	7.35–7.45
–Venous	7.36–7.41	7.36–7.41
Phosphatase, serum alkaline	20–130 IU/L at 37°C	20–130 U/L at 37°C
Phosphorus, serum		
–Adults	2.3–4.7 mg/dL	0.74–1.52 mmol/L
–Children	4.0–7.0 mg/dL	1.29–2.26 mmol/L
Potassium, plasma	3.7–5.1 mEq/L	3.7–5.1 mmol/L
Prolactin, serum		
–Male	<20 ng/mL	<20 µg/L
–Female	<25 ng/mL	<25 µg/L
Prostate specific antigen, serum	<4 ng/mL (male)	
Proteins, serum		
–Total	6.0–8.5 g/dL	60–85 g/L
–Albumin	3.2–5.0 g/dL	32–50 g/L
–Globulin	2.3–4.2 g/dL	23–42 g/L
Protoporphyrin, erythrocytes	15–50 mg/dL	0.27–0.89 µmol/L
Pyruvate, whole blood	0.3–0.9 mg/dL	34–102 µmol/L
Sodium, plasma	135–145 mEq/L	135–145 mmol/L
Sulfhemoglobin, whole blood	Negative	Negative

continued

Continued

Component	Conventional Units	SI Units
Testosterone, serum total		
–Male	300–1,200 ng/dL	10.4–41.6 nmol/L
–Female	30–90 ng/dL	1.0–3.1 nmol/L
Thyroid hormone tests, serum		
–Thyroxine, total (T4)	5.5–12.0 µg/dL	71–154 nmol/L
–Thyroxine, free (free T_4)	0.9–2.3 ng/dL	12–30 pmol/L
–T_3 resin uptake	25–38 relative % uptake	Relative uptake fraction: 0.25–0.38
–Thyrotropin (TSH)	0.5–5 µIU/mL	0.5–5 µIU/L
–Triiodothyronine (T_3)	80–200 mg/dL	1.23–3 of nmol/L
Troponin I, serum	<0.06 ng/mL	<0.06 µg/L
Troponin T, serum	<0.2 µg/L	<0.2 µg/L
Urea nitrogen (BUN), serum	7–25 mg/dL	2.5–8.9 mmol/L
Uric acid, serum		
–Male	4.0–8.5 mg/dL	0.24–0.51 mmol/L
–Female	2.5–7.5 mg/dL	0.15–0.45 mmol/L
Vitamin B_{12}, serum	160–950 pg/mL	118–701 pmol/L
Vitamin C, plasma	0.6–1.6 mg/dL	34–91 µmol/L
Xylose absorption, serum (doses: adults 25 g D-xylose; children 0.5 g D-xylose/kg)	25–40 mg/dL between 1 and 2 h; in malabsorption, the maximum is ≅ 10 mg/dL	1.67–2.66 mmol/L between 1 and 2 h; in malabsorption, the maximum is ≅ 0.67 mmol/L
Zinc, serum	50–150 µg/dL	7.7–23.0 µmol/L

[a] The lower limit for the vitamin B_{12} serum reference range is variable, depending on the methodology used, and has not been unequivocally established.

Representative urine test values

Acetoacetic acid, random	Negative	Negative
Acetone	Negative	Negative
Albumin		
–Random	Negative	Negative
–24-h	<35 mg/d	0.035 g/d
δ-Aminolevulinic acid, random		
–Adult	0.1–0.6 mg/dL	8–46 µmol/L
–Children	<0.5 mg/dL	<38 µmol/L
Bence Jones protein, random	Negative	Negative
Bilirubin, qualitative random	Negative	Negative
Blood, random occult	Negative	Negative
Calcium, 24 h (average diet)	100–250 mg/d	2.5–6.2 mmol/d
Catecholamines, 24 h		
–Epinephrine	<20 µg/d	<110 nmol/d
–Norepinephrine	<50 µg/d	<296 nmol/d
–Metanephrines	<1.6 mg/d	0.5–8.7 µmol/d
Concentration test, random after fluid restriction	>850 mOsm/kg	>850 mmol/kg
Copper, 24 h	<60 µg/d	<0.94 µmol/d
Creatinine, 24 h		
–Male	20–26 mg/kg/d 1.0–2.0 g/d	177–230 µmol/kg/d 8.8–17.7 mmol/d
–Female	14–22 mg/kg/d 0.8–1.8 g/d	124–195 µmol/kg/d 7.1–15.9 mmol/d
Cystine, qualitative random	Negative	Negative
Dehydroepiandrosterone, 24 h		
–Male	0.2–2.0 mg/d	0.7–6.9 µmol/d
–Female	0.2–1.8 mg/d	0.7–6.2 µmol/d
Epinephrine, 24 h	<20 µg/d	<110 nmol/d
Estrogens, 24 h		
–Male	5–30 µg/d	17–104 nmol/d
–Female		
Ovulation	28–100 µg/d	97–347 nmol/d
Pregnancy	≤45,000 µg/d	≤156 µmol/d
Postmenopausal	≤10 µg/d	≤35 nmol/d
N-formininoglutamic acid (FIGLU), 24 h	<3 mg/d	<17.2 µmol/d
Follicle-stimulating hormone, 24 h		
–Adult male	<22 IU/d	<22 IU/d

continued

Continued

–Prepubertal female	<5 IU/d	<5 IU/d
–Adult female	<30 IU/d	<30 IU/d
–Midcycle adult female	2 × baseline	2 × baseline
–Postmenopausal female	2–3 × normal cycle levels	2–3 × normal cycle levels
Glucose, qualitative random	Negative	Negative
Glucose, quantitative 24 h	<120 mg/d	<0.67 mmol/d
11-Hydroxyandrosterone, 24 h		
–Male	0.1–0.8 mg/d	0.3–2.6 µmol/d
–Female	<0.5 mg/d	<1.6 µmol/d
11-Ketoandrosterone, 24 h		
–Male	0.2–1.0 mg/d	0.7–3.3 µmol/d
–Female	0.2–0.8 mg/d	0.7–2.6 µmol/d
Lead, 24 h	<90 µg/d	<0.43 µmol/d
Magnesium, 24 h	6.0–10 mg/dL	3.0–4.5 mmol/d
Myoglobin, random qualitative	Negative	Negative
Osmolality, random	500–800 mOsm/ kg water	500–800 mmol/kg
pH, random	4.6–8.0	4.6–8.0
Phosphorus, random	0.9–1.3 g/d	29–42 mmol/d
Porphobilinogen, 24 h	<1.0 mg/d	<4.4 µmol/d
Potassium, 24 h	40–70 mEq/d	40–70 mmol/d
Pregnancy tests	Positive in pregnancy or tumors that produce chorionic gonadotropin	Positive in pregnancy or tumors that produce chorionic gonadotropin
Protein		
–Random	Negative	Negative
–24 h	30–150 mg/d	30–150 mg/d
Sodium, 24 h	75–200 mEq/d	75–200 mmol/d
Specific gravity, random	1.016–1.022 (normal fluid intake)	1.016–1.022 (normal fluid intake)
Uric acid, 24 h	250–750 mg/d	1.5–4.5 mmol/d
Urobilinogen, 24 h	0.05–2.5 mg/d	0.1–4.2 µmol/d
Uroporphyrins, 24 h	10–30 µg/d	12–36 nmol/d
Vanillylmandelic acid (VMA), 24 h	1.5–9.0 mg/d	7.6–45.4 µmol/d
Volume, total 24 h	600–1,600 mL/d	0.6–1.6 L/d

Representative coagulation test values

Bleeding time	2–8 min (varies dramatically because of method and instrument used)	2–8 min (varies dramatically because of method and instrument used)
Activated partial thromboplastin time (aPTT)	Commonly 24–36 s	Commonly 24–36 s
Antithrombin, functional	80–120 U/dL	800–1,200 U/L
Clot lysis time, euglobulin	>90 min at 37°C	>90 min at 37°C
Coagulation factors	0.50–1.50 μ/mL	500–1,500 U/L
D-dimer	<250 ng/mL	<250 μg/L
Fibrinogen	200–400 mg/dL	2.0–4.0 g/L
Plasminogen, functional	80–120 U/dL	800–1,200 U/L
Protein C	0.6–1.3 μ/mL	700–1,400 U/L
Protein S	0.6–1.3 μ/mL	700–1,400 U/L
Prothrombin time (PT)	Usually 10–13 s; varies with reagents	Usually 10–13 s; varies with reagents
Thrombin time	Usually 17–25 s, varies with reagents	Usually 17–25 s, varies with reagents
5 M Urea	Clot insoluble at 24 h	Clot insoluble at 24 h
von Willebrand factor, immunologic or ristocetin cofactor activity	50–150 U/dL	50–150 U/dL

Representative complete blood count (CBC) values

Tests	Conventional Units		SI Units	
Erythrocyte Tests (Adult Values)				
–Red cell count				
—Male	$4.5–6.0\ 10^6/\mu L$		$4.5–6.0\ 10^{12}/L$	
—Female	$4.3–5.5\ 10^6/\mu L$		$4.3–5.5\ 10^{12}/L$	
–Hemoglobin				
—Male	14–18 g/dL		140–180 g/L	
—Female	12–16 g/dL		120–160 g/L	
–Hematocrit			Volume fraction	
—Male	40%–50%		0.40–0.50	
—Female	36%–46%		0.36–0.46	
–Mean corpuscular volume (MCV)	$80–98\ \mu m^3$		80–98 fL	
–Mean corpuscular hemoglobin (MCH)	27–32 pg		27–32 pg	
–Mean corpuscular hemoglobin concentration (MCHC)	33%–36%		Concentration: fraction 0.33–0.36	
–Miscellaneous tests				
—Hemoglobin A_2	1%–3% of total hemoglobin		0.01–0.03 of total hemoglobin	
—Hemoglobin F	<2%		<0.02	
—Reticulocyte count	0.5%–1.5% 25,000– 75,000 cells/μL		0.005–0.015 $25–75 \times 10^9/L$	
—Sedimentation rate (ESR)				
—Male:				
<50 y	<15 mm/h		<15 mm/h	
50–80 y	<20 mm/h		<20 mm/h	
>80 y	<30 mm/h		<30 mm/h	
—Female:				
<50 y	<20 mm/h		<20 mm/h	
50–80 y	<30 mm/h		<30 mm/h	
>80 y	<40 mm/h		<40 mm/h	
White Cell Tests (Adult Values)				
–White cell count	$4.5–11.5 \times 10^3/\mu L$		$4.5–11.5 \times 10^9/L$	
–White cell differential	*Percent*	*Absolute counts*	*Fraction range:*	*Absolute counts*
—Segmented neutrophils	40%–70%	$2.0–8.0 \times 10^3/\mu L$	0.40–0.70	$2.0–8.0 \times 10^9/L$
—Bands	0%–5%	$0–0.6 \times 10^3/\mu L$	0–0.05	$0–0.6 \times 10^9/L$
—Eosinophils	0%–5%	$0–0.6 \times 10^3/\mu L$	0–0.05	$0–0.6 \times 10^9/L$
—Basophils	<1%	$0–0.2 \times 10^3/\mu L$	0–0.02	$0–0.2 \times 10^9/L$
—Lymphocytes	20%–50%	$1.0–5.0 \times 10^3/\mu L$	0.20–0.50	$1.0–5.0 \times 10^9/L$
—Monocytes	0%–8%	$0–1.0 \times 10^3/\mu L$	0–0.08	$0–1.0 \times 10^9/L$
Platelet Count (Adult Values)	140,000–400,000/μL		$140–400 \times 10^9/L$	

Representative pediatric red blood cell (RBC) test values

Age	RBC count (× 10⁶/μL)	Hemoglobin (g/dL)	Hematocrit (%)	Mean Corpuscular Volume (fL)
1 d	3.9–6.6	15–23	44–66	98–122
2–6 d	4.3–6.6	14–22	42–66	90–140
2–3 wk	3.7–6.1	13–21	39–62	86–124
1 mo	3.1–5.5	10.5–18.5	31–54	85–124
2 mo	2.8–5.0	9.0–14.5	28–50	77–110
3–6 mo	3.0–4.6	9.5–14	29–44	74–105
0.5–2 y	3.6–5.2	1.5–13.5	32–42	68–90
2–6 y	3.9–5.2	11.5–13.5	34–40	75–92
6–12 y	4.0–5.2	11.5–15.5	35–45	77–95
12–18				
–Male	4.5–5.3	13.0–16.0	37–49	78–98
–Female	4.1–5.1	12.0–16.0	36–46	78–102

Selected representative pediatric chemistry values

Test	Birth–1 wk	2 wk–2 y	2–12 y	12–18 y
Albumin (g/dL)	2.0–5.0	3.0–5.0	3.3–5.0	3.3–5.0
Alk phosphatase (U/L)	<300	<270	<400	<500 (male growth spurt; <225 after) <350 (female growth spurt; <160 after)
ALT/SGPT (U/L)	<60	<50	<48	<48
AST/SGOT (U/L)	<70	<60	<45	<40
Bicarbonate (CO_2)	17–24	20–28	20–29	20–32
Bilirubin (mg/dL)				
–Total	<12.0 (peak at 3–5 d)	0–1.3	0–1.3	0–1.3
–Direct	0–0.4	0–0.4	0–0.4	0–0.4
–Indirect	<12.0 (peak at 3–5 d)	0–1.2	0–1.2	0–1.2
BUN (mg/dL)	4–15	5–18	8–21	8–25
Calcium (mg/dL)	7.0–12.0	10.0–12.0	9.0–11.0	9.0–11.0
Chloride (mEq/L)	95–109	95–109	95–109	95–109
Creatinine (mg/dL)	0.3–1.0	0.2–0.6	0.3–1.0	0.7–1.3
GGT (U/L)	<260	<120	<60	<55 (male) <35 (female)
Globulin (g/dL)	1.0–2.7	1.2–3.0	1.3–3.4	2.1–4.1
Glucose (mg/dL)	30–110	60–110	70–120	70–120
LDH (U/L)	<500	<500	<250	<200
Magnesium (mEq/L)	1.2–2.0	1.2–2.0	1.2–2.0	1.2–2.0
Phosphorus (mg/dL)	5.0–8.0	4.0–8.0	3.0–6.0	2.5–4.5
Potassium (mEq/L)	3.5–5.5	3.9–5.5	3.5–5.5	3.5–5.3
Protein, total (g/dL)	4.5–7.5	4.5–7.5	5.5–8.0	6.5–8.0
Sodium (mEq/L)	135–145	135–145	135–145	135–145
Uric acid (mg/dL)	1.0–9.0	2.0–8.0	2.0–8.0	4.0–8.0 (male) 2.5–7.5 (female)

AST/SGOT, aspartate aminotransferase/serum glutamic-oxaloacetic transaminase; ALT/SGPT, alanine aminotransferase/serum glutamate pyruvate transaminase; BUN, blood urea nitrogen; GGT, gamma glutamyltransferase; LDH, lactase dehydrogenase. (Adapted from: Jacobs DS, Editor-in-Chief, DeMott WR, Grady HJ, Horvat RT, Huestis DW, Kasten Jr BL. *Laboratory test handbook*, 4th ed. Hudson (Cleveland, OH): Lexi-Comp, Inc., 1996; and Henry JB. *Clinical diagnosis and management by laboratory methods*, 19th ed. Philadelphia: WB Saunders Company, 1996.)

Subject Index

Note: Page numbers followed by *f* indicate figures; those followed by *t* indicate tables.